Proceedings of the 11th World Congress on Pain

Editors

Herta Flor, PhD
*Department of Clinical and Cognitive Neuroscience,
University of Heidelberg, Central Institute of Mental Health,
Mannheim, Germany*

Eija Kalso, MD, PhD
*Institute of Clinical Medicine, University of Helsinki; Pain Center,
Department of Anesthesiology, Intensive Care Medicine, Emergency
Medicine, and Pain Medicine, Helsinki University Central Hospital,
Helsinki, Finland*

Jonathan O. Dostrovsky, PhD
*Department of Physiology, University of Toronto,
Toronto, Ontario, Canada*

IASP PRESS® • SEATTLE

Library of Congress Cataloging-in-Publication Data

World Congress on Pain (11th : 2005: Sydney, N.S.W.)
 Proceedings of the 11th World Congress on Pain / editors, Herta Flor, Eija Kalso, Jonathan
  O. Dostrovsky. p. ; cm.
 Includes bibliographical references and index.
 ISBN 0-931092-60-4
1. Pain--Congresses. I. Flor, Herta. II. Kalso, Eija, 1955- III. Dostrovsky, Jonathan O. IV.
International Association for the Study of Pain. V. Title. VI. Title: Proceedings of the
Eleventh World Congress on Pain.
 [DNLM: 1. Pain--Congresses. WL 704 W927p 2006]
 RB127 W675 2005
 616'.0472--dc22
                           2006041820

Published by:

IASP Press
International Association for the Study of Pain
111 Queen Anne Ave N, Suite 501
Seattle, WA 98109-4955, USA
Fax: 206-283-9403
www.iasp-pain.org
www.painbooks.org

Printed in the United States of America

Contents

Contributing Authors

Preface

The field of pain is growing at an enormous rate, and much progress has been made on the elucidation of basic mechanisms, innovative approaches to assessment and treatment, and awareness of the problem of pain in health policy. This exponential growth was evident at the 11th World Congress on Pain, held in Sydney, Australia, August 21–26, 2005. The congress attracted more than 4,800 professionals from all disciplines involved in pain and provided a an exciting forum for scientific discourse. The congress featured a full day of refresher courses that are published in a separate volume edited by Douglas Justins (*Pain 2005—An Updated Review: Refresher Course Syllabus*). The scientific sessions included 20 plenary lectures, 82 workshops or minisymposia, and 1,725 free communications. Only a small fraction of the many interesting contributions and topics could be selected for this volume, which contains a total of 75 chapters organized into 9 sections with 20 plenary lectures, 26 workshop contributions, and 29 papers based on free communications. The editors have attempted to provide the reader with a broad range of cutting-edge topics in the field of pain, topics that address basic research as well as clinical applications and health policy issues. The international focus of IASP is evident from the broad range of countries represented in the speakers' affiliations.

Due to the location of the congress in Sydney, we attracted a number of contributions on pain assessment and management in Asia and the Pacific. Part I includes some of these contributions as well as the addresses of the outgoing (Michael R. Bond) and incoming (Troels S. Jensen) presidents, the John Loeser Distinguished Lecture on narrative medicine by Rita Charon, and discussions of ethical and educational issues in the field of pain. Part II presents many important advances on molecular and cellular mechanisms of pain, ranging from ion channels to the role of cytokines in pain. A special focus of this congress was the many central changes that take place as a consequence of pain such as neurodegenerative processes, glial activation, or altered descending inhibition and facilitation. These are included in Part III, Nociceptive Pathways and Central Processing, which also contains the John J. Bonica Lecture on spinal cord nociceptive pathways by William D. Willis. Part IV contains contributions on the imaging of pain, ranging from preterm infants to dynamic aspects of pain processing and the central consequences of repetitive pain exposure. Part V focuses on opioid mechanisms and treatment, ranging from the role of reward circuitry in pain processing to the efficacy of opioid treatment in various pain conditions and the analysis of side effects. Part VI presents new insights into the role of psychological and psychosocial factors and addresses gender issues as well as epidemiological perspectives. Part VII discusses specific clinical syndromes such as pain related to spinal cord injury or postherpetic neuralgia, as well as pain conditions that are less in the focus of pain research such as obstetric pain, urogenital pain, and pain in multiple sclerosis. Part VIII focuses on pain assessment and outcome measurement and deals, for example, with the challenges of pain assessment in children, the elderly, and mentally impaired persons, clinical decision making, and prospective approaches. Part IX, Psychological Interventions, Occupational Therapy, and Physical Approaches, presents nonpharmacological treatment approaches to chronic pain that range from behavioral treatments of cancer pain to the use of movement therapies, TENS, and interventions such as weight loss.

This congress was characterized by many innovative approaches to basic mechanisms, assessment, and treatment of pain, and we hope that we can provide the reader with a taste of the excitement and lively scientific discourse that characterized the Sydney meeting.

HERTA FLOR
EIJA KALSO
JONATHAN O. DOSTROVSKY

Acknowledgments

The editors of this volume and the officers and members of the Council of the International Association for the Study of Pain express their appreciation to the many individuals whose efforts were so important to the success of the 11th World Congress on Pain and this book.

We wish first to thank our colleagues on the Scientific Program Committee: Ralf Baron, Allan I. Basbaum, Michael R. Bond, Geert Crombez, Samuel F. Dworkin, Maria Fitzgerald, Cynthia Goh, Geoffrey K. Gourlay, Kazuo Hanaoka, Anthony K.P. Jones, Louisa E. Jones, Douglas M. Justins, Robert G. Large, Frank Porreca, Maureen J. Simmonds, Olaitan A. Soyannwo, Horacio Vanegas, and Judith H. Watt-Watson. Their hard work and dedication created the Congress's very successful scientific program, which in turn created this volume.

We are grateful to everyone in Sydney who worked to make the Congress a success. We wish to thank Geoffrey K. Gourlay, chair of the Local Arrangements Committee, and his colleagues, Michael R. Bond, Milton Cohen, Michael J. Cousins, Paul Glare, David Gronow, Amal Helou, Robyn Quinn, and Philip Siddall, who planned the non-scientific aspects of the Congress. Tour Hosts oversaw registration and all on-site details, while the staff of the Sydney Convention and Exhibition Centre consistently attended to all the Congress's needs.

We extend our special gratitude to IASP Honorary Member Louisa Jones, retiring after 32 years as IASP Executive Officer, during which she has organized every one of the IASP World Congresses. Her guiding hand will be greatly missed. We are especially grateful to Elizabeth Twiss, Coordinator, Meetings and Publications, for her invaluable effort in organizing the Congress. We thank the IASP office staff: Susan Couch, Yaa Cuguano, Marleda Di Pierri, Kathleen Havers, Karen Lauderback, Kris Lukkarila, Jane Milliken, Keith Peterson, and especially IASP Press Production Editor Elizabeth Endres and Desktop Technician Dale Schmidt for their dedicated work in preparing this book for publication.

Finally, we wish to thank all the speakers and delegates whose ideas, energy, and enthusiasm made both the IASP 11th World Congress on Pain and this resulting volume so exciting and valuable. It has been our pleasure and privilege to oversee this compilation of what was presented and discussed at the 11th World Congress.

On behalf of the members and Council of IASP, the editors acknowledge and express their special appreciation for the financial support given to the 11th World Congress on Pain and related IASP programs by the following:

Amgen (USA)
Boots Healthcare (UK)
Cephalon (USA)
Elan Pharmaceuticals (USA)
Endo Pharmaccuticals (USA)
GlaxoSmithKline (USA)
Grünenthal (Germany)
Janssen Pharmaceutica (Belgium)
Medtronic (USA)
Merck & Co., Inc. (USA)
Pfizer Global Pharmaceuticals (UK)
Purdue/Mundipharma/Napp Independent Associated Companies (USA)
Scan/Design by Inger and Jens Bruun Foundation, USA
SchwarzPharma (Germany)
SP Hersh/MICC Educational Fund

Part I

IASP, the 11th World Congress, and Perspectives on Pain

Proceedings of the 11th World Congress on Pain,
edited by Herta Flor, Eija Kalso, and Jonathan O.
Dostrovsky, IASP Press, Seattle, © 2006.

1

Outgoing President's Address

Michael R. Bond

Development and Alumni Office, University of Glasgow,
Glasgow, United Kingdom

The 30th anniversary of the International Association for the Study of Pain (IASP)'s first World Congress was celebrated at the 11th World Congress in Sydney by the publication of *The Paths of Pain 1975–2005,* edited by Harold Merskey, John D. Loeser, and Ronald Dubner. This volume provides a broad-based historical record of the many advances in pain research and clinical practice during the past 30 years. Despite those advances, however, it is clear that the benefits of the progress made by scientists and pain clinicians have not yet been incorporated into the clinical practice of many physicians, nurses, and other health professionals. For example, a major epidemiological study of over 30,000 individuals in 12 European countries revealed that chronic pain, with a mean duration of 7 years, was a major cause of disability and distress, and in a proportion of cases, 20% of the doctors concerned did not regard the pain as a problem. Relatively few of the individuals surveyed had been to a pain clinic (Breivik et al. 2005). The extent of acute and chronic pain in developing countries is unknown but can be inferred from the prevalence of known painful diseases, such as cancer, HIV/AIDS, and sickle cell anemia, and from the fact that in some of those parts of the world there are many victims of local wars and other forms of civil commotion. Figures released by the World Health Organization (WHO) in 2002 show that in the period 1990 to 2020 there will be a significant increase in illnesses and degenerative disorders that cause pain, especially in the elderly. Regarding specific conditions and diseases, the incidence of new cancer cases and cancer deaths was projected to almost double in that period in developing countries. In addition, the problem of HIV/AIDS, which has reached epidemic proportions in South Africa, India, and elsewhere, is associated with severe pain of the neuropathic type in its late stages and will greatly increase the extent of pain and suffering in those countries. On the basis of such evidence, unrelieved pain clearly remains a problem worldwide (Breivik and Bond 2004). Chronic pain disrupts quality of life and may become a disease in its own right; ethically, we appreciate that pain treatment should be a human right (Brennan and Cousins 2004).

ACTION BY IASP

The observations quoted above provide good reasons for IASP to redouble its work in support of basic and clinical research. In addition, it is equally important that the association continues to increase its aid to developing countries to sponsor the education of those concerned with pain management, to foster research, and to persuade governments and health agencies to take a greater interest in this aspect of suffering.

The main barriers in both developed and developing countries against better pain treatment include lack of education for undergraduates and postgraduates, the failure of governments and health providers to supply the resources needed for pain relief, which often is not given high priority, the uneven distribution of those resources that are available, and the influence of ethnic and cultural differences in attitudes to pain relief. In developing countries, treatment may be hampered by fears associated with the use of opioids and the reluctance of pharmaceutical companies to produce pain-relieving drugs at affordable prices.

SPECIFIC INITIATIVES

Since its foundation, IASP has disseminated research and clinical information through the publication of its journal *PAIN,* a range of curricula, and other publications, and IASP Press has published books since 1994. The *Core Curriculum for Professional Education in Pain* has been revised and is available both online (www.iasp-pain.org) and as a softbound volume (Charlton 2005).

At the time of the 10th World Congress on Pain in 2002, there was awareness of a need to increase existing aid programs for developing countries, as shown in Table I. A specific budget for aid for developing countries has been established, and there has been an increase in educational grants. In particular, a

Table I
IASP aid programs for developing countries

Visiting lectureships and consultancies
Adopt-a-Library program (copies of all publications are sent to libraries in developing and currency-restricted countries)
Grants for translation of IASP publications into local languages
Adopt-a-Member program
Grants for travel to world congresses

program of grants for educational development was introduced in 2005 that provided three grants on the basis of competition among chapters in Latin America. The funds were granted for one year to groups in Chile, Brazil, and Mexico. The number of grants will be increased to 10 per year, and application will be open to all IASP members in developing countries, in contrast to the restricted distribution during the pilot year in progress. Separate educational grants have been given since 2002 to Kenya and Nigeria, and IASP contributed to a major WHO project in six African countries focusing on cancer, HIV/AIDS, and palliative care. In 2005, IASP's first award for excellence was given for basic and clinical research in developing countries.

IASP GLOBAL DAY AGAINST PAIN

A very different type of initiative was launched in 2004 following the example of the European Federation of IASP Chapters (EFIC), which held its first European Week Against Pain in October 2001. IASP decided to initiate a Global Day Against Pain in collaboration with EFIC and WHO in October 2004. The theme of that event, held in Geneva, was "Pain Treatment Should be a Human Right." It has been decided to continue the Global Day in years to come and to make that day the first of a complete year against specific types of pain. For example in the year 2005–2006, the topic is "Pain in Children." The purpose of the Global Day is to stimulate all members and chapters to make local efforts to bring the topic to the attention of health professionals, health service providers, the media, and the general public, with a view to improving local knowledge, local resources, and as a consequence, pain relief around the world. Evidence from the first Global Day events revealed that these goals were achieved by many chapters.

INTERACTION WITH THE WORLD HEALTH ORGANIZATION

IASP has been a nongovernmental organization affiliate of WHO for many years. The association played a major part through Kathleen Foley and Vittorio Ventafridda in the development of the WHO analgesic ladder for the treatment of cancer pain. In recent years, the level of interaction has increased significantly, principally through the actions of Harald Breivik. In addition to collaborating with the WHO African Project and the launch of the Global Day, IASP has emphasized the need for WHO to promote more strongly the relief of chronic noncancer pain, especially in developing countries. This effort has resulted in IASP being invited to contribute to the writing and production of the publication *Neurological Disorders: Public Health Challenges.* This volume will contain a chapter dealing with pain in neurological disorders and represents the first step in what it is hoped will be further WHO publications focusing upon noncancer pain.

NEXT STEPS

Progress has been made toward the goals set at the time of the 10th World Congress in 2002 and in particular, toward my intention as incoming president to improve pain treatment in developing countries. This goal was to be achieved by greater use of IASP's resources, including its chapters, and by collaborating with WHO and other nongovernmental organizations. To some extent, the past three years have constituted a period of exploration of these possibilities, and ahead lies the task of strengthening and broadening existing programs as well as developing new ones. The steps that need to be taken are outlined in Table II.

Plans for the future will not be directed solely at the objectives mentioned in Table II. The incoming president, Troels Jensen, intends to build further upon the contribution of IASP to basic and clinical research. Therefore, the parallel streams of activity always present in the work of IASP will continue to flow even more strongly.

CONCLUSIONS

When concluding his period of office in 2002, Barry Sessle stated that for pain, IASP has become the "gold standard reference society" at an international level. During the past three years, the activities of IASP have been extended further, especially in the direction of the needs of developing countries.

I feel honored to have had the responsibility of leading IASP as president for three years. I am grateful to many people for their support, without which I

Table II
Developing countries: the next steps for IASP

Increase IASP's budget for programs in developing countries
Extend educational grants worldwide
Develop existing and new distance learning packages via the IASP Web site
Develop a pain management training grant program
Consider a developing countries research support program
Provide further awards for clinical management and for research
Continue to work with the World Health Organization
Continue the Global Day and Global Year Against Pain

could not have completed my task, and I thank especially the officers of IASP, the members of Council and of the many committees and task forces, particularly the Task Force on Developing Countries. I would like to thank Louisa Jones and her staff at the IASP Secretariat, without whom none of us could cope with the myriad functions of IASP. I wish my successor, Troels Jensen, every success during his presidency and I know that with him as leader, IASP will continue to flourish and to increase the scope of its work for all those who suffer pain.

REFERENCES

Breivik H, Bond MJ. Why pain control matters in a world full of killer diseases. *Pain: Clin Updates* 2004 XII:4.

Breivik H, Collett B, Ventafridda V, Cohen R, Gallacher D. Survey of chronic pain in Europe: prevalence, impact on daily life, and treatment. *Eur J Pain* 2005; Aug 8.

Brennan F, Cousins MJ. Pain relief as a human right. *Pain: Clin Updates* 2004; XII:5.

Charlton JE (Ed). *Core Curriculum for Professional Education in Pain,* 3rd ed. Seattle: IASP Press, 2005.

Merskey H, Loeser JD, Dubner R (Eds). *The Paths of Pain 1975–2005.* Seattle: IASP Press, 2005.

World Health Organization. *Innovative Care for Chronic Conditions: Building Blocks for Action—Global Report.* Geneva: World Health Organization, 2002.

Correspondence to: Sir Michael R. Bond, MD, PhD, Development and Alumni Office, University of Glasgow, No. 2 The Square, Glasgow G12 8QQ, United Kingdom. Email: m.bond@admin.gla.ac.uk.

Proceedings of the 11th World Congress on Pain,
edited by Herta Flor, Eija Kalso, and Jonathan O.
Dostrovsky, IASP Press, Seattle, © 2006.

2

Incoming President's Address: To Study Pain

Troels Staehelin Jensen

Department of Neurology and Danish Pain Research Center, Aarhus, Denmark

I would like to begin by thanking the members of the International Association for the Study of Pain (IASP) for the confidence they have shown by selecting me as president. It is an honor, a privilege, and a pleasure to work for an association devoted to the study of pain. It is with feelings of humility that I accept this position, following in the footsteps of so many brilliant and dedicated persons who have all—each in his or her own way— helped shape our association into the well-respected scientific society full of vitality, dynamics, and energy that we celebrate today.

In particular, I would like to recognize the great leadership shown by Sir Michael Bond in the three years of his presidency. It has been a wonderful experience to work with Michael, Barry Sessle, Fernando Cervero, and Russell Portenoy on the Executive Committee, as well as the rest of the IASP Council, the various IASP committees, and the IASP task forces. I would like to extend special thanks to the Scientific Program Committee, headed by Herta Flor, and to the Local Arrangements Committee, headed by Geoffrey Gourlay, for helping us make this congress an unforgettable success. I know from my own experience the immense workload associated with these tasks. All these successes would not have been possible without the very capable, hard-working, and friendly staff at the IASP secretariat, under the exemplary leadership of our Executive Officer Louisa Jones.

A BIT OF HISTORY

What is the reason for IASP's success? The answer can be found in our history. French dramatist Jean Anouilh stated in his 1937 play *Le Voyageur sans Baggage:* "Without knowing the history we carry on, we don't understand ourselves." Although the history of IASP is well known to some of you, a large group of younger members may not know the story, or may know only parts of it, and they deserve to know how IASP evolved. Let us take a look at our history, which goes back approximately 30 years.

The first milestone came in 1973, at the Providence Heights Conference Center, Issaquah, Washington, just outside Seattle, where the founder of our Association, John J. Bonica, gathered a group of dedicated individuals to hold the first comprehensive multidisciplinary meeting on pain. Dr. Bonica opened the meeting with the statement: "Pain is a major human concern influencing every aspect of life: it is the most common symptom of disease which compels patients to seek medical counsel." And he noted further: "Pain is a malefic force which often imposes severe emotional, physical, and economic stresses on the patient, on his family, and on society." The truth and depth of these words cannot be overstated, and for many of us, I believe, they represent the essence of what characterizes the chronic pain patient. After the Issaquah meeting that marked the beginning of IASP, things moved quickly. The first world congress took place in Florence in 1975 under the presidency of one of France's greatest scientists, Denise Albe-Fessard. A series of congresses followed in Montreal, Edinburgh, Seattle, Hamburg, and Adelaide, as the field of pain studies flourished and produced a stream of scientific papers. From the start, the growth of the association has been steady in almost all aspects: the number of IASP members, the number of IASP chapters, the number of delegates at world congresses, the increase in money disbursed, and the increase in income. The membership is now stabilizing at around 7,000 members, coming from a variety of fields and specialties including neuroscience, anesthesiology, neurology, neurosurgery, psychology, nursing, rehabilitation medicine, physical therapy, and dentistry. The last 30 years of IASP's history are beautifully displayed in the anniversary book (Merskey et al. 2005), which was presented to all delegates at the 11th World Congress on Pain. Many of the contributors to the anniversary book attended that first congress 30 years ago. They are to be commended for their remarkable contributions, both to the field of pain research and to this historic landmark in IASP's history.

Not only has IASP grown in terms of knowledge and publications, it has also spread its activities to almost every corner of the world. For an international organization like ours, dissemination of knowledge is crucial, so I would like to discuss in more detail the IASP chapters, which are essential elements of our association. The formation of local chapters throughout the world has been a key factor in the dissemination of new information about pain. The formation of chapters provides a means for effective liaisons with governments, patient groups, and the media, and the chapters are a crucial part of the new initiative, the IASP Global Day Against Pain, which brings pain into focus in all parts of the world. I encourage all chapters to participate by organizing local events on this day to increase awareness of pain.

As shown in Fig. 1, the number of chapters has increased: we are now up to 63 chapters, and others are in the process of formation. IASP has established a chapter liaison position within the Council in order to promote and strengthen collaboration with the chapters. Although the chapters are organizationally and financially independent, IASP does provide aid, such as sending IASP Press books and other publications, providing grants for translations, and arranging for visiting lecturers. IASP further supports the chapters by sending the journal *PAIN* and various IASP Press books to more than 100 libraries in developing countries and in currency-restricted parts of the world.

But this effort is not enough: we should do more. It is important that IASP officers visit the chapters, participate in their activities, and provide information about IASP resources; the councillors and I will participate in such activities. Correspondence and communication between the national chapters and IASP, and between IASP headquarters and the members of the chapters, must be strengthened. In several countries, both in developed and less developed parts of the world, chapter members are not joining IASP. For example, in the People's Republic of China there are close to 6,000 members of the Chinese Association for the Study of Pain, but only 27 members of IASP.

Research and education are central to the activities of IASP. A number of publications are produced by our organization. Two initiatives are in the forefront: our flagship journal *PAIN* and IASP Press. Originally under the leadership of Patrick Wall, *PAIN* next enjoyed the joint leadership of Patrick Wall and Ronald Dubner, followed by a short period with Ron Dubner acting as single chief editor. *PAIN* is now under the fine leadership of Allan Basbaum. Not only has it proven to be the leading pain journal in terms of scientific content, impact factor, and number of manuscript pages, but *PAIN* is also a source of significant revenue for IASP. A new contract has been signed with our publisher Elsevier, and the future looks prosperous. I would like to extend my sincere gratitude to Allan Basbaum and his field and associate editors for the great job they have done. The economic freedom created by the surplus from the journal makes IASP strong, independent, and able to accomplish its scientific and educational goals.

Another important educational activity is IASP Press, which began under the skillful leadership of Howard Fields and is now under the excellent direction of Editor-in-Chief Catherine Bushnell. An increased number of new books appeared this year, and more are scheduled for next year to fulfill the Press's mission of providing our members with timely, high-quality publications relevant to pain. I notice with satisfaction that these new books have colorful and attractive dust covers, which can only help in disseminating IASP's message.

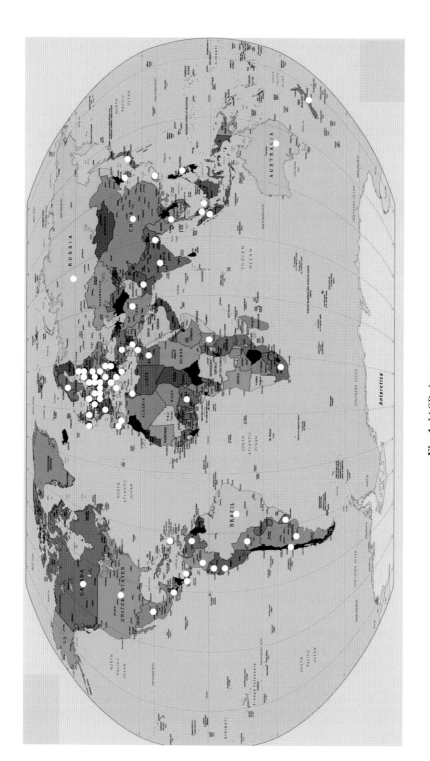

Fig. 1. IASP chapters.

WORLD CONGRESSES AND SPECIAL INTEREST GROUPS

The triennial world congresses represent, of course, the core of IASP's scientific and educational goals. If there is one thing that characterizes these congresses, it is the vitality and enthusiasm with which participants from a wide spectrum of disciplines present and discuss all scientific and clinical aspects of pain, seasoned with joy and good humor, and enlivened by remarkable receptions. These congresses, like all other aspects of IASP activities, have grown throughout the years, from about 700 participants in 1975 to over 5,000 participants in 2005. The 2005 congress boasts the highest number of scientific presentations ever submitted or accepted, with more than 1,800 registered abstracts.

The world congresses cover all aspects of pain ranging from molecular biology to cognitive processing of pain, but the science moves much faster and encompasses much more than can be fully covered in a triennial congress. The formation of IASP special interest groups (SIGs) is an important element filling the gaps between the different interests of the members and the long duration between the world congresses. The SIGs were formed to allow our members to stay within IASP while focusing on specific topics or areas of pain; they also hold meetings and symposia under the auspices of IASP. The SIGs have had varying success rates: some have been scientifically very strong and have attracted a lot of members, while others have chosen topics that attract fewer members but are still very important. IASP intends to follow existing SIGs closely and support them as much as possible, while also encouraging the formation of new groups. This year has seen applications for the formation of three new SIGs: one on acute pain, one on pain in older persons, and one on

Table I
IASP Special Interest Groups (SIGs) and time of formation

Pain in Childhood (1989)
Pain and the Sympathetic Nervous System (PSNS) (1990)
Clinical-Legal Issues in Pain (CLIP) (1994)
Systematic Reviews in Pain Relief (1996)
Placebo (1997)
Sex, Gender, and Pain (1997)
Pain of Urogenital Origin (PUGO) (1998)
Neuropathic Pain (NeuP) (1999)
Orofacial Pain (1999)
Pain and Movement (2000)
Torture, Organized Violence, and War (2004)
Acute Pain (2005)
Pain in Older Persons (2005)
Pain and Pain Management in Non-Human Species (2005)

pain and pain management in nonhuman species. I encourage members who are active in specific areas to encourage colleagues to join the relevant SIGs, or even to start up new ones. The SIGs may be thought of as scientific spearheads for IASP, allowing us to be dynamic and up-to-date on specific topics while not losing our comprehensive multidisciplinary overview.

WHY IS IASP SUCCESSFUL?

One of the reasons for IASP's success is that we are an honest organization with a very clear goal. IASP has stayed independent of industry and other bodies for years. As stated in the bylaws for the association, our main purpose is to foster and encourage research in pain mechanisms, to improve management of acute and chronic pain, and to promote education and training in pain. These goals are to be achieved by bringing together scientists, physicians, and other health care professionals who have an interest in pain research and management. Surely we all agree with this very simple—but also very demanding—goal of joining forces on a major issue: fighting pain, which threatens not only our bodies, but also our souls and our human dignity. The pain and suffering that surround us remind all of us to go out and do something about it, and to join forces. This was the vision promoted by our founder, John J. Bonica, and it has been upheld by our leaders and members throughout our history.

IASP is special in the sense that it has succeeded in gathering enthusiastic people from the basic and clinical sciences, from a variety of disciplines and from various countries, seeking to understand and to increase our knowledge about pain. This goal can only be possible with a multidisciplinary approach, as John J. Bonica originally proposed. Let us take advantage of this long-lasting marriage between the basic and clinical sciences in our battle against pain.

MY MEETING WITH PAIN AND IASP

Having discussed the history of IASP, I would now like to turn briefly to my own history. My interest in pain was awakened 25 years ago, when I first met Patrick Wall at a small neurosurgery meeting in my hometown. I knew almost nothing about pain, but I had started a clinical project on sequelae after amputation and was working at the same time at my university's neuropharmacological department on the pharmacology of spinal nociceptive reflex activity. Pat advised me on my clinical project and encouraged me to continue my basic research by going abroad to learn more. This suggestion led me to Tony L. Yaksh, who at that time was at the Mayo Clinic. Working with Dr. Yaksh and experiencing the ambience that surrounded him has been an inspiration to me ever since. Together with Tony, I explored opioid- and glutamate-sensitive areas of the brain that were of interest in modulating spinal nociceptive behavior. I was also fortunate at that time to know Fred Kerr, a neurosurgeon and neuroanatomist at Mayo, next door to us (his technician, Ms. Margareth Mourning, performed the histological sections for us, which enabled me to talk at length with Fred). Fred had a marvellous ability to integrate basic discoveries with clinical observations, trying to see the potential clinical relevance—or lack thereof—in each new scientific discovery, and asking simple basic-science questions dictated by a clinical observation. This ability to unite the basic and clinical sciences, which Fred shared with other great scientists such as William K. Livingston, William Noordenbos, and Patrick Wall, encapsulates what I believe is the key element of our association, something I try to keep as the guiding star for my own work and science. I hope IASP can and will continue along this path.

The power to unravel the mechanisms of pain that results from combining basic and clinical scientific approaches became clear to me at the first IASP meeting I attended, the 5th World Congress in Seattle in 1984. The energy, the enthusiasm, and the dynamics were self-evident when I came in late in the afternoon and heard a discussion session with Howard Fields and several others. I knew then that IASP was something I just had to belong to.

FUTURE DIRECTIONS FOR IASP

Having talked about the past and touched on the present, it is time to consider the future. Where does IASP want to go—and where do I want to take IASP in the next three years? IASP has developed into a large international organization. Advances have been made, but there are still tasks to be undertaken. A summary of what I consider important tasks for the next three years is shown in Table II and will briefly be described below.

Young Investigator Program. Our organization has proven to be the leading pain organization in terms of scientific activity, scientific quality, members, publications, connections to other societies, and educational activities. This position needs to be maintained and extended. IASP is extraordinary in one particular aspect: the number of basic scientists is high, with currently close to 1,000 members coming from different basic disciplines, and the number of clinical scientists is also extensive. The main aim of IASP is to foster and encourage research on pain. For the last few decades, activities have depended on dedicated individuals who have worked as officers, speakers, organizers, or participants in workshops, mini-symposia, educational courses, and SIGs.

Table II
IASP Activities in 2005–2008

Young Investigator Program
Reinforcement of IASP activities
Strengthening of contact to Chapters
Strengthening and expansion of Special Interest Groups
Recruitment of new members
IASP publications
Journal *PAIN*
IASP Press
Education and the Web
Education in developing countries

We need new blood to gradually take over many of these functions, and many young people are ready to step onto the stage if invited. Many of these young investigators and trainees have very limited resources to go to congresses and other meetings, to visit other laboratories and research units, or to obtain funding for their work. It may not quite be like Hans Christian Andersen's fairy tale *The Little Match Girl*, where the young investigators are standing outside the door wanting to get inside, but unable to afford it—but the analogy is there. Young investigators from the basic and clinical sciences represent the bread and butter of IASP. We need to support these people, and IASP's strong financial situation makes it possible to do so. I propose that we support these young investigators, including those who are not yet members of IASP, in joining us, in the expectation that in the future they will keep the association strong, dynamic, and vital. Considerable resources should be devoted to improving conditions for these young investigators and also to recruiting new young members, because if we do not recruit these bright young minds, others will. I suggest the formation of an ad hoc committee to start a program aimed at improving conditions for young investigators, which would include financial support to participate in IASP congresses, an increase in the number of existing grants, the creation of funds for exchange visits between laboratories, and an increase in funds for research and educational materials. This program may involve interactions with industry in order to create funds, based of course on completely unrestricted grants. With the scientific reputation surrounding IASP, I believe such a program will be possible and will, if successful, make a great difference for the future of pain research, for IASP, and for the young investigators. I am not a specialist in economics, but I am sure that investing in these young investigators is better than putting our money in the bank. I see this young investigator program as our most important task for the coming years, but there are of course other efforts that can and should be made.

New members. Our association is multidisciplinary, but some specialties such as rheumatology, cardiology, and orthopedic and general surgery are very weakly represented in our society, despite pain's importance to these disciplines. Recruitment of members from these disciplines needs consideration. IASP already has 7,000 members and, as was very wisely said by our esteemed former president, Jean-Marie Besson, "Our goal has never been to recruit new members at all costs" (Besson 2000). What we need are people with enthusiasm for the aims of our association who will encourage research on pain mechanisms and pain syndromes.

Contact with chapters and special interest groups. Communications between IASP and the local chapters should be strengthened. The SIGs also need support and close follow-up by IASP, and in this context a new program to assist the SIGs and the chapters should be considered.

Education. Improvement in education and in the dissemination of new information about pain is a major goal for IASP. Over the years, members have produced valuable educational materials. Some of this material needs to be updated, and undoubtedly there are many young and new members who can be recruited to this type of work. Access to the Web represents an inexhaustible resource for delivering up-to-date educational material to our members and our chapters. Therefore, the resources allocated to the IASP Web page should be increased. *PAIN* and IASP Press need to be maintained and strengthened.

Education in developing countries. During my predecessor's time in office, IASP initiated a program to improve pain management and other pain-related activities in developing countries, with an initial focus on Latin America. This program will take time to establish and is demanding. This effort needs to be continued for the next three years, in collaboration with the World Health Organization (WHO). Sir Michael Bond will continue the program in developing countries, and as the next WHO liaison, he will also have the opportunity to convince people outside our association about the importance of pain and its treatment in the developing world.

CONCLUDING REMARKS

Let me conclude this chapter with a few caveats. The last few years have seen the formation of new societies, the introduction of federations of IASP chapters, and the launching of new journals with pain as their main focus. Some may consider these bodies and journals as threats to the existence of IASP. I do not share this fear—on the contrary. The more focus and interest we have on pain, the better. However, the focus has to be scientifically solid and evidence-based. This is particularly important for an experience like pain, subjective and variable as it is, and in principle not measurable by any physiological method. Pain patients are at risk of being taken advantage of by those making unethical claims for unproven therapies. IASP should guard patients against these deceptive approaches.

Some may say we do not need more science in pain; we need more clinical approaches and "how-to" advice. However, allow me to remind you of the name of our association: our mission is to *study* pain. We are already surrounded by many other societies that teach clinicians how to do things. It is my clear conviction that clinicians—whether engaged in research or not—are sincerely interested in learning new scientific information. As the leading society in pain, we should be at the forefront in providing new and scientifically solid information. This work will not be easy, and there is no magic bullet that will "cure" chronic pain. But by *studying* pain, by putting one small brick on top of the next, we will eventually gain knowledge that can be used to help patients. By encouraging basic and clinical scientists to join forces, I am confident that we will make progress in our understanding of pain to the benefit of our patients. I wish you welcome to three more years with IASP.

REFERENCES

Besson JM. President's address to the 9th World Congress on Pain: basic researchers and clinicians must unite in the fight against pain. In: Devor M, Rowbotham MC, Wiesenfeld-Hallin Z (Eds). *Proceedings of the 9th World Congress on Pain,* Progress in Pain Research and Management, Vol. 16. Seattle: IASP Press, 2000, pp 1–7.
Jensen TS. Pain: from molecules to suffering. *Nat Rev Neurosci* 2005; 6:505.
Merskey H, Loeser JD, Dubner R (Eds). *The Paths of Pain 1975–2005*. Seattle: IASP Press, 2005.

Correspondence to: Prof. Troels Staehelin Jensen, MD, PhD, Department of Neurology and Danish Pain Research Center, Aarhus University Hospital, DK- 8000 Aarhus C, Denmark. Tel: 45-8949-4137; Fax: 45-8949-3269; email: tsjensen@ ki.au.dk.

Proceedings of the 11th World Congress on Pain, edited by Herta Flor, Eija Kalso, and Jonathan O. Dostrovsky, IASP Press, Seattle, © 2006.

3

Suffering, Storytelling, and Community: An Approach to Pain Treatment from Columbia's Program in Narrative Medicine[1]

Rita Charon

Program in Narrative Medicine, Columbia University, New York, New York, USA

John Loeser is a pioneer and a visionary. He recognized a long time ago the need for a narrative approach to the person in pain, realizing that the health care professional—whether neurosurgeon, anesthesiologist, physical therapist, acupuncturist, or psychiatrist—needs to richly and powerfully *imagine* what the individual patient suffers, what ordeal he or she endures. Only on the grounds of clinically and affectively accurate knowledge can the caregiver deliver that which is needed and that which will help. And only when the pain patient is *recognized*—not only for all that he suffers but for all who he is—will healing occur.

Pain exposes deep problems of meaning. The pain I want to consider is chronic, unremitting, and untreatable pain—the kind that plagues us in pain medicine, our challenge. Unlike such acute pain as renal colic or postoperative pain, this kind of chronic pain is, in the end, often unresponsive to our usually effective modalities.

Severe chronic pain is our contemporary central dilemma—it *stands for* our most impenetrable dilemmas of unnameable and unfixable and unwarranted suffering. From metastatic cancer to whatever fibromyalgia will turn out to be, it is the pain one lives one's life around. Chronic pain is today's equivalent to other time's tragedies—widespread epidemics in one age, the crisis of faith in another—a devastation that comes, unannounced, to those who have done nothing to deserve it. It probably stands for death or for sacrificial suffering

---

[1] The John Loeser Distinguished Lecture.

that occurs randomly to some and spares the rest of us—epidemiologically speaking—the need to suffer ourselves.

Those who treat pain patients work on behalf of the whole culture. You must have great courage to do this work—this daily, personally costly work of facing suffering, usually without having the wherewithal to cure it or even relieve it. In treating those with chronic pain, we come to know the pain and we come to know its meaning. Our work endows us with wisdom, not just about particular diseases or particular patients, but about human life. This work inflicts on us our own brand of misery, that of countenancing suffering beyond our power to end it. Instead of choosing it, it chooses us, and we now have to fulfill our duties toward having been called. Whether chosen or not, this work makes us philosophers and sages. Wherever in the spectrum of pain medicine you are, you cannot escape the person in pain. Whether you work in a pain clinic or in a basic science laboratory examining PET scans, your work is never limited solely to the amygdala or the anterior cingulate gyrus. By virtue of having dedicated yourself to the mystery of pain, you are on the frontier of mind/body, of definition of self, of the convergence of the physical and the mental and the spiritual. You are examining urgent and challenging questions that today are being asked by science and by culture.

I want to bring to your attention some dimensions of pain that might not be center stage in the departments of neurosurgery or anesthesia or pharmacology but that repay study. Chronic pain involves *loss*—loss of health, loss of pleasure, loss of joy, loss of function, loss of the ordinary things that one who has no pain can do. Chronic pain involves *trauma*—something destructive or damaging has happened, although what has happened to cause the pain is often a mystery. Chronic pain has a *plot*—it has a career, a past, a present, and a future, even if the future is not in sight. Like any career, it accrues experience and mastery along the way and, like any plot, it unfolds gradually to reveal meaning.

To tolerate loss, human beings remember what has been lost—in obituaries, funerals, memorials, commemorations. We preserve traces of what has been lost in *memory*. We *mourn* (Freud 1957; Spiegel 1997; Derrida 2001). We keep the lost alive, even after it has gone away. Through memory, we say: *it is not gone.* We use language, pictures, and sensory data to store memory—in letters, conversations, diaries, dreams, and imagination as well as through literature, religion, ritual, and art. Memory enables the bereaved to preserve that which has been lost so that he or she can endure the loss and carry on. Although lost, the thing lost is still part of self. It is not forgotten. The lost survives.

To survive trauma, human beings give its testimony—eye-witness accounts, news reports, depositions, trial proceedings, claims. We *bear witness* to what happened (Felman and Laub 1992; LaCapra 1994; Caruth 1996; Pham et al. 2004). Through bearing witness we say: *it happened.* We do this when we register what we have gone through in settings like support groups or public hearings. More formally, we bear witness through history, journalism, and the law. These forms of testimony enable the survivor to declare that trauma has happened so that he or she can outlast the trauma and persist. Although it happened, the trauma does not erase the self. Despite the trauma, the self survives.

If chronic pain combines loss with trauma, then pain patients need to commemorate their lost health and to bear witness to the trauma that happened. Both commemorating loss and bearing witness to trauma are accomplished by *telling* of them, and so pain, too, must be told. Here, then, is my hypothesis. Pain patients have to tell the story of their pain in order to get better. This is where the plot of pain comes in. Telling the story of the pain—its past, present, and future—combines memory and bearing witness, enabling the sufferer to behold not only the reality of the pain but its meaning.

Telling the story of pain is not easy. We know that it is difficult to remember pain when it is gone and to remember the absence of pain when pain is present. This complicates the memory work in commemorating what has been lost and requires expert assistance. We also know that in the case of chronic pain, it is often difficult to know what happened to bring it about. This complicates the bearing witness to the trauma and also requires expert assistance.

These complexities mean that the plot of the pain is contested. What caused it? When did it start? How has it lived in my life? What has it done to my life? When will it end? And so the means of telling of pain will be contested: the telling might take place in language, in pictures, perhaps in some cases directly through the body in performance or movement of some kind. The listener must know how to listen for the story of pain.

This is where narrative medicine comes in. Narrative medicine is what we call medicine practiced with the narrative competence to receive and honor other people's stories—how to attend to stories, to absorb them, respect them, understand their surface and deep meanings, how to enter them, to let them transform their tellers and listeners (Charon 2001). By learning how to elicit stories from patients, receive them fully, and interpret them accurately, doctors and nurses and therapists can improve the effectiveness of their care. Narrative medicine lets us attend to patients fully, lets us represent that which they emit to us, and then, as a consequence of our attention and representation, lets us affiliate with them and with colleagues in new and therapeutically consequential ways.

I find myself having adopted new clinical routines in my practice as a result of what I have learned in narrative medicine. When I meet with new patients, I no longer go through the standard drill of eliciting the history of present illness, the past medical history, social history, family history, and review of systems.

Instead, I say these sentences: "I will be your doctor, and so I need to know a lot about your body and your health and your life. Please tell me what you think I should know about your situation." I do not write anything down or enter things in the computer while the patient answers. Instead, I sit still, gazing at the patient, trying very, very hard to absorb every aspect of what the patient tells. The first time I did this, I had no idea what to expect. The patient, a Dominican man in his fifties who had come in with concerns about chest pain and joint pain, chose to start his narration with the death of his father 20 years ago, the death of his brother 10 years ago, and the difficulty he was having being a father to his teen-age son. And then he started to cry. I asked him why he was weeping. He answered, "Nobody ever let me do this before" (Charon 2004).

What I have learned since having adopted this routine about a year ago is that if patients are given the chance to frame their own illnesses, they do so eloquently and often gratefully. I learn something I would not otherwise have learned by giving a patient this opportunity to tell of the illness in whatever way seems right. What I learn is not only about symptoms or diseases but about how the illness fits in with the rest of life. Ordinarily, I learn a great deal about bodily complaints as well as about home and work and life. I learn what the patient considers to have been the beginning of the illness, and I often learn what the patient thinks will happen in its future. I learn what the patient fears in relation to the illness and what helps him or her to cope with it. This knowledge is unavailable unless one asks for it, and I have found that what I learn during this first narrative account by the patient is pivotal in what I choose to do and in which order. While the patient is changing into a gown in preparation for the physical exam, I write down as close a representation as I can produce of what the patient says during this initial recitation, not sanitizing the report into the format of a medical note but reproducing the order of topics and often the actual words the patient used in talking. I give the patient a copy of that part of my note at the close of the first visit. In this way, the patient and I together can remember where we started our work. Patients often refer to this note later on in treatment, confirming to me the power of simply giving them back their own words.

Not only patients but their caregivers have urgent narratives of illness to tell or to write. My Program in Narrative Medicine at Columbia sponsors several writing seminars for health care professionals. We find that doctors, nurses, and social workers value the opportunity to write about their practice, not in the technical language and format of the medical chart but in ordinary language in stories or poems. In Narrative Oncology, for example, I meet twice a month for an hour at a time with oncologists, nurses, and social workers who staff the in-patient oncology service at Presbyterian Hospital. The health care professionals come to the lunch-time seminar with something they have written about a particular patient. Over sandwiches and cookies, they read to one another what they have written. (We met with hospital counsel at the start of our work to ensure that we were fully complying with the Health Insurance Portability and Accountability Act and with our own commitment to maintain patient confidentiality.) Over time, these professionals have strengthened their capacity to represent their powerful experiences with severely ill patients. By virtue of increasing their ability to represent what their patients endure in illness and what they themselves go through in caring for them, they are better able to attend to what the patients tell them. They *understand* more accurately and with more empathy what patients say. We hypothesize (and are seeking funding to demonstrate) that this simple and inexpensive intervention will improve individual health care professional well-being, will strengthen the cohesion of the health care team, and will increase patient satisfaction on the unit (Klein 2003). Similar writing groups have taken root in pediatric oncology, the AIDS/HIV clinic, the neonatal intensive care unit, and the primary care internal medicine residency.

Narrative medicine has been learning about the power of telling of suffering—by trauma survivors, the dying, or the bereaved. We have been working with oral historians, chaplains, psychoanalysts, and people in trauma studies to learn about bearing witness and giving testimony. To be able to give testimony about one's suffering and to have others bear witness to that testimony is not only a relief for the teller and an education for those who listen, but the transaction between teller and listener is a healing one. Attentive listening to pain or suffering can help the sufferer to see the pain whole, to contain it, to give shape to it. Once the story of pain of suffering is uttered or written, it can be gazed at, apprehended, perhaps understood freshly by virtue of its form, now, as a story or narrative (Morris 1997; Anderson and MacCurdy 2000; Hartman 2002).

These methods work not only for catastrophic trauma like rape or the Holocaust or September 11, 2001. It is as important for someone who has undergone non-catastrophic trauma like migraine headaches or spinal stenosis. Perhaps it is even more important in chronic pain than in remote trauma, because in chronic pain, there is a possibility for improvement. Chronic pain is always there—its mysterious presence in every day complicates simple actions, cancels pleasure. But unlike the suffering related to trauma, chronic pain seems sometimes to have come from nowhere. Many of my patients with pain cannot really say with certainty what caused the pain or when it started. And so their tellings of their suffering are a more difficult task than that faced by the rape survivor, who at least knows what must be told.

In chronic pain, the tellings may be even more chaotic or unsystematic than the remembrances of trauma. The longer the pain or distress has lasted, the more time might be needed to tell it fully in all its details. The more obscure are the origins of the suffering, the more urgent it is for the telling and discovery to proceed.

Health care professionals are not, as a matter of course, equipped with skills of attention, but we are developing methods of training them how to bear witness to their patients' narratives of illness and pain. It often does not feel like one is "doing" something when one listens attentively to another's story. Doctors, anyway, get fidgety unless we roll up our sleeves and *do* something to fix the situation. Nurses, chaplains, and social workers are better able to equate attentive listening with caring. But all of us can learn to listen and confirm with power and generosity.

We think it is critical that the doctors, nurses, and therapists themselves do the work of listening to patients' narratives of pain. The listening is central to the treatment. Unless the neurosurgeon or the radiation oncologist or physical therapist knows what the patient endures, he or she cannot provide effective care. It is not enough for the patients' family or friends to hear the patients out. Nor is it sufficient for members of a support group or an electronic chat room to hear of their pain. The hearing has got to be done by those in charge of the treatment, because the treatment will depend on the knowledge gained. The hearing out is, indeed, a central part of treatment. Such listening is a prelude to action, for without it, the caregiver will not learn all that might help the patient's pain. The listening is done not only because it is necessary and generous; it is done because it will lead directly to action.

The biggest dividend for the patient and for those who care for the patient of narrative methods is that telling plots let us look into the future. Yes, there have been losses. Yes, there have been traumas. But the patient's most serious commitment is to look clearly at the present, at the *now*, and to look toward the future. Where am I now? Who have I become? What will happen to me? Once the past that preceded the pain has been mourned and once the pain's sources have been acknowledged, the patient's present and future can be envisioned. Narrative methods can help to bring our patients to the point of active choice—how, now, shall I live my life despite my current health status? Instead of the fruitless search for cure in more and more outlandish sectors, the patient can be encouraged to accept whatever limitations are inevitable and to make realistic and productive choices for the rest of life, toward a chosen future.

Narrative medicine holds out hope not only for improving individual pain patients' situations but also for nourishing the communities that form, always, in the wake of genuine telling and attentive listening. Patients, families, and health care professionals affiliate, by virtue of narrative work, into communities who recognize one another and who support one another's health. Here, then, is comfort for our misery as we care for pain patients. Our stories, too, can productively be told.

I would like to propose a narrative writing exercise that anyone reading this chapter can try. I invite you to write a paragraph about a patient's pain. Think of a pain patient in your care who moves you particularly—to sadness, to triumph, to disappointment, to rage, to love. Think of someone whose pain seems to govern much of his or her life. Try to evoke the presence of that patient in your imagination. First, try to describe the patient in words. Think of the last time you saw the patient. Write down what you see when you imagine the patient as you saw him or her the last time.

When I did this exercise myself in preparation for this essay, here is what I wrote:

"She is clutching the arm crutches, covered with foam rubber so as to limit the hand pain caused by all her weight on the crutches. She moves slowly, taking forever to get to my office not so far from the waiting room, She seems more downcast than usual. Her only request is for brand name Prozac because the generic doesn't work. How little it seems to be that I can do for her."

This paragraph contains a physical description of the patient's posture, her presence, her altered mobility. We see the slowness caused by her pain, the way time has been changed by her pain. We see her mood, spoken almost through her physical posture of downcastness. And then we hear the nihilist realization that there is so little the doctor can do.

Next, please imagine your patient talking directly to you, telling you the story of his or her pain. What would the patient say if you said, "Tell me the story of your pain"? Can you imagine it? Can you tolerate hearing it? Can you hear it clearly enough that you can write it down? Here is what I wrote, imagining the voice of the patient I described above:

"It's like it keeps moving around and around. It used to be just in my legs. Then my arms and hands. Of course, always my head. I can't even walk like I used to. Soon, I will need a wheelchair even in the house. I cannot imagine a time before the pain. I think I was born with it. That's what cerebral palsy means, right? I was never a person without pain. How unfair it all is."

We hear what she has lost—mobility, independence, confidence in her power. We hear about the trauma—a trauma of birth, an unfair trauma. And we hear the plot, including the pain's time course—its past (or perhaps more accurately the absence of past, for the patient cannot picture a time when she had what was lost, an innocence from pain), its present (contained in its physical geography), and its future (it will only worsen).

By reading your own sentences, you begin to see what aspects of pain you yourself are porous to. Do your sentences include what the patient lost? Do they include the trauma? Do they contain the plot of the patient's pain? What about your own interior responses to this patient? Simply reading closely what you yourself wrote will give you some sense of how you approach this patient in pain and what you are curious to learn about him or her.

You are by no means guaranteed to be right when you imagine the patient's story of pain, although those of us who do such narrative writing a lot have discovered that such writing grants us access to knowledge we do not realize we possess (Anderson 1998). This exercise generates hypotheses; it does not test them. You test the hypotheses generated by talking with the patient. The next time you see the patient you have just written about, you will have thought about him or her in a new way. You will have tried to inhabit his or her inner reality. You will have imagined some things about his or her experience or thoughts or feelings. When you see the patient the next time, you will be curious to learn whether or not you were right. In the process of testing your hypotheses, you will engage the patient in conversation perhaps a little different from the ones you ordinarily have. This simple writing exercise may invest you in learning more about this patient, or at least in learning different kinds of things about him or her. If nothing else, the exercise may prompt you to ask this patient to tell you the story of his or her pain.

Unlike taking the clinical history using conventional methods, narrative medicine methods mobilize the health care professional's imagination in generating clinical hypotheses. Our narrative methods attend to multiple registers as patients convey or emit that which they know or feel or fear, perhaps enabling patients to reveal more fully all that is entailed in this history of pain. These methods actively try to bridge the divides between patients and professionals by shifting the locus of control toward the patient, inviting the patient to, in effect, *authorize* the full story of pain, however he or she chooses to tell it. We think that such methods might round out that which we health care professionals come gradually to know about our patients. Many teams, at Columbia and elsewhere, are hoping to test these methods, hypothesizing that such aspects of care as adherence with treatment recommendations, sturdiness of the therapeutic relationship, the patient's own sense of agency or effectiveness in controlling pain, fidelity to a treatment team, ability to make realistic plans for the future, and positive involvement of other members of a support circle (family, friends, colleagues) might improve by virtue of these methods. Simply allowing patients to feel more fully heard, including being heard fully by themselves, may well have practical consequences in how clinical problems are framed and what kinds of solutions are sought. Simultaneously, the health care professional using these methods might feel more fully nourished by the practice, realizing the dividends for the patient of skilled attentive listening.

Narrative medicine for pain gives us a means to capture the loss of health, the trauma of hurt, and the *now* of life. By skillfully opening up our patients' narratives of health and illness, by knowing what to listen *for*, we can encourage patients to look toward and to create a future, however chronic is the pain, that they can choose to live.

REFERENCES

Anderson CM. "Forty acres of cotton waiting to be picked": medical students, storytelling, and the rhetoric of healing. *Lit Med* 1998; 17:280–297.

Anderson CM, MacCurdy MM (Eds). *Writing and Healing: Toward an Informed Practice*. New York: National Council of Teachers of English, 2000.

Derrida J. *The Work of Mourning*. Chicago: University of Chicago Press, 2001.

Caruth C. *Unclaimed Experience: Trauma, Narrative, and History*. Baltimore: Johns Hopkins University Press, 1996.

Charon R. Narrative medicine: a model for empathy, reflection, profession, and trust. *JAMA* 2001; 286:1897–1902.

Charon R. Narrative and medicine. *N Engl J Med* 2004; 350:862–864.

Felman S, Laub D. *Testimony: Crises of Witnessing in Literature, Psychoanalysis, and History*. New York: Routledge, 1992.

Freud S. Mourning and melancholia. In: *Standard Edition of the Complete Psychological Works of Sigmund Freud*, Vol. 14. London: Hogarth Press, 1957, pp 237–258.

Hartman G. *Scars of the Spirit: The Struggle against Inauthenticity*. New York: Palgrave/Macmillan, 2002.

Klein J. Narrative Oncology: medicine's untold stories. *Oncology Times* 2003; February 25:10,13.

LaCapra D. *Representing the Holocaust: History, Theory, Trauma*. Ithaca: Cornell University Press, 1994.

Morris D. Voice, genre, and moral community. In: Kleinman A, Das V, Lock M (Eds). *Social Suffering*. Berkeley: University of California Press, 1997.

Pham PN, Weinstein HM, Longman T. Trauma and PTSD symptoms in Rwanda: implications for attitudes toward justice and reconciliation." *JAMA* 2004; 292:602–612.

Spiegel M, Tristman R (Eds). *The Grim Reader: Writings on Death, Dying, and Living On*. New York: Anchor Books/Doubleday, 1997.

Correspondence to: Prof. Rita Charon, MD, PhD, Program in Narrative Medicine, Columbia University, 630 West 168th Street, New York, NY 10032, USA. Email: rac5@columbia.edu.

Proceedings of the 11th World Congress on Pain, edited by Herta Flor, Eija Kalso, and Jonathan O. Dostrovsky, IASP Press, Seattle, © 2006.

4

Interprofessional Pain Education: Models, Issues, and Possibilities

Judy Watt-Watson,[a] Kate Seers,[b] and Jenny Strong[c]

[a]Faculty of Nursing and Centre for the Study of Pain, University of Toronto, Toronto, Ontario, Canada; [b]Royal College of Nursing Institute, Radcliffe Infirmary, Oxford, United Kingdom; [c]Department of Occupational Therapy, School of Health and Rehabilitation Sciences, University of Queensland, Brisbane, Queensland, Australia

Inadequate practitioner knowledge about pain management continues to be documented despite the availability of both the core curriculum (Charlton 2005) and discipline-specific curricula of the International Association for the Study of Pain (IASP). Moreover, pain education for health professionals at all levels has been identified as a means of changing ineffective pain management practices (Sessle 2003). Effective pain management can require approaches that exceed the expertise of one profession; therefore, a team of health professionals who understand each other's role and expertise is essential. This understanding is the foundation for effective collaboration in the management of complex problems, particularly for patients with persistent pain. Ideally, trainees and practitioners from diverse professions should have opportunities to work together to develop a shared understanding of effective pain management approaches and the contributions that each profession can make. However, students in health professional programs usually have few collaborative learning experiences, despite evidence that these opportunities help them to balance socialization into their own profession with learning about interprofessional collaboration. This chapter will present three diverse, interprofessional initiatives to develop, implement, and evaluate pain education for health care professionals. Watt-Watson reports on the University of Toronto, Canada, Centre for the Study of Pain Curriculum Committee's integrated pain curriculum, a requirement for pre-licensure students from six health science faculties. Strong's interprofessional pain course was developed as an elective for occupational therapy and physical therapy students at Queensland University, Brisbane, Australia. Seers used a work-based interprofessional approach to examine the impact of an educational intervention with ward staff on postoperative patient pain outcomes at the Royal College of Nursing Institute, Oxford, United Kingdom.

AN INTEGRATED, INTERPROFESSIONAL PAIN EDUCATION MODEL FOR PRE-LICENSURE HEALTH SCIENCE STUDENTS

Deficiencies in pain knowledge have been reported for almost two decades within a variety of health professional groups including medicine, pharmacy, and nursing (Lebovitz et al. 1997; Furstenberg et al. 1998; Poyhia and Kalso 1998; Watt-Watson et al. 2001; Simpson et al. 2002); occupational therapy (Unruh 1995; Strong et al. 1999; Gough et al. 2002); and physical therapy (Scudds and Solomon 1995). Moreover, students have lacked important pain knowledge at graduation (Unruh 1995; Rochman 1998; Wilson et al. 1998; Strong et al. 1999; Simpson et al. 2002). Pain curricula have been developed by the IASP that are both core and discipline specific. The challenge is to use these curricula as a basis for integrating pain content into pre-licensure health science programs despite their time constrictions and priority biases.

We found no published data describing interprofessional pain management as a required course for pre-licensure/undergraduate students in health science faculties in Canada or elsewhere. To address this shortcoming, the University of Toronto Centre for the Study of Pain established an Interfaculty Pain Curriculum Committee with representatives from its unique partnership of four health science faculties: dentistry, medicine, nursing, and pharmacy. The departments of physical therapy and occupational therapy are included in the faculty of medicine. A survey to determine the pain content in our current curricula pointed to variability and gaps across the six faculties or departments. Therefore, the committee developed a 20-hour pain education program for 540 pre-licensure students in March 2002, based on the IASP curriculum guidelines. The learning objectives for students are outlined in Table I. The students, almost all of whom were "second-entry-students" with a previous degree, were in either their second or third year. This intensive interprofessional learning experience was mandatory for all students from the six health science disciplines and aimed to promote collaborative practice for patient-centered pain management. The pain curriculum was developed using an iterative design, partnering with experts in research, education, and information technology. The curriculum is discussed in more detail elsewhere (Watt-Watson et al. 2004a).

Teaching strategies included large and small groups, standardized patients (actors role-playing pain patients), manuals, and clinician facilitators. Sessions were both multiprofessional (large groups) and interprofessional (small groups)

Table I
Learning objectives for students

1. To describe current theories of the anatomical, pathophysiological, and psychological bases of pain and pain relief:
   Describe the evolution of pain theories.
   Describe the mechanisms involved in peripheral and central nociceptive transmission and modulation.
   Discuss pain and suffering.

2. To describe the World Health Organization model of consequences of chronic problems related to physical impairment, activity limitation, and social participation:
   Describe differences between the three dimensions of functioning and disablement.
   Discuss how pain prevention can reduce treatment complications and the potential for chronic pain.
   Identify individual rehabilitation goals that would include remediation, compensation, and prevention as appropriate for each person with chronic pain.

3. To complete a comprehensive pain assessment:
   Identify the goals of pain assessment and management.
   Identify common misbeliefs that limit effective assessment and management.
   Describe various factors influencing individuals' pain expression and clinicians' responses.
   Recognize the differences in pain assessment related to duration and complexity.
   Outline the components of a comprehensive pain history.
   Apply several established assessment tools with clinical utility, both uni- and multidimensional.

4. To describe strategies for planning, intervention, and monitoring pain management in a manner that reflects both their collaborative and discipline-specific roles:
   Describe the available resources: local, national, international
   Describe the integrated and distinct roles of each professional.
   Describe methods of integrated and comprehensive delivery of pain management care.

Source: Adapted from Watt-Watson et al. (2004, p 142).

during five mornings in a 1-week period. The multiprofessional sessions were used to present core content related to the prevalence of pain, common clinical challenges, and mechanisms of nociceptive and neuropathic pain. In addition, a panel of patients with pain related to cancer, multiple sclerosis, trauma, or complex regional pain shared their stories and responded to students' questions. The interprofessional small group sessions focused on developing assessment and management plans for a cancer patient case. Students were assigned to 23 interprofessional groups, which were again divided into smaller interprofessional teams of about eight participants to work on action-based assigned tasks related to the patient case. Each group was assigned an actor trained to play a scripted cancer patient with pain, in order to help students work through assessment and management issues in a context that was as realistic as possible. The smaller group sessions provided opportunities for students to learn from each other about expertise the professions held in common, as well as about their unique

role. The 63 clinician facilitators representing the professions involved were assigned to each small group to act as resources for students. The facilitators had
experience managing pain and working with groups and were required to have
attended a 2- hour orientation session. Manuals with resources, question guides,
and key publications were developed for both students and facilitators.

We evaluated process and content across the five mornings using the Pain
Knowledge and Beliefs Questionnaire (PKBQ) pre- and post-tests and the
Daily Content and Process Questionnaire (DCPQ). Data were analyzed by total
response for the PKBQ, paired Student t-tests were used to compare matched
pre- and post-test scores, and unpaired t-tests were used to compare unmatched
pre- and post-test scores. Descriptive analyses were completed for the DCPQ.
In addition, faculty-specific examinations were also used to evaluate students'
learning, but these were not the responsibility of this committee.

Test scores showed an improvement in students' knowledge and beliefs
about pain and the need for interprofessional collaboration for effective pain
management. Mean scores and standard deviations for correct responses on
the PKBQ were 26.5 (SD = 4.56) for the pre-test (i.e., 66% correct) and 33.0
(SD = 3.36) for the post-test (i.e., 83% correct), with a statistically significant
mean difference of 6.53 using a pooled standard deviation (4.22); t (df = 545)
= 181.28 ($P < 0.001$). The DCPQ daily summary ratings of exceeding or meeting expectations for the curriculum ranged from 74% to 92%; the highest daily
ratings were for the small group sessions. In particular, students reported that
the small, interprofessional sessions gave them the opportunity not only to work
through assessment and management plans for a pain patient, but also to work
collaboratively with other professionals in the process.

Outcomes were generally less favorable for the multiprofessional sessions,
particularly regarding the amount and degree of complexity of the neurophysiology content. This variability may reflect students' diverse backgrounds from
their first degree, the stage they had reached in their pre-licensure program, and
the diversity of faculty teaching styles, some being more case based than lecture
based. Students asked for greater clinical application in all sessions, including
more discussion and modeling of interprofessional roles in the context of pain
management. Therefore, changes implemented for subsequent years included
a greater clinical focus for all sessions including the basic science components,
more evidence to support management strategies, including pharmacology,
and some choice in sessions to accommodate the variety of student interests.
The challenge of diverse interests was also evident in the choice of focus for
the case study. Not all students found the cancer patient case relevant to their
current experience or to their perceived future practice, particularly those from
dentistry and rehabilitation sciences (i.e., occupational and physical therapy).
Therefore, the case study for the following years has focused on a person with
chronic noncancer pain.

In summary, students' overall ratings of the pain curriculum indicated that we were successful in integrating profession-specific learning goals concerning pain into an interfaculty curriculum. Students also made statistically and pedagogically significant changes in pain knowledge and beliefs. Moreover, students' feedback indicated that interprofessional collaboration was an important component of the pain curriculum and was fostered by an increase in understanding of other practitioners' roles and expertise. We have continued to offer this unique and valuable learning opportunity with some modifications every year since 2002.

DEVELOPING AN ELECTIVE INTERPROFESSIONAL PAIN COURSE FROM IASP CURRICULA

We developed an interprofessional elective pain course, based upon the IASP curriculum, for occupational therapists and physiotherapists at the University of Queensland (Strong et al. 2003). The course was first developed as a 14-hour lecture series on topics such as pain as survival, the medical model, the epidemiology and sociology of pain, and peripheral and central processing of pain. The following year, the course was expanded to a 28-hour program that included lectures and interactive student-led seminars dealing with questions such as: "Why are people with cancer pain continuing to receive inadequate pain management?" In addition to the lecture topics covered in the smaller course, we added material about pain in children, in people unable to communicate their pain, and in patients with HIV/AIDS.

We were interested in determining whether participation in the course made a difference in the students' knowledge and attitudes about pain and in their attitudes toward people with pain. The revised Pain Knowledge and Attitudes Questionnaire (R-PKAQ) was used as the measurement tool in a pre-test/post-test study (Unruh 1995). The R-PKAQ consists of 69 items measuring generic knowledge of pain across six subscales: the physiological basis of pain, the psychological components of pain, assessment and management strategies, lifespan issues, cognitive-behavioral applications, and pharmacological management principles. Participants were required to score each statement on the questionnaire using the following response categories: strongly disagree, disagree, uncertain, agree, and strongly agree.

Forty-one students drawn from occupational therapy, physical therapy, dentistry, and science enrolled in the elective course in the first, or pilot, year. Twenty-two students completed the pre- and post-course R-PKAQs, which represented just over 50% of the entire group. For the following 2 years, a total of 35 students (from human movements, occupational therapy, physical therapy and social work) enrolled in the expanded course, with 22 students completing the R-PKAQ.

The first year pilot had pre-test total scores that ranged from 25 to 53, with a mean of 39.9 correct responses out of 59 questions. Students were most knowledgeable about the physiological basis of pain (mean = 76% correct) and psychological factors of pain perception (mean = 74% correct) and least knowledgeable about pharmacological management of pain (mean = 32% correct). Post-test total scores ranged from 36 to 56, with a mean of 46.9 correct responses. We measured improvements in mean test scores across all six subscales, with the greatest improvement on the pharmacological pain management subscale (mean = 45% correct).

Pre-test total scores for the expanded course ranged from 19 to 51, with a mean of 34.7 correct out of 59. As in the pilot group, students were most knowledgeable about the physiological basis of pain (mean = 69% correct) and least knowledgeable about pharmacological management of pain (mean = 27.6% correct). Post-test total scores ranged from 28 to 56, with a mean of 43.4. Improvements in mean test scores occurred across all subscales. Again, as seen in the pilot group, the largest improvement for the expanded course was seen on the pharmacological pain management subscale (mean = 43% correct).

We used analysis of variance (ANOVA) to compare the means of the subscale test scores for each cohort and from pre- to post-tests, as well as considering a three-factor interaction between subscale, trial, and timing of test. Both cohorts demonstrated significant improvement in scores from pre- to post-testing ($F = 14.10$, df = 1,461, $P < 0.0001$). Results revealed no significant differences between the subscales of the pilot cohort compared to the expanded course cohort ($P = 0.065$) and no significant interaction effect between the three factors ($P = 0.91$).

To test the hypothesis that the students' knowledge improved, as measured by the proportion of correct items, we used a logistic regression model including subscale as a factor and pre-score as a covariate, as well as a subscale by pre-score interaction term. To allow for possible correlations between students' performances across the subscales, the model included a random term for students. We fitted this generalized linear mixed model using a Penalized Quasi-Likelihood routine. Results generally supported the ANOVA findings, although students' knowledge of psychological factors of pain perception ($t = -2.05$, df = 461, $P = 0.04$) and cognitive-behavioral pain methods ($t = -2.64$, df = 461, $P = 0.008$) were found to differ significantly between the two cohorts, with scores lower in the expanded cohort group than the pilot group. However, significant improvement in post-course knowledge scores was found in five of the six subscales measured, regardless of course. Increased knowledge was evident for the physiological basis of pain ($t = 2.12$, df = 461, $P = 0.03$), pain assessment and measurement ($t = 2.27$, df = 461, $P = 0.02$), psychological factors of pain perception ($t = 2.68$, df = 461, $P = 0.007$), cognitive-behavioral pain methods ($t = 2.05$, df = 461, $P = 0.04$), and pharmacological pain management ($t = 3.41$, df = 461, $P = 0.0007$). Knowledge of developmental changes in pain perception did not improve significantly for either group.

Students demonstrated an increase of 13.8% in the mean final score on the R-PKAQ and showed statistically significant gains in five out of six domains of pain knowledge. Completion of both elective pain courses, based on the IASP curriculum for students of occupational therapy and physical therapy, improved pain knowledge on the R-PKAQ. Students' pain knowledge increased significantly in the following areas: pharmacological pain management, physiological aspects, pain assessment and measurement, cognitive-behavioral pain methods, and psychological pain issues. These subscales of the R-PKAQ reflect important interprofessional aspects of pain knowledge and management; therefore, we found these results encouraging.

The lack of a control group in this study was a limitation, since we cannot conclude that the improvement in knowledge of pain amongst participants was due to course participation. Furthermore, given the poorer performance of students in the expanded course relative to the shorter course in the areas of psychological pain issues and cognitive-behavioral pain methods, both the content and delivery of the course should be examined. Additionally, since we found that students in the shorter course had a greater baseline knowledge in all pain domains according to their pre-course scores, closer attention in further studies should be given to students' prior knowledge of pain and experience with pain patients.

In summary, data from this study supported earlier findings that a pain course can improve pain knowledge in the short term. Student knowledge increased regardless of course length. However, the long term impact of improved pain knowledge on pain management practices still needs to be evaluated. It will be important to follow up with practicing health professionals who have received pain education to demonstrate whether the knowledge is retained and transferred to practice over a longer time period.

EVALUATING PATIENT OUTCOMES AFTER WORK-BASED EDUCATION WITH PRACTITIONERS

Practitioner education models are often profession-specific and do not always evaluate outcomes for patient care. We carried out a study to assess whether implementing evidence-based pain management after a work-based interprofessional education intervention would improve postoperative pain outcomes. The study is discussed in more detail elsewhere (Seers et al. 2004).

Postoperative pain continues to be a problem for patients, with 30–60% experiencing moderate to severe pain after surgery (Dolin et al. 2002; Watt-Watson et al. 2004b). Although relevant high-quality research exists (e.g., Moore et al. 2003), these data have not necessarily been implemented in practice. Therefore, this study aimed to promote the use of evidence-based pain management in practice through using research on the most effective way to implement this evidence (Bero et al. 1998; University of York NIH Centre for Review and Dissemination 1999; Grimshaw et al. 2004). Health professionals working on four surgical wards in an orthopedic National Health Service Trust hospital were involved in deciding the focus of the study. As a result of a baseline audit that revealed that postoperative pain was a problem, the investigators decided to focus on the prescribing of postoperative oral analgesics. A wide range of analgesics and doses were being utilized, but practices were not always based on good research evidence from analgesic league tables that clearly show that some analgesics are more effective than others. This evidence is described as a number needed to treat, i.e., the number of patients in moderate to severe pain who need to receive the active drug in order for one patient to achieve at least 50% relief of pain compared with placebo over a 4–6-hour treatment period after surgery (Moore et al. 2003).

The study design included a baseline audit of pain and oral analgesic usage for patients ($n = 120$) on four surgical wards, as well as a randomized controlled trial to look at the effects of a ward-based learning intervention on pain outcomes 3 months after the intervention. The four wards were randomized to received either the intervention ($n = 2$ wards) or to act as the control ($n = 2$ wards). Control wards continued with their usual practices of analgesic administration. For the intervention wards, strategies used to encourage the use of more effective implementation practices included interactive educational sessions using multifaceted rather than single interventions, reminder systems (a laminated piece of paper showing the algorithm), and audit and feedback (University of York NIH Centre for Review and Dissemination 1999). However, as Grimshaw et al. (2004) concluded when reviewing guideline implementation strategies, evidence does not clearly show which strategies are effective under different circumstances. Grimshaw's team recommended that decision makers would need to use "considerable judgement" and that more research was needed to "estimate the efficiency of dissemination and implementation strategies in the presence of different barriers and effect modifiers." The intervention involved four interactive educational sessions that included feedback of audit baseline data and discussion about next steps; discussion of systematic reviews, analgesic league tables, and choice of analgesics; discussion of the principles of evidence-based health care and its relevance to practice; and a facilitation and change workshop (facilitated by a person with change management expertise).

Additional support and teaching were provided, including Internet access for researching evidence on analgesic usage. The teaching sessions were open to members of the health care team, but they always included a nurse from each ward taking part in the study. We planned sessions to take place over a 6-week period for 60–90 minutes each, excluding the half-day facilitation and change workshop. The health professionals involved chose to implement an oral analgesic algorithm and made decisions about which analgesics they would use based on the concept of number needed to treat.

Results at 3 months after the intervention did not demonstrate any significant difference in postoperative pain or analgesic use between the intervention and control groups. However, both the intervention and control wards significantly increased their use of algorithm drugs and decreased their use of non-algorithm drugs during the study. The control wards also changed their practices during the control period. While staff on the experimental and control wards were encouraged not to discuss the study, we could not determine whether they complied with this request.

We partly explained why both the control and experimental wards changed by considering factors such as contamination between experimental and control wards, some other unknown change in advice to ward staff, and staff being disappointed that they were not in the intervention group and thus becoming more active in pain management. We found planned staff attendance at ward-based teaching sessions very challenging to enforce, because of redeployment at short notice to cover various urgent incidents or staff sickness on the wards, in addition to a rapid staff turnover. These problems meant that sessions had to be repeated frequently, which was difficult to schedule. Staff did genuinely want to improve pain relief, but these practicalities of day-to-day care made moving toward evidence-based practice very difficult.

Additional challenges included difficulties in standardizing the intervention, given the wide variations in the amount and level of teaching and discussion required. A randomized controlled trial may be an unrealistic method to evaluate complex changes in a large organization, although Hawe et al. (2004) argue that the function and process of the intervention should be standardized and not the components themselves. Also, while analgesic league tables are helpful, they have limitations, especially when the primary trials are conducted on people under 65 years old and lack data on adverse effects. The culture of the ward appeared to be important, but it was not assessed and needs to be considered in future work, and the nurses who participated on the team were sometimes quite junior, making it difficult for them to introduce change on the ward. Our aim to involve a range of health care professionals in the sessions was hard to achieve because of competing demands on their time in the ward environment, and because different professions tended to have separately scheduled training programs. The interprofessional input came mainly from the acute pain steering group, which consisted of nursing, anesthetics, surgery, pharmacy, physiotherapy and hospital management staff, rather than in the individual sessions.

In summary, suggestions for future work include a broader approach to design and inclusion of the context of care, which may provide more meaningful answers. Analgesic league tables need to be used with care until further data are available for the older population. Other forms of evidence, such as clinical experience and patient preferences, remain key factors in managing pain. Ward-based learning has many challenges, but staff reported that they valued it as a way of improving care.

CONCLUSION

Despite the continuing problem of ineffective pain management practices, pain educational programs for health professionals are inadequate, especially for pre-licensure students. Interprofessional pain educational opportunities are minimally referenced in the literature, despite the collaborative approaches needed for many people experiencing pain. We have reported on three different initiatives from three different countries that have had success in changing health professionals' knowledge and beliefs about pain. However, evaluating patient-centered outcomes beyond the education intervention itself is complex and requires further investigation. Interprofessional collaboration should benefit from a better understanding of each other's roles and the development of interdisciplinary curricula.

ACKNOWLEDGMENTS

Support is acknowledged from: (a) the University of Toronto Centre for the Study of Pain Curriculum Committee, collaborators of Judy Watt-Watson; (b) Dawn Carroll, now at Pfizer, formerly at the Royal College of Nursing Institute (RCNI) and the Oxford Pain Research Group, University of Oxford; Sarah Richards, clinical nurse specialist in pain, Teresa Saunders, research assistant, RCNI; Nicola Crichton, statistician, RCNI and London South Bank University, collaborators of Kate Seers; and (c) Pamela Meredith, Ross Darnell, Marlene Chong, and Patricia Ross, collaborators of Jenny Strong.

REFERENCES

Bero LA, Grilli R, Grimshaw JM, et al. On behalf of Cochrane Effective Practice and Organisation of Care Review Group. Closing the gap between research and practice: an overview of systematic reviews of interventions to promote the implementation of research findings. *BMJ* 1998; 317:465–468

Charlton JE (Ed). *Core Curriculum for Professional Education in Pain,* 3rd ed. Seattle: IASP Press, 2005.

Dolin SJ, Cashman JN, Bland JM. Effectiveness of acute postoperative pain management: I. Evidence from published data. *Br J Anaesth* 2002; 89:409–423.

University of York NHS Centre for Reviews and Dissemination. Getting evidence into practice. *Effective Health Care Bull* 1999; 5(1):1–16.

Furstenberg C, Ahles TA, Whedon MB, et al. Knowledge and attitudes of health-care providers toward cancer pain management: a comparison of physicians, nurses, and pharmacists in the State of New Hampshire. *J Pain Symptom Manage* 1998; 16:335–349.

Gough L Strong J, New F. The current status of pain curricula for selected health professionals in Australia and New Zealand. *Focus Health Prof Educ Multi-disciplinary J* 2002; 4:57–68.

Grimshaw JM, Thomas RE, MacLennan G, et al. Effectiveness and efficiency of guideline dissemination and implementation strategies. *Health Technol Assess* 2004; 8:1–102.

Hawe P, Shiell A, Riley T. Complex interventions: how "out of control" can a randomised controlled trial be? *BMJ* 2004; 328:1561–1563.

Lebovitz A, Florence I, Bathina R, et al. Pain knowledge and attitudes of health care providers: practice characteristic differences. *Clin J Pain* 1997; 13:237–243.

Moore A, Edwards J, Barden J, McQuay H. *Bandolier's Little Book of Pain.* Oxford: Oxford University Press, 2003.

Poyhia R, Kalso E. Pain related undergraduate teaching in medical facilities in Finland. *Pain* 1999; 79:121–125.

Rochman DL. Students' knowledge of pain: a survey of four schools. *Occup Ther Int* 1998; 5:140–154.

Scudds R, Solomon P. Pain and its management: a new pain curriculum for occupational therapists and physical therapists. *Physiother Can* 1995; 47:77–78.

Seers K, Crichton N, Carroll D, Richards S, Saunders T. Evidence based postoperative pain management in nursing: is a randomised controlled trial the most appropriate design? *J Nurs Manag* 2004; 12:183–189.

Sessle B. Outgoing President's address: issues and initiatives in pain education, communication and research. In: Dostrovsky J, Carr DB, Koltzenburg M (Eds). *Proceedings of the 10th World Congress on Pain,* Progress in Pain Research and Management, Vol. 24. Seattle: IASP Press, 2003, pp 3–12.

Simpson K, Kautzman L, Dodd S. The effects of a pain management education program on the knowledge level and attitudes of clinical staff. *Pain Manag Nurs* 2002; 3:87–93.

Strong J, Tooth L, Unruh A. Knowledge about pain among newly graduated occupational therapists: relevance for curriculum development. *Can J Occup Ther* 1999; 66:221–228.

Strong J, Meredith P, Darnell R, Chong M, Roche PM. Does participation in a pain course based on the IASP curriculum guidelines change student knowledge about pain? *Pain Res Manage* 2003; 8:137–142.

Unruh A. Teaching student occupational therapists about pain: a course evaluation. *Can J Occup Ther* 1995; 62:30–36.

Watt-Watson J, Stevens B, Streiner D, Garfinkel P, Gallop R. Relationship between pain knowledge and pain management outcomes for their postoperative cardiac patients. *J Adv Nurs* 2001; 36:535–545.

Watt-Watson J, Hunter J, Pennefather P, et al. An integrated undergraduate curriculum, based on IASP curricula, for six health science faculties. *Pain* 2004a; 110:140–148.

Watt-Watson J, Stevens B, Katz J, et al. Impact of a pain education intervention on postoperative pain management. *Pain* 2004b; 109:73–85.

Wilson J, Brockopp G, Kryst S, Steger H, Witt W. Medical students' attitudes towards pain before and after a brief course on pain. *Pain* 1992; 50:251–256.

Correspondence to: Judy Watt-Watson, RN, PhD, Faculty of Nursing, University of Toronto, 155 College Street, Suite 215, Toronto, ON, Canada M5T 1P8. Fax: 416-978-8222; email: j.watt.watson@utoronto.ca.

Proceedings of the 11th World Congress on Pain,
edited by Herta Flor, Eija Kalso, and Jonathan O.
Dostrovsky, IASP Press, Seattle, © 2006.

5

Ethical Challenges in Pain Management

Allen H. Lebovits[a] and Rollin M. Gallagher[b,c]

[a]Departments of Anesthesiology and Psychiatry, Pain Management Center, New York University Medical Center, New York, New York, USA; [b]Center for Pain Medicine, Research and Policy, University of Pennsylvania School of Medicine, Philadelphia, Pennsylvania, USA; [c]Pain Service, Department of Anesthesiology, Philadelphia Veterans Affairs Medical Center, Philadelphia, Pennsylvania, USA

The Hippocratic Oath, which focuses primarily on the perception of physicians' behavior, has provided the foundational principles of medical ethics since the times of ancient Greece, but the horrors of World War I, followed by the Nazi regime's misuse of medical experimentation, exposed the need for additional principles to guide practice. The Nuremberg Code of 1947, written to preserve the rights of patients in all medical settings, including prisoners of war, was strengthened by the World Medical Association's Declaration of Helsinki in 1964. The exposure of the Tuskegee syphilis study, in which African American veterans with syphilis were left untreated to study the course of the disease, led to the Belmont Report in 1978, which created the United States' National Policy on Ethics and Human Subject Research. Subsequently, Foley and colleagues published the World Health Organization's analgesic ladder, providing a single, easily understood, worldwide standard for pain care (World Health Organization 1990). By creating a standard for treating cancer pain, the ladder also raised medical consciousness of pain, creating a performance touchstone for providers in all countries. In the United States, the Department of Veterans Affairs established pain as the fifth vital sign, assuring that pain would be routinely evaluated in this nationwide system of more than 150 hospitals and hundreds of clinics. The Joint Commission on Accreditation of Healthcare Organizations followed suit, developing performance standards for pain assessment and management that all U.S. health care institutions must meet to achieve accreditation.

As the specialty of pain management continues to grow and develop, increasingly complex ethical challenges are emerging. Increasing economic pressures and advancing technologies place the pain practitioner in the midst of new conflicts and challenges. A survey of the memberships of the American

Academy of Pain Medicine and the American Pain Society suggests significant concern on the part of pain specialists regarding ethical dilemmas in the daily practice of pain management (Ferrell et al. 2001). More journals are devoting sections and special issues to the area of ethics and pain. Professional organizations and pain societies have developed ethical guidelines and principles, recognizing that ethics education promotes quality control among pain management professionals, which in turn enhances pain control (Wynia et al. 1999; AAPM Council on Ethics 2005; Sullivan et al. 2005).

Hamaty (2001) has noted significant concerns about the physician's role in today's medical practice, remarking that he or she stands alone in the struggle to obtain proper care for the patient and is stonewalled by inconsistent social standards and reining economic forces. Today's physician is forced to stand painfully by as his or her controlling health care institution, which is not held to the same code of ethics, condones the withholding of treatment or allows improper treatment. Physicians, according to Hamaty, are reluctant entrepreneurs in a commercialized, amoral health care system. They may see the patient's self-direction compromised by captivating media offerings, such as Internet assurances of miracle cures. They are faced with the moral implications of progress in genetic engineering, which promises to impose more tension on those responsible for allocating resources. Physicians, Hamaty believes, are part of a culture where self-governance is immune to morality and law, part of a society that assigns no value to controlling one's behavior through a life of virtue and adherence to an oath.

BIOETHICAL PRINCIPLES IN PAIN MANAGEMENT

Five bioethical principles are commonly encountered in the practice of pain management. These principles are beneficence, nonmaleficence, autonomy, justice, and double effect.

Beneficence is defined as the physician's duty to "take positive steps to help others and not just refrain from harmful acts" (Sullivan 2001). The International Association for the Study of Pain has published ethical standards that extend the obligation of the pain specialist to "a moral responsibility to those patients" in which "preventing or alleviating such pain is not merely a matter of charity or doing good (beneficence) but carries a duty to prevent harm (nonmaleficence)" (Charlton 2005, p. 27).

The American Medical Association (2002) has stated: "A physician shall recognize a responsibility to participate in activities contributing to the improvement of the community and the betterment of health." Of course, this responsibility also applies to specialists in pain medicine. We do have a responsibility for public health because pain is one of the major public health problems in our society. Our social responsibilities in this regard include educating patients, the public, and policy makers, with the aim of creating policies that foster improved care for pain, for the greater good of society. Social responsibility has led to the development of several organizations that advocate for empowerment of patients; changes in policy have been developed over the last few years to accomplish this goal.

Casarett and Karlawish (2001) discuss beneficence in designing research. Beneficence is defined as the use of data to improve patient care. To this end: (1) The intervention selected for a clinical trial should have a reasonable chance of success for meaningful improvement over other interventions. (2) The design should be valid. (3) The research should have value and should have the potential to improve the health of future patients. (4) Risks and burdens should be minimized. (5) Volunteerism should be protected, and opportunities to withdraw should be provided.

Nonmaleficence is the obligation of physicians "not to inflict harm on patients intentionally or carelessly" (Sullivan 2001). Examples of not adhering to nonmaleficence might include failure to provide adequate analgesia to neonates undergoing painful procedures or overly aggressive pain procedures that may provide short-term relief but are associated with severe long-term problems. Similarly, the principle of nonmaleficence is tested when initiating beneficial therapies that cannot be continued in the patient's home or in alternate care settings due to expense or the need for sophisticated delivery systems.

Autonomy comes from the Greek *autos nomos,* or self-rule. It is defined as "personal rule of the self, free from ... controlling interferences by others ... that prevent meaningful choice" (Beauchamp and Childress 1994). Autonomy requires "independence from a controlling influence and ... a capacity for intentional action" (Sullivan 2001). The classic example of autonomy would include obtaining the patient's consent for a medical intervention (infants and the cognitively impaired present specific challenges). Unrelieved chronic pain may impair patient autonomy through the patient's development of dependency on drugs and on the physicians who prescribe them.

Justice is described as the "fair, equitable, and appropriate distribution in society of a privilege, benefit or service" (Sullivan 2001). Disparities in care based on racial origin, gender, and socioeconomic status are examples of lack of justice. In a study of emergency room care, Hispanics were half as likely as white non-Hispanics to receive analgesics for fractures; when they were treated with opioids for fractures, Hispanics were given two-thirds the dose of morphine that white patients received (Todd et al. 1993, 2000). Patients treated in outpatient cancer clinics with a majority of patients from ethnic minorities were three times more likely to be undertreated for their pain (Cleeland et al. 1994).

Double effect occurs when the primary intent (of an intervention) may have undesirable and unintended secondary effects; however, "an action to secure a desired effect can be justified even if it has predictable, unwanted associated effects" (Emanuel 2001). The classic example of the double effect principle is opioid administration for the desired effect of pain control, despite the drug's possible secondary effects of respiratory depression that might hasten death in terminal cancer patients.

ETHICAL DILEMMAS IN CHRONIC PAIN MANAGEMENT

It is important to understand that the nature of chronic pain and the system in which we practice often lead to ethical dilemmas (Lebovits 2001). The inherent difficulty of "curing" chronic pain goes against the traditional medical model of the doctor healing the patient. Lack of education and understanding about the fact that it may be impossible to cure the patient's presenting problem can lead practitioners as well as patients to be overly aggressive in their approaches. Even when the pain specialist is focused on the "management" of pain rather than its "cure," patient expectations of a cure can lead to conflicts with doctors and inevitable disappointment with treatment, even if there is improvement in pain and functionality.

Additional ethical challenges arise when chronic pain patients have psychological problems. Such problems might have existed prior to the pain condition, but they also may develop as reactions to the pain or to the lack of relief. When iatrogenic injuries occur, anger, fueled by litigation, can add to depression or somatization. With traumatic injuries such as accidents, patients can also present with post-traumatic stress disorder. The result of this concurrent psychopathology is that the patient's physical pain might not be taken seriously enough. If pain is considered to be "in the patient's head," it might not be treated at all or might be treated psychiatrically, rather than medically. Alternatively, patients might receive overly aggressive medical treatment because their depression or somatization disorder might amplify their pain, suffering, or illness behavior. The ethical dictum of nonmaleficence, or doing no harm, is strongly tested under these conditions. A careful interdisciplinary evaluation of the patient can be beneficial in solving this often very perplexing problem. Mental health professionals specially trained in pain management need to be integral members of the interdisciplinary evaluation of patients who present to the pain clinic.

End-of-life issues pose enormously challenging ethical dilemmas for the pain practitioner. In a survey of over 1,000 pain specialists, management of pain at the end of life was ranked first when participants were asked to list in descending order the ethical challenges of pain management (Ferrell et al. 2001).

Pain is one of the most common reasons for assisted suicide or euthanasia and is often a significant issue in palliative care, so it places the pain practitioner at the forefront of these very difficult issues. The ethical bind of the "double effect" principle is often encountered in palliative care, when the need for pain control requires drugs that have adverse effects or secondary effects such as hastening death. Having a palliative care team can alleviate the pain specialist's burden in dealing with these ethical complexities.

Most interventions employed today by pain centers use unproven methods that have not been scientifically demonstrated to be efficacious. Adding to the confusion, many adjuvant pharmacological agents commonly used in pain patients, such as gabapentin or tricyclic antidepressants, although demonstrated to be effective for pain in clinical trials, are not approved as analgesics by national regulatory agencies such as the U.S. Food and Drug Administration. Additionally, we lack well-designed outcome studies related to regional anesthesia, psychological interventions, or rehabilitation. Even more troubling, however, is the growing popularity and acceptance by the medical community of scientifically unproven complementary techniques, which are often used for pain (Eisenberg et al. 1993, 1998). The ethical quandary is exacerbated by practitioners who not only fail to tell the patient that the intervention is scientifically unproven but present it in a manner that would suggest otherwise. The problem of lack of therapeutic standards of care, however, is being remedied by the recent development of practice guidelines by the American Pain Society (2002, 2005a,b) for disease-specific states such as arthritis, cancer, and fibromyalgia.

The vulnerable, often desperate nature of many pain patients makes them very susceptible to trying anything that all-to-willing practitioners might offer. Aggressive interventions may represent compassionate efforts or at times they might be taking advantage of a vulnerable patient, even when practitioners believe they are acting in the patient's best interest. This severely tests the bioethical principle of nonmaleficence. The International Association for the Study of Pain's ethical guidelines for pain management (Charlton 2005) recognize the existence of other "vulnerable" groups of patients with pain such as those who cannot communicate verbally (infants, the elderly, those in an intensive care unit), cancer patients, dying patients, and economically disadvantaged patients. This latter group, in particular, tests the ethical principle of "justice" in terms of equal access to health care for all patients.

The physician's primary professional duty is to the patient, but because pain specialists are often in the role of consultant, conflicts of interest may arise, such as when a patient is referred to them for a procedure such as a nerve block that they do not believe to be in accordance with usual standards of care or normal practice. The referral source may even forbid consultation with a psychiatrist or psychologist (AAPM Council on Ethics 2005).

The preceding issue becomes more pronounced when one considers the increasing economic pressures of pain clinics. The advent of "managed care" in the United States, with its limitations on reimbursement and its rejections of authorization or lengthy delays in obtaining it, has changed the practice of pain management. This policy has increased the incentive to perform more invasive and profitable interventions. These economic pressures may not always conform with the best interest of the patient. Patients with low back pain may be referred for an unnecessary MRI scan, nerve block, or psychotherapy to produce practice revenue. The ethical conflict occurs when physicians maximize their income by providing any medical intervention that will be reimbursed, while ignoring the greater societal burden of unnecessarily higher cost and the other treatment needs of the patient. The ethical principle of nonmaleficence may be seriously taxed with this conflict. Different reimbursement rates for different patients and for different procedures is not in the best interest of all patients and calls into question the bioethical principle of justice. Do providers spend more time, provide better care, and give more attention to more profitable patients or do all patients receive "just" care—the equal right and access to all available treatment modalities? Are more profitable interventions such as spinal cord stimulators and implantable pumps always used judiciously, by appropriately trained practitioners, and only when necessary?

Many patients with chronic pain are involved in litigation as a result of the conditions of the onset of their pain, which frequently is the result of a motor vehicle or work-related accident. Such accidents may cause disabling impairments so that patients must fight for worker's compensation as well as health care coverage. Many states have a "de facto" requirement that patients obtain legal representation in order to seek these benefits. However, this process can also powerfully reinforce, both consciously or subconsciously, pain perception, illness behavior, and health care utilization. The litigation process may work against the goals of treatment, facilitating the overutilization of the health care system, interfering with the patient's commitment to return to work (until the case is over), and fostering dependency needs and helplessness on the part of the patient. The ethical dilemma becomes both how to evaluate the salience of these effects on pain and pain behavior and whether or how to treat the patient in the face of such a powerful reinforcer of pain behavior. Additionally, litigation may place the clinician, particularly the mental health specialist, in an ethically challenging dual relationship of advocating (for or against) the patient in court and also treating the patient.

The worker's compensation system in the United States, which basically pays the patient to have pain—in other words, pain becomes their new job—presents the pain provider with many ethical conflicts. For example, does one treat a patient for whom authorization has been delayed or denied, characteristic occurrences for patients under worker's compensation? Accurate diagnosis and treatment are often delayed. Compensation providers are often asked to give an "independent" evaluation of the patient that will determine the necessity of treatment, but these providers, paid by compensation, often offer a "subjective" opinion. Delays and difficulties in returning to work also complicate the recovery of the pain patient.

SOLUTIONS

Personal and professional experiences help physicians to answer the various ethical questions that come our way from day to day. Collegial associations can provide support and clarity of analysis for the physician who, immersed in an ethical quandary, cannot see the larger perspective—the proverbial "can't see the forest for the trees." Our own poignant clinical encounters help forge our own personal ethics. It is to be hoped that future generations of doctors will learn these lessons in training and be more capable of integrating ethical reasoning into clinical decision-making. Unfortunately, because of the increasingly important, albeit often unconscious, role of factors such as preservation of employment and income in determining physician behavior, the need to train physicians in ethical reasoning is increasingly critical to our identity as a respected, autonomous profession.

It is important to recognize the importance of ethics in pain medicine. Ethical analysis can clarify the clinician's duties and responsibilities in the doctor-patient relationship, even when it is complicated by a dysfunctional health care delivery system (Gallagher 2001). It is "a roadmap that allows us to keep practicing in the face of an increasingly complex—and often confusing … environment without losing our way and ending in … jail, or forced retirement" (Dubois 2005).

REFERENCES

AAPM Council on Ethics. Ethics Charter from American Academy of Pain Medicine. *Pain Med* 2005; 6:203–212.

American Medical Association. Principles of medical ethics. In: *Code of Medical Ethics, 2002–2003 Edition.* Chicago: AMA Press, 2002, p xiv.

American Pain Society. *Guideline for the Management of Pain in Osteoarthritis, Rheumatoid Arthritis, and Juvenile Chronic Arthritis.* Glenview, IL: American Pain Society, 2002.

American Pain Society. *Guideline for the Management of Cancer Pain in Adults and Children.* Glenview, IL: American Pain Society, 2005a.

American Pain Society. *Guideline for the Management of Fibromyalgia Syndrome Pain in Adults and Children.* Glenview, IL: American Pain Society, 2005b.

Beauchamp TL, Childress JF. *Principles of Biomedical Ethics,* 4th ed. Oxford: Oxford University Press, 1994.

Casarett DJ, Karlawish J. Beyond informed consent: the ethical design of pain research. *Pain Med* 2001; 2:138–146.

Charlton JE (Ed). Ethical standards in pain management and research. In: Charlton JE (Ed). *Core Curriculum for Professional Education in Pain,* 3rd ed. Seattle: IASP Press, 2005, pp 27–31.

Cleeland CS, Gonin R, Hatfield AK, et al. Pain and its treatment in outpatients with metastatic cancer. *N Engl J Med* 1994; 330:592–596.

Dubois MY. The birth of an ethics charter for pain medicine. *Pain Med* 2005; 6(3):201–202.

Eisenberg DM, Kessler RC, Foster C, et al. Unconventional medicine in the United States: prevalence, costs, and patterns of use. *N Engl J Med* 1993; 328:246–252.

Eisenberg DM, Davis RB, Ettner SL, et al. Trends in alternative medicine use in the United States, 1990–1997: results of a follow-up survey. *JAMA* 1998; 280:1569–1575.

Emanuel L. Ethics and pain management. *Pain Med* 2001; 2:112–116.

Ferrell BR, Novy D, Sullivan MD, et al. Ethical dilemmas in pain management. *J Pain* 2001; 2:171–180.

Gallagher RM. Ethics in pain medicine: good for our health, good for the public health. *Pain Med* 2001; 2(2):87–88.

Hamaty D. Pain medicine's role in the restoration and reformation of medical ethics. *Pain Med* 2001; 2:117–120.

Lebovits AH. Ethics and pain: why and for whom? *Pain Med* 2001; 2:92–96.

Sullivan M. Ethical principles in pain management. *Pain Med* 2001; 2:106–111.

Sullivan M, Terman GW, Peck B, et al. American Pain Society position statement on the use of placebos in pain management. *J Pain* 2005; 6:215–217.

Todd KH, Samaroo N, Hoffman JR. Ethnicity as a risk factor for inadequate emergency department analgesia. *JAMA* 1993; 269:1537–1539.

Todd KH, Deaton C, D'Adamo AP, Goe L. Ethnicity and analgesic practice. *Ann Emerg Med* 2000; 35:11–16.

World Health Organization. *Cancer Pain Relief and Palliative Care.* Geneva: World Health Organization, 1990.

Wynia MK, Latham SR, Kao AC, et al. Medical professionalism in society. *N Engl J Med* 1999; 341:1612–1616.

Correspondence to: Allen H. Lebovits, PhD, Departments of Anesthesiology and Psychiatry, NYU Pain Management Center, 317 East 34th Street, Suite 902, New York, NY 10016, USA. Fax: 212-685-5365; email: allen.lebovits@med.nyu.edu.

Proceedings of the 11th World Congress on Pain,
edited by Herta Flor, Eija Kalso, and Jonathan O.
Dostrovsky, IASP Press, Seattle, © 2006.

6

Pain Management in Asia

Ramani Vijayan

Department of Anesthesiology, University of Malaya, Kuala Lumpur, Malaysia

Asia is the most heavily populated continent and is home to more than half the world's population (World Fact Book 2005). It is a heterogeneous mixture of countries in various stages of economic development. Only Japan, Hong Kong, and Singapore have high scores on the Human Development Index, which measures achievements in terms of life expectancy, educational attainment, and adjusted real income, while other Asian countries fall into the "developing country" category (United Nations Development Program 2004).

Asia has a rich diversity of cultural and religious groups, each with its own beliefs and values, which can sometimes create barriers in pain management. Large discrepancies in health care access exist between wealthy urban populations and the rural poor. Governments must grapple with poverty, disaster, and unrest, and thus the focus of health care services is on diseases such as tuberculosis and malaria and on maternal and child health, emerging cardiovascular problems, trauma services, and cancer treatment.

Pain management has therefore been given low priority in terms of government funding. Medical curricula also reflect the perceived lack of importance of pain management. Flourishing traditional practices have often filled this vacuum in Asia. Chinese medicine shops and acupuncture clinics are common in Singapore and Kuala Lumpur, and Ayurvedic medicine clinics are extremely popular in India.

The last two decades, however, have seen tremendous changes in the economies of several countries, including the "tiger economies" of Asia (Singapore, Thailand, Malaysia, South Korea, and Taiwan) and the emerging economic powerhouses of China and India. Rising standards of living have brought improvements in the level of education and an awareness that pain has not been dealt with adequately.

This chapter highlights some of the problems and achievements of selected Asian countries with regard to cancer pain, chronic pain, and acute pain management.

CANCER PAIN MANAGEMENT

Of the approximately 11 million new cancer patients diagnosed in the world each year, a large proportion live in Asia, and most will require morphine at some stage. In the absence of published data, morphine consumption is often taken as a marker of adequacy of pain management in a given country. Data from 1999 show that Asia, with a population of 3.6 billion, consumes just over 5% of the amount of morphine used by the developed world (Fig. 1). If Japan and South Korea are excluded, the figure is a meager amount, indicating that pain control has probably not been achieved in a large proportion of the population.

REASONS FOR INADEQUATE CANCER PAIN MANAGEMENT IN ASIA

Liu et al. (2001) conducted a survey to collect nationwide basic data about cancer-related pain in China. Sixty cancer patients in each province were randomly selected to participate in this survey. Two structured questionnaires were designed (one for patients and one for physicians) and were used to assess pathophysiology, types of pain, and methods used for pain management. The results showed that 61.6% of patients (958/1555) had various types of cancer-related pain, with the majority of the pain (85.1%) caused by advanced cancer. The major reasons (64.4%) for poor management were patients' concerns about addiction, their reluctance to report pain, or their refusal to use opioid analgesics

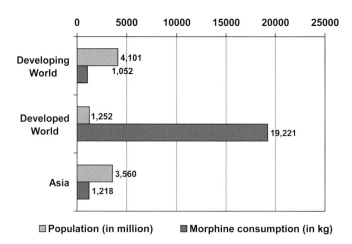

Fig. 1. Availability and use of morphine in 1999 in Asia and other developing countries compared to the developed world; data are from the International Narcotics Control Bureau (2000/2001).

until the pain became unbearable; other reasons were physicians' failure to prescribe opioids and their lack of knowledge about pain management (26.8%), a shortage of various kinds of opioids (16.2%), and unavailability of opioids and strict regulations restricting their use (16.1%).

Patients' and caregivers' concerns about opioids were found to be significant barriers to pain control in Taiwan (Lin 2000). A survey conducted among doctors in Manila showed that despite a strong awareness of the usefulness of opioids, there tended to be hesitancy in prescribing them (Javier et al. 2001). Less than 15 kg of the annual International Narcotics Control Bureau allocation of 87 kg is consumed in the Philippines. Inadequate access to potent opioids for large numbers of patients in India, particularly in rural areas, has been highlighted repeatedly over the last two decades (Koshy et al. 1998). Lack of proper education in cancer pain management and the stigma attached to using opioids were issues noted in South Korea (Yun et al. 2003). In addition, bureaucracy in the legal and administrative systems was reported to hamper an adequate supply of drugs in South Korea (Han 2001). Barriers to effective pain relief appear to be universal—fear of addiction on the patient's part (perhaps reminded about the moral degradation associated with opium addiction in China in the 19th century), lack of knowledge about opioids, and strict regulations for obtaining and prescribing potent opioids. All of the surveys mentioned above emphasized the need to educate patients and their caregivers in order to break down one of the major barriers to pain control. Removing bureaucratic hurdles in order to provide adequate availability of potent opioids was another universal requirement.

ATTEMPTS TO IMPROVE THE SITUATION

With 1.8 million new patients with cancer per year in China, the survey by Liu et al. (2001) prompted the Chinese government to undertake a top-down initiative (Huang 2001). Educational programs were initiated with government support, with a promise to improve the availability of morphine. National guidelines were published and educational activities instituted in hospitals in major cities. With this support from the government, the consumption of morphine for medical purposes has increased significantly in China since the mid-1990s (Fig. 2), although there is still room for improvement with annual per capita use at only 0.11 mg, compared to the world average of 5.8 mg and 28.9 mg in the United States (International Narcotics Control Bureau 2001).

The situation in India has been a cause of concern since strict regulations were passed to prevent drug diversion in 1985; morphine use plummeted to an all-time low in 1997 (International Narcotics Control Bureau data from 1989/1999). Due to this alarming trend, the Indian Association of Palliative

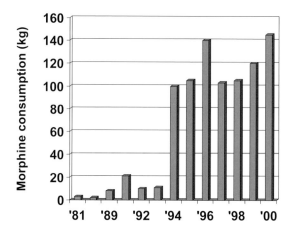

Fig. 2. Changing trends in morphine consumption in China. Morphine consumption is shown in kilograms. Data are from the International Narcotics Control Bureau (2000/2001).

Care, along with the World Health Organization Collaborative Center for Policy Studies, undertook a series of initiatives (Joranson 1998). First, they convened a committee to study regulatory requirements to obtain morphine, and then they conducted a series of workshops throughout India to mobilize support for easing restrictions. These initiatives have led to some simplification of licensing regulations. In addition, small groups of workers, the most well-known being the anesthesiologists who founded the Palliative Care Clinic in Calicut, Kerala (www.aphn.org), have demonstrated that it is possible to bring palliative care to rural India without any problems of drug diversion (Sureshkumar et al. 1996; Ajithakumari et al. 1997; Seamark et al. 2000).

A 10-day foundation course for physicians interested in palliative care was introduced in Kerala in 1997, followed by a more comprehensive 6-week basic course beginning in 2001. These programs were conducted with the help of Robert Twycross from Oxford University (www.aphn.org). Pain clinics in the United Kingdom have helped provide palliative care courses to help educate doctors in Kerala, and many doctors from neighboring countries have also been trained. Education centers for clinicians involved in palliative care are now being established in other parts of India. Sri Lanka, facing similar problems, also recruited the help of a U.K. cancer pain center to establish a cancer pain clinic (Williams et al. 2001).

ASIA PACIFIC HOSPICE NETWORK

The Asia Pacific Hospice Palliative Care Network (APHN) evolved over a series of meetings from 1995 to 2001, the first hosted in Japan by the Life

Planning Centre. Delegates from countries in the Asia Pacific region were invited. The aim was to provide an opportunity to share experiences, frustrations, knowledge, and concerns for the future regarding palliative care. Some of these concerns included the need to gain medical and patient acceptance for the concept of hospice, problems relating to the availability of appropriate analgesic drugs, and issues relating to funding of services. Other specific issues included the need for culturally relevant education and the need to maintain voluntary and community involvement in hospice programs.

The APHN was registered in 2001 as a nongovernmental organization with 13 countries in the Asia Pacific region as members. The main objectives of APHN are: (1) to facilitate development of palliative care programs, (2) to promote professional and public education, (3) to foster research and collaborative activities, (4) to enhance communication and dissemination of information among members, and (5) to encourage cooperation with other relevant professional or public organizations. APHN has been active in the last few years in providing education to health care professionals providing palliative care for patients, particularly those in the more disadvantaged segment of society (www. aphn.org).

CHRONIC NONCANCER PAIN MANAGEMENT

Data on the prevalence of chronic noncancer pain in Asia are sparse. A telephone survey of 1,000 people in Hong Kong showed that 10.8% of those surveyed had suffered persistent pain for more than 3 months (Ng et al. 2002). The prevalence of chronic pain in the Asian region may well be similar to that in Australia (Blyth et al. 2001), which is around 15–20% of the population. The concept of a pain clinic and a pain specialist is relatively new in Asia. The physician of first contact—whether an orthopedic surgeon, rheumatologist, neurologist, general practitioner, or general physician—often manages chronic pain. In addition, as mentioned above, many patients favor alternative medicine and are willing to try acupuncture or herbs for chronic pain management.

However, the last decade has seen considerable interest in several Asian countries in setting up pain clinics of all varieties, from the single-modality nerve block clinic to multidisciplinary pain management centers offering many modalities of therapy. Anesthesiologists have taken the lead in setting up such pain clinics. An example of such a center is the pain management clinic of the All India Institute of Medical Sciences in Delhi, India, which caters to the greater Delhi area with its nearly 60 million inhabitants. It is run by a team of doctors from the department of anesthesiology, who see about 1,300 patients per month. Pain management includes sophisticated interventional techniques such as implantation of spinal cord stimulators. The institute conducts collaborative research and is now becoming a venue for pain management training and referral. Demand for such centers is growing, and many clinics have been established in major cities throughout India. This type of management may not be available to all because of the size of the population, but a large number of middle-income earners now have access to treatment.

Hong Kong has six pain clinics in the public sector: three of them conduct pain management programs about two to three times per year, with a full complement of physicians, physiotherapists, psychologists, occupational therapists, and nurses (Chen et al. 2004; Lee et al. 2005; see Nicholas et al., this volume). Singapore has excellent pain management and palliative care services at the Singapore General Hospital and National Cancer Centre, respectively. Thailand has a few pain clinics, with the Pain Clinic in Siriraj Hospital, Bangkok, being the first to be established; traditional medicine, which includes acupuncture and Thai massage, is incorporated into the treatment of chronic pain (Chaudakshetrin and Ketuman 2002). Malaysia now has eight pain clinics in public hospitals, which treat chronic cancer and non-cancer pain.

ACUTE POSTOPERATIVE PAIN MANAGEMENT

In most parts of Asia, surgeons have traditionally managed postoperative pain. As was found in several studies previously conducted in developed countries (Owen et al. 1990), postoperative pain management has probably been inadequate. One survey was conducted in Malaysia in which all patients undergoing elective surgery over a 3-week period were interviewed 24 hours after surgery (Vijayan et al 1994a). Forty-seven percent of patients complained of moderate to severe pain over the past 24 hours. This study prompted the establishment of the first acute pain service in Malaysia in Kuala Lumpur in 1992 (Vijayan et al. 1994b).The classical paper by Ready et al. (1988) on an anesthesiology-based acute pain service was a catalyst for the establishment of such services in many of the major hospitals in East and Southeast Asia. These services have used techniques such as patient-controlled analgesia and epidural analgesia; they are involved in the education of nurses and physicians in addition to research. Many acute pain services are now nurse-based, anesthesiologist-directed services; they have markedly improved the standard of patient care in their institutions (Shah 1997; Tsui et al. 1997; Wong et al. 1997; Hung et al. 2002; Ng and Goh 2002).

EDUCATION AND TRAINING

Creating awareness of the importance of pain control and providing training in pain management techniques are important if the goal is to reach pain sufferers in the population at large. Chapters of the International Association for the Study of Pain in different countries of Asia have played important roles in this endeavor over the last decade. Two regional groups have been established: the South Asian Regional Pain Society (Bangladesh, India, Pakistan, and Sri Lanka) was formed in 2001, and the Association of South East Asian Pain Societies was formed in 2004. The main objectives of these two regional societies are to pool the expertise and resources of member countries for educational activities. They help organize meetings in Asia and bring in well-known clinicians from around the world so that local delegates who are unable to travel overseas can benefit from their expertise.

Recent international conferences in Asia include the fifth East West Pain Conference, held in China in 2004; the Global Update on Pain conference, held in Mumbai, India, in 2000; the Triumph over Acute Postoperative Pain conference in Manila in 2002; New Paradigms in Pain Management in Kuala Lumpur in 2004; Asia against Pain in Singapore in 2004; and the 6th Asia Pacific Hospice conference in Seoul in 2005. Workshops for nurses continue to be helpful in training them to manage acute pain after surgery. Locally produced guidelines, newsletters, Web sites, and public forums are other ways in which the message of pain management is being promoted.

CONCLUSION

Asia is a continent with a vast population. Pain management was given little priority in the past. However, thanks to the dynamism shown by a new generation of professionals, problems are being tackled to improve pain management. There is still a long way to go, but the first steps have been taken. There appears to be a glimmer of hope for pain management in Asia.

REFERENCES

Ajithakumari K, Sureshkumar K, Rajagopal MR. Palliative home care: the Calicut experience. *Palliat Med* 1997; 11:451–454.

Blyth FM, March LM, Barnbic AJ, et al. Chronic pain in Australia. A prevalence study. *Pain* 2001; 89:127–134.

Chaudakshetrin P, Ketuman P. Anesthetic pain management in Siriraj Hospital: a retrospective review. *J Med Assoc Thai* 2002; 3(Suppl):S858–865.

Chen PP, Chen J, Gin T, et al. Out-patient chronic pain service in Hong Kong: prospective study. *Hong Kong Med J* 2004; 10:150–155.

Javier FO, Magpantay LA, Espinosa EL, Harder SM, Unite MA. Opioid use in chronic pain management in the Philippines. *Eur J Pain* 2001; 5(Suppl A):83–85.

Han T. Opioids in cancer and non-cancer pain management in Korea: the past, present and future. *Eur J Pain* 2001; 5(Suppl A):73–78.

Huang Y. Current status of pain management in China: an overview. *Eur J Pain* 2001; 5(Suppl A):67–71.

Hung CT, Lau LL, Chan CK, et al. Acute pain services in Hong Kong: facilities, volume and quality. *Hong Kong Med J* 2002; 8:196–201.

International Narcotics Control Bureau. *Report of the International Narcotics Control Bureau, 2001.* Available at: www.incb.org/incb/annual_report.

Joranson DE. A proposal to simplify Indian narcotic drugs and psychotropic substances act (NDPS) to improve cancer patient access to pain medications. *Ind J Palliat Care* 1998; 4:12–15.

Koshy RC, Rhodes D, Devi S, Grossman SA. Cancer pain management in developing countries: a mosaic of complex issues resulting in inadequate analgesia. *Support Care Cancer* 1998; 6:430–437.

Lee S, Chen PP, Lee A, et al. A prospective evaluation of health-related quality of life in Hong Kong Chinese patients with chronic non-cancer pain. *Hong Kong Med J* 2005; 11:174–180.

Lin CC. Barriers to the analgesic management of cancer pain: a comparison of attitudes of Taiwanese patients and family caregivers. *Pain* 2000; 88:7–14.

Liu Z, Lian Z, Zhou W, Mu Y, et al. National survey on prevalence of cancer pain. *Chin Med Sci J* 2001; 16:175–178.

Ng JM, Goh MH. Problems related to epidural analgesia for postoperative pain control. *Ann Acad Med Singapore* 2002; 31:509–515.

Ng KF, Tsui SL, Chan WS. Prevalence of common chronic pain in Hong Kong adults. *Clin J Pain* 2002; 18:275–281.

Owen H, McMillan V, Rogowski D. Postoperative pain therapy: a survey of patients' expectations and experiences. *Pain* 1990; 41: 303–307.

Ready LB, Oden R, Chadwick HS, et al. Development of an anesthesiology-based postoperative pain management service. *Anesthesiology* 1988; 68:100–106.

Seamark D, Ajithakumari K, Burn G, et al. Palliative care in India. *J R Soc Med* 2000; 93:292–295.

Shah MK. Acute pain service in Kandang Kerbau Hospital 1994—a first year's experience. *Singapore Med J* 1997; 38:375–378.

Sureshkumar K, Rajagopal MR. Palliative care in Kerala. Problems at presentation in 440 patients with advanced cancer in a South Indian state. *Palliat Med* 1996; 10:293–298.

Tsui SL, Irwin MG, Wong CM, et al. An audit of the safety of an acute pain service. *Anaesthesia* 1997; 52:1042–1047.

Vijayan R, Delilkan AE. First year's experience with an acute pain service: University Hospital, Kuala Lumpur. *Med J Malaysia* 1994; 49:385–400.

Vijayan R, Tay KH, Tan LB, Loganathan. Survey of postoperative pain in University Hospital, Kuala Lumpur. *Singapore Med J* 1994; 35:502–504.

United Nations Development Program. *Human Development Report 2004.* Available at: http://hdr.undp.org/2004.

Williams JE, Chandler A, Ranwala R, Desilva BS, Amarsinghe I. Establishing a cancer pain clinic in a developing country: effect of a collaborative link project with a UK cancer pain centre. *J Pain Symptom Manage* 2001; 22:872–878.

World Fact Book. *Rank Order of Population.* Available at: www.cia.gov/cia/publications/factbook.

Wong LT, Koh LH, Kaur K, Boey SK. A two-year experience on an acute pain service in Singapore. *Singapore Med J* 1997; 38:209–213.

Yun YH, Heo DS, Lee IG, et al. Multicenter study of pain and its management in patients with advanced cancer in Korea. *J Pain Symptom Manage* 2003; 25:430–437.

Correspondence to: Professor Ramani Vijayan, FFARCS, FRCA, FANZCA, Department of Anaesthesiology, Faculty of Medicine, University of Malaya, 50603 Kuala Lumpur, Malaysia. Email: ramani@um.edu.my.

Proceedings of the 11th World Congress on Pain,
edited by Herta Flor, Eija Kalso, and Jonathan O.
Dostrovsky, IASP Press, Seattle, © 2006.

7

Pain Relief on a Shoestring Budget: Experience from Kerala, India

Gayatri Palat and M.R. Rajagopal

*Department of Pain and Palliative Medicine, Amrita Institute
of Medical Sciences, Kochi, Kerala, India*

Over two-thirds of about 100 million people who could benefit from pain relief live in developing countries (Stjernsward and Clark 2003). The vast population, poverty, and lack of access to pain relief centers contribute to this high pain burden. In India, approximately two million people are estimated to be in pain from cancer alone. We have no reliable statistics, and therefore the actual number of people suffering from various chronic pain conditions is unknown, but it is estimated that less than 1% of them have access to pain relief.

Traditionally throughout the world, anesthesiologists have led the field of pain therapy. Their familiarity with analgesics, nerve blocks, and multidisciplinary work makes them particularly suited to work with pain patients. But on the negative side are criticisms against many anesthesiologists that they have leaned heavily toward invasive procedures, with inadequate attention to optimal pharmacotherapy or psychosocial support. Such a bias, if it were true, would compromise both the quality and availability of pain management.

The introduction of the World Health Organization (WHO) analgesic ladder (1986) revolutionized cancer pain management in most of the developed world (Zech et al. 1995). It is now accepted that the ladder is applicable, with suitable adaptations, to many chronic pain conditions. The fact that it is a low-cost system is most relevant to the developing world, but that is where it is most lacking too. Paradoxically, high-technology modalities of diagnosis and management such as magnetic resonance imaging (MRI) scanners and linear accelerators are often available in the poorer countries, but not the low-cost modalities such as simple analgesics, which could relieve much unnecessary pain. Clearly the problem is not mainly a lack of resources, but rather the lack of a system that could deliver available resources to the needy. It is in this context that the success of the pain relief network in Kerala becomes relevant.

THE KERALA EXPERIENCE IN PAIN TREATMENT

Kerala is a tiny overpopulated state on the southwest coast of India. It accounts for about 1% of the geographical area and 3% of the population of the country. In 1994, a pain and palliative care service was started based in a government medical college hospital in the city of Calicut (Sureshkumar and Rajagopal 1996). The clinic was run by doctors in the department of anesthesiology in their spare time, in one tiny room outside the operating theaters. It was supported by a nongovernmental organization called the Pain and Palliative Care Society, which was started by some anesthesiologists along with socially motivated laypersons and other professionals (Rajagopal and Kumar 1999). Over the next 10 years, this service became the model for about 50 pain and palliative care services spread over various parts of the state (Fig. 1). Centrally located

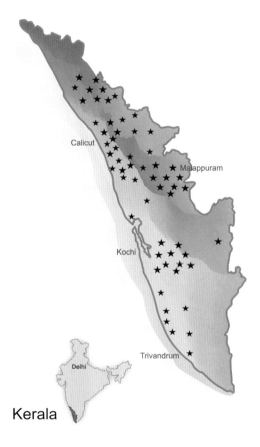

Fig. 1. Geographic distribution of pain clinics in Kerala, India. Although the state is not uniformly covered, coverage is better than in most parts of India.

referral centers cater to patients who need specialized care. They also provide education on pain and palliative care to doctors, nurses, and volunteers.

PAIN MANAGEMENT IN THE HOME SETTING

In the absence of an effective socialized system of health care delivery, and in the context of poor roads and difficult transport systems, it would be impossible for most patients to travel to distant referral centers (Seamark et al. 2000). The majority need the means of pain relief at their homes, not in hospitals, and so the system provides treatment at home whenever possible (Ajithakumari et al. 1997).

Each of the centers has the services of at least one doctor and nurse who have at least 6 weeks' training in the fundamentals of pain evaluation and in the use of the WHO ladder. Records of evaluation include a body chart and pain ratings as a numerical score from 0 to 10. Non-opioids, opioids, and adjuvant analgesics are prescribed as required and titrated to achieve optimal pain relief over the next few days. Thereafter, the patient receives a 2-week supply of analgesics, including oral morphine. A study of 1,723 patients receiving oral morphine in this way over a period of 2 years brought to light no diversion or misuse (Rajagopal et al. 2001).

Outpatient clinics are conducted in a central place in each of these establishments. Patients who can easily travel to these clinics are encouraged to do so. For those who are too sick or who cannot afford to travel to the clinic, most of the centers have developed home visit systems (Fig. 2). Volunteers often act as a link between patients and professionals. Volunteers are not required to work regular hours, which gives them enough flexibility to combine this work with their regular means of livelihood. The volunteers go through a structured training program of at least 16 hours of classroom sessions, followed by practical training in the field. They are taught how to evaluate pain on follow-up visits and are trained in evaluating adverse effects of drugs, breakthrough pain, or other symptoms. With this system in place, the professional's visit to the patient can be reduced to once a week, or sometimes less.

The system is based largely on locally raised resources from the community. Individual nongovernmental organizations are formed in towns and villages, and local enthusiasts keep the system going. Most families lose much of their livelihood when a family member is too sick to work, and the cost of initial treatment impoverishes them further. Giving them prescriptions never helps because they cannot afford to fill them, so poor patients are given all drugs free of charge. The money comes from donations; each center has devised ways of raising the necessary funds.

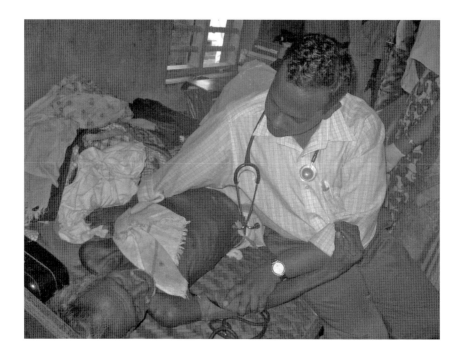

Fig. 2. A physician makes a home visit to a patient. Most patients in these humble homes would not have found it easy to see a doctor unless the doctor visited the patient at home.

Simple pharmacotherapy according to the WHO ladder is effective in relieving at least 80% of cancer pain and a smaller percentage of other chronic pain (Walker 1988). The minority who do not obtain enough relief have access to the services of referral centers, mostly attached to major institutions. These usually provide inpatient treatment for patients who have difficult pain or other symptoms and for those who need invasive procedures.

COMBINING PAIN RELIEF AND PALLIATIVE CARE SERVICES

Pain services and palliative care services function as two parallel systems in the West. Since these services were virtually nonexistent in most parts of India, it was considered necessary to develop both together in Kerala. This has turned out to be a huge advantage. Pain relief according to the WHO ladder remains accessible not only to those with cancer pain, but also to those with chronic noncancer pain. In addition, psychosocial support has become closely integrated to chronic pain treatment, as indeed it should be.

OPIOID AVAILABILITY

India, a country that legally grows poppy, manufactures opium, and exports it to the developed world, nevertheless shares with the rest of the developing world the problem of lack of availability of opioids for pain relief. Fear of addiction and abuse led to the very complex Narcotic Substances and Psychotropic Substances Act of 1986, which steadily decreased opioid availability. A poor reporting system by the government of India leaves us with inadequate data, but going by the quantity of morphine powder sold to manufacturers by the Government Opium and Alkaloid factory, the consumption of morphine reached an all-time low in 1998. Unfortunately, this matter comes under the purview of individual state governments, each of which has a different system of licensing, thus complicating matters still further. The initiative of the WHO Collaborating Center at Madison-Wisconsin, working with Indian palliative care workers, led to action by the government of India, which instructed all states to simplify their narcotic regulations. Most states initially failed to accept these instructions, but continued work with state governments has led to simplification of narcotic regulations in 13 of India's 28 states. Since 1999, as evidenced by the report from the government of India to the International Narcotics Control Bureau, morphine consumption has been on the rise (Fig. 3; Joranson et al. 2002). Simplification of narcotic regulations, unfortunately, has not improved opioid availability in all of these 13 states. It is becoming more and more apparent that unless the medical community is trained in the principles of pain relief, fear of analgesics will continue to result in a lot of unnecessary pain.

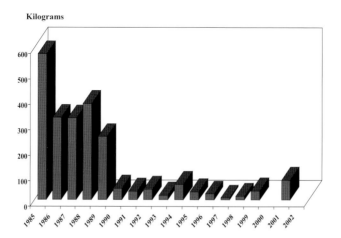

Fig 3. Consumption of morphine in India, 1985–2002, as reported to the International Narcotics Control Bureau (with permission from the Pain and Policy Studies Group, Madison, Wisconsin, USA).

EDUCATION OF PROFESSIONALS

Pain and its relief do not form part of undergraduate or postgraduate medical and nursing education in most of the country. Major pain relief centers mostly concentrate on teaching invasive procedures to anesthesiologists, so that pain pharmacotherapy continues to remain virtually unknown by most of the medical profession. Kerala has made significant progress in this matter. Pain relief is taught to medical students in two medical colleges in the state. Certificate courses of 4–6 weeks' duration in pain and palliative care are available to doctors and nurses in three major institutions in Kerala. Those who complete these courses are incorporating the fundamentals of pain relief into their clinical practice, and most doctors with the pain and palliative care certificate now have access to oral morphine.

The Amrita Institute of Medical Sciences in Kochi, Kerala, has pioneered a postgraduate educational program at the next level. This institute, a constituent of a university, has established a full-time postgraduate 2-year residential diploma in pain and palliative medicine. The course is designed to create a corps of teacher-practitioners who will be well versed in pharmacotherapy as well as invasive procedures, and who will combine pain relief with management of other symptoms and with psychosocial support and rehabilitation where possible.

PUBLIC AWARENESS

Part of the success of the pain relief program in Kerala can be attributed to the fact that it became part of a public movement. Awareness of the needs and possibilities of pain relief empowered the public to seek referrals to pain clinics, and public awareness forced doctors to learn more. Active involvement of journalists in the movement, frequent write-ups in the press, programs in the visual media, and awareness sessions for students and for socially active groups were the major tools of change (Rajagopal and Palat 2002). Wherever volunteers became a strong force, public awareness soon followed. One of the main messages conveyed at the public awareness sessions was that chronic pain is not only a medical problem, but also a social problem, and therefore the community had to get involved.

GOVERNMENT POLICY

Action in India in the field of pain relief has mostly come from nongovernmental agencies. The government of India declared in 1991 that pain relief should be an integral part of cancer care, but the policy did not become a reality. Systematic pain education is not yet part of the medical or nursing curricula. While action by nongovernmental organizations is no doubt valuable, unless pain treatment becomes part of government policy, it will be difficult to achieve coverage over a large and resource-poor country like India. However, things are slowly changing, and encouragement from India's Ministry of Health and Family Welfare has been a major factor in incorporating pain relief programs in more and more cancer centers.

SUMMARY AND CONCLUSIONS

The huge pain burden in the developing world can be significantly reduced by realistic measures aimed at inexpensive yet effective options, as has been shown by the success of the 12-year-old movement in Kerala. Nongovernmental agencies in which medical professionals work hand in hand with volunteers ensure pain relief in the home setting, with oral pharmacotherapy as the fundamental modality. Inpatient treatment and invasive procedures in referral centers serve as a back-up for this system. Improved awareness, advocacy, and work with central and state governments have facilitated improved opioid availability, better pain education for professionals, and changing government policy. Simple and cost-effective measures with strong roots in the community can achieve a significant reduction in pain burden even in resource-poor countries.

REFERENCES

Ajithakumari K, Sureshkumar K, Rajagopal MR. Palliative home care: the Calicut experience. *Palliat Med* 1997; 11:451–454.

Joranson DE, Rajagopal MR, Gilson AM. Improving access to opioid analgesics for palliative care in India. *J Pain Symptom Manage* 2002; 26:152–159.

Rajagopal MR, Kumar S. A model for delivery of palliative care in India: the Calicut experiment. *J Palliat Care* 1999; 15:44–49.

Rajagopal MR, Palat G. Kerala, India: status of cancer pain relief and palliative care. J Pain Symptom Manage 2002; 24:191–193.

Rajagopal MR, Joranson DE, Gilson AM. Medical use, misuse and diversion of opioids in India. *Lancet* 2001; 358:139–143.

Seamark D, Ajithakumari K, Burn G, et al. Palliative care in India. *J R Soc Med* 2000; 93;292–295.

Stjernsward J, Clark D. Palliative care: a global perspective. In: Doyle D, Hanks GW, et al. (Eds). *Oxford Textbook of Palliative Medicine,* 3rd ed. New York: Oxford University Press, 2003.

Sureshkumar K, Rajagopal MR. Palliative care in Kerala: problems at presentation in 440 patients with advanced cancer in a South Indian state. *Palliat Med* 1996; 10:293–298.

Walker VA. Evaluation of WHO analgesic guidelines for cancer pain in a hospital based palliative care unit. *J Pain Symptom Manage* 1988; 3:145–149.

World Health Organization. *Cancer Pain Relief.* Geneva: World Health Organization, 1986.

Zech DFJ, Grond S, Lynch J, Hertel D, Lehman KA. Validation of World Health Organisation guidelines for cancer pain relief. A 10 year prospective study. *Pain* 1995; 63: 65–76.

Correspondence to: Gayatri Palat, DA, DNB, Department of Pain and Palliative Medicine, Amrita Institute of Medical Sciences, Kochi 682026, Kerala, India. Email: gpalat@gmail.com.

Proceedings of the 11th World Congress on Pain,
edited by Herta Flor, Eija Kalso, and Jonathan O.
Dostrovsky, IASP Press, Seattle, © 2006.

8

Understanding the Role of Culture in Pain: Assessing Pain from a Maori Perspective

Jane E. Magnusson[a,b] and Joyce A. Fennell[c]

Departments of [a] Sport and Exercise Science, [b] Psychology, and [c] Psychological Medicine, University of Auckland, Auckland, New Zealand

Chronic pain presents with considerable difficulties and complexities for those who suffer from it, as well as for those who treat it. Physiological mechanisms cannot account for all aspects of pain, nor can physiological or pharmacological treatments relieve all pain. The complex and multidimensional nature of pain necessitates investigation of numerous factors that contribute to the experience of pain and its impact on patients' lives. Commonly recognized elements of the pain experience include sensory, emotional, motivational, and social factors. Within each of these factors are many subtle and complex aspects that contribute to the perception and experience of pain. For example, culture could be considered an aspect of how social factors influence pain. Many psychological and anthropological studies have shown that culture can play an essential role in how individuals perceive and respond to pain (Melzack and Wall 1996).

CULTURE AND PAIN

Among the factors that determine how a person perceives, experiences, and responds to pain, culture represents an important influence. The values, beliefs, norms, and practices that are shared by members of the same cultural group represent a significant force in shaping beliefs and behaviors (Davidhizar and Giger 2004). Culture gives meaning to the pain experience and influences the way it is expressed, as shown in studies that have reported that attitudes and responses to pain vary by cultural group (Kazarian and Evans 2001). While not all differences in pain experiences are due to cultural differences (Melzack and

Wall 1996), the influence of culture on a patient's perception and experience of pain needs to be considered because it may influence the assessment and treatment of pain.

MEASURING THE EXPERIENCE OF PAIN

Although the experience of pain is universal among persons of all ages, cultures, and socioeconomic status (Bjorklund and Bergstrom 2000), assessment of pain has yet to adequately take into account the diversity found within this universal construct. When studying pain behaviors and the reporting of pain experiences, it is important to be aware of cultural or ethnic influences and to acknowledge individual differences. This is especially true with regard to the use of assessment and measurement tools.

To better understand how people perceive and experience pain, most studies use some form of questionnaire or pain measure. While this is done to provide a standardized and objective measure of the person's subjective experience, there are some concerns with regard to how we assess pain in different cultures. For example, to better understand the influence of culture on pain, one approach has been to use well-established measures with different cultural and ethnic groups. While this approach attempts to keep the measurement of the experience of pain within the standardized norms of the measure used, it does not take into account differences in how people perceive and report pain as influenced by their culture and language. To use a standardized assessment measure in another culture, one must translate that measure into the appropriate language. However, due to the subtleties of language and how people refer to personal experiences such as pain, it is not clear that merely translating measures from one language to another adequately captures the experiences of different cultures, each of which may use unique words and phrases to describe pain.

The subjective and complex nature of health issues such as pain, suffering, wellness, and quality of life creates significant difficulties for measurement. Translating a health measure into another language assumes the cross-cultural equivalence of the construct being assessed, which may not always be appropriate. For example, the Medical Outcomes Study Short Form-36 (Ware and Sherbourne 1992) is one of the most widely used health outcome measures, yet it was found to be unsuitable for Pacific people and for older Maori in New Zealand because it did not adequately measure the construct of quality of life of these cultural groups (Scott et al. 2000). Hence, we need health measures that are based upon culturally appropriate health constructs. An example of how this can be done comes from the World Health Organization (WHO), which used a "bottom-up" approach in the development of its quality of life measure by asking groups of patients, health professionals, and healthy people to define the construct. The WHO then generated the questions that were deemed to measure the agreed domains of the construct within various cultures (Power et al. 1999).

ASSESSING PAIN IN DIFFERENT CULTURES: THE IMPORTANCE OF LANGUAGE

Just as numerical scales (pain rated from 0–10) and verbal scales (e.g., mild, moderate, severe) capture only the intensity aspect of pain, and even then in a manner that does not lend itself to gaining insight into the person's experience, so too are questionnaires at risk of inadequately capturing the diversity of pain experiences in different cultures. It is essential that we have assessment measures that enable individuals to convey their experiences if we are to understand the many aspects of their pain and its impact on their life. Without such knowledge, we miss out on information that could facilitate the assessment and treatment of pain and suffering. If we are to understand a person's experience, he or she must be allowed to express it, which requires language, but it is often language that can fail to capture the essence of the person's experiences.

The importance of language as a means to capture and convey one's perceptions and experiences exists in all cultures. The language of the indigenous people of New Zealand, the Maori, is called te Reo and has been returning to popular use since the 1970s, which saw a revitalization of the Maori culture. We wanted to study the experience of pain within the Maori culture, so we needed to understand pain from a Maori perspective. To accomplish this objective, it would not be adequate to simply translate existing pain and disability measures into te Reo Maori. We needed to do this work in consultation with those who best understand the Maori perspective of health, the Maori elders (*kaumatua*) and Maori health care providers.

MAORI PERSPECTIVES OF HEALTH

In a manner consistent with the widely accepted biopsychosocial view of health and wellness, the traditional Maori view of health is multidimensional, incorporating a balance between four interacting dimensions—spiritual, emotional or mental, physical, and family health. The most widely recognized Maori model of health, *te whare tapa wha* (Durie 1985, 1998), likens these dimensions to the four supporting walls of a house in that the integrity of all four dimensions is required for a sound whole.

With regard to the experience of pain, while there is a growing body of literature on the influence of culture on the experience of pain, little has been published about Maori perspectives on pain. One article by Thompson (1989) provided a brief description of the relationship among *mamae* (pain), *mauri* (life force), and *wairua* (spiritual force), in which *mamae* was described as a spiritual force that splits or restrains the *mauri* or the *wairua*. Thompson's (1989) account demonstrates the universality of the destructive impact that pain can have on people's lives.

ASSESSING PAIN FROM A MAORI PERSPECTIVE

To better understand the Maori perspective of pain, we asked *kaumatua* and Maori health care providers (physicians, nurses, physiotherapists, and midwives) to complete a survey containing descriptive pain-related words and phrases. Participants were asked to provide feedback regarding the suitability of words and phrases typically used to describe symptoms of pain and pain-related disability. Participants were also asked to provide words or phrases (in English or te Reo Maori) representing characteristics of pain that had not been included. Additionally, we conducted interviews with *kaumatua* and Maori health care providers to gain insight into the experience of pain from a Maori perspective. This was the first step in establishing what words and phrases would be appropriate in the development of a pain assessment measure for Maori. Approval for this research was obtained from the University of Auckland Human Participants Ethics Committee as well as from the *kaumatua*. As it can be difficult for non-Maori (*Pakeha*) researchers to undertake studies involving Maori, it was essential that the *kaumatua* supported this work.

Of the 61 descriptive statements provided regarding the experience of pain, 56 (92%) were endorsed by 65% or more of the participants. Examples of these statements are: "I feel stressed because of my pain," "My pain makes me frustrated," and "I avoid being around people when I'm in pain." Of the 123 pain descriptors provided, 77 (63%) were endorsed by 100% of the participants; 65% of the participants endorsed all of the descriptors. Examples of these descriptors in various categories include: Sensory: stabbing, excruciating, tender. Emotional: confused, helpless, exhausted, terrified. Cognitive: annoying, irritating, desperate, worried. Social: forgotten, misunderstood, isolated, unsupported. Table I presents a sample of alternative words provided by respondents.

From the interviews we conducted with 24 *kaumatua* and 7 Maori health care providers, themes of the universality of pain and its impact on people's lives emerged. For example, when asked to describe pain from a Maori perspective, a *kaumatua* commented: "What do you mean Maori pain? I've never

Table I
A sample of additional pain descriptors
provided by Maori respondents

Sensory	Emotional	Cognitive	Social
Boring	Angry	Suicidal	Dependent
Bruised	Crappy	Useless	Despair
Constant	Shattered	Unthinkable	Left out
Sprained	Stuffed	Unconscious	Restless
Sticking	Broken	Delirium	Quarrelsome

heard of cultural pain, I thought pain was a human experience." Similarly, a Maori health care provider stated: "I have worked with a number of Maori patients and their *whanau* who have experienced pain. I can think of a group of words which are very much the common parlance—burning, stabbing, tearing, ripping, aching—and the pain might have a quality of being intermittent, pervasive, fluctuating or consistent in intensity, or building over certain periods, alleviated by some things and exacerbated by other things, and I can't really think of anything particularly unusual that would differentiate Maori patients from non-Maori patients in the language that they used."

CONCLUSIONS

The results of our surveys and interviews with *kaumatua* and Maori health care providers show that as with many cultures, Maori perceive pain as a multidimensional experience that affects them in physiological, psychological, and spiritual ways. The clinical implications of this study are that using established descriptive words and phrases in addition to those provided by respondents is an important component to treating pain from a multidimensional perspective and would be appropriate within the Maori culture.

While there is clearly a commonality among cultures with regard to the experience of pain, it is valuable to understand each culture's perceptions and experiences of pain before assessing and treating patients with pain. Our findings with the Maori of New Zealand demonstrate that while commonly used and widely accepted descriptors of pain are appropriate to use when assessing Maori pain patients, it would be of considerable benefit to include additional words that capture aspects of the pain experience that may be specific to that culture. Once a survey has been developed that includes these additional items, further studies need to be undertaken with Maori pain patients to further explore the experience of pain within this cultural group.

ACKNOWLEDGMENTS

We are grateful for the support of our Maori cultural advisors, the *kaumatua* and the Maori health care providers.

REFERENCES

Bjorklund K, Bergstrom S. Is pelvic pain in pregnancy a welfare complaint? *Acta Obstet Gynecol Scand* 2000; 79:24–30.

Davidhizar R, Giger JN. A review of the literature on care of clients in pain who are culturally diverse. *Int Nurs Rev* 2004; 51:47–55.

Durie MH. A Maori perspective of health. *Soc Sci Med* 1985; 205:483–486.

Durie MH. *Whaiora: Maori Health Development*, 2nd ed. Auckland: Oxford University Press, 1998.

Kazarian SS, Evans DR (Ed). *Handbook of Cultural Health Psychology*. San Diego: Academic Press, 2001.

Melzack R, Wall PD. *The Challenge of Pain,* 2nd ed. New York: Penguin, 1996.

Power M, Harper A, Bullinger M. The World Health Organization WHOQOL-100. *Health Psychol* 1999; 18:495–505.

Scott KM, Sarfati D, Tobias MI, Haslett SJ. A challenge to the cross-cultural validity of the SF-36 health survey. *Soc Sci Med* 2000; 51:1655–1664.

Thompson NA. A Maori perspective of pain. *New Zealand Pain Soc J* 1989; Apr:4–5.

Ware JE Jr, Sherbourne CD. The MOS 36-item short-form health survey (SF-36). *Med Care* 1992; 30:473–483.

Correspondence to: Jane E. Magnusson, PhD, Department of Sport and Exercise Science, University of Auckland, Private Bag 92019, Auckland, New Zealand. Email: j.magnusson@auckland.ac.nz.

Part II

Molecular and Cellular Aspects of Pain

Proceedings of the 11th World Congress on Pain,
edited by Herta Flor, Eija Kalso, and Jonathan O.
Dostrovsky, IASP Press, Seattle, © 2006.

9

Ion Channels: Recent Advances and Clinical Applications

Michael S. Gold

Department of Biomedical Sciences, Dental School; Program in Neuroscience; and Department of Anatomy and Neurobiology, Medical School, University of Maryland, Baltimore, Maryland, USA

Pain is a multidimensional phenomenon dependent on a complex interaction between several regions of the cerebral cortex that, in the case of tissue injury are activated by sensory input. Underlying this complexity are ion channels, which are single proteins or protein complexes that enable the movement of ions (Na^+, K^+, Ca^{2+}, and Cl^-) across lipid membranes. Thus, understanding the ion channels that underlie pain may enable more effective treatments of pain.

Neural activity is the electricity in the nervous system. This electricity is caused by the movement of charged particles and provides the basis for recordings made with electroencephalography (EEG) or electromyography (EMG). However, unlike the electricity in a house, which depends on the movement of electrons through wires, the electricity in the nervous system depends on the movement of ions across the membranes of neurons. The driving force for this movement arises from forces acting on ions in solution. These forces are the diffusion of ions down concentration gradients and electrical forces resulting from the repulsive and attractive properties of the ions. Because the cell membrane is a lipid structure, charged molecules like ions cannot diffuse through the membrane. Thus, the only way ions can move across a membrane is with the assistance of specialized proteins in the membrane. These proteins may actively transport ions across the membrane, as is the case of ion pumps and exchangers, or they may allow the passive transport of ions through pores or channels in the protein structure. The focus of this chapter is on the role of these ion channels in pain transmission.

The specific protein structures that form ion channels confer unique properties to the channel, such as when, how, and for how long the channels are opened and closed and which ions are able to pass through them. These properties serve as the basis for classifying most ion channels. Thus, voltage-gated ion channels are opened and closed by changes in membrane potential, while ligand-gated ion channels are opened or closed following binding of a molecule, such as a neurotransmitter, to receptors on the ion channel protein. Moreover, channels are most often selective for a specific ion or ions (e.g., sodium ion channels are selective for Na^+). Thus, a voltage-gated Na^+ channel would be a channel selective for Na^+ that is opened and closed by changes in membrane potential.

The relationship between ion channels and pain is readily appreciated if one considers the actions of local anesthetics such as lidocaine. Application of lidocaine to a nerve blocks voltage-gated Na^+ channels. These channels are necessary for electrical activity in a nerve. Thus, the block of Na^+ movement through voltage-gated Na^+ channels results in the block of neural activity and the block of pain. However, lidocaine blocks voltage-gated Na^+ channels in neurons. As a result, lidocaine not only blocks pain, but it blocks light touch, proprioception, and other sensations arising from the body. While this type of anesthesia is desirable for localized surgical interventions, it is not optimal for pain relief.

It has become clear over the last several decades not only that ion channels are critical for the transmission of pain "messages," but that changes in ion channels contribute to increases in pain following injury. Identification of specific ion channels critical both for the expression of pain and for increases in pain following injury has yielded a number of potential targets for the treatment of pain. The focus of this chapter will be on the factors that influence whether or not a particular ion channel is likely to be a viable target for the development of novel therapeutic interventions for the treatment of pain. These factors will be highlighted by focusing on three ion channels for which there are compelling links to pain (although half a dozen other excellent examples could have been used). These ion channels are expressed in subpopulations of primary afferent neurons. An important advantage to selectively blocking activity in specific subpopulations of primary afferent neurons is that such selectivity may provide pain relief in the absence of deleterious side effects associated with drugs that affect the central nervous system (CNS) and other sensory afferents. Finally, it is important to note that the decision to focus on the ion channels in primary afferent neurons does not mean that various ion channels within the CNS may not also be potential therapeutic targets.

ION CHANNELS IN PRIMARY AFFERENT NEURONS

Several major events are necessary for primary afferents to rapidly signal the presence of tissue-damaging stimuli to the CNS. Ion channels play critical roles in each of these steps. As depicted in Fig. 1, the first step in this process involves stimulus transduction, whereby energy from the environment (i.e., thermal, mechanical or chemical) is converted into an electrical signal. A number of specialized ion channels have been identified that underlie transduction. These include thermoreceptors, such as TRPV1 (Caterina et al. 1999), TRPV3 (Peier et al. 2002b), and TRPM8 (McKemy et al. 2002; Peier et al. 2002a), which open or close in response to changes in temperature; mechanoreceptors, such as the epithelial Na$^+$ channel ENaC (Askwith et al. 2001) and the K$^+$ channel TRAAK (Maingret et al. 1999), which respond to mechanical stimuli; and chemoreceptors such as the ATP receptor P2X$_3$ (Chen et al. 1995) and the serotonin receptor 5HT$_3$ (Maricq et al. 1991), which respond to chemical stimuli. Opening or, as in the case of TRAAK, closing these channels enables a relative increase in the movement of positively charged ions, primarily Na$^+$ and Ca^{2+}, into the neuron, resulting in membrane depolarization.

The depolarization that results from the transduction event provides the driving force for the second step in the afferent signaling process: spike initiation.

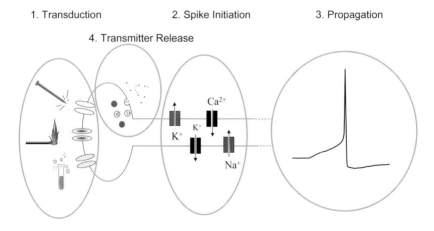

Fig. 1. Four steps necessary for rapid signaling in sensory neurons. (1) Transduction: Unique proteins that respond to mechanical, thermal and chemical stimuli are depicted. (2) Spike initiation: the depolarization resulting from stimulus transduction opens voltage-gated ion channels. If the depolarization is large enough, an action potential will result. (3) Action potential propagation: The process underlying spike initiation is repeated along the axon. Different types of voltage-gated channels may underlie spike initiation and action potential propagation. (4) Transmitter release: membrane depolarization in both peripheral and central terminals will drive the activation of voltage-gated Ca^{2+} channels (only the peripheral terminal is shown). These channels enable Ca^{2+} influx (not shown), which triggers transmitter release.

The change in membrane potential initiated by the transduction event causes voltage-gated ion channels to open or close in response to the change in membrane potential. If the depolarization reaches a critical threshold, widespread activation of voltage-gated Na^+ channels occurs, driving a feed-forward reaction that underlies the very rapid membrane depolarization associated with an action potential. The feed-forward reaction occurs because Na^+ ions flowing into the neuron depolarize the membrane, which triggers more voltage-gated Na^+ channels to open, which enables more Na^+ influx, and so on. The entire depolarization phase of an action potential can occur in less than a millisecond.

Once the action potential is initiated, and the change in membrane potential is sufficient to activate nearby voltage-gated Na^+ channels, the process is repeated along the neural membrane. The successful repetition of this process, called action potential propagation, is the third critical step of rapid afferent signaling. The fourth and final step occurs when the action potential invades the afferent terminals in the peripheral and central nervous systems. Voltage-gated Ca^{2+} channels in the terminals are activated by the invading action potential, enabling Ca^{2+} influx. In turn, Ca^{2+} influx triggers the release of neurotransmitters, which initiates the same process in subsequent neurons in the pathway. While rapid signaling to the CNS depends on this fourth step, a neurotransmitter also can be released from peripheral terminals, a process that contributes to neurogenic inflammation (Sluka et al. 1995).

Changes in ion channels that underlie each of these steps have been described in the presence of injury. For example, inflammatory mediators such as nerve growth factor (NGF; Shu and Mendell 2001), prostaglandin E_2 (PGE_2, Pitchford and Levine 1991), and bradykinin (Cesare and McNaughton 1996; Vellani et al. 2001) increase TRPV1-mediated currents and decrease the temperature at which these channels are activated. These changes appear to reflect an increase in the number of channels as well as changes in channel properties, resulting in the facilitation of thermal transduction and inflammatory hyperalgesia. Similarly, inflammatory mediators decrease K^+ channels, which appear to be critical for attenuating the excitability of primary afferents (Nicol et al. 1997). The result is a decrease in action potential threshold and an increase in the number of action potentials evoked in response to suprathreshold stimuli. This increase in afferent excitability should result in an increase in pain associated with inflammation. While the impact of changes in action potential propagation on nociception have yet to be clearly defined, evidence indicates that inflammation is associated with an increase in axonal conduction velocity (Djouhri and Lawson 2001). An increase in axonal conduction velocity may contribute to an increase in the afferent barrage impinging on the CNS. Finally, inflammatory mediators increase voltage-gated Ca^{2+} currents in sensory neurons (Borgland et al. 2002), a change that may contribute to inflammatory-mediator-induced increases in evoked neurotransmitter release (Hingtgen and Vasko 1994; Hingtgen et al. 1995). Together, these observations indicate that changes in ion channels throughout the primary afferent may contribute to increased pain associated with tissue injury.

POINTS OF CONVERGENCE

The number of channels that may contribute to increased pain associated with injury raises a number of questions. Primary among these, from a therapeutic perspective, is the question of which ion channels to target. Should one try and block the ion channels responsible for the increase in excitability, or would it be better to target the ion channels unique to the afferent populations that are responsible for the problem signal? Or is it possible to identify ion channels that are not directly involved in signaling tissue injury, but may provide a way to access afferents responsible for the problem signal?

I would suggest that the primary rationale for identification of a putative therapeutic target is to consider whether or not the ion channel in question functions at a point of convergence. Points of convergence are readily identified when one considers the steps depicted in Fig. 1. For example, it is clear that an ion channel that mediates the actions of PGE_2 would not be at a point of convergence if PGI_2, serotonin, and tumor necrosis factor α all increase the excitability of afferents by modulating ion channels that function in parallel with that modulated by PGE_2. Conversely, ion channels underlying spike initiation or action potential propagation clearly function at points of convergence because blocking these channels will prevent action potential generation and block the flow of neural activity into the CNS. Evidence that such an approach should be feasible comes from the observation that specific ion channels not only are differentially distributed among sensory neurons, but are differentially distributed within sensory neurons. Thus, not only is it possible to selectively target ion channels in specific populations of neurons, but more importantly, one can target channels that subserve specific functions. That this approach has yet to be more successful reflects a number of factors, not the least of which are relatively recent data indicating that the role of specific ion channels may change in response to the immediate demands of the neuron (see Gold et al. 2003). The result of this plasticity is that a number of factors, including the target of innervation (skin, muscle, or joint), the type of injury (inflammatory versus neuropathic), time (both duration of injury and history of injured tissue), and sex or gonadal status all impact the relative involvement of specific ion channels. The following examples are not only promising targets that illustrate the potential impact of attacking points of convergence, but they illustrate the impact of these complicating factors.

P2X$_3$ RECEPTORS

Adenosine triphosphate (ATP) and adenosine are purines that are endogenous ligands for a family of receptors called purinoceptors. Adenosine acts at P1 receptors, and ATP acts at P2 receptors. P2 receptors are divided into P2X and P2Y receptors, based on whether they directly couple to ion channels (P2X) or to second-messenger pathways (P2Y). There are multiple receptor subtypes within each of these major classes of purinoceptors, and several receptor subtypes within each of the classes are involved in either the transmission or modulation of nociceptive information (Liu and Salter 2005). Given that the focus of this chapter is on ion channels, I will address the role of P2X receptors in nociception.

Members of the P2X receptor family that play critical roles in nociception include P2X$_4$, P2X$_7$, and P2X$_3$ receptors. P2X$_4$ receptors are expressed in activated microglia in the spinal cord following peripheral nerve damage (Tsuda et al. 2003) or spinal cord injury (Schwab et al. 2005). Activation of these receptors appears to be critical for nerve-injury-induced increases in the expression of nociceptive behaviors (Tsuda et al. 2003), and it may contribute to the manifestation of inflammatory pain as well (Guo et al. 2005). P2X$_7$ receptors are primarily expressed in immune cells and appear to be involved in the release of pronociceptive cytokines, in particular interleukin-1β. Changes in nociceptive behaviors associated with either inflammation or nerve injury are significantly attenuated in mice lacking P2X$_7$ receptors (Chessell et al. 2005). However, it is the P2X$_3$ receptor that appears to be the key player in primary afferent signaling of pain.

The observation that an injection of ATP into skin is immediately painful (Keele and Armstrong 1964) suggested that primary afferents express an ATP receptor that underlies the rapid activation of afferents. That the P2X$_3$ receptor might underlie the rapid activation of nociceptive afferents was suggested by the observation that this receptor is highly expressed in nociceptive afferents (Chen et al. 1995). Compelling support for this suggestion was obtained in an *in vitro* experiment involving the co-culture of primary afferent neurons and keratinocytes (Cook and McCleskey 2002). Crushing the keratinocytes close to afferent processes, as would occur with tissue damage, resulted in action potential generation in the afferent. Importantly, of all the mediators released from the damaged cell that could have activated the afferent (such as amino acids, protons, or peptides), ATP appeared to be the mediator solely responsible for this effect. The pharmacological signature of the receptor underlying this action of ATP was that of a P2X$_3$ homomer (i.e., a receptor consisting of only P2X$_3$-receptor subunits) or a P2X$_3$/P2X$_2$ heteromultimer (i.e., a receptor consisting of P2X$_3$- and P2X$_2$-receptor subunits). That the P2X$_3$ receptor is critical for the response to tissue damage is consistent with the observation that the response to formalin injection (which is overtly tissue damaging) is significantly attenuated in mice lacking this receptor (Cockayne et al. 2000; Souslova et al. 2000).

The $P2X_3/P2X_2$ heteromultimer is likely to play a critical role in mediating ATP-evoked pain. This suggestion is based on the observation that homomultimers of $P2X_3$ desensitize very rapidly, while the heteromultimer has a significant sustained component (McCleskey and Gold 1999). The importance of $P2X_2$ receptors in nociceptive signaling is also suggested by the finding that the $P2X_2/P2X_3$ double knockout mouse has a diminished response to noxious stimuli (Cockayne et al. 2005).

There are at least three reasons to focus on the $P2X_3$ receptor. First, the receptor appears to be expressed nowhere else in the body other than primary afferent neurons and is primarily localized to nociceptive afferents (North 2004). Thus, antagonizing or attenuating the expression of this receptor should selectively prevent the activation of a subpopulation of afferents largely responsible for signaling the presence of tissue damage. Second, this receptor has been shown to play a critical role in inflammatory hyperalgesia. Inflammation appears to induce changes in receptor properties, resulting in an increase in ATP-evoked current (Xu and Huang 2002). Direct administration of a $P2X_3$ agonist appears to be painful (Dai et al. 2004), particularly in the presence of inflammation (Hamilton et al. 1999). Furthermore, selectively blocking the receptor with antagonists (Dai et al. 2004; Wu et al. 2004) or knocking down expression of the receptor with antisense oligodeoxynucleotides (Barclay et al. 2002; Honore et al. 2002) will result in a profound reduction in inflammatory hyperalgesia. Third, this receptor plays a critical role in nociceptive behavior associated with nerve injury. The receptor appears to contribute to nerve-injury-induced pain behavior via an upregulation in the uninjured neighbors of afferents injured following a partial nerve injury (Tsuzuki et al. 2001; Obata et al. 2003). The difference between nerve injury and inflammation with respect to the role of $P2X_3$ receptors illustrates the point that the type of injury influences the role of specific ion channels to changes in nociception. Similar to inflammation, however, antagonizing the receptor (McGaraughty et al. 2003; Wu et al. 2004) or knocking it down (Barclay et al. 2002; Honore et al. 2002) will significantly attenuate nerve-injury-induced nociceptive behavior. Thus, the receptor is in the right subpopulation of afferents and appears to contribute to both inflammatory and neuropathic pain.

As a first pass, focusing on $P2X_3$ receptors as a potential therapeutic target may appear to contradict the notion that therapeutic interventions are likely to be most efficacious if the target functions at a point of convergence. Because these ion channels are primarily responsive to ATP, they function as chemoreceptors in primary afferent neurons. Thus, antagonizing this receptor should leave thermoreceptors and mechanoreceptors intact. However, recent evidence indicates that, at least within visceral structures, $P2X_3$ channels appear to function at a point of convergence. Blocking the channel in visceral structures such as the bladder and colon is able to attenuate responses to noxious thermal, mechanical, and chemical stimuli.

P2X$_3$ receptors are able to function at a point of convergence in the bladder and colon because epithelial cells in these structures appear to be the cells primarily responsible for transducing environmental stimuli (Fig. 2). These cells store ATP and release it in a Ca^{2+}-dependent fashion (Birder et al. 2003; Wynn et al. 2003). This release is triggered by a variety of stimuli including stretch, changes in temperature, and chemical stimuli (Birder 2005). In other words, the epithelial cells in the bladder and colon transduce the stimulus, so the afferents that innervate these structures simply need a $P2X_3$ receptor in order to respond to a wide array of stimuli. Thus, even though these visceral afferents express a number of different channels involved in transduction (Brierley et al. 2005; Dang et al. 2005), preclinical data suggest that attenuating $P2X_3$ receptor activity either pharmacologically (Wynn et al. 2003) or with molecular biological approaches (Cockayne et al. 2000; Vlaskovska et al. 2001) effectively reduces behavioral responses to noxious stimulation of these structures. ATP release from the bladder epithelium may also mediate normal micturition reflexes, as mice lacking $P2X_3$ receptors urinate infrequently (Cockayne et al. 2000). Given

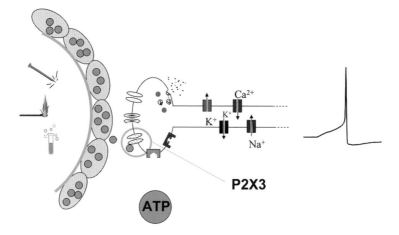

Fig. 2. Stimulus transduction in afferents innervating hollow organ structures (i.e., the bladder and colon) may occur in epithelial cells. These cells are able to store and release adenosine triphosphate (ATP) in a Ca^{2+}-dependent manner. Epithelial cells have been shown to release ATP in response to thermal, mechanical, and chemical stimuli. Stimulus-dependent release of ATP from epithelial cells will activate afferent terminals expressing $P2X_3$ receptors. In these afferents, the $P2X_3$ receptor becomes a point of convergence for the transduction of a wide array of stimuli.

that keratinocytes also release ATP (Mizumoto et al. 2003), a similar mechanism may underlie the efficacy of $P2X_3$-receptor antagonists against thermal and mechanical stimulation of cutaneous tissue following tissue injury. Such a mechanism may also explain warm-coding deficits in $P2X_3$-deficient mice, given that a warm receptor, TRPV3, is expressed in keratinocytes (Peier et al. 2002b).

$NA_V1.8$

Voltage-gated Na^+ channels are composed of an α-subunit, with up to two β-subunits (Catterall 2002). Although there are multiple types of α-subunits, with unique biophysical and pharmacological properties, each contains everything necessary for a functional channel including a voltage-sensor, ion channel, and inactivation gate (part of the protein that mediates channel inactivation observed following channel activation). Nine α-subunits have been cloned that clearly function as voltage-gated channels (Table I). A 10th α-subunit, called Na_X, has also been identified that appears to be a distant relative of the other nine and is thought to function as a sodium ion transport molecule as opposed to a voltage-gated ion channel (Catterall et al. 2003). The α-subunits are differentially distributed throughout the body (Table I) as well as within individual cells. Eight of the nine α-subunits are expressed in sensory neurons, with the majority of sensory neurons expressing multiple α-subunits (Black et al. 1996). The β-subunits appear to primarily influence membrane expression and biophysical properties of the α-subunits (Isom 2000). All four β-subunits are expressed in sensory neurons (Table I).

Voltage-gated Na^+ channels play a critical role in mediating the rapid depolarization associated with the upstroke of the action potential, and for many years it was believed that this was their only function. Modulation of action potential waveform and spike patterns was thought to be controlled by K^+ channels. More recently, however, investigators have begun to appreciate that Na^+ channels also contribute to changes in excitability because the biophysical properties, distribution, and expression pattern of these channels are surprisingly malleable (Lai et al. 2004). A number of α-subunits and at least one β-subunit may contribute to pain following injury (Lai et al. 2004) (Table I).

The α-subunit $Na_V1.3$ has received considerable attention for its potential role in mediating neuropathic pain. This α-subunit is regulated in the peripheral nervous system such that it is normally only expressed during development. Following tissue injury in the adult, however, there is a dramatic upregulation of $Na_V1.3$ (Waxman et al. 1994). The upregulation of this channel, its distribution in injured afferents, and its biophysical properties suggest that this subunit

Table I
Sodium channels in sensory neurons

Name	Gene	Previous Names	Major Site of Expression	Present in Primary Afferent	Change with Injury*
Alpha Subunits					
$Na_V1.1$	*SCN1A*	Rat Brain I	CNS, PNS	Moderate level	↓ (NI) – (I)
$Na_V1.2$	*SCN2A*	Rat Brain II/IIA	CNS, glia	Low level	↓ (NI) – (I)
$Na_V1.3$	*SCN3A*	Rat Brain III	CNS, glia	Development	↑ (NI) ↑ (I)
$Na_V1.4$	*SCN4A*	μ1, SkM1	Skeletal Muscle	No	NA
$Na_V1.5$	*SCN5A*	μ2, SkM2, H1	Cardiac muscle	Development	?? (NI) ?? (I)
$Na_V1.6$	*SCN8A*	NaCh6, CerIII, PN4, CSC-1	CNS, PNS, glia, axons, nodes of Ranvier	High level	↓ (NI) – (I)
$Na_V1.7$	*SCN9A*	PN1, HNe-Na, NaS	PNS, glia	High level	↓ (NI) ↑ (I)
$Na_V1.8$	*SCN10A*	PN3, SNS, SNS1	PNS	High level	↓ (NI)† ↑ (I)
$Na_V1.9$	*SCN11A*	PN5, NaN, SNS2	PNS	High level	↓ (NI) ↑ (I)‡
Na_x	*SCN6A, SCN7A*	HNaV2.1, NaG, SCL-11	Heart, uterus, glia	High level	↑ (NI) ?? (I)
Beta Subunits					
β1/1A	β1/1A	β1/1A	CNS, PNS	Medium and large	No
β2	β2	β2	CNS, PNS	Small, medium, and large	No
β3	β3	β3	CNS, PNS	Small	↑ (NI)
β4	β4	β4	CNS, PNS	Medium and large	??

Source: Data are from Waxman et al. (1994), Dib-Hajj et al. (1996), Tanaka et al. (1998), Coward et al. (2001), Kim et al. (2001, 2002), Abdulla and Smith (2002), Takahashi et al. (2003), Black et al. (2004), and Rush and Waxman (2004).
* NI = nerve injury and refers to changes in subunits in injured neurons; I = inflammation. ↑ = increase; ↓ = decrease; – = no change; ?? = data not available.
† Increases and decreases refer to changes in mRNA in most cases. For $Na_V1.9$, the increase observed was in current density after application of an inflammatory mediator.
‡ There is one observation suggesting that $Na_V1.8$-mediated current may be increased following nerve injury (Abdulla and Smith 2002).

plays a major role in mediating ongoing activity in injured afferents (Waxman et al. 1999). However, a recent antisense knockdown study suggests that $Na_V1.3$ contributes little to nerve-injury-induced changes in pain behavior (Lindia et al. 2005). In contrast, $Na_V1.3$ is also upregulated in the spinal cord following spinal cord injury, a change that appears to contribute to the associated pain (Hains et al. 2003, 2004).

$Na_V1.7$ is another α-subunit that has received a lot of attention. This α-subunit is only expressed in the peripheral nervous system, but it can be found in both afferents and efferents. It appears to be present in afferent terminals, where it is likely to contribute to spike initiation (Toledo-Aral et al. 1995). Particularly exciting was the discovery that mutations of this channel appear to be responsible for the symptoms of a hereditary disorder referred to as erythermalgia or erythromelalgia (Yang et al. 2004). This disorder is characterized by the presence of intense pain in distal appendages. The mutations in $Na_V1.7$ render the channel more excitable (Dib-Hajj et al. 2005). Results from $Na_V1.7$ knockout mice suggest that this channel contributes to both acute pain processing and inflammatory pain (Nassar et al. 2004).

Despite these compelling data on $Na_V1.3$ and $Na_V1.7$, the $Na_V1.8$ channel is of particular interest for several reasons. First, like $P2X_3$, $Na_V1.8$ is in the right place. The subunit is only expressed in primary afferent neurons (Akopian et al. 1996; Sangameswaran et al. 1996) and is preferentially expressed in nociceptive afferents (Djouhri et al. 2003). The channel is localized in terminals and cell bodies of nociceptive afferents, which enables the channel to play a critical role in spike initiation (Brock et al. 1998). Second, the subunit has biophysical properties that enable it to sustain action potential generation in the face of prolonged membrane depolarization, as might be observed in the presence of tissue injury with the sustained release of inflammatory mediators (Lai et al. 2004). Third, there is evidence to suggest that $Na_V1.8$ contributes to both the initiation and maintenance of inflammatory hyperalgesia. $Na_V1.8$ channels are modulated by a number of inflammatory mediators, including PGE_2 (England et al. 1996; Gold et al. 1996), 5HT (Gold et al. 1996; Cardenas et al. 1997), adenosine (Gold et al. 1996), endothelin (Zhou et al. 2001), NGF (Zhang and Nicol 2004), and epinephrine (Khasar et al. 1999), in a manner consistent with an increase in excitability. This modulation is antagonized by mediators that block the initiation of inflammatory hyperalgesia (Gold and Levine 1996; Yang and Gereau 2004). Knockdown of the subunit prevents the development of inflammatory hyperalgesia (Khasar et al. 1998) and the sensitization of bladder afferents (Yoshimura et al. 2001). Finally, $Na_V1.8$ knockdown reverses hyperalgesia associated with persistent inflammation (Porreca et al. 1999).

$Na_V1.8$ is also of interest because there is evidence that the subunit contributes to the initiation and maintenance of neuropathic pain (Lai et al. 2002; Gold et al. 2003). Knockdown of the subunit prior to partial nerve injury prevents the development of mechanical hypersensitivity, and knockdown of the subunit after the development of mechanical hypersensitivity will reverse this nociceptive behavior. That this channel may contribute to pain associated with other forms of neuropathy is suggested by the increase in $Na_V1.8$-mediated current in a model of diabetic neuropathy (Hirade et al. 1999).

In addition to the compelling data in support of a role for $Na_V1.8$ in both inflammatory and neuropathic pain and the evidence that the channel normally functions at a point of convergence, there are several additional reasons to focus on this subunit. First, the subunit appears to contribute to neuropathic and inflammatory pain in unique ways. Second, injury-induced changes in the pattern of expression of this channel also illustrate the impact of time on the role of ion channels in pain. Third, preliminary data from our laboratory suggest that expression of this channel, at least in specific subpopulations of neurons, is influenced by the sex and gonadal state of the animal.

As mentioned above, in naive tissue, $Na_V1.8$ appears to be present in nociceptive terminals, where it contributes to spike initiation (Brock et al. 1998; Strassman and Raymond 1999). In the presence of inflammation, a number of inflammatory mediators are released that appear to induce phosphorylation of $Na_V1.8$, resulting in an increase in current and more rapid gating (opening and inactivating) of the channel (Fitzgerald et al. 1999). Inflammatory mediators also appear to be able to increase expression of the channel (Tanaka et al. 1998; Black et al. 2004), which would further facilitate spike initiation in the afferent terminals.

In contrast, nerve injury results in a distinctly different pattern of changes in $Na_V1.8$. There is an initial decrease in $Na_V1.8$ expression in the cell body of injured afferents (Dib-Hajj et al. 1996; Cummins and Waxman 1997; Decosterd et al. 2002), with no detectable accumulation of channel protein at the site of injured axons (Gold et al. 2003). However, in the uninjured neighboring afferents, there appears to be a redistribution of $Na_V1.8$ to unmyelinated and thinly myelinated axons (Gold et al. 2003). This redistribution of $Na_V1.8$ results in functional channels that can sustain action potential conduction. While it is possible that this redistribution of $Na_V1.8$ contributes to spike initiation in these axons, I believe that these channels contribute to the expression of neuropathic pain behavior by enabling transmission of activity generated at peripheral terminals or ectopic sites to the CNS.

Time-dependent changes in the distribution of $Na_V1.8$ following nerve injury suggests that the contribution of specific ion channels to pain may be quite dynamic. As mentioned above, at early time points following nerve injury, there is a redistribution of $Na_V1.8$ to uninjured axons, with a loss of this subunit in injured neurons (Gold et al. 2003). However, data obtained from neuropathic pain patients suggests that at later time points (more than 6 months) after traumatic nerve injury, there is an increase in $Na_V1.8$ in neuromas formed at sites of nerve injury (Coward et al. 2000). Thus, in contrast to data obtained less than 14 days after traumatic nerve injury, at later time points this subunit may contribute to neuropathic pain via an aberrant accumulation in injured fibers.

Finally, we have obtained preliminary data suggesting that expression of $Na_V1.8$ may be influenced by the sex and the hormone levels of the animal. Pain associated with temporomandibular disorder occurs with a higher incidence, severity, and duration in women than in men (LeResche 1997). We initiated a series of studies in an effort to identify mechanisms that may contribute to this sex difference in the expression of this pain syndrome (Flake et al. 2005). Results from one of these studies indicated that the $Na_V1.8$-mediated current density was lower in temporomandibular joint afferents from female rats than from males (Flake and Gold 2003). Interestingly, this difference appeared to reflect the presence of testosterone in males because it was reversed with castration and reinstated with testosterone replacement.

KCNQ CHANNELS

The number and diversity of K^+ channels surpass those of any other kind of ion channel. These channels are involved in regulating all aspects of neuronal excitability and neural signaling, including determination of threshold for spike initiation, the spike duration, the number and timing of subsequent action potentials, and the duration of a burst of action potentials (Korn and Trapani 2005). Multiple K^+ channels contribute to the regulation of each of these properties as well as many others. Therefore, it is not surprising to find that K^+ channels have been implicated in mediating increases in afferent excitability following tissue injury. While the specific subunits have yet to be identified, there is evidence that a delayed rectifier type of K^+ channel is acutely modulated by a number of inflammatory mediators, including PGE_2 (Nicol et al. 1997) and NGF (Zhang and Nicol 2004). Furthermore, in the presence of persistent inflammation of specific tissues, specific subsets of K^+ channels are downregulated. For example, persistent inflammation of both the bladder (Yoshimura and de Groat 1999) and the stomach (Dang et al. 2004) results in a decrease in an A-type (or inactivating) K^+ current. In contrast, persistent inflammation of the ileum results in decreases in both A-type and sustained K^+ currents (Stewart et al. 2003). All of these changes in K^+ currents are associated with dramatic increases in afferent excitability (Yoshimura and de Groat 1999; Moore et al. 2002). Interestingly, similar changes in K^+ currents have been described following nerve injury (Everill and Kocsis 1999).

That K$^+$ channels might provide valuable targets for the treatment of pain is suggested by the observation that like P2X$_3$ and Na$_V$1.8, these channels are differentially distributed both within and between neurons (Rasband et al. 1998). This differential distribution raises the possibility that specific channels in the right location may provide an avenue to decrease excitability following tissue injury. The differential distribution of K$^+$ channels within neurons has been clearly demonstrated in neurons of the CNS. For example, the voltage-gated K$^+$ channel K$_V$2.1 is localized to the cell body and proximal dendrites but is not expressed in distal dendrites or axons of hippocampal neurons (Misonou et al. 2004). Consequently, the channel is in a critical location to influence activity generated in distal dendrites.

Pharmacological manipulation of two distinct classes of K$^+$ channels in sensory neurons provides proof in principle that this approach can be used to decrease neuronal excitability. One of the channels studied was a Ca^{2+}-modulated K$^+$ channel that appears to regulate action potential duration and spike adaptation in sensory neurons (Zhang et al. 2003). Selectively opening the channel by applying the compound NS1619 decreased the number of action potentials evoked in response to depolarizing current injection (Zhang et al. 2003). A second channel studied with a selective channel opener in sensory neurons underlies a current referred to as IK$_{(M)}$ because of its sensitivity to the cholinergic agonist muscarine. IK$_{(M)}$ is a non-inactivating voltage-dependent current that is active at subthreshold membrane potentials. When IK$_{(M)}$ is inhibited by muscarine, the result is an increase in neuronal excitability. Channels underlying IK$_{(M)}$ are members of the KCNQ family, of which KCNQ$_2$, KCNQ$_3$, and KCNQ$_5$ are present in sensory neurons. Retigabine is a KCNQ$_{2/3}$ channel opener currently in clinical trials for the treatment of epilepsy. Application of this compound to sensory neurons results in membrane hyperpolarization and in a decrease in excitability (Passmore et al. 2003). Based on these observations, one would predict that either potassium channel opener should attenuate both inflammation and nerve-injury-induced pain.

Consistent with this prediction, results with retigabine in animal models of both inflammatory and neuropathic pain have been promising. Systemic administration of retigabine significantly attenuated inflammation-induced mechanical hypersensitivity, as assessed in a load-bearing assay, and reduced the spinal hyperexcitability observed following nerve injury (Passmore et al. 2003). In a second study, nerve-injury-induced hypersensitivity to pinprick, but not to von Frey hairs, was attenuated by retigabine (Blackburn-Munro and Jensen 2003), suggesting that the channel is present at higher densities in specific subpopulations of nociceptive afferents.

SUMMARY AND CONCLUSIONS

Recent advances in our understanding of the neurobiology of ion channels continue to underscore the conclusion that ion channels are necessary not only for perception of pain, but also for the initiation and maintenance of increased pain observed following tissue injury. Ion channels play such an instrumental role in pain following tissue injury because the biophysical properties, distribution, and relative density of many different ion channels are dynamically regulated. Several factors influence the nature of this plasticity and therefore are critical for determining the relative contribution of a given ion channel to pain associated with tissue injury. These factors include target of innervation, type of injury, time both in respect to the history of the neuron (the subject's age and any previous injury) and time elapsed since the injury, and the sex or hormonal status of the injured organism. As a result of our increased understanding of neural signaling and the neural plasticity that occurs in response to tissue injury, a number of ion channels have been identified that function at points of convergence. Identification of such ion channels provides hope that it may be possible to selectively and effectively treat pain with minimal side effects. Indeed, preclinical results with novel compounds targeting channels that function at points of convergence, such as $P2X_3$, $Na_V1.8$, and KCNQ, has yielded promising results, suggesting that novel therapeutic interventions for the treatment of pain are on the horizon.

ACKNOWLEDGMENTS

Some of the work discussed in this chapter was supported by NIH grants 1P50 AR049555, and P01 NS41384. I would also like to thank Dr. Michael Morgan for helpful discussions during the preparation of this manuscript.

REFERENCES

Abdulla FA, Smith PA. Changes in Na^+ channel currents of rat dorsal root ganglion neurons following axotomy and axotomy-induced autotomy. *J Neurophysiol* 2002; 88:2518–2529.

Akopian AN, Sivilotti L, Wood JN. A tetrodotoxin-resistant voltage-gated sodium channel expressed by sensory neurons. *Nature* 1996; 379:257–262.

Askwith CC, Benson CJ, Welsh MJ, Snyder PM. DEG/ENaC ion channels involved in sensory transduction are modulated by cold temperature. *Proc Natl Acad Sci USA* 2001; 98:6459–6463.

Barclay J, Patel S, Dorn G, et al. Functional downregulation of P2X3 receptor subunit in rat sensory neurons reveals a significant role in chronic neuropathic and inflammatory pain. *J Neurosci* 2002; 22:8139–8147.

Birder LA. More than just a barrier: urothelium as a drug target for urinary bladder pain. *Am J Physiol Renal Physiol* 2005; 289:F489–F495.

Birder LA, Barrick SR, Roppolo JR, et al. Feline interstitial cystitis results in mechanical hypersensitivity and altered ATP release from bladder urothelium. *Am J Physiol Renal Physiol* 2003; 285:F423–F429.

Black JA, Dib-Hajj S, McNabola K, et al. Spinal sensory neurons express multiple sodium channel alpha-subunit mRNAs. *Brain Res Mol Brain Res* 1996; 43:117–131.

Black JA, Liu S, Tanaka M, Cummins TR, Waxman SG. Changes in the expression of tetrodotoxin-sensitive sodium channels within dorsal root ganglia neurons in inflammatory pain. *Pain* 2004; 108:237–247.

Blackburn-Munro G, Jensen BS. The anticonvulsant retigabine attenuates nociceptive behaviours in rat models of persistent and neuropathic pain. *Eur J Pharmacol* 2003; 460:109–116.

Borgland SL, Connor M, Ryan RM, Ball HJ, Christie MJ. Prostaglandin E$_2$ inhibits calcium current in two sub-populations of acutely isolated mouse trigeminal sensory neurons. *J Physiol* 2002; 539(Pt 2):433–444.

Brierley SM, Carter R, Jones W III, et al. Differential chemosensory function and receptor expression of splanchnic and pelvic colonic afferents in mice. *J Physiol* 2005; 567(Pt 1):267–281.

Brock JA, McLachlan EM, Belmonte C. Tetrodotoxin-resistant impulses in single nociceptor nerve terminals in guinea-pig cornea. *J Physiol (Lond)* 1998; 512(Pt 1):211–217.

Cardenas CG, Del Mar LP, Cooper BY, Scroggs RS. 5HT4 receptors couple positively to tetrodotoxin-insensitive sodium channels in a subpopulation of capsaicin-sensitive rat sensory neurons. *J Neurosci* 1997; 17:7181–7189.

Caterina MJ, Rosen TA, Tominaga M, Brake AJ, Julius D. A capsaicin-receptor homologue with a high threshold for noxious heat. *Nature* 1999; 398:436–441.

Catterall WA. Molecular mechanisms of gating and drug block of sodium channels. *Novartis Found Symp* 2002; 241:206–218; discussion 218–232.

Catterall WA, Striessnig J, Snutch TP, Perez-Reyes E. International Union of Pharmacology. XL. Compendium of voltage-gated ion channels: calcium channels. *Pharmacol Rev* 2003; 55:579–581.

Cesare P, McNaughton P. A novel heat-activated current in nociceptive neurons and its sensitization by bradykinin. *Proc Natl Acad Sci USA* 1996; 93:15435–15439.

Chen CC, Akopian AN, Sivilotti L, et al. A P2X purinoceptor expressed by a subset of sensory neurons [see comments]. *Nature* 1995; 377:428–431.

Chessell IP, Hatcher JP, Bountra C, et al. Disruption of the P2X7 purinoceptor gene abolishes chronic inflammatory and neuropathic pain. *Pain* 2005; 114:386–396.

Cockayne DA, Hamilton SG, Zhu QM, et al. Urinary bladder hyporeflexia and reduced pain-related behaviour in P2X3-deficient mice. *Nature* 2000; 407:1011–1015.

Cockayne DA, Dunn PM, Zhong Y, et al. P2X2 knockout mice and P2X2/P2X3 double knockout mice reveal a role for the P2X2 receptor subunit in mediating multiple sensory effects of ATP. *J Physiol* 2005; 567(Pt 2):621–639.

Cook SP, McCleskey EW. Cell damage excites nociceptors through release of cytosolic ATP. *Pain* 2002; 95:41–47.

Coward K, Plumpton C, Facer P, et al. Immunolocalization of SNS/PN3 and NaN/SNS2 sodium channels in human pain states. *Pain* 2000; 85:41–50.

Coward K, Aitken A, Powell A, et al. Plasticity of TTX-sensitive sodium channels PN1 and brain III in injured human nerves. *Neuroreport* 2001; 12:495–500.

Cummins TR, Waxman SG. Downregulation of tetrodotoxin-resistant sodium currents and upregulation of a rapidly repriming tetrodotoxin-sensitive sodium current in small spinal sensory neurons after nerve injury. *J Neurosci* 1997; 17:3503–3514.

Dai Y, Fukuoka T, Wang H, et al. Contribution of sensitized P2X receptors in inflamed tissue to the mechanical hypersensitivity revealed by phosphorylated ERK in DRG neurons. *Pain* 2004; 108:258–266.

Dang K, Bielefeldt K, Gebhart GF. Gastric ulcers reduce A-type potassium currents in rat gastric sensory ganglion neurons. *Am J Physiol Gastrointest Liver Physiol* 2004; 286:G573–G579.

Dang K, Bielefeldt K, Gebhart GF. Differential responses of bladder lumbosacral and thoracolumbar dorsal root ganglion neurons to purinergic agonists, protons, and capsaicin. *J Neurosci* 2005; 25:3973–3984.

Decosterd I, Ji RR, Abdi S, Tate S, Woolf CJ. The pattern of expression of the voltage-gated sodium channels Na(v)1.8 and Na(v)1.9 does not change in uninjured primary sensory neurons in experimental neuropathic pain models. *Pain* 2002; 96:269–277.

Dib-Hajj S, Black JA, Felts P, Waxman SG. Down-regulation of transcripts for Na channel alpha-SNS in spinal sensory neurons following axotomy. *Proc Natl Acad Sci USA* 1996; 93:14950–14954.

Dib-Hajj SD, Rush AM, Cummins TR, et al. Gain-of-function mutation in $Na_v1.7$ in familial erythromelalgia induces bursting of sensory neurons. *Brain* 2005; 128(Pt 8):1847–1854.

Djouhri L, Lawson SN. Increased conduction velocity of nociceptive primary afferent neurons during unilateral hindlimb inflammation in the anaesthetised guinea-pig. *Neuroscience* 2001; 102:669–679.

Djouhri L, Fang X, Okuse K, et al. The TTX-resistant sodium channel Nav1.8 (SNS/PN3): expression and correlation with membrane properties in rat nociceptive primary afferent neurons. *J Physiol* 2003; 550(Pt 3):739–752.

England S, Bevan S, Docherty RJ. PGE_2 modulates the tetrodotoxin-resistant sodium current in neonatal rat dorsal root ganglion neurons via the cyclic AMP-protein kinase A cascade. *J Physiol (London)* 1996; 495:429–440.

Everill B, Kocsis JD. Reduction in potassium currents in identified cutaneous afferent dorsal root ganglion neurons after axotomy. *J Neurophysiol* 1999; 82:700–708.

Fitzgerald EM, Okuse K, Wood JN, Dolphin AC, Moss SJ. cAMP-dependent phosphorylation of the tetrodotoxin-resistant voltage- dependent sodium channel SNS. *J Physiol (Lond)* 1999; 516(Pt 2):433–446.

Flake NM, Gold MS. Sex differences in voltage-gated Na^+ currents in sensory neurons innervating the rat temporomandibular joint. *J Dent Res* 2003; 82(B):1181.

Flake NM, Bonebreak DB, Gold MS. Estrogen and inflammation increase the excitability of rat temporomandibular joint afferent neurons. *J Neurophysiol* 2005; 93:1585–1597.

Gold MS, Levine JD. DAMGO inhibits prostaglandin E_2-induced potentiation of a TTX-resistant Na^+ current in rat sensory neurons in vitro. *Neurosci Lett* 1996; 212:83–86.

Gold MS, Reichling DB, Shuster MJ, Levine JD. Hyperalgesic agents increase a tetrodotoxin-resistant Na+ current in nociceptors. *Proc Natl Acad Sci USA* 1996; 93:1108–1112.

Gold MS, Weinreich D, Kim CS, et al. Redistribution of $Na_v1.8$ in uninjured axons enables neuropathic pain. *J Neurosci* 2003; 23:158–166.

Guo LH, Trautmann K, Schluesener HJ. Expression of P2X4 receptor by lesional activated microglia during formalin-induced inflammatory pain. *J Neuroimmunol* 2005; 163:120–127.

Hains BC, Klein JP, Saab CY, et al. Upregulation of sodium channel $Na_v1.3$ and functional involvement in neuronal hyperexcitability associated with central neuropathic pain after spinal cord injury. *J Neurosci* 2003; 23:8881–8892.

Hains BC, Saab CY, Klein JP, Craner MJ, Waxman SG. Altered sodium channel expression in second-order spinal sensory neurons contributes to pain after peripheral nerve injury. *J Neurosci* 2004; 24:4832–4829.

Hamilton SG, Wade A, McMahon SB. The effects of inflammation and inflammatory mediators on nociceptive behaviour induced by ATP analogues in the rat. *Br J Pharmacol* 1999; 126:326–332.

Hingtgen CM, Vasko MR. Prostacyclin enhances the evoked-release of substance P and calcitonin gene-related peptide from rat sensory neurons. *Brain Res* 1994; 655:51–60.

Hingtgen CM, Waite KJ, Vasko MR. Prostaglandins facilitate peptide release from rat sensory neurons by activating the adenosine 3',5'-cyclic monophosphate transduction cascade. *J Neurosci* 1995; 15:5411–5419.

Hirade M, Yasuda H, Omatsu-Kanbe M, Kikkawa R, Kitasato H. Tetrodotoxin-resistant sodium channels of dorsal root ganglion neurons are readily activated in diabetic rats. *Neuroscience* 1999; 90:933–939.

Honore P, Kage K, Mikusa J, et al. Analgesic profile of intrathecal P2X$_3$ antisense oligonucleotide treatment in chronic inflammatory and neuropathic pain states in rats. *Pain* 2002; 99:11–19.

Isom LL. I. Cellular and molecular biology of sodium channel beta-subunits: therapeutic implications for pain? I. Cellular and molecular biology of sodium channel beta-subunits: therapeutic implications for pain? *Am J Physiol Gastrointest Liver Physiol* 2000; 278:G349–G353.

Keele CA, Armstrong D. *Substances Producing Pain and Itch.* Baltimore: Williams and Wilkins, 1964.

Khasar SG, Gold MS, Levine JD. A tetrodotoxin-resistant sodium current mediates inflammatory pain in the rat. *Neurosci Lett* 1998; 256:17–20.

Khasar SG, McCarter G, Levine JD. Epinephrine produces a beta-adrenergic receptor-mediated mechanical hyperalgesia and in vitro sensitization of rat nociceptors. *J Neurophysiol* 1999; 81:1104–1112.

Kim CH, Oh Y, Chung JM, Chung K. The changes in expression of three subtypes of TTX sensitive sodium channels in sensory neurons after spinal nerve ligation. *Brain Res Mol Brain Res* 2001; 95:153–161.

Kim CH, Oh Y, Chung JM, Chung K. Changes in three subtypes of tetrodotoxin sensitive sodium channel expression in the axotomized dorsal root ganglion in the rat. *Neurosci Lett* 2002; 323:125–128.

Korn SJ, Trapani JG. Potassium channels. *IEEE Trans Nanobioscience* 2005; 4:21–33.

Lai J, Gold MS, Kim CS, et al. Inhibition of neuropathic pain by decreased expression of the tetrodotoxin-resistant sodium channel, Na$_V$1.8. *Pain* 2002; 95:143–152.

Lai J, Porreca F, Hunter JC, Gold MS. Voltage-gated sodium channels and hyperalgesia. *Annu Rev Pharmacol Toxicol* 2004; 44:371–397.

LeResche L. Epidemiology of temporomandibular disorders: implications for the investigation of etiologic factors. *Crit Rev Oral Biol Med* 1997; 8:291–305.

Lindia JA, Kohler MG, Martin WJ, Abbadie C. Relationship between sodium channel Na$_V$1.3 expression and neuropathic pain behavior in rats. *Pain* 2005; 117:145–153.

Liu XJ, Salter MW. Purines and pain mechanisms: recent developments. *Curr Opin Investig Drugs* 2005; 6:65–75.

Maingret F, Fosset M, Lesage F, Lazdunski M, Honore E. TRAAK is a mammalian neuronal mechano-gated K$^+$ channel. *J Biol Chem* 1999; 274:1381–1387.

Maricq AV, Peterson AS, Brake AJ, Myers RM, Julius D. Primary structure and functional expression of the 5HT3 receptor, a serotonin-gated ion channel. *Science* 1991; 254:432–437.

McCleskey EW, Gold MS. Ion channels of nociception. *Annu Rev Physiol* 1999; 61:835–856.

McGaraughty S, Wismer CT, Zhu CZ, et al. Effects of A-317491, a novel and selective P2X3/P2X2/3 receptor antagonist, on neuropathic, inflammatory and chemogenic nociception following intrathecal and intraplantar administration. *Br J Pharmacol* 2003; 140:1381–1388.

McKemy DD, Neuhausser WM, Julius D. Identification of a cold receptor reveals a general role for TRP channels in thermosensation. *Nature* 2002; 416:52–58.

Misonou H, Mohapatra DP, Park EW, et al. Regulation of ion channel localization and phosphorylation by neuronal activity. *Nat Neurosci* 2004; 7:711–718.

Mizumoto N, Mummert ME, Shalhevet D, Takashima A. Keratinocyte ATP release assay for testing skin-irritating potentials of structurally diverse chemicals. *J Invest Dermatol* 2003; 121:1066–1072.

Moore BA, Stewart TM, Hill C, Vanner SJ. TNBS ileitis evokes hyperexcitability and changes in ionic membrane properties of nociceptive DRG neurons. *Am J Physiol Gastrointest Liver Physiol* 2002; 282:G1045–G1051.

Nassar MA, Stirling LC, Forlani G, et al. Nociceptor-specific gene deletion reveals a major role for Nav1.7 (PN1) in acute and inflammatory pain. *Proc Natl Acad Sci USA* 2004; 101:12706–12711.

Nicol GD, Vasko MR, Evans AR. Prostaglandins suppress an outward potassium current in embryonic rat sensory neurons. *J Neurophysiol* 1997; 77:167–176.

North RA. P2X3 receptors and peripheral pain mechanisms. *J Physiol* 2004; 554(Pt 2):301–308.

Obata K, Yamanaka H, Fukuoka T, et al. Contribution of injured and uninjured dorsal root ganglion neurons to pain behavior and the changes in gene expression following chronic constriction injury of the sciatic nerve in rats. *Pain* 2003; 101:65–77.

Passmore GM, Selyanko AA, Mistry M, et al. KCNQ/M currents in sensory neurons: significance for pain therapy. *J Neurosci* 2003; 23:7227–7236.

Peier AM, Moqrich A, Hergarden AC, et al. A TRP channel that senses cold stimuli and menthol. *Cell* 2002a; 108:705-715.

Peier AM, Reeve AJ, Andersson DA, et al. A heat-sensitive TRP channel expressed in keratinocytes. *Science* 2002b; 296:2046–2049.

Pitchford S, Levine JD. Prostaglandins sensitize nociceptors in cell culture. *Neurosci Lett* 1991; 132:105–108.

Porreca F, Lai J, Bian D, et al. A comparison of the potential role of the tetrodotoxin-insensitive sodium channels, PN3/SNS and NaN/SNS2, in rat models of chronic pain. *Proc Natl Acad Sci USA* 1999; 96:7640–7644.

Rasband MN, Trimmer JS, Schwarz TL, et al. Potassium channel distribution, clustering, and function in remyelinating rat axons. *J Neurosci* 1998; 18:36–47.

Rush AM, Waxman SG. PGE_2 increases the tetrodotoxin resistant $Na_v1.9$ sodium current in mouse DRG neurons via G proteins. *Brain Res* 2004; 1023:264–271.

Sangameswaran L, Delgado SG, Fish LM, et al. Structure and function of a novel voltage-gated, tetrodotoxin-resistant sodium channel specfic to sensory neurons. *J Biol Chem* 1996; 271:5953–5956.

Schwab JM, Guo L, Schluesener HJ. Spinal cord injury induces early and persistent lesional P2X4 receptor expression. *J Neuroimmunol* 2005; 163:185–189.

Shu X, Mendell LM. Acute sensitization by NGF of the response of small-diameter sensory neurons to capsaicin. *J Neurophysiol* 2001; 86:2931–2938.

Sluka KA, Willis WD, Westlund KN. The role of dorsal root reflexes in neurogenic inflammation. *Pain Forum* 1995; 4:141–149.

Souslova V, Cesare P, Ding Y, et al. Warm-coding deficits and aberrant inflammatory pain in mice lacking P2X3 receptors. *Nature* 2000; 407:1015–1017.

Stewart T, Beyak MJ, Vanner S. Ileitis modulates potassium and sodium currents in guinea pig dorsal root ganglia sensory neurons. *J Physiol* 2003; 552(Pt 3):797–807.

Strassman AM, Raymond SA. Electrophysiological evidence for tetrodotoxin-resistant sodium channels in slowly conducting dural sensory fibers. *J Neurophysiol* 1999; 81:413–424.

Takahashi N, Kikuchi S, Dai Y, et al. Expression of auxiliary beta subunits of sodium channels in primary afferent neurons and the effect of nerve injury. *Neuroscience* 2003; 121:441–450.

Tanaka M, Cummins TR, Ishikawa K, et al. SNS Na⁺ channel expression increases in dorsal root ganglion neurons in the carrageenan inflammatory pain model. *Neuroreport* 1998; 9:967–972.

Toledo-Aral J, Brehm P, Halegoua S, Mandel G. A single pulse of nerve growth factor triggers long-term neuronal excitability through sodium channel gene induction. *Neuron* 1995; 14:607–611.

Tsuda M, Shigemoto-Mogami Y, Koizumi S, et al. P2X4 receptors induced in spinal microglia gate tactile allodynia after nerve injury. *Nature* 2003; 424:778–783.

Tsuzuki K, Kondo E, Fukuoka T, et al. Differential regulation of $P2X_3$ mRNA expression by peripheral nerve injury in intact and injured neurons in the rat sensory ganglia. *Pain* 2001; 91:351–360.

Vellani V, Mapplebeck S, Moriondo A, Davis JB, McNaughton PA. Protein kinase C activation potentiates gating of the vanilloid receptor VR1 by capsaicin, protons, heat and anandamide. *J Physiol* 2001; 534(Pt 3):813–825.

Vlaskovska M, Kasakov L, Rong W, et al. P2X3 knock-out mice reveal a major sensory role for urothelially released ATP. *J Neurosci* 2001; 21:5670–5677.

Waxman SG, Kocsis JD, Black JA. Type III sodium channel mRNA is expressed in embryonic but not adult spinal sensory neurons, and is reexpressed following axotomy. *J Neurophysiol* 1994; 72:466–470.

Waxman SG, Dib-Hajj S, Cummins TR, Black JA. Sodium channels and pain. *Proc Natl Acad Sci USA* 1999; 96:7635–7639.

Wu G, Whiteside GT, Lee G, et al. A-317491, a selective P2X3/P2X2/3 receptor antagonist, reverses inflammatory mechanical hyperalgesia through action at peripheral receptors in rats. *Eur J Pharmacol* 2004; 504:45–53.

Wynn G, Rong W, Xiang Z, Burnstock G. Purinergic mechanisms contribute to mechanosensory transduction in the rat colorectum. *Gastroenterology* 2003; 125:1398–1409.

Xu GY, Huang LY. Peripheral inflammation sensitizes P2X receptor-mediated responses in rat dorsal root ganglion neurons. *J Neurosci* 2002; 22:93–102.

Yang D, Gereau RW 4th. Group II metabotropic glutamate receptors inhibit cAMP-dependent protein kinase-mediated enhancement of tetrodotoxin-resistant sodium currents in mouse dorsal root ganglion neurons. *Neurosci Lett* 2004; 357:159–162.

Yang Y, Wang Y, Li S, et al. Mutations in *SCN9A,* encoding a sodium channel alpha subunit, in patients with primary erythermalgia. *J Med Genet* 2004; 41:171–174.

Yoshimura N, de Groat WC. Increased excitability of afferent neurons innervating rat urinary bladder after chronic bladder inflammation. *J Neurosci* 1999; 19:4644–4653.

Yoshimura N, Seki S, Novakovic SD, et al. The involvement of the tetrodotoxin-resistant sodium channel $Na_V1.8$ (PN3/SNS) in a rat model of visceral pain. *J Neurosci* 2001; 21:8690–8696.

Zhang XF, Gopalakrishnan M, Shieh CC. Modulation of action potential firing by iberiotoxin and NS1619 in rat dorsal root ganglion neurons. *Neuroscience* 2003; 122:1003–1011.

Zhang YH, Nicol GD. NGF-mediated sensitization of the excitability of rat sensory neurons is prevented by a blocking antibody to the p75 neurotrophin receptor. *Neurosci Lett* 2004; 366:187–192.

Zhou QL, Strichartz G, Davar G. Endothelin-1 activates ET_A receptors to increase intracellular calcium in model sensory neurons. *Neuroreport* 2001; 12:3853–3857.

Correspondence to: Michael S. Gold, PhD, University of Maryland Dental School, 666 W. Baltimore Street, Room 5-A-12, Baltimore, MD 21201, USA. Fax: 410-706-0865; email: mgold@umaryland.edu.

Proceedings of the 11th World Congress on Pain,
edited by Herta Flor, Eija Kalso, and Jonathan O.
Dostrovsky, IASP Press, Seattle, © 2006.

10

Pain and Neuroplastic Changes in the Dorsal Root Ganglia

Koichi Noguchi

*Department of Anatomy and Neuroscience, Hyogo College of Medicine,
Nishinomiya, Japan*

Originally, the term "neuronal plasticity" referred to the variability of the strength of a signal transmitted through a synapse. Synaptic plasticity is believed to be a fundamental mechanism of memory and learning. The term "neuroplastic changes" has been used recently to mean that the nervous system changes dynamically in a variety of ways following various stimuli that continue for a significant period. Two molecular mechanisms for neuronal plasticity have been revealed by a number of previous studies. The first mechanism involves modification of the intracellular signal transduction system, typically protein phosphorylation, resulting in an altered sensitivity of the channel or receptor protein, or affecting transcription. This pattern of change is rapid and has a short time course. The second mechanism involves changes in gene expression, which are reflected by changes in the levels of synthesis of key proteins in both terminals and primary afferents. This mechanism can be triggered by altered intracellular signal transduction and shows a prolonged time course.

There are many kinds of intracellular signal transduction systems in the nervous system. This chapter will focus on mitogen-activated protein kinase (MAPK), a family of serine/threonine kinases that are activated by phosphorylation of threonine and tyrosine residues. Much evidence indicates that the MAPK cascade plays important roles in transducing extracellular stimuli into intracellular responses. Within the MAPK family, I will describe data on extracellular signal-regulated kinases (ERKs) and p38 MAPK. These MAPKs were originally known as regulators of cell proliferation and survival, but recent findings strongly suggest that MAPK has a major role in regulating neuronal plasticity.

In the last few years researchers have identified a number of channels, including the transient receptor potential (TRP) channels, that are known to have important roles in the pain transduction system. Natural stimuli, including noxious heat, cold, and mechanical stimuli, activate channel proteins located on the membrane in the nerve terminals and generate action potentials. These action potentials are then transmitted to spinal cord through the primary afferent fibers. The action potentials also affect gene expression in the cell bodies of primary afferents that are located in the dorsal root ganglion (DRG). The changes in gene expression alter the production of many kinds of proteins. The increased proteins synthesized in the DRG are transported to the peripheral and central nerve terminals, causing changes in the sensitivity and excitability of afferents in a number of pain conditions.

NEUROPLASTIC CHANGES IN THE DORSAL ROOT GANGLIA AFTER NOXIOUS STIMULATION

ERK ACTIVATION

Much attention has focused on the signal transduction mechanisms of primary afferent neurons responsible for the modulation of pain transmission. Inflammatory mediators, such as prostaglandin E_2, serotonin, epinephrine, and nerve growth factor (NGF), produce hyperalgesia through activation of protein kinase A (PKA) or protein kinase C (PKC) in primary afferent neurons (Gold et al. 1998; Khasar et al. 1999). Recent studies have shown that the ERK cascade acts in epinephrine-induced hyperalgesia and that the Ras-MEK-ERK pathway is activated independently of PKA or PKC (Aley et al. 2001; Dina et al. 2003). Furthermore, NGF injected into peripheral tissue increases labeling of phosphorylated ERK (p-ERK) in DRG neurons that contain tyrosine kinase A (trkA) (Averill et al. 2001; Delcroix et al. 2003). However, only a few studies have investigated the signal transduction involved in the activity-dependent plasticity of primary afferent neurons (Fields et al. 1997; Fitzgerald 2000). My colleagues and I have demonstrated activity-dependent activation of ERK in DRG neurons by determining that phosphorylation of ERK in primary afferent neurons occurs in response to noxious stimulation of the peripheral tissue or to electrical stimulation of the peripheral nerve (Dai et al. 2002). We detected phospho-ERK immunoreactivity in the DRG after natural noxious stimulation and found a stimulus intensity-dependent increase in labeled cell size and in the number of activated neurons in a C- and Aδ-fiber population. Immunohistochemical double labeling with p-ERK/TRPV1 and a pharmacological study demonstrated that noxious heat stimulation induced pERK in primary afferents in a TRPV1-dependent manner. Capsaicin injection into the skin also significantly increased pERK labeling in peripheral fibers and terminals in the skin, which was prevented by a MAPK/ERK kinase (MEK) inhibitor, U0126. Behavioral experiments showed that U0126 dose-dependently attenuated thermal hyperalgesia after capsaicin injection. These results suggest that the activation of ERK pathways in DRG neurons is involved in peripheral sensitization in acute pain conditions. The phosphorylation of ERK in DRG neurons after noxious stimulation might be useful for examining the activation state of each neuron that contains various pain-related molecules (Dai et al. 2002).

p38 ACTIVATION

A recent report demonstrated that TRPV1, formerly known as the vanilloid receptor-1, is regulated by NGF-induced activation of the ERK/MAPK pathway in DRG neurons in vitro (Bron et al. 2003). On the other hand, Ji and colleagues (2002) showed that p38 MAPK activation in the DRG is required for NGF-induced increases in TRPV1 expression and that it contributes to the maintenance of inflammatory pain hypersensitivity. p38, a MAPK that operates through a separate intracellular cascade, functions as a mediator of cellular stresses such as inflammation and apoptosis (Widmann et al. 1999; Shi and Gaestel 2002). An activity-dependent p38 activation occurs in neurons (Mao et al. 1999), and p38 exerts effects in the hippocampus that oppose that of ERK (Bolshakov et al. 2000)

In a recent report on the contribution of p38 MAPK to nociception and pain hypersensitivity, we demonstrated very rapid phosphorylation of p38 MAPK in DRG neurons that were participating in the transmission of noxious signals (Mizushima et al. 2005). Capsaicin injection induced phosphorylated p38 (p-p38) in small- to medium-diameter sensory neurons with a peak 2 minutes after the injection. Furthermore, we examined p-p38 labeling in the DRG after noxious thermal stimulation and found a stimulus-intensity-dependent increase in the size and number of labeled neurons. Most of these p-p38-immunoreactive neurons were small or medium-sized and coexpressed TRPV1 and p-ERK. Intrathecal administration of the p38 inhibitor FR167653 reversed the thermal hyperalgesia produced by the capsaicin injection, suggesting that the activation of p38 pathways in primary afferents by noxious stimulation in vivo may be involved in the development of thermal hyperalgesia. In addition, we found that noxious cold stimulation of the rat hindpaw induced phosphorylation of ERK and p38 in different populations in DRG neurons (unpublished observations). Therefore, ERK and p38 probably have similar and distinct roles, which may be dependent on the pain states evoked by different stimuli. Alternatively, there may be cross-talk between the ERK and p38 pathways (Torocsik and Szeberenyi 2000). On the other hand, p-p38 is constitutively expressed in ~15% of the neurons, as stated above, while very few neurons are labeled for p-ERK in the naive DRG, indicating that the activation of p38 may be a less accurate reflection of activity than that of ERK. However, the characteristics of p-p38 labeling in DRG neurons after noxious stimulation suggest that the labeling is, at least in part, correlated with the activation state of the primary afferent neurons. We believe that p-p38 and p-ERK are very useful indicators of the activated DRG neurons after noxious stimulation in vivo (Fig. 1).

LONG-TERM CHANGES IN THE DORSAL ROOT GANGLIA ASSOCIATED WITH TISSUE INFLAMMATION AND PERIPHERAL NERVE INJURY

TRPA1 EXPRESSION AFTER TISSUE INFLAMMATION

Tissue inflammation and peripheral nerve injury induce a variety of changes in gene expression in DRG neurons by altering the intracellular signal transduction cascade. Prolonged alterations in the excitability of primary afferents, synaptic transmission, and protein synthesis and release occur, resulting in

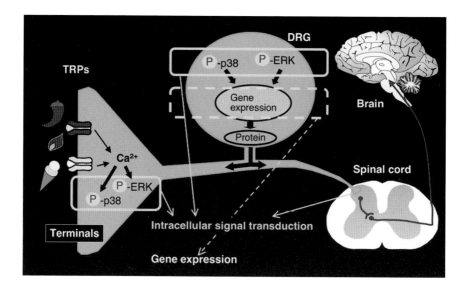

Fig. 1. Phosphorylation of mitogen-activated protein kinases, extracellular signal-regulated kinase (ERK) and p38, after noxious stimuli, and the effect on gene expression in primary afferents. There are two known molecular mechanisms for neuronal plasticity in primary afferents. The first mechanism involves modification of the intracellular signal transduction system, typically a chain process of protein phosphorylation, resulting in the altered sensitivity of channel or receptor protein. Noxious stimuli (capsaicin, heat, and cold) induced phosphorylation of ERK and p38 in dorsal root ganglia (DRG), nerve terminals, and the spinal dorsal horn. The second mechanism involves changes in gene expression and can be triggered by altered intracellular signal transduction.

extended pain responses. There are many reports regarding gene expression in the DRG after tissue inflammation. A number of molecules, including neuropeptides such as substance P and calcitonin gene-related peptide (CGRP), growth factors, cytokines, and neurotransmitters, have increased expression in the DRG after tissue inflammation. Here I discuss new findings from my laboratory on one member of the TRP channel family, TRPA1. Previous studies indicate that TRPA1 is a candidate as a transducer of noxious cold. This channel is activated by temperatures below 18°C and is expressed in small or medium-sized DRG neurons (Kobayashi et al. 2005). There are some controversial issues regarding the electrophysiological properties of receptors activated by cold stimuli. Therefore, we studied the role of TRPA1 on cold pain hypersensitivity by examining changes in its expression (Obata et al. 2005).

In situ hybridization histochemistry revealed that TRPA1 mRNA was expressed in $32.4 \pm 1.8\%$ of DRG neurons in naive control rats. Tissue inflammation induced a significant increase in the percentage of TRPA1 mRNA-positive neurons in the ipsilateral DRG at days 1 and 3 ($44.1 \pm 2.9\%$ and $42.0 \pm 2.2\%$, respectively). Thereafter, the levels gradually declined, returning to normal by day 7. This upregulation corresponded well with the development and maintenance of the cold hypersensitivity induced by complete Freund's adjuvant (CFA). Cutaneous nociceptors can be divided into two broad groups: NGF-responsive, trkA-expressing neurons and GDNF-responsive, c-ret-expressing neurons. Double labeling showed that TRPA1 heavily colocalized with trkA after inflammation and that TRPA1-expressing neurons coexpressed substance P, CGRP, and TRPV1. Rats with peripheral inflammation were either treated intrathecally with an antisense oligodeoxynucleotide targeting TRPA1, or with a missense oligodeoxynucleotide, beginning 12 hours before CFA injection. We found that the CFA-induced increase in the number of paw lifts on a cold plate was significantly less in the TRPA1 antisense group than in the missense oligodeoxynucleotide group. These data suggest that the TRPA1 increase in DRG neurons in tissue inflammation is necessary for cold hypersensitivity (Obata et al. 2005).

AXOTOMY-INDUCED ALTERATION IN GENE EXPRESSION

Peripheral nerve injury changes the expression of neurotransmitters, neuromodulators, growth factors, their receptors and transcriptional factors, and neuroactive molecules in primary afferent neurons. A recent study using a cDNA microarray chip revealed changes in the expression of hundreds of genes in the DRG at the same time after peripheral nerve injury (Xiao et al. 2002). The genes that are upregulated after peripheral nerve injury include those expressing the neuropeptides cholecystokinin, galanin, neuropeptide Y, and vasoactive intestinal polypeptide, the G-protein coupled receptors cholecystokinin B and the adrenoceptor α_{2A}, the calcium channel subunit $\alpha_2\delta$, the growth-associated protein GAP43, basic fibroblast growth factor, and many others. However, few of these genes have been reported to be involved in the central sensitization at the central terminals in the dorsal horn. Some of the molecules upregulated in the DRG after peripheral nerve injury that have nociceptive roles in the dorsal horn are described next.

The voltage-gated calcium channel subunit $\alpha_2\delta$ is upregulated in injured DRG neurons, and this channel is well known to be involved in mediating the effects of gabapentin, a popular drug for neuropathic pain (Luo et al. 2001, 2002). Other subunits, α_{1B} and β_3, were reported not to change in expression in the DRG. Another ion channel that is upregulated after nerve injury is the TTX-sensitive sodium channel $Na_V1.3$, which is normally expressed in embryonic, but not in adult, DRG neurons (Waxman et al. 1994).

The majority of molecules expressed in DRG neurons show downregulation following axotomy. For example, substance P, CGRP, and TRPV1 decrease in small and medium-sized trkA-containing DRG neurons. However, axotomy induces a dynamic phenotypic change in gene expression in large DRG neurons such that substance P and CGRP mRNA and protein are newly expressed and transported to lamina III–IV dorsal horn neurons and to dorsal column nuclei in the medulla (Noguchi et al. 1995; Miki et al. 1998). The increased neuropeptides in lamina III–IV and in the dorsal column nuclei may have a role in the alteration in the excitability of neurons in this area. However, the possible role of excitatory neuropeptides in large DRG neurons in mediating pain remains to be explored.

ERK ACTIVATION AND GENE EXPRESSION

The involvement of the ERK pathway in the neurotrophin-dependent survival and differentiation of developing peripheral neurons has been characterized in detail (Klesse and Parada 1999; Miller and Kaplan 2001; Patapoutian and Reichardt 2001). For example, the high-affinity receptor for NGF, trkA, can signal through at least six different pathways, one of which is a MAPK pathway (i.e., the ERK pathway; Finkbeiner 2000; Chang and Karin 2001). In this pathway, activated receptors induce guanosine triphosphate (GTP) loading and activation of the small G-protein Ras. In turn, Ras-GTP recruits a three-tiered enzyme cascade in which a MAPK kinase (Raf) phosphorylates MEK, which phosphorylates and activates ERK (English et al. 1999). However, very little is known about how the ERK pathway is responsible for the maintenance of the nociceptive phenotype of adult sensory neurons and for the changes after peripheral inflammation and nerve injury. Furthermore, it is not clear what role these changes play in generating pain hypersensitivity (Woolf and Costigan 1999; Ji and Woolf 2001). Inflammation and nerve injury lead to altered gene transcription and protein synthesis in DRG neurons (Hokfelt et al. 1994; Noguchi et al. 1995; Fukuoka et al. 1998; Alvares and Fitzgerald 1999; Woolf and Salter 2000; Fukuoka and Noguchi 2002). For example, synthesis of brain-derived neurotrophic factor (BDNF) is known to increase in trkA-expressing small and medium-sized DRG neurons after inflammation (Apfel et al. 1996; Michael et al. 1997; Kerr et al. 1999; Mannion et al. 1999; Thompson et al. 1999; Obata et al. 2002), whereas after nerve injury, the increase in BDNF occurs in the axotomized medium- to large-diameter DRG neurons (Cho et al. 1988; Tonra et al. 1998; Li et al. 1999; Michael et al. 1999; Zhou et al. 1999b; Obata et al. 2003a).

Recently, we have shown that the activation of ERK regulates gene expression of BDNF in primary afferent neurons after peripheral inflammation and sciatic nerve transection (Obata et al. 2003a). Peripheral inflammation induced an increase in the phosphorylation of ERK, mainly in trkA-containing small- to medium-diameter DRG neurons 1 day after CFA injection. Treatment with the MEK inhibitor U0126 reversed both the CFA-induced pain hypersensitivity and the increase in p-ERK and BDNF in DRG neurons. In contrast, axotomy activated ERK, mainly in medium-sized and large DRG neurons and in satellite glial cells at 3, 7, and 14 days after the nerve lesion. U0126 suppressed the axotomy-induced autotomy behavior and reversed the increase in p-ERK and BDNF. To elucidate whether alterations of endogenous NGF can trigger changes in the phosphorylation of ERK and in BDNF expression similar to those seen after peripheral inflammation and axotomy, we administered intrathecal injections of rat recombinant beta-NGF or anti-NGF. In this test, NGF increased the number of p-ERK- and BDNF-labeled cells, mainly small neurons, whereas anti-NGF induced an increase in p-ERK and BDNF in some medium- to large-diameter DRG neurons. These findings suggest that the activation of ERK in the primary afferents occurs in different populations of DRG neurons after peripheral inflammation and axotomy, respectively, through alterations in the target-derived NGF and that it contributes to persistent inflammatory and neuropathic pain, via transcriptional regulation of BDNF expression (Obata et al. 2003a).

ACTIVATION OF OTHER MAP KINASES

Recent reports have demonstrated that not only peripheral inflammation but also axotomy induces p38 activation in small DRG neurons (Ji et al. 2002; Kim et al. 2002; Jin et al. 2003; Schafers et al. 2003a). A p38 inhibitor, SB203580, reduced inflammation-induced thermal hyperalgesia as well as mechanical allodynia induced by L5 spinal nerve ligation (SNL) (Ji et al. 2002b; Jin et al.

2003; Schafers et al. 2003a,b). Considering that ERK activation occurs in different populations of DRG neurons after peripheral inflammation and axotomy, ERK and p38 are likely to play distinct roles in pain states evoked by several different mediators and pathological conditions.

In addition to ERK and p38, other MAPK pathways, such as the Jun N-terminal kinase (JNK)/SAPK or ERK5 pathway, also may be activated by inflammation or nerve injury (Kenney and Kocsis 1998; Ma et al. 2001; Watson et al. 2001). Peripheral axotomy induces long-term activation of JNK and stress-activated protein kinase (SAPK) in DRG neurons. Long-lasting JNK/SAPK activation and c-Jun expression may participate in gene regulation (Kenney and Kocsis 1998; Fernyhough et al. 1999; Hou et al. 2003). Furthermore, phosphorylation of JNK/SAPK, as well as of ERK and p38, plays a role in primary sensory afferents, contributing to the development of tolerance to opioid-induced analgesia (Ma et al. 2001). Watson and colleagues (2001) reported that not only ERK, but also ERK5, mediate nuclear responses following direct cell body stimulation by NGF, whereas during retrograde signaling, endocytosed tyrosine kinases activate ERK5. These findings suggest that JNK/SAPK and ERK5, as well as ERK and p38, play important roles in the generation of pain hypersensitivity.

CHANGES IN PRIMARY AFFERENTS
IN NEUROPATHIC PAIN MODELS

Several animal models have been introduced to represent chronic pain following nerve injury. Chronic constriction injury (CCI) of the sciatic nerve (Bennett and Xie 1988), partial sciatic nerve ligation (Seltzer et al. 1990), L5 and L6 spinal nerve ligation (SNL) (Kim and Chung 1992), and spared nerve injury (Decosterd and Woolf 2000) have been widely used. All of these neuropathic pain models are made by partial nerve injury, where some primary afferents are axotomized and the others are spared. CCI of the rat sciatic nerve produces various symptoms similar to the clinical features of human causalgia and reflex sympathetic dystrophy. Behavioral signs in the CCI model include hyperalgesia to heat stimulation, as well as allodynia to cold and mechanical stimulation (Attal et al. 1990). Among neuropathic pain models, the L5 SNL model is unique because the L4 DRG neurons are clearly separated from the axotomized L5 DRG neurons. The underlying pathological mechanism of the abnormal behavioral features of neuropathic pain in animals has been identified at every level of the nociceptive pathways. Hyperalgesia and allodynia after nerve injury not only result from an increase in the sensitivity of primary afferent nociceptors at the site of injury, but also depend on central changes in synaptic excitability. There is ample evidence for sensitization of spinal dorsal horn cells and for facilitation of spinal reflexes initiated by repetitive or prolonged noxious afferent input after peripheral nerve injury.

ROLE OF UNINJURED PRIMARY AFFERENTS IN NEUROPATHIC PAIN

In previous studies, much attention has been focused on the directly damaged primary afferents and their influence on the activity of dorsal horn neurons. For example, nerve-injury-induced pain has been closely linked to activation of spontaneous and persistent abnormal discharge from ectopic foci, primarily observed in Aβ fibers (Devor and Wall 1990; Koltzenburg et al. 1994; Devor and Seltzer 1999). Moreover, A fibers have been suggested to drive central sensitization (Scholz and Woolf 2002). However, recent electrophysiological experiments using the partial nerve injury model have suggested that the uninjured C-fiber afferents are functionally important in the maintenance of neuropathic pain (Ali et al. 1999; Michaelis et al. 2000; Wu et al. 2001; Schafers et al. 2003a,b). Furthermore, changes have been reported in the molecular phenotype of undamaged small DRG neurons in these partial nerve injury models. For example, substance P, CGRP, BDNF, and TRPV1 increase in the intact small neurons (Ma and Bisby 1998; Fukuoka et al. 2001; Hudson et al. 2001; Obata et al. 2003a, 2004a). NGF levels are increased in adjacent uninjured primary afferents, leading to the upregulation of BDNF in injured neurons (Fukuoka et al. 2001). Local application of anti-NGF antibody to the L4 spinal nerve adjacent to the L5 SNL site prevented the development of thermal hyperalgesia for 5 days after ligation. We also found that L5 SNL activated p38 MAPK in trkA-expressing small to medium-sized DRG neurons in the uninjured L4 DRG (Fig. 2). Moreover, intrathecal injection of anti-NGF on the DRG cell bodies reduced the SNL-induced upregulation of BDNF and TRPV1 expression in the L4 DRG (Obata et al. 2004b). These findings suggest that NGF-mediated increased excitability of uninjured primary afferent neurons, including upregulation of gene expression of several molecules, may be an important aspect of peripheral sensitization because presumably the stimuli applied to the peripheral tissue must be transferred to the spinal cord through the uninjured primary afferents.

MAPK ACTIVATION IN NON-NEURONAL CELLS

The activation of spinal cord glial cells, including microglia and astrocytes, has been implicated in the pathogenesis of pain (Meller et al. 1994; Watkins et al. 1997, 2001a,b; DeLeo and Yezierski 2001; Tsuda et al. 2003). Proinflammatory cytokines released from glial cells produce pain hypersensitivity,

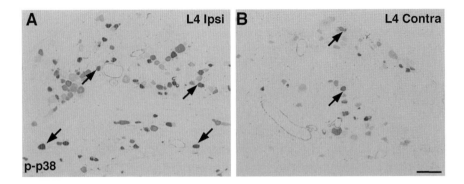

Fig. 2. Photomicrographs showing phosphorylated p38 MAPK immunoreactivity in the ipsilateral (A) and contralateral (B) L4 dorsal root ganglia (DRG) at 7 days after L5 spinal nerve ligation surgery. There was an increase in the number of p-p38-immunoreactive neurons (arrows), but not in the number of satellite glial cells, in the ipsilateral L4 DRG. Scale bar: 100 µm. (From Obata et al. 2004.)

and microglia and astrocytes are activated in the spinal cord after peripheral inflammation and nerve injury and in cancer models (Fu et al. 1999; Sweitzer et al. 1999; Winkelstein et al. 2001; Mantyh et al. 2002). Phosphorylated p38 is present constitutively in non-neuronal cells in the spinal cord, and peripheral inflammation induces only a modest increase in p-p38 levels (Ji et al. 2002). In contrast, peripheral axotomy activates p38 in spinal microglia (Nomura et al. 2001; Kim et al. 2002; Jin et al. 2003). p38 inhibitors diminish inflammation-induced hyperalgesia and pain hypersensitivity in the sciatic inflammatory neuropathy model by blocking spinal p38 activation (Watkins et al. 1997; Milligan et al. 2000, 2003; Svensson et al. 2003a,b). On the other hand, ERK and JNK/SAPK, but not p38, are phosphorylated in astrocytes in the spinal cord after partial nerve injury (Ma and Quirion 2002), whereas dorsal rhizotomy induces ERK activation in spinal microglia and oligodendrocytes (Cheng et al. 2003).

In the DRG, p-ERK expression was upregulated in satellite glial cells that surrounded, in particular, the larger-diameter neuronal somata after sciatic nerve transection (Obata et al. 2003b). In addition, peripheral axotomy induces p38 activation in satellite cells surrounding neurons in the DRG (Jin et al. 2003). These findings emphasize the importance of glial cells and glial-neuronal interactions in the DRG, as well as in the spinal cord, after peripheral axotomy (McLachlan and Hu 1998; Ramer et al. 1999; Zhou et al. 1999a; Hu and McLachlan 2002).

CONCLUSIONS

This chapter has described neuroplastic changes in primary afferent neurons and their possible role in mediating nociceptive, inflammatory, and neuropathic pain. I first described the rapid increase of phospho-ERK and p38 MAPK after noxious stimulation in primary afferent neurons and showed how the activation of MAPK in the cell body and nerve terminals may be involved in the rapid changes in the sensitivity of primary afferent after noxious stimulation. My collaborators and I believe that the rapid changes in the intracellular signal transduction cascade are important in the early phase of peripheral sensitization.

Tissue inflammation and peripheral nerve injury also induce a variety of neuroplastic changes. For instance, the increased expression of TRPA1 may be involved in cold hyperalgesia in inflamed tissue. We found that in the L5 SNL model of neuropathic pain, there are dynamic changes in gene expression and signal transduction molecules in neighboring intact primary afferent neurons, as well as in the axotomized neurons. Increased expression of a neuromodulator, BDNF, and of the thermosensitive channel TRPV1, in DRG neurons may be involved in the modulation of spinal cord neurons and in the peripheral sensitization to the specific stimuli in the neuropathic model. We believe that a number of neuroplastic changes occur in the DRG after peripheral nerve injury and that these changes are important pathological alterations that result in neuropathic pain.

All of the conditions described here produce a variety of neuroplastic changes in DRG cell bodies and nerve terminals. All these changes are involved in altering pain behavior in specific ways. Understanding these changes is important in our efforts to understand and study the mechanisms of a variety of pain conditions. The clarification of these mechanisms may contribute to the development of new approaches for the treatment of chronic pain.

REFERENCES

Aley KO, Martin A, McMahon T, et al. Nociceptor sensitization by extracellular signal-regulated kinases. *J Neurosci* 2001; 21:6933–6939.

Ali Z, Ringkamp M, Hartke TV, et al. Uninjured C-fiber nociceptors develop spontaneous activity and alpha-adrenergic sensitivity following L6 spinal nerve ligation in monkey. *J Neurophysiol* 1999; 81:455–466.

Alvares D, Fitzgerald M. Building blocks of pain: the regulation of key molecules in spinal sensory neurones during development and following peripheral axotomy. *Pain* 1999; Suppl 6: S71–85.

Apfel SC, Wright DE, Wiideman AM, et al. Nerve growth factor regulates the expression of brain-derived neurotrophic factor mRNA in the peripheral nervous system. *Mol Cell Neurosci* 1996; 7:134–142.

Attal N, Jazat F, Kayser V, Guilbaud G. Further evidence for 'pain-related' behaviours in a model of unilateral peripheral mononeuropathy. *Pain* 1990; 41:235–251.

Averill S, Delcroix JD, Michael GJ, et al. Nerve growth factor modulates the activation status and fast axonal transport of ERK 1/2 in adult nociceptive neurones. *Mol Cell Neurosci* 2001; 18:183–196.

Bennett GJ, Xie YK. A peripheral mononeuropathy in rat that produces disorders of pain sensation like those seen in man. *Pain* 1988; 33:87–107.

Bolshakov VY, Carboni L, Cobb MH, Siegelbaum SA, Belardetti F. Dual MAP kinase pathways mediate opposing forms of long-term plasticity at CA3-CA1 synapses. *Nat Neurosci* 2000; 3:1107–1112.

Bron R, Klesse LJ, Shah K, Parada LF, Winter J. Activation of Ras is necessary and sufficient for upregulation of vanilloid receptor type 1 in sensory neurons by neurotrophic factors. *Mol Cell Neurosci* 2003; 22:118–132.

Chang L, Karin M. Mammalian MAP kinase signalling cascades. *Nature* 2001; 410:37–40.

Cheng XP, Wang BR, Liu HL, et al. Phosphorylation of extracellular signal-regulated kinases 1/2 is predominantly enhanced in the microglia of the rat spinal cord following dorsal root transection. *Neuroscience* 2003; 119:701–712.

Cho HJ, Basbaum AI. Increased staining of immunoreactive dynorphin cell bodies in the deafferented spinal cord of the rat. *Neurosci Lett* 1988; 84:125–130.

Dai Y, Iwata K, Fukuoka T, et al. Phosphorylation of extracellular signal-regulated kinase in primary afferent neurons by noxious stimuli and its involvement in peripheral sensitization. *J Neurosci* 2002; 22:7737–7745.

Decosterd I, Woolf CJ. Spared nerve injury: an animal model of persistent peripheral neuropathic pain. *Pain* 2000; 87:149–158.

Delcroix JD, Valletta JS, Wu C, et al. NGF signaling in sensory neurons: evidence that early endosomes carry NGF retrograde signals. *Neuron* 2003; 39:69–84.

DeLeo JA, Yezierski RP. The role of neuroinflammation and neuroimmune activation in persistent pain. *Pain* 2001; 90:1–6.

Devor M, Seltzer Z. Pathophysiology of damaged nerves in reaction to chronic pain. In: Wall PD, Melzack R (Eds). *Textbook of Pain.* London: Churchill Livingstone, 1999, pp 129–164.

Devor M, Wall PD. Cross-excitation in dorsal root ganglia of nerve-injured and intact rats. *J Neurophysiol* 1990; 64:1733–1746.

Dina OA, McCarter C, de Coupade C, Levine JD. Role of the sensory neuron cytoskeleton in second messenger signaling for inflammatory pain. *Neuron* 2003; 39:613–624.

English J, Pearson G, Wilsbacher J, et al. New insights into the control of MAP kinase pathways. *Exp Cell Res* 1999; 253:255–270.

Fernyhough P, Gallagher A, Averill SA. Aberrant neurofilament phosphorylation in sensory neurons of rats with diabetic neuropathy. *Diabetes* 1999; 48:881–889.

Fields RD, Eshete F, Stevens B, Itoh K. Action potential-dependent regulation of gene expression: temporal specificity in Ca^{2+}, cAMP-responsive element binding proteins, and mitogen-activated protein kinase signaling. *J Neurosci* 1997; 17:7252–7266.

Finkbeiner S. CREB couples neurotrophin signals to survival messages. *Neuron* 2000; 25:11–14.

Fitzgerald EM. Regulation of voltage-dependent calcium channels in rat sensory neurones involves a Ras-mitogen-activated protein kinase pathway. *J Physiol* 2000; 527(Pt 3):433–444.

Fu KY, Light AR, Matsushima GK, Maixner W. Microglial reactions after subcutaneous formalin injection into the rat hind paw. *Brain Res* 1999; 825:59–67.

Fukuoka T, Noguchi K. Contribution of the spared primary afferent neurons to the pathomechanisms of neuropathic pain. *Mol Neurobiol* 2002; 26:57–67.

Fukuoka T, Tokunaga A, Kondo E, et al. Change in mRNAs for neuropeptides and the GABA(A) receptor in dorsal root ganglion neurons in a rat experimental neuropathic pain model. *Pain* 1998; 78:13–26.

Fukuoka T, Kondo E, Dai Y, Hashimoto N, Noguchi K. Brain-derived neurotrophic factor increases in the uninjured dorsal root ganglion neurons in selective spinal nerve ligation model. *J Neurosci* 2001; 21:4891–900.

Gold MS, Levine JD, Correa AM. Modulation of TTX-R INa by PKC and PKA and their role in PGE2-induced sensitization of rat sensory neurons in vitro. *J Neurosci* 1998; 18:10345–10355.

Hokfelt T, Zhang X, Wiesenfeld-Hallin Z. Messenger plasticity in primary sensory neurons following axotomy and its functional implications. *Trends Neurosci* 1994; 17:22–30.

Hou L, Li W, Wang X. Mechanism of interleukin-1 beta-induced calcitonin gene-related peptide production from dorsal root ganglion neurons of neonatal rats. *J Neurosci Res* 2003; 73:188–197.

Hu P, McLachlan EM. Macrophage and lymphocyte invasion of dorsal root ganglia after peripheral nerve lesions in the rat. *Neuroscience* 2002; 112:23–38.

Hudson LJ, Bevan S, Wotherspoon G, et al. VR1 protein expression increases in undamaged DRG neurons after partial nerve injury. *Eur J Neurosci* 2001; 13:2105–2114.

Ji RR, Woolf CJ. Neuronal plasticity and signal transduction in nociceptive neurons: implications for the initiation and maintenance of pathological pain. *Neurobiol Dis* 2001; 8:1–10.

Ji RR, Samad TA, Jin SX, Schmoll R, Woolf CJ. p38 MAPK activation by NGF in primary sensory neurons after inflammation increases TRPV1 levels and maintains heat hyperalgesia. *Neuron* 2002; 36:57–68.

Jin SX, Zhuang ZY, Woolf CJ, Ji RR. p38 mitogen-activated protein kinase is activated after a spinal nerve ligation in spinal cord microglia and dorsal root ganglion neurons and contributes to the generation of neuropathic pain. *J Neurosci* 2003; 23:4017–4022.

Kenney AM, Kocsis JD. Peripheral axotomy induces long-term c-Jun amino-terminal kinase-1 activation and activator protein-1 binding activity by c-Jun and junD in adult rat dorsal root ganglia in vivo. *J Neurosci* 1998; 18:1318–1328.

Kerr BJ, Bradbury EJ, Bennett DL, et al. Brain-derived neurotrophic factor modulates nociceptive sensory inputs and NMDA-evoked responses in the rat spinal cord. *J Neurosci* 1999; 19:5138–5148.

Khasar SG, Lin YH, Martin A, et al. A novel nociceptor signaling pathway revealed in protein kinase C epsilon mutant mice. *Neuron* 1999; 24:253–260.

Kim SH, Chung JM. An experimental model for peripheral neuropathy produced by segmental spinal nerve ligation in the rat. *Pain* 1992; 50:355–363.

Kim SY, Bae JC, Kim JY, et al. Activation of p38 MAP kinase in the rat dorsal root ganglia and spinal cord following peripheral inflammation and nerve injury. *Neuroreport* 2002; 13:2483–2486.

Klesse LJ, Parada LF. Trks: signal transduction and intracellular pathways. *Microsc Res Tech* 1999; 45:210–216.

Kobayashi K, Fukuoka T, Obata K, et al. Distinct expression of TRPM8, TRPA1 and TRPV1 mRNAs in rat primary afferent neurons with A-delta/C-fibers and colocalization with Trk receptors. *J Comp Neurol* 2005; 493:596–606.

Koltzenburg M, Torebjork HE, Wahren LK. Nociceptor modulated central sensitization causes mechanical hyperalgesia in acute chemogenic and chronic neuropathic pain. *Brain* 1994; 117:579–591.

Li WP, Xian C, Rush RA, Zhou XF. Upregulation of brain-derived neurotrophic factor and neuropeptide Y in the dorsal ascending sensory pathway following sciatic nerve injury in rat. *Neurosci Lett* 1999; 260:49–52.

Luo ZD, Chaplan SR, Higuera ES, et al. Upregulation of dorsal root ganglion $\alpha_2\delta$ calcium channel subunit and its correlation with allodynia in spinal nerve-injured rats. *J Neurosci* 2001; 21:1868–1875.

Luo ZD, Calcutt NA, Higuera ES, et al. Injury type-specific calcium channel alpha 2 delta-1 subunit up-regulation in rat neuropathic pain models correlates with antiallodynic effects of gabapentin. *J Pharmacol Exp Ther* 2002; 303:1199–1205.

Ma W, Bisby MA. Increase of preprotachykinin mRNA and substance P immunoreactivity in spared dorsal root ganglion neurons following partial sciatic nerve injury. *Eur J Neurosci* 1998; 10:2388–2399.

Ma W, Quirion R. Partial sciatic nerve ligation induces increase in the phosphorylation of extracellular signal-regulated kinase (ERK) and c-Jun N-terminal kinase (JNK) in astrocytes in the lumbar spinal dorsal horn and the gracile nucleus. *Pain* 2002; 99:175–184.

Ma W, Zheng WH, Powell K, Jhamandas K, Quirion R. Chronic morphine exposure increases the phosphorylation of MAP kinases and the transcription factor CREB in dorsal root ganglion neurons: an in vitro and in vivo study. *Eur J Neurosci* 2001; 14:1091–1104.

Mannion RJ, Costigan M, Decosterd I. Neurotrophins: peripherally and centrally acting modulators of tactile stimulus-induced inflammatory pain hypersensitivity. *Proc Natl Acad Sci USA* 1999; 96:9385–9390.

Mantyh PW, Clohisy DR, Koltzenburg M, Hunt SP. Molecular mechanisms of cancer pain. *Nat Rev Cancer* 2002; 2:201–209.

Mao Z, Bonni A, Xia F, Nadal-Vicens M, Greenberg ME. Neuronal activity-dependent cell survival mediated by transcription factor MEF2. *Science* 1999; 286:785–790.

McLachlan EM, Hu P. Axonal sprouts containing calcitonin gene-related peptide and substance P form pericellular baskets around large diameter neurons after sciatic nerve transection in the rat. *Neuroscience* 1998; 84:961–965.

Meller ST, Dykstra C, Grzybycki D, Murphy S, Gebhart GF. The possible role of glia in nociceptive processing and hyperalgesia in the spinal cord of the rat. *Neuropharmacology* 1994; 33:1471–1478.

Michael GJ, Averill S, Nitkunan A, et al. Nerve growth factor treatment increases brain-derived neurotrophic factor selectively in TrkA-expressing dorsal root ganglion cells and in their central terminations within the spinal cord. *J Neurosci* 1997; 17:8476–8490.

Michael GJ, Averill S, Shortland PJ, Yan Q, Priestley JV. Axotomy results in major changes in BDNF expression by dorsal root ganglion cells: BDNF expression in large trkB and trkC cells, in pericellular baskets, and in projections to deep dorsal horn and dorsal column nuclei. *Eur J Neurosci* 1999; 11:3539–3551.

Michaelis M, Liu X, Janig W. Axotomized and intact muscle afferents but no skin afferents develop ongoing discharges of dorsal root ganglion origin after peripheral nerve lesion. *J Neurosci* 2000; 20:2742–2748.

Miki K, Fukuoka T, Tokunaga A, Noguchi K. Calcitonin gene-related peptide increase in the rat spinal dorsal horn and dorsal column nucleus following peripheral nerve injury: up-regulation in a subpopulation of primary afferent sensory neurons. *Neuroscience* 1998; 82:1243–1252.

Miller FD, Kaplan DR. On Trk for retrograde signaling. *Neuron* 2001; 32:767–770.

Milligan ED, Mehmert KK, Hinde JL. Thermal hyperalgesia and mechanical allodynia produced by intrathecal administration of the human immunodeficiency virus-1 (HIV-1) envelope glycoprotein, gp120. *Brain Res* 2000; 861:105–116.

Milligan ED, Twining C, Chacur M, et al. Spinal glia and proinflammatory cytokines mediate mirror-image neuropathic pain in rats. *J Neurosci* 2003; 23:1026–1046.

Mizushima T, Obata K, Yamanaka H, et al. Activation of p38 MAPK in primary afferent neurons by noxious stimulation and its involvement in the development of thermal hyperalgesia. *Pain* 2005; 113:51–60.

Noguchi K, Kawai Y, Fukuoka T, Senba E, Miki K. Substance P induced by peripheral nerve injury in primary afferent sensory neurons and its effect on dorsal column nucleus neurons. *J Neurosci* 1995; 15:7633–7643.

Nomura H, Furuta A, Suzuki SO, Iwaki T. Dorsal horn lesion resulting from spinal root avulsion leads to the accumulation of stress-responsive proteins. *Brain Res* 2001; 893:84–94.

Obata K, Tsujino H, Yamanaka H, et al. Expression of neurotrophic factors in the dorsal root ganglion in a rat model of lumbar disc herniation. *Pain* 2002; 99:121–132.

Obata K, Yamanaka H, Dai Y, et al. Differential activation of extracellular signal-regulated protein kinase in primary afferent neurons regulates brain-derived neurotrophic factor expression after peripheral inflammation and nerve injury. *J Neurosci* 2003a; 23:4117–4126.

Obata K, Yamanaka H, Fukuoka T, et al. Contribution of injured and uninjured dorsal root ganglion neurons to pain behavior and the changes in gene expression following chronic constriction injury of the sciatic nerve in rats. *Pain* 2003b; 101:65–77.

Obata K, Yamanaka H, Dai Y, et al. Differential activation of MAPK in injured and uninjured DRG neurons following chronic constriction injury of the sciatic nerve in rats. *Eur J Neurosci* 2004a; 20:2881–2895.

Obata K, Yamanaka H, Kobayashi K. Role of mitogen-activated protein kinase activation in injured and intact primary afferent neurons for mechanical and heat hypersensitivity after spinal nerve ligation. *J Neurosci* 2004b; 24:10211–10222.

Obata K, Katsura H, Mizushima T, et al. TRPA1 induced in sensory neurons contributes to cold hyperalgesia after inflammation and nerve injury. *J Clin Invest* 2005; 115:2393–2401.

Patapoutian A, Reichardt LF. Trk receptors: mediators of neurotrophin action. *Curr Opin Neurobiol* 2001; 11:272–280.

Ramer MS, Thompson SW, McMahon SB. Causes and consequences of sympathetic basket formation in dorsal root ganglia. *Pain* 1999; Suppl 6:S111–120.

Schafers M, Svensson CI, Sommer C, Sorkin LS. Tumor necrosis factor-alpha induces mechanical allodynia after spinal nerve ligation by activation of p38 MAPK in primary sensory neurons. *J Neurosci* 2003a; 23:2517–2521.

Schafers M, Lee DH, Brors D, Yaksh TL, Sorkin LS. Increased sensitivity of injured and adjacent uninjured rat primary sensory neurons to exogenous tumor necrosis factor-alpha after spinal nerve ligation. *J Neurosci* 2003b; 23:3028–3038.

Scholz J, Woolf CJ. Can we conquer pain? *Nat Neurosci* 2002; 5(Suppl):1062–1067.

Seltzer Z, Dubner R, Shir Y. A novel behavioral model of neuropathic pain disorders produced in rats by partial sciatic nerve injury. *Pain* 1990; 43:205–218.

Shi Y, Gaestel M. In the cellular garden of forking paths: how p38 MAPKs signal for downstream assistance. *Biol Chem* 2002; 383:1519–1536.

Svensson CI, Hua XY, Protter AA, Powell HC, Yaksh TL. Spinal p38 MAP kinase is necessary for NMDA-induced spinal PGE(2) release and thermal hyperalgesia. *Neuroreport* 2003a; 14:1153–1157.

Svensson CI, Marsala M, Westerlund A, et al. Activation of p38 mitogen-activated protein kinase in spinal microglia is a critical link in inflammation-induced spinal pain processing. *J Neurochem* 2003b; 86:1534–1544.

Sweitzer SM, Colburn RW, Rutkowski M, DeLeo JA. Acute peripheral inflammation induces moderate glial activation and spinal IL-1-beta expression that correlates with pain behavior in the rat. *Brain Res* 1999; 829:209–221.

Thompson SW, Bennett DL, Kerr BJ, Bradbury EJ, McMahon SB. Brain-derived neurotrophic factor is an endogenous modulator of nociceptive responses in the spinal cord. *Proc Natl Acad Sci USA* 1999; 96:7714–7718.

Tonra JR, Curtis R, Wong V, et al. Axotomy upregulates the anterograde transport and expression of brain-derived neurotrophic factor by sensory neurons. *J Neurosci* 1998; 18:4374–4383.

Torocsik B, Szeberenyi J. Anisomycin uses multiple mechanisms to stimulate mitogen-activated protein kinases and gene expression and to inhibit neuronal differentiation in PC12 phaeochromocytoma cells. *Eur J Neurosci* 2000; 12(2):527–532.

Tsuda M, Shigemoto-Mogami Y, Koizumi S, et al. P2X4 receptors induced in spinal microglia gate tactile allodynia after nerve injury. *Nature* 2003; 424:778–783.

Watkins LR, Martin D, Ulrich P, Tracey KJ, Maier SF. Evidence for the involvement of spinal cord glia in subcutaneous formalin induced hyperalgesia in the rat. *Pain* 1997; 71:225–235.

Watkins LR, Milligan ED, Maier SF. Glial activation: a driving force for pathological pain. *Trends Neurosci* 2001a; 24:450–455.

Watkins LR, Milligan ED, Maier SF. Spinal cord glia: new players in pain. *Pain* 2001b; 93:201–205.

Watson FL, Heerssen HM, Bhattacharyya A, et al. Neurotrophins use the Erk5 pathway to mediate a retrograde survival response. *Nat Neurosci* 2001; 4:981–988.

Waxman SG, Kocsis JD, Black JA. Type III sodium channel mRNA is expressed in embryonic but not adult spinal sensory neurons, and is reexpressed following axotomy. *J Neurophysiol* 1994; 72:466–470.

Widmann C, Gibson S, Jarpe MB, Johnson GL. Mitogen-activated protein kinase: conservation of a three-kinase module from yeast to human. *Physiol Rev* 1999; 79:143–180.

Winkelstein BA, Rutkowski MD, Sweitzer SM, Pahl JL, DeLeo JA. Nerve injury proximal or distal to the DRG induces similar spinal glial activation and selective cytokine expression but differential behavioral responses to pharmacologic treatment. *J Comp Neurol* 2001; 439:127–139.

Woolf CJ, Costigan M. Transcriptional and posttranslational plasticity and the generation of inflammatory pain. *Proc Natl Acad Sci USA* 1999; 96:7723–7730.

Woolf CJ, Salter MW. Neuronal plasticity: increasing the gain in pain. *Science* 2000; 288:1765–1769.

Wu G, Ringkamp M, Hartke TV, et al. Early onset of spontaneous activity in uninjured C-fiber nociceptors after injury to neighboring nerve fibers. *J Neurosci* 2001; 21:RC140.

Xiao HS, Huang QH, Zhang FX, et al. Identification of gene expression profile of dorsal root ganglion in the rat peripheral axotomy model of neuropathic pain. *Proc Natl Acad Sci USA* 2002; 99:8360–8365.

Zhou XF, Deng YS, Chie E, et al. Satellite-cell-derived nerve growth factor and neurotrophin-3 are involved in noradrenergic sprouting in the dorsal root ganglia following peripheral nerve injury in the rat. *Eur J Neurosci* 1999a; 11:1711–1722.

Zhou XF, Chie ET, Deng YS, et al. Injured primary sensory neurons switch phenotype for brain-derived neurotrophic factor in the rat. *Neuroscience* 1999b; 92:841–853.

Correspondence to: Koichi Noguchi, MD, PhD, Department of Anatomy and Neuroscience, Hyogo College of Medicine, 1-1 Mukogawa-cho, Nishinomiya 663-8501, Japan. Email: noguchi@hyo-med.ac.jp.

Proceedings of the 11th World Congress on Pain,
edited by Herta Flor, Eija Kalso, and Jonathan O.
Dostrovsky, IASP Press, Seattle, © 2006.

11

Control of Activity: Relationship between Excitatory and Inhibitory Receptors Expressed by Nociceptors

Istvan Nagy,[a] Peter Reeh,[b] Giulio Srubek Tomassy,[b,c] and Peter Santha[a,d]

[a]Department of Anaesthetics, Pain Medicine and Intensive Care, Faculty of Medicine, Imperial College London, Chelsea and Westminster Hospital, London, United Kingdom; [b]Department of Physiology and Pathophysiology, University of Erlangen-Nuremberg, Erlangen, Germany; [c]Department of Cell Biology, University of Rome "La Sapienza," Rome, Italy; [d]Department of Physiology, University of Szeged, Szeged, Hungary

Primary sensory neurons (PSNs) express various membrane molecules, including transducers, ion channels, and receptors. These receptors respond to different signaling molecules that are produced and released by various non-neuronal and neuronal cells in pathological conditions both at the periphery and in the spinal cord (Bhave and Gereau 2004; Nagy 2004; Vanegas and Schaible 2004). Activation of some of the receptors, such as the bradykinin B2 receptor (Liang et al. 2001) or the vanilloid type 1 transient receptor potential ion channel (TRPV1; Nagy and Rang 1999), increases the discharge activity of the cells and may evoke post-translational and transcriptional changes that sensitize the neurons, causing a prolonged increase in their activity and excitability (Bhave and Gereau 2004). Activation of other receptors, such as that of the cannabinoid 1 (CB1) receptor (Ahluwalia et al. 2003a) or the muscarinic M2 receptor (Dussor et al. 2004), however, reduces the activity and sensitivity of the cells. Since sensitized nociceptors initiate and maintain changes in second-order neurons that result in prolonged or chronic pain sensations (Ji et al. 2003), controlling the activity of the excitatory and inhibitory receptors on nociceptors has been proposed as a means to relieve pathological pain. Here we discuss some of complex relationships between the excitatory and inhibitory receptors of nociceptors, which should be considered when designing therapeutic approaches for pain relief.

ANANDAMIDE-RESPONSIVE RECEPTORS ON NOCICEPTIVE
PRIMARY SENSORY NEURONS

Anandamide, found in various tissues (Di Marzo et al. 1994), activates at least two receptors expressed by PSNs: the inhibitory CB1 receptor (Devane et al. 1992) and the excitatory TRPV1 receptor, which is sensitive to capsaicin, noxious heat, and protons (Zygmunt et al. 1999). While the CB1 receptor binds anandamide at an extracellular site (Song and Bonner 1996), TRPV1 binds it at an intracellular binding domain (Jordt and Julius 2002). Activation of the CB1 receptor lessens the activity and excitability of nociceptors by reducing cyclic adenosine monophosphate (cAMP) levels and voltage-gated Ca^{2+} currents and by increasing K^+ currents (Mackie and Hille 1992; Daedwyler et al. 1993; Ahluwalia et al. 2003a). Activation of TRPV1 activates nociceptors by producing depolarizing currents (Caterina et al. 1997; Nagy and Rang 1999). TRPV1 activity evokes a burning pain sensation (Carpenter and Lynn 1981). This channel is essential for the development of inflammatory heat hyperalgesia (Caterina et al. 2000; Davis et al. 2000) and inflammatory bladder hyperreflexia (Silva et al. 2004).

Virtually all TRPV1-expressing PSNs, which comprise the great majority of the nociceptive cells, also express the CB1 receptor (Ahluwalia et al. 2000). In naive cultured PSNs, anandamide activates both the CB1 receptor and TRPV1 (Ahluwalia et al. 2003a). Although both receptors respond to anandamide at low nanomolar concentrations, below ~300 nM anandamide the CB1 receptor-mediated inhibitory effects, while above 1 μM anandamide the TRPV1 receptor-mediated excitatory effects are evident as the net effect.

Given that CB1-receptor activation reduces cAMP activity, the recent finding that blocking the activity of the cAMP-dependent protein kinase A reduces TRPV1-mediated currents (Sathianathan et al. 2003; Sing et al. 2005) suggests that CB1-receptor activation might inhibit TRPV1 activity. Here we report that anandamide indeed reduces capsaicin-evoked whole-cell currents in a proportion of naive capsaicin-sensitive cultured PSNs in a CB1-receptor-mediated fashion (Fig. 1A,B). However, in parallel with this inhibitory effect, anandamide seems to reduce the capsaicin-evoked desensitization. Nevertheless, these data indicate that activation of the CB1 receptor by anandamide could diminish the activity and excitability of TRPV1 and of TRPV1-expressing nociceptors, thus reducing inflammatory heat hyperalgesia and bladder hyperactivity.

Recent evidence shows that the relationship between the CB1 and TRPV1 receptors and their endogenous ligand, anandamide, could be more complex than the data described above may suggest. Ahluwalia et al. (2003a) showed that the excitatory potency and efficacy of anandamide is significantly increased in inflammatory conditions. Furthermore, Ahluwalia et al. (2003b) also showed

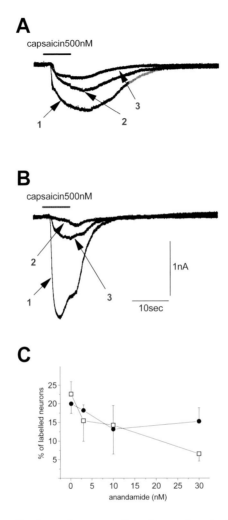

Fig. 1. (A,B) Whole-cell voltage-clamp recordings from cultured primary sensory neurons (PSNs) taken from adult rats. Recordings were taken at –60 mV holding potential with physiological intracellular and bath solutions. Capsaicin (500 nM) was applied every 2 minutes. (A) Currents evoked by three consecutive capsaicin applications. All applications were made in control bath solution. Note the distinctive desensitization of the responses. (B) Currents evoked by three consecutive capsaicin applications. The first and third applications were performed in control bath solution, while the second application was performed in the presence of anandamide (10 nM), beginning after the return of the current to baseline after the first capsaicin application. Anandamide reduced the capsaicin-evoked response and also reduced desensitization. (C) Cultured PSNs taken from adult rats were incubated in the presence of capsaicin (500 nM) and $CoCl_2$ for 5 minutes at 37°C either in the absence or presence of anandamide (10–30 nM), bradykinin (10 μM), and prostaglandin E_2 (10 μM). Anandamide concentration-dependently reduced the capsaicin-evoked cobalt uptake in naive cultured PSNs (open squares). In the presence of bradykinin and prostaglandin E_2, anandamide failed to reduce capsaicin-evoked cobalt uptake (closed circles).

that following Ca^{2+}-influx, TRPV1-expressing cultured PSNs produce anandamide in an amount that is sufficient to activate TRPV1 receptors. Since activation of various excitatory receptors in nociceptors, such as the bradykinin or prostaglandin receptors, induces Ca^{2+} influx (Linhart et al. 2003), these findings indicate that anandamide might contribute to TRPV1 activation, and thus to the development of inflammatory heat hyperalgesia and bladder hyperactivity.

In order to test this hypothesis, Dinis et al. (2004) measured bladder activity in naive rats and in rats injected by cyclophosphamide, which induces severe cystitis accompanied by increased bladder contractions both in humans and laboratory animals. Their data show that cyclophosphamide injection increased the anandamide content of the bladders, and that the time course of the increase correlated with the development of bladder hyperreflexia. Anandamide applied onto the serosal surface of naive bladders increased the frequency of bladder contractions in a concentration- and TRPV1-dependent manner, and in contrast to resiniferatoxin, anandamide did not desensitize TRPV1. The potency of anandamide in naive conditions could be significantly increased by blocking the CB1 receptor. Moreover, the excitatory effect of exogenously applied anandamide could be replicated by applying a blocker of the fatty acid amide hydrolyse, which is responsible for anandamide hydrolysis. The same treatment of inflamed bladders either had no effect or increased the bladder contractions further. Data from this study also suggest that the inhibitory efficacy of CB1-receptor activation could be reduced in inflammation; since in contrast to the sensitizing effect of the CB1-receptor antagonist in the bladder of naive rats, the compound had no effect in the inflamed bladder. Here we also report that in the presence of the inflammatory mediators bradykinin and prostaglandin E_2, anandamide could no longer decrease the capsaicin-evoked activity of TRPV1 in PSNs (Fig. 1C).

These latter data are in conflict with those showing that local application of anandamide reduces inflammatory heat hyperalgesia (Richardson et al. 1998). However, it is well documented that at the periphery, anandamide may evoke antinociception through mechanisms independent of the CB1 receptors expressed by PSNs (Farquhar-Smith and Rice 2003). The relationships between TRPV1 and the CB1 receptor and between these receptors and anandamide are further complicated by the findings that CB1-receptor activation can enhance the activity of TRPV1 in CB1-receptor- and TRPV1-receptor-overexpressing human embryonic kidney cells (Hermann et al. 2003). Furthermore, the anandamide membrane transporter (Di Marzo et al. 1994), which can be involved in either the release of anandamide produced in PSNs or the uptake of anandamide produced by non-neuronal cells, is expressed by PSNs (Price et al. 2005). We lack data on whether or not CB1-receptor activation has TRPV1-sensitizing effects, and on how the activity of anandamide membrane transporter is changed in PSNs during pathological events. Nevertheless, the available data indicate that anandamide might amplify rather than reduce the nociceptive signal in PSNs in pathological conditions.

NICOTINIC NOCICEPTION, MUSCARINIC ANTINOCICEPTION

Administration of acetylcholine (ACh), or its synthetic analogue carbachol, to primary nociceptive nerve endings in isolated rat or mouse skin preparations results in a biphasic response. An initial excitatory and weakly sensitizing effect is followed by a profound, long-lasting desensitization to noxious heat and mechanical stimulation (Bernardini et al. 2001b). These events match the acute burning pain sensation followed by a "certain numbness" produced by intradermally administered ACh in humans (Keele and Armstrong 1964). Pharmacological dissection of the two phases showed that the transient excitatory effects and the sustained desensitizing effects are mediated by nicotinic (Flores et al. 1996) and muscarinic type 2 (M2) acetylcholine receptors, respectively (Bernardini et al. 2002). Consistent with these results, the M2-preferring agonist arecaidine proved to be more potent than the nonselective muscarine in evoking the antinociceptive effect (Bernardini et al. 2001a). However, since M2-receptor activation reduces the heart rate and the conduction velocity of electrical impulses in the heart, the potent M2-receptor-mediated antinociception could be considered for use as an analgesic only if the M2 receptor in cardiomyocytes were different from that expressed by neurons. Although sequencing and comparing rat M2-receptor mRNAs from cardiac and nervous tissues indicated four distinct nucleotide differences that would translate into amino acid sequence differences at the protein level, no such differences were found in humans (H. Hofmann and A. Siegling, unpublished data). However, locally restricted elevation of the ACh level appears to be a viable way to utilize M2-mediated antinociception. For example, intra-articular administration of the cholinesterase inhibitor neostigmine has been successfully used to reduce postoperative pain in patients with knee arthroscopy (Yang et al. 1998). This approach requires an ACh source in the vicinity of sensory terminals.

In recent years, many non-neuronal cell types have been shown to synthesize and release ACh, including glial and immune cells, as well as epithelial cells in the human airways and alimentary tract (Wessler et al. 1997, 1998, 1999). In the skin, epidermal keratinocytes and dermal fibroblasts have been shown to produce, store, and secrete ACh (Grando et al. 1993; Buchli et al. 1999), which seems to function as a short-distance paracrine mediator controlling the proliferation, migration, adhesion, differentiation and apoptosis of the cells (Grando 1997). Since intraepidermal bare nerve endings establish intimate contacts with keratinocytes, it is possible that the sensitivity of these nociceptors could be modulated by ACh released from the epidermis.

We studied ACh release from keratinocytes using whole-skin explants treated with dispase in order to gain flaps of intact epidermis with keratinocytes in tissue-typical conjunction (Tschachler et al. 2004). ACh release was measured using a luminometric assay (Bernardini et al. 2004). Warm or noxious temperatures, the ultrapotent TRPV1 agonist resiniferatoxin (RTX), and buffer solutions of pH 5.7 or 6.1 were employed as potential stimuli. We found that noxious temperatures (44°–50°C, Fig. 2) evoked significant and graded release of ACh by an amount up to three times higher than that of stable constitutive baseline secretion. This ACh release was largely dependent on extracellular calcium, since the baseline was lowered to 40% and the heat response abolished at 50°C in a calcium-free solution with 10 µM EGTA added. RTX (at concentrations of 10^{-8}–10^{-6} M) also evoked a concentration-dependent increase of the epidermal ACh release (Fig. 3). As RTX is a phorbol ester, we also studied the effect of phorbol 12-myristate 13-acetate (PMA, 10^{-6} M), but found no effect on ACh release. This finding indicates that the RTX effect was due not to protein

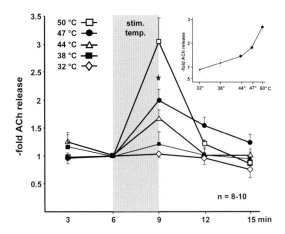

Fig. 2. Stimulated acetylcholine (ACh) release from explants of neonatal rat epidermis in response to warm and hot temperature stimulation. Only noxious temperatures (44°–50°C) caused significant increases over baseline (large dots in inset graph; Wilcoxon test) that were temperature-dependent (asterisk; *U*-test) and calcium-dependent (see text). The skin was isolated from the trunk of neonate Wistar rats and left floating for 3 hours at 37°C on top of a physiological solution containing the proteolytic enzyme dispase. The epidermis could then be mechanically separated in total from the corium, keeping the basement membrane intact (Tschachler et al. 2004). The epidermal flaps were washed for 30 minutes at 32°C and then passed through a series of five incubations lasting 3 minutes each. During the third incubation, the preparations were stimulated by warm or noxiously hot temperatures. The basal and stimulated ACh content of the incubation fluid was determined using a luminometric assay, as recently described in detail (Bernardini et al. 2004).

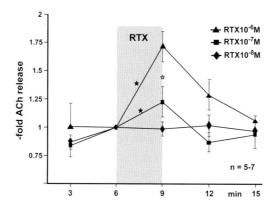

Fig. 3. Stimulated acetylcholine (ACh) release from explants of neonatal rat epidermis in response to the capsaicin receptor (TRPV1) agonist resiniferatoxin (RTX 10^{-8}–10^{-6}M), which caused significant increases over baseline (full asterisks; Wilcoxon test) that were concentration-dependent (blank asterisk; U-test). For methods, see Fig. 2.

kinase C but, presumably, to TRPV1 activation. In addition to noxious heat and RTX, TRPV1 is also responsive to protons (Caterina et al. 1997). Thus, it was a surprise that the epidermal ACh release was almost abolished at pH 6.1 and reduced by 60% at pH 5.7. After 6 minutes of washout, the level of ACh release recovered to baseline. This pH dependency could relate to proton-induced inhibition of ACh storage and/or release in the keratinocytes; however, this assumption awaits further experimentation. Although the data show that the intact epidermis releases ACh upon stimulation, our measurements do not allow us to estimate the concentration "seen" by intra- or subepidermal nerve endings. However, this information would be essential because similar to anandamide, the effect of ACh on nociceptors also depends on its concentration; lower concentrations induce sustained M2-receptor-mediated desensitizing effects, whereas higher concentrations evoke the nicotinic receptor-mediated excitatory effect (Steen et al. 1993; Bernardini et al. 2001b).

Recent studies have demonstrated, and our work fully confirms, that keratinocytes respond to certain sensory stimuli in much the same way as primary afferent nerve fibers. Noxious and innocuous temperatures, which evoke inward currents and increases in intracellular calcium, seem to evoke responses in keratinocytes, as do mechanical and chemical stimuli such as capsaicin and protons (Inoue et al. 2002; Peier et al. 2002; Chung et al. 2004; Koizumi et al. 2004). The temperature and chemical sensitivities of keratinocytes result from the expression of three subtypes of TRPV channels by these cells. While TRPV4 and TRPV3 account for sensitivity to warmth and higher temperatures, respectively, TRPV1 is responsible for noxious heat and capsaicin/proton responsiveness.

I. NAGY ET AL.

The epidermal ACh release in the experiments described in this chapter was induced by the TRPV1 agonist RTX and by noxious heat. Our data did not allow us to determine the possible involvement of TRPV3 in warmth-induced ACh release (e.g., at 38°C, Fig. 2). Protons are reported to raise the calcium level in keratinocytes in a TRPV1-dependent manner (Inoue et al. 2002). Given that ACh release was found to be calcium-dependent, protons should have enhanced this secretion through TRPV1 activation. The observed inverse proton response, i.e., suppression of ACh release, may therefore be due to a proton block further downstream in the cascade of the release mechanism.

In conclusion, the first biochemical analysis of constitutive ACh release from intact isolated epidermis revealed major stimulatory and depressant effects of noxious heat and chemical stimulations, part of which involve the capsaicin receptor TRPV1 expressed in keratinocytes. Whether the effects of released ACh extend to cutaneous sensory nerves expressing nicotinic as well as M2 muscarinic receptors remains to be elucidated.

ACKNOWLEDGMENT

P. Santha has been supported by the Marie Curie Intra-European Fellowship, MEIF-CT-2003 500960, received from the European Union.

REFERENCES

Ahluwalia J, Urban L, Capogna M, et al. Cannabinoid 1 receptors are expressed in nociceptive primary sensory neurons. *Neuroscience* 2000; 100:685–688.

Ahluwalia J, Urban L, Bevan S, et al. Anandamide regulates neuropeptide release from capsaicin-sensitive primary sensory neurons by activating both the cannabinoid 1 receptor and the vanilloid receptor 1 in vitro. *Eur J Neurosci* 2003a; 17:2611–2618.

Ahluwalia J, Yaqoob M, Urban L, et al. Activation of capsaicin-sensitive primary sensory neurones induces anandamide production and release. *J Neurochem* 2003b; 84:585–591.

Bernardini N, Reeh PW, Sauer SK. Muscarinic M2 receptors inhibit heat-induced CGRP release from isolated rat skin. *Neuroreport* 2001a; 12:2457–2460.

Bernardini N, Sauer SK, Haberberger R, et al. Excitatory nicotinic and desensitizing muscarinic (M2) effects on C-nociceptors in isolated rat skin. *J Neurosci* 2001b; 21:3295–3302.

Bernardini N, Roza C, Sauer SK, et al. Muscarinic M2 receptors on peripheral sensory nerve endings—a molecular target for antinociception. *J Neurosci* 2002; 22(RC229):1–5.

Bernardini N, Tomassy GS, Tata AM, Augusti-Tocco G, Biagioni S. Detection of basal and potassium-evoked acetylcholine release from embryonic DRG explants. *J Neurochem* 2004; 88:1533–9153.

Bhave G, Gereau RW IV. Posttranslational mechanisms of peripheral sensitization. *J Neurobiol* 2004; 61:88–106.

Buchli R, Ndoye A, Rodriguez JG, et al. Human skin fibroblasts express m2, m4, and m5 subtypes of muscarinic acetylcholine receptors. *J Cell Biochem* 1999; 74:264–277.

Carpenter SE, Lynn B. Vascular and sensory responses of human skin to mild injury after topical treatment with capsaicin. *Br J Pharmacol* 1981; 73:755–758.

Caterina MJ, Schumacher MA, Tominaga M, et al. The capsaicin receptor: a heat-activated ion channel in the pain pathway. *Nature* 1997; 389:816–824.

Caterina MJ, Leffler A, Malmberg AB, et al. Impaired nociception and pain sensation in mice lacking the capsaicin receptor. *Science* 2000; 288:306–313.

Chung MK, Lee H, Mizuno A, et al. TRPV3 and TRPV4 mediate warmth-evoked currents in primary mouse keratinocytes. *J Biol Chem* 2004; 279:21569–21575.

Daedwyler SA, Hampson RE, Bennet BA, et al. Cannabinoids modulate potassium current in cultured hippocampal neurons. *Recept Channels* 1993; 1:121–134.

Davis JB, Gray J, Gunthrope MJ, et al. Vanilloid receptor-1 is essential for inflammatory thermal hyperalgesia. *Nature* 2000; 405:183–187.

Devane WA, Hanus L, Breuer A, et al. Isolation and structure of a brain constituent that binds to the cannabinoid receptor. *Science* 1992; 258:1946–1949.

Di Marzo V, Fontana A, Cadas H, et al. Formation and inactivation of endogenous cannabinoid anandamide in central neurons. *Nature* 1994; 372:686–691.

Dinis P, Charrua A, Avelino A, et al. Anandamide-evoked activation of the vanilloid receptor 1 contributes to the development of bladder hyperreflexia and nociceptive transmission to spinal dorsal horn neurons in cystitis. *J Neurosci* 2004; 24:11253–11263.

Dussor GO, Helesic G, Hargreaves KM, et al. Cholinergic modulation of nociceptive responses in vivo and neuropeptide release in vitro at the level of the primary sensory neuron. *Pain* 2004; 107:22–32.

Farquhar-Smith WP, Rice AS. A novel neuroimmune mechanism in cannabinoid-mediated attenuation of nerve growth factor-induced hyperalgesia. *Anesthesiology* 2003; 99:1391–1401.

Flores CM, DeCamp RM, Kilo S, et al. Neuronal nicotinic receptor expression in sensory neurons of the rat trigeminal ganglion: demonstration of alpha 3 beta 4, a novel subtype in the mammalian nervous system. *J Neurosci* 1996; 16:7892–7901.

Grando SA. Biological functions of keratinocyte cholinergic receptors. *J Investig Dermatol Symp Proc* 1997; 2:41–48.

Grando SA, Kist DA, Qi M, et al. Human keratinocytes synthesize, secrete and degrade acetylcholine. *J Invest Dermatol* 1993; 101:32–36.

Hermann H, De Petrocellis L, Bisogno T, et al. Dual effect of cannabinoid CB1 receptor stimulation on a vanilloid VR1 receptor-mediated response. *Cell Mol Life Sci* 2003; 60:607–616.

Inoue K, Koizumi S, Fuziwara S, et al. Functional vanilloid receptors in cultured normal human epidermal keratinocytes. *Biochem Biophys Res Commun* 2002; 291:124–129.

Ji RR, Kohno T, Moore KA, et al. Central sensitization and LTP: do pain and memory share similar mechanisms? *Trends Neurosci* 2003; 26:696–705.

Jordt SE, Julius D. Molecular basis for species-specific sensitivity to "hot" chili peppers. *Cell* 2002; 108:421–430.

Keele CA, Armstrong D (Eds). *Substances Producing Pain and Itch*. London: Edward Arnold, 1964.

Koizumi S, Fujishita K, Inoue K et al. Ca^{2+} waves in keratinocytes are transmitted to sensory neurons: the involvement of extracellular ATP and P2Y2 receptor activation. *Biochem J* 2004; 380:329–338.

Liang YF, Haake B, Reeh PW. Sustained sensitization and recruitment of rat cutaneous nociceptors by bradykinin and a novel theory of its excitatory action. *J Physiol* 2001; 532:229–239.

Linhart O, Obreja O, Kress M. The inflammatory mediators serotonin, prostaglandin E2 and bradykinin evoke calcium influx in rat sensory neurons. *Neuroscience* 2003; 118:69–74.

Mackie K, Hille B. Cannabinoids inhibit N-type calcium channels in neuroblastoma-glioma cells. *Proc Natl Acad Sci USA* 1992; 89:3825–3829.

Nagy I. Sensory processing: primary afferent neurons/DRG. In: Evers, Maze M (Eds). *Anesthetic Pharmacology: Physiologic Principles and Clinical Practice*. Philadelphia: Churchill Livingstone, 2004, pp 187–197.

Nagy I, Rang HP. Similarities and differences between the responses of rat sensory neurons to noxious heat and capsaicin. *J Neurosci* 1999; 19:10647–10655.

Peier AM, Reeve AJ, Andersson DA, et al. A heat-sensitive TRP channel expressed in keratinocytes. *Science* 2002; 296:2046–2049.

Price TJ, Patwardhan AM, Flores CM, et al. A role for the anandamide membrane transporter in TRPV1-mediated neurosecretion from trigeminal sensory neurons. *Neuropharmacology* 2005; 49:25–39.

Richardson JD, Kilo S, Hargreaves KM. Cannabinoids reduce hyperalgesia and inflammation via interaction with peripheral CB1 receptors. *Pain* 1998; 75:111–119.

Sathianathan V, Avelino A, Charrua A, et al. Insulin induces cobalt uptake in a sub-population of rat cultured primary sensory neurons. *Eur J Neurosci* 2003; 18:2477–2486.

Silva A, Charrua A, Dinis, P Cruz, F. TRPV1 knockout mice do not develop bladder overactivity during acute chemical bladder inflammation. *Soc Neurosci Abstracts* 2004; 34:288.16.

Song ZH, Bonner TL. A lysine residue of the cannabinoid receptor is critical for receptor recognition by several agonists but not WIN55212-2. *Mol Pharmacol* 1996; 49:891–896.

Steen KH, Reeh PW. Actions of cholinergic agonists and antagonists on sensory nerve endings in rat skin, *in vitro*. *J Neurophysiol* 1993; 70:397–405.

Tschachler E, Reinisch CM, Mayer C, et al. Sheet preparations expose the dermal nerve plexus of human skin and render the dermal nerve end organ accessible to extensive analysis. *J Invest Dermatol* 2004; 122:177–182.

Vanegas H, Schaible HG. Descending control of persistent pain: inhibitory or facilitatory? *Brain Res Brain Res Rev* 2004; 46:295–309.

Wessler I, Reinheimer T, Klapproth H, et al. Mammalian glial cells in culture synthesize acetylcholine. *Naunyn Schmiedebergs Arch Pharmacol* 1997; 356:694–697.

Wessler I, Kirkpatrick CJ, Racke K. Non-neuronal acetylcholine, a locally acting molecule, widely distributed in biological systems: expression and function in humans. *Pharmacol Ther* 1998; 77:59–79.

Wessler I, Kirkpatrick CJ, Racke K. The cholinergic "pitfall": acetylcholine, a universal cell molecule in biological systems, including humans. *Clin Exp Pharmacol Physiol* 1999; 26:198–205.

Yang LC, Chen LM, Wang CJ, et al. Postoperative analgesia by intra-articular neostigmine in patients undergoing knee arthroscopy. *Anesthesiology* 1998; 88:334–339.

Zygmunt PM, Petersson J, Andersson DA, et al. Vanilloid receptors on sensory nerves mediate the vasodilator action of anandamide. *Nature* 1999; 400:452–457.

Correspondence to: Istvan Nagy, MD, PhD, Department of Anaesthetics, Intensive Care and Pain Medicine, Faculty of Medicine, Imperial College London, Chelsea and Westminster Hospital, 369 Fulham Road, London, SW10 9NH, United Kingdom. Fax: 44-(0)20-8237-5109; email: i.nagy@imperial.ac.uk.

Proceedings of the 11th World Congress on Pain,
edited by Herta Flor, Eija Kalso, and Jonathan O.
Dostrovsky, IASP Press, Seattle, © 2006.

12

Onset of Ectopic Firing in the Chung Model of Neuropathic Pain Coincides with the Onset of Tactile Allodynia

Michael Tal,[a,b] Junesun Kim,[d] Seung Keun Back,[d] Heung Sik Na,[d] and Marshall Devor[b,c]

[a]Department of Anatomy and Cell Biology, Hadassah Medical School, [b]Center for Research on Pain, and [c]Department of Cell and Animal Biology, Institute of Life Sciences, Hebrew University of Jerusalem, Israel; [d]Department of Physiology, Korea University College of Medicine, Seoul, South Korea

Patients with traumatic and other neuropathies frequently report that pain is evoked by light touch or brush stimuli on the skin. Similar hypersensibility is inferred in animal models of neuropathic pain in which brisk paw withdrawal is observed in response to skin contact with calibrated von Frey monofilaments that exert forces to which the animal is indifferent prior to undergoing nerve injury. It was once believed that this "tactile allodynia" is due to the sensitization of sensory endings of C-fiber mechanonociceptors in the skin. However, an alternative hypothesis has arisen in light of the lack of evidence that nociceptor endings in fact come to respond to the weak forces that evoke tactile allodynia (Koltzenburg et al. 1994; Banik and Brennan 2004; Tsuboi et al. 2004; Shim et al. 2005) and the plethora of evidence that the impulses that evoke tactile allodynia are carried centrally on low-threshold mechanoreceptive Aβ fibers (Campbell et al. 1988; Torebjork et al. 1992). Specifically, it is now widely accepted that tactile allodynia in neuropathy results from abnormal spinal processing of Aβ-fiber input due to a central hyperexcitability, a state termed "central sensitization" (Woolf 1983; Gracely et al. 1992). Central sensitization, in turn, is thought to be induced and dynamically maintained by neuroactive chemical mediators, such as substance P, that are normally present exclusively in afferent C fibers. There are two competing hypotheses on the source of these mediators in neuropathy. By one account they are released in the spinal cord from uninjured C fibers that become spontaneously active due to an interaction with injured, degenerating afferents within shared nerve trunks (Li et al. 2000). By the second account, the mediators are released from injured, spontaneously active A fibers that begin to synthesize them as a result of neuropathic phenotypic switching (Liu et al. 2000a; Weissner et al. 2006). These hypotheses are not mutually exclusive.

The neural process underlying central sensitization is unknown. Nerve injury induces a large number of changes in the central nervous system; there are now at least 50 competing hypotheses vying for attention, and additional ones continue to appear at frequent intervals (Costigan et al. 2002; Devor 2006). Moreover, it is not yet certain that the critical nerve-injury-evoked central changes are necessarily dependent upon ectopic afferent impulse discharge in peripheral afferents. In only a few instances has it been determined whether nerve conduction block prevents the development of a specific central change. This chapter describes a study in which we tried to answer this question in a more general manner. We argue that if central sensitization and the resulting tactile allodynia are indeed triggered by abnormal afferent input, then this input ought to appear just before, or simultaneously with, the tactile allodynia.

METHODS

ANIMALS AND SURGERY

Experiments were carried out using adult male C3H and CBA strain mice (20–30 g). Initial stock was purchased from the Jackson Laboratories (C3H/HeJ, CBA/J), or in the case of the C3H mice used for electrophysiological recording, from Harlan Laboratories (C3H/HeN, a strain that originated as C3H/HeJ). Experiments were carried out using these animals or their offspring bred in our local university colonies. All procedures were approved by the institutional animal care and use committee of the Life Sciences Institute, Hebrew University of Jerusalem, or the Korea University College of Medicine, Seoul.

Tactile allodynia was induced by partial denervation of the hindpaw using the method of Kim and Chung (1992). Briefly, for animals intended for behavioral assessment we first obtained preoperative baseline data. Animals were then anesthetized with enflurane (0.5–2.0%), and the skin was cleansed. The L5 spinal nerve was then exposed, tightly ligated with 6-0 silk, and cut across with microsurgical scissors about 8 mm from the corresponding dorsal root ganglia (DRG). The wound was closed in layers. Recovery was uneventful. For animals intended for electrophysiological assessment, the surgical procedure was similar except that the anesthetic used was chloral hydrate (400 mg/kg i.p.), and often both L4 and L5 spinal nerves were cut, without ligation.

BEHAVIORAL PHENOTYPING

The behavioral phenotype was assessed in two groups of animals from each of the two mouse strains. The first group of each strain was tested for tactile (mechanical), cold, and heat sensitivity and spontaneous pain behavior one day preoperatively (day −1) and then again 1, 4, 7, 14, and 28 days postoperatively (dpo). The second group of each strain was tested for tactile response only, preoperatively and at 2–3-hour intervals over the first 24 hours postoperatively (hpo).

Tactile sensitivity (von Frey test). Mice were brought from the animal colony and placed under transparent plastic boxes (55 × 95 × 50 mm) on a metal mesh floor (3 × 3 mm mesh). They were then left alone for at least 20 minutes of acclimation before sensory testing began. Tactile (mechanical) sensitivity was assessed by measuring the force just sufficient to elicit a brisk paw-withdrawal response to graded mechanical stimuli using a series of nylon von Frey monofilaments with logarithmically increasing stiffness (0.20, 0.69, 1.57, 3.92, 9.80, 19.60, 39.20, and 58.80 mN, equivalent to 0.02, 0.07, 0.16, 0.4, 1.0, 2.0, 4.0, and 6.0 g). The 50% withdrawal threshold was determined using the up-down method (Chaplan et al. 1994). In brief, we began by determining the most sensitive spot on the hindpaw by probing various areas using the filament with initial bending force of 0.4 g. If no paw-withdrawal response was elicited, the process was repeated with the next stiffest filament. If there was a response, the sensitive spot was then touched once with the next weaker stimulus. Lack of withdrawal led to presentation of the next stronger stimulus again, and a positive response led to presentation of the next weaker stimulus. Stimuli were presented at intervals of several seconds.

Thermal sensitivity: withdrawal from cold and heat stimuli. A drop of 15°C water was delicately placed on the lateral plantar surface of the hindpaw, using a length of polyethylene tubing connected to a syringe. The tubing did not touch the skin. Responses were recorded from 0.5 to 20 seconds after the stimulation. The criterion for a positive response in this test, interpreted as cold allodynia, was a brisk paw withdrawal or a clear supraspinal sign such as paw shaking or licking and vocalization. The test was repeated five times on each paw at 5-minute intervals. Frequency of paw withdrawal was calculated as the number of paw withdrawals/total trials × 100%.

Heat sensitivity was assessed using the rat "plantar test" apparatus as described by Hargreaves et al. (1988). Animals were habituated to the apparatus, which consisted of three individual Perspex boxes on an elevated glass table. A mobile radiant heat source under the table was focused on the hindpaw. The heat intensity was adjusted to obtain an average paw-withdrawal latency of about 6 seconds (IR 70 heat setting on the apparatus), and the cut-off time was set at 15 seconds to prevent tissue damage. Three heat stimuli were given for each paw at an interval of 5–10 minutes. Mean paw-withdrawal latency for each paw was calculated.

Spontaneous pain. The same "plantar test" apparatus was used, but animals were observed passively, without stimulation. After 20 minutes of adaptation, the cumulative time that the mouse held any foot off the floor over the following 3 minutes was recorded. The time of lifts associated with locomotion or body repositioning was not counted. Since the duration of foot lifts of less than 1 second were difficult to measure accurately, such lifts were scored as 0.36 seconds each. This value was obtained by accurately measuring 100 such foot lifts, and averaging. Spontaneous paw-lifting behavior was taken as an indicator of ongoing pain or dysesthesia.

ELECTROPHYSIOLOGICAL TESTING

The intensity of ectopic spontaneous impulse discharge generated in the spinal nerve end neuroma and associated DRG was assessed at close intervals following spinal nerve transection. For assessment of the effects of acute nerve cut (0–3 hpo), the anesthesia induced for neurectomy was maintained with re-peated doses of chloral hydrate at ~60 mg/kg/h (i.p.). For survival intervals of >3 hpo the animals were allowed to recover from the anesthesia under which the nerve had been cut, and they were then re-anesthetized for electrophysi-ological assessment (chloral hydrate, 400 mg/kg, followed by ~60 mg/kg/h, i.p.). Measurements of ectopic afferent discharge were made within 3-hour time windows as indicated in the Results section below.

Spontaneous ectopic discharge was quantified using the teased fiber record-ing method. Briefly, small bundles of axons (microfilaments) were teased from the L4 or L5 dorsal root, in continuity with the DRG and neuroma peripherally but cut centrally, and adhered to an Ag/AgCl recording electrode referenced to a nearby indifferent electrode. Each microfilament was observed passively for at least 1 minute, and a spike-triggered delay-line and a multispike detector system were used to determine the number of distinct spontaneously active axons that were present in each microfilament. We also evaluated spike waveform, firing frequency, and discharge pattern, and used this information to identify active af-ferents as A or C fibers using criteria given in Liu et al. (2000a). In our previous studies using these methods (in rats) we determined the percentage of axons that fired spontaneously by dividing the number of spontaneously active axons per microfilament by the total number of axons present in each microfilament. The denominator was obtained by stimulating the nerve just central to the neuroma, and gradually increasing the stimulation current to saturation while counting the number of all-or-none spikes evoked. However, the short conduction distance in mice with spinal nerves cut precluded use of this method in the present study.

As an alternative, using a separate sample of 75 dorsal root microfilaments from three nerve-intact mice, we stimulated the sciatic nerve and counted the number of axons contained in each microfilament. These microfilaments contained a mean of 10.4 ± 7.2 A fibers and 8.7 ± 5.5 (resolvable) C fibers (mean $\pm$ SD). In rats, 58.7% of afferents teased from the L4 and L5 dorsal roots run in the sciatic nerve (Devor et al. 1985). Assuming a similar value for mice, the dorsal root microfilaments contained on average about 18 A fibers and 15 C fibers. These values were used in calculating the percentage of afferents with spontaneous firing.

At all postoperative time points, to assure that recording conditions were satisfactory and that the segment recorded from had indeed been cut, we occasionally sampled microfilaments from the L3 or L6 dorsal root. These microfilaments always contained spontaneously active muscle spindle afferents, easily recognizable by their $A\beta$ spike waveform, characteristic tonic firing pattern, and response to muscle stretching. They also contained axons that responded to gentle brushing of hindlimb skin. No such responses were encountered in dorsal roots of which the spinal nerve had previously been cut.

STATISTICAL ANALYSIS

The significance of changes from tactile and thermal baseline were tested using Friedman's repeated ANOVA and the Mann-Whitney U test. Changes in ectopic firing were evaluated using two-way Student's t-tests. Criterion for significance was $P < 0.05$. Means are given $\pm$ SE (standard error of the mean), or where indicated, $\pm$ SD (standard deviation).

RESULTS

ONSET OF TACTILE ALLODYNIA

In both mouse strains, paw-withdrawal threshold fell sharply by 24 hpo, from baseline values of 2.87 ± 0.33 g (C3H, $n = 25$) and 3.73 ± 0.53 g (CBA, $n = 11$) to <0.5 g ($P < 0.05$; Fig. 1). Tactile allodynia remained stable at this level for the duration of the 28-day testing period.

In light of this result, we examined a second group of C3H and CBA mice ($n = 9$ for both strains). These were checked one day preoperatively and then at 10 time points from 3 to 24 hpo (Fig. 2). At 3 and 6 hpo there was a minor increase in response threshold (hypoalgesia), but the change was not statistically significant ($P > 0.05$). Response threshold first fell below the baseline level between 8 and 11 hpo, and then continued to fall gradually until 20 hpo, at which time it stabilized.

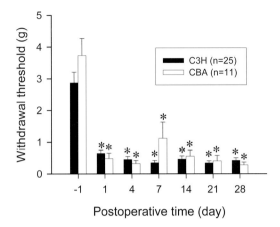

Fig. 1. Development of mechanical hypersensitivity in C3H and CBA mice in the Chung model of neuropathic pain (* indicates $P < 0.05$, Friedman repeated ANOVA, versus 1 day preoperatively).

We considered the possibility that the early stage of hypoalgesia at 3–6 hpo may reflect residual sedation from the general anesthesia used for nerve surgery. To test this hypothesis, additional mice of the CBA strain underwent sham surgery in which the spinal nerves were exposed but not cut ($n = 6$). We reasoned that residual anesthetic sedation should affect nerve-injured and sham-operated mice equally. In fact, significant early hypoalgesia occurred in the nerve-injured CBA mice compared to sham-operated mice ($P < 0.01$). Hypoalgesia in the sham-operated controls was not significantly different after surgery compared to 24 hours prior to surgery, suggesting that the early hypoalgesia is a real effect of the nerve injury (Fig. 2).

ONSET OF COLD ALLODYNIA AND HEAT HYPERSENSITIVITY

Both cold and heat hypersensitivity were less striking than tactile allodynia in terms of the percentage change from baseline. Moreover, these symptoms progressed gradually over the 28 days of postoperative observation. For both cold and heat, a significant increase in sensitivity was present by 1 dpo (Fig. 3A,B).

SPONTANEOUS PAIN

Spontaneous pain, inferred from the duration of spontaneous lifting of the paw, increased sharply in the first 24 hours after nerve injury and then gradually declined from 7 to 28 dpo, especially in CBA mice. Spontaneous paw lifting was the only measure in which C3H and CBA mice differed markedly (Fig. 3C).

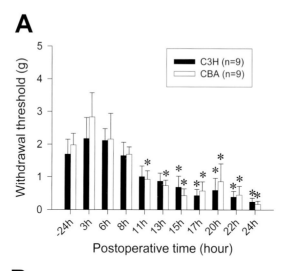

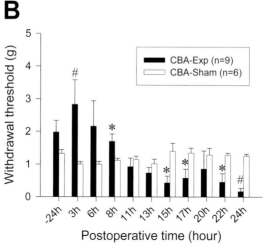

Fig. 2. Rapid emergence of tactile hypersensitivity within the first 24 hours after L5 spinal nerve ligation and cut. Upper graph: * $P < 0.05$, Friedman repeated ANOVA, versus 24 hours preoperatively. Lower graph: # $P < 0.01$, * $P < 0.05$, Mann-Whitney U test, versus sham.

ONSET OF SPONTANEOUS ECTOPIC DISCHARGE

Estimates of the incidence of spontaneous ectopic discharge were made in 20 C3H and 17 CBA mice over the first 24 hours following spinal nerve injury. In these animals we sampled from a total of 529 microfilaments, 14 ± 6 SD microfilaments per mouse, containing about 250 myelinated (A) fibers and 210 (resolvable) unmyelinated (C) fibers per mouse, for a total of roughly 9,500

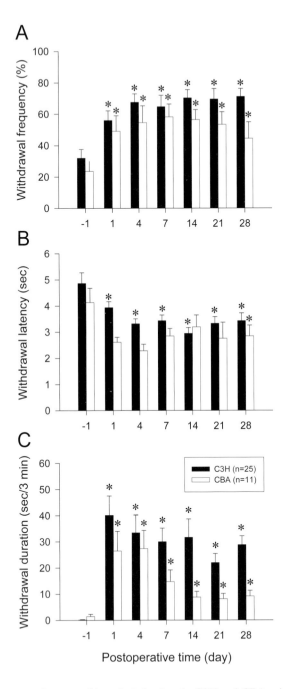

Fig. 3. Development of neuropathic pain behaviors in C3H and CBA mice in the Chung model of neuropathy. (A) Cold and (B) heat hypersensitivity, and (C) a behavioral marker of spontaneous pain (*$P < 0.05$, Friedman repeated ANOVA, versus 1 day preoperatively).

A and 8,000 C fibers overall. In the time intervals 0–3 hpo and 4–7 hpo there was very little ectopic activity (< 1% of A fibers sampled, no active C fibers). In both C3H and CBA mice, activity increased significantly in the 7–10 hpo time window ($P < 0.01$) and continued to increase in the 11–14 hpo time window ($P < 0.01$ compared to 7–10 hpo). By 14–17 hpo, the mean percentage of fibers with spontaneous activity appeared to reach a peak of ~12% of A fibers, and this level was maintained at least until 24 hpo (Fig. 4). In the majority of fibers, discharge was either tonic or bursting, with instantaneous firing rates typically in the range of 20 ± 10 (SD) impulses per second. The remainder fired at relatively slow rates (< 1–5 impulses per second) with an irregular interspike interval. Remarkably, all spontaneously active fibers were A fibers, as assessed by spike shape criteria (Liu et al. 2000a). No spontaneously active C fibers were noted. Firing frequency and pattern and time of onset were the same in C3H and CBA mice.

DISCUSSION

Tactile allodynia in the Chung model of neuropathic pain emerges rapidly following spinal nerve section. Many previous studies in mice have reported the presence of tactile allodynia at the first postoperative time interval checked,

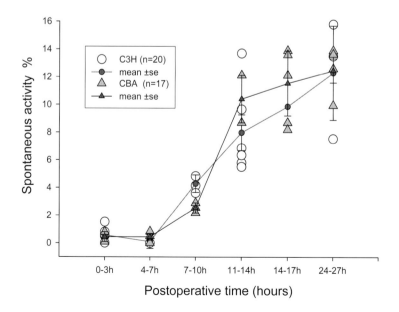

Fig. 4. Ectopic spontaneous discharge develops within hours of transection of the spinal nerve in the Chung model of neuropathic pain in both C3H and CBA mice.

1 dpo. Testing at closer intervals, we found that it emerges in the time window 8–11 hpo. This window is earlier than in rats, in which we first detected tactile allodynia at 16–24 hpo (Liu et al. 2000a). It is likely that the critical factor is distance from the nerve injury site to the associated DRG. When hindlimb afferents are cut across still further from the DRG, in sciatic nerve tributaries at the level of the popliteal fossa (in rats), tactile allodynia reaches maximal values several days later (Decosterd and Woolf 2000). Likewise, the kinetics and magnitude of phenotypic switching of gene expression in axotomized DRG neurons depend prominently on the distance to the cut.

The earliest time window in which ectopic firing in injured afferents was significantly elevated was 7–10 hpo. The fraction of cut afferents with ongoing discharge continued to increase thereafter, reaching a maximum at about 20 hpo. This time frame matches closely with both the time of onset of tactile allodynia measured behaviorally, and the time to reach peak sensitivity. A similar match, although delayed in time, has been reported previously in rats (Liu et al. 2000a; Sun et al. 2005).

Afferent ectopic discharge in dorsal root microfilaments in continuity with the DRG originates alternatively in the spinal nerve-end neuroma and in the DRG itself. We were unable to distinguish these two sources in the experiments in this study. Earlier work in rats, however, indicated that about 25% of the activity originates in the neuroma, and 75% in the DRG (Liu et al. 2000a). It is important to note that all of the spontaneous discharge observed was carried in A fibers. This conclusion must be stated with some caution, however, because the identification of afferent type was based primarily on waveform criteria. The short propagation distances in the present experiment, and the need to stimulate at relatively high power (current × pulse width) to activate C fibers, precluded direct measurement of axonal conduction velocity.

The absence of spontaneous ectopic activity in C fibers in these mice is consistent with our previous observations in rats in which conduction velocity *was* measured, and with the observations of a number of other groups (Liu et al. 2000a,b). Taken together, these results imply that axotomized A fibers can evoke central sensitization and/or directly drive spinal pain-signaling neurons. Although we were not aware of the possibility of ongoing C-fiber activity at extremely low firing frequencies in our earlier studies, we were aware of this possibility here, and we did not see such activity. Systematic recordings of spontaneous C-fiber activity were not made from uninjured axons in neighboring L3 and 6 dorsal roots because these fibers remained connected to the skin and deep tissues. In such recordings we do not know how to distinguish ongoing discharge originating in normal cutaneous thermosensitive afferents, or deep thermo-, mechano-, or chemosensitive afferents, from pathophysiological discharge that arises ectopically due to the spinal nerve injury (Li et al. 2000; Wu et al. 2001). Partly denervated tissue is likely to be warmer than normal due to sympathectomy and neurogenic edema, and it contains a soup of inflammatory mediators. These conditions could evoke discharge in intact afferent endings that is not easily distinguished from ectopia. Either, of course, could contribute to central sensitization.

On the assumption that tactile allodynia is dependent on the emergence of central sensitization, central sensitization must also be in place within 8–11 hpo. This rapid onset time puts a severe constraint on the cellular mechanism underlying the central sensitization (Devor 2001, 2006). For example, do inhibitory GABAergic neurons die, do Aβ afferent terminals sprout into the superficial layers of the dorsal horn, or are microglia and astrocytes activated within this time frame? Some changes in gene expression in DRG neurons occur within hours of nerve injury, but others do not. A useful way of screening hypothetical mechanisms of central sensitization is to compare the time of onset of the process in question with that of tactile allodynia.

ACKNOWLEDGMENT

Supported by the German-Israel Foundation for Research and Development (GIF), a Korean-Israeli Research Cooperation grant, and the European Community's 6th Framework Program (project LSHM-CT-2004-502800 Pain Genes). The manuscript reflects only the authors' views. The European Community is not liable for any use that may be made of the information contained therein.

REFERENCES

Banik RK, Brennan TJ. Spontaneous discharge and increased heat sensitivity of rat C-fiber nociceptors are present in vitro after plantar incision. *Pain* 2004; 112:204–213.

Campbell JN, Raja SN, Meyer RA, MacKinnon SE. Myelinated afferents signal the hyperalgesia associated with nerve injury. *Pain* 1988; 32:89–94.

Chaplan SR, Bach FW, Pogrel JW, Chung JM, Yaksh TL. Quantitative assessment of tactile allodynia evoked by unilateral ligation of the fifth and sixth lumbar nerves in the rat. *J Neurosci Methods* 1994; 53:55–63.

Costigan M, Befort K, Karchewski L, et al. Replicate high-density rat genome oligonucleotide microarrays reveal hundreds of regulated genes in the dorsal root ganglion after peripheral nerve injury. *BMC Neurosci* 2002; 3:16–28.

Decosterd I, Woolf CJ. Spared nerve injury: an animal model of persistent peripheral neuropathic pain. *Pain* 2000; 87:149–158.

Devor M. Neuropathic pain: what do we do with all these theories? *Acta Anaesthesiol Scand* 2001; 45:1121–1127.

Devor M. Central changes after nerve injury. In: Willis W, Schmidt R (Eds). *Encyclopedic Reference of Pain*. Berlin: Springer Verlag, 2006, in press.

Devor M, Govrin-Lippmann R, Frank, Raber P. Proliferation of primary sensory neurons in adult rat dorsal root ganglion and the kinetics of retrograde cell loss after sciatic nerve section. *Somatosens Res* 1985; 3:139–167.

Gracely R, Lynch S, Bennett G. Painful neuropathy: altered central processing, maintained dynamically by peripheral input. *Pain* 1992; 51:175–194.

Hargreaves K, Dubner R, Brown F, Flores C, Joris J. A new and sensitive method for measuring thermal nociception in cutaneous hyperalgesia, *Pain* 1988; 32:77–88.

Kim SH, Chung JM. An experimental model for peripheral neuropathy produced by segmental spinal nerve ligation in the rat. Pain 1992; 50:355–363.

Koltzenburg M, Kees S, Budweiser S, Ochs G, Toyka KV. The properties of unmyelinated nociceptive afferents change in a painful chronic constriction neuropathy. In: Gebhart G, Hammond D, Jensen T (Eds). *Proceedings of the 7th World Congress on Pain,* Progress in Pain Research and Management, Vol. 2. Seattle: IASP Press, 1994, pp 511–521.

Li Y, Dorsi M, Meyer R, Belzberg A. Mechanical hyperalgesia after an L5 spinal nerve lesion in the rat is not dependent on input from injured nerve fibers. *Pain* 2000; 85.

Liu C-N, Wall PD, Ben-Dor E, et al. Tactile allodynia in the absence of C-fiber activation: altered firing properties of DRG neurons following spinal nerve injury. *Pain* 2000a; 85:503–521.

Liu X, Eschenfelder S, Blenk K-H, Jänig W, Habler H-J. Spontaneous activity of axotomized afferent neurons after L5 spinal nerve injury in rats. *Pain* 2000b; 84:309–318.

Shim B, Kim DW, Kim BH, et al. Mechanical and heat sensitization of cutaneous nociceptors in rats with experimental peripheral neuropathy. *Neuroscience* 2005; 132:193–201.

Sun Q, Tu H, Xing GG, Han JS, Wan Y. Ectopic discharges from injured nerve fibers are highly correlated with tactile allodynia only in early, but not late, stage in rats with spinal nerve ligation. *Exp Neurol* 2005; 191:128–136.

Torebjork H, Lundberg L, LaMotte R. Central changes in processing of mechanoreceptive input in capsaicin-induced secondary hyperalgesia in humans. *J Physiol (Lond)* 1992; 448:765–780.

Tsuboi Y, Takeda M, Tanimoto T, et al. Alteration of the second branch of the trigeminal nerve activity following inferior alveolar nerve transection in rats. Pain 2004; 111:323–334.

Weissner W, Winterson BJ, Stuart-Tilley A, Devor M, Bove GM. Time course of substance P expression in dorsal root ganglia following complete spinal nerve transection. *J Comp Neurol* 2006; in press.

Woolf CJ. Evidence for a central component of postinjury pain hypersensitivity. Nature 1983; 306:686–688.

Wu G, Ringkamp M, Hartke, et al. Early onset of spontaneous activity in uninjured C-fiber nociceptors after injury to neighboring nerve fibers. *J Neurosci* 2001; 21:RC140.

Correspondence to: Prof. Michael Tal, Department of Anatomy and Cell Biology, Hebrew University-Hadassah Medical School, Ein Kerem, Jerusalem, Israel. Email: talm@cc.huji.ac.il.

Proceedings of the 11th World Congress on Pain,
edited by Herta Flor, Eija Kalso, and Jonathan O.
Dostrovsky, IASP Press, Seattle, © 2006.

13

Cytokine-Induced Pain: From Molecular Mechanisms to Human Pain States

Claudia Sommer,[a] Linda Sorkin,[b] and Michaela Kress[c]

*[a]Department of Neurology, University of Würzburg, Würzburg, Germany;
[b]Anesthesiology Research Laboratory, University of California San Diego,
La Jolla, California, USA; [c]Department of Physiology and Medical Physics,
Institute of Physiology, Medical University of Innsbruck, Innsbruck, Austria*

MOLECULAR MECHANISMS OF PROINFLAMMATORY CYTOKINES IN THE PERIPHERY

Cytokines are small proteins with a molecular mass lower than 30 kDa. In vivo concentrations are in the range of a few picograms to nanograms per milliliter. Cytokines are produced on demand and have a short life span and therefore travel only over short distances. Their binding is specific, with binding constants between 10^{-12} and 10^{-10} M, and requires receptor molecules on the cell surfaces. In spite of the redundancy and pleiotropy of the cytokine network, specific actions of individual cytokines and endogenous control mechanisms have been identified. The proinflammatory cytokines tumor necrosis factor-alpha (TNF-α) and the interleukins IL-1β and IL-6 play an important role in plastic changes of nociceptors (Watkins and Maier 1999).

TNF-alpha is generally accepted as the prototypic proinflammatory cytokine due to its role in initiating the cascade of activation of other cytokines and growth factors in the inflammatory response. Intraplantar injection of TNF-α in rats induces mechanical allodynia and thermal hyperalgesia (Cunha et al. 1992; Perkins and Kelly 1994; Woolf et al. 1997). TNF-α has also been linked to the generation and maintenance of neuropathic pain (Wagner and Myers 1996; Sommer and Schäfers 1998; Wagner et al. 1998; Sommer et al. 2001), where it may lower mechanical activation thresholds (Junger and Sorkin 2000). In vitro,

TNF-α elicits neuronal discharges in dorsal root ganglion (DRG) neurons; injured as well as neighboring uninjured afferent neurons exhibit an increased sensitivity to TNF-α (Schäfers et al. 2003b). TNF-α seems to affect nociceptors directly; in vitro preparations can be sensitized to heat, which largely excludes secondary effects (Opree and Kress 2000; Schäfers et al. 2003b). TNF-α binds to TNF receptor 1 (TNFR1) and TNF receptor 2 (TNFR2), and the effects associated with experimental hyperalgesia largely seem to depend on TNFR1 (Vogel et al. 2000), which is in line with an upregulation of TNFR1 following experimental chronic constriction injury or inflammation (Shubaycv and Myers 2000; Parada et al. 2003; Li et al. 2004; Ohtori et al. 2004). Downstream of the receptor, mechanical hyperalgesia induced by TNF-α is mediated via p38 mitogen-activated protein (MAP) kinase (Ji et al. 2002; Milligan et al. 2003; Schäfers et al. 2003d; see Fig. 1). Simultaneous or consecutive activation of further kinases, mobilization of Ca^{2+}, and induction of nitric oxide synthases may further contribute to the sensitizing effects that TNF-α has on nociceptors

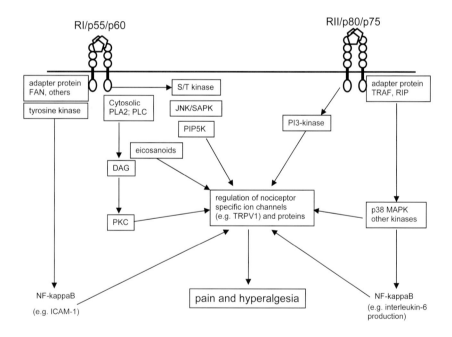

Fig. 1. Diagram of tumor necrosis factor (TNF) membrane receptor subtypes and their downstream signaling molecules: FAN (factor associated with neutral SMase activation), PLA_2 (phospholipase A_2), PLC (phospholipase C), TRAF (tumor necrosis factor receptor-associated factor), RIP (receptor-interacting protein) DAG (diacylglycerol), SAPK (stress-activated protein kinase), JNK (c-Jun N-terminal kinases), PI3K (phosphatidylinositol 3-kinase), and ICAM-1 (intercellular adhesion molecule), targeting ion channels such as the capsaicin receptor TRPV1.

in vitro (Opree and Kress 2000; Pollock et al. 2002; Abe et al. 2003). TNF-α and IL-1β also induce the functional expression of cyclooxygenase-2 receptors, but not of prostaglandin E_2 (PGE_2) receptors, in DRG cells in culture, suggesting that cytokine-induced sensitization can occur secondary to prostaglandin production, but not secondary to alterations in PGE_2 receptors (Fehrenbacher et al. 2005).

IL-1-beta can be produced by many cell types (Watkins and Maier 1999); major cellular sources in the context of pain include glial cells and both sympathetic and sensory neurons (Freidin et al. 1992; Copray et al. 2001). Expression of IL-1 receptor type I (IL-1RI) mRNA in sensory neurons suggests a possible autocrine or paracrine influence of IL-1β on sensory processing (Copray et al. 2001; Obreja et al. 2002a). Inflammatory hyperalgesia was prevented by experimental administration of endogenous IL-1 receptor antagonist (IL-1ra), and neutralizing antibodies to IL-1 receptors reduced pain-associated behavior in mice with experimental neuropathy (Sommer et al. 1999; Cunha et al. 2000). The peripheral pronociceptive IL-1 action is likely mediated by a complex signaling cascade and by secondary production of nitric oxide, bradykinin, or prostaglandins, which may account for sensitization or excitation of nociceptors (Ferreira et al. 1988; Fukuoka et al. 1994; Perkins and Kelly 1994; Fu and Longhurst 1999; Inoue et al. 1999). Initial evidence for a more direct action of IL-1β on nociceptors came from an in vitro preparation in which brief exposure to IL-1β facilitated heat-evoked release of calcitonin gene-related peptide (CGRP; Opree and Kress 2000). In addition, IL-1β induced a sensitization of heat-activated inward currents (I_{heat}) in sensory neurons. This heat sensitization was independent of G-protein-coupled receptors or rises of intracellular Ca^{2+}, but was mediated by the activation of protein kinase C and tyrosine kinase. In addition, IL-1β-induced c-Src kinase activation regulated preprotachykinin gene expression and substance P secretion in rat sensory ganglia (Igwe 2003).

IL-6. Most experimental studies reported pro-inflammatory and pronociceptive roles for IL-6 (Oka et al. 1995; Poole et al. 1995; DeLeo et al. 1996). In neuropathic mice, nerve injury correlates well with upregulated IL-6 levels and with development of thermal hyperalgesia and allodynia (DeLeo et al. 1996; Murphy et al. 1999; Okamoto et al. 2001). IL-6 knockout mice present with reduced thermal hyperalgesia after carrageenan inflammation or nerve constriction (Xu et al. 1997; Murphy et al. 1999; Zhong et al. 1999). Antisera neutralizing endogenous IL-6 inhibit lipopolysaccharide -induced hyperalgesia (Ferreira et al. 1993). In most systems including sympathetic neurons, IL-6 effects depend on the presence of the soluble IL-6 receptor (sIL-6R) (März et al. 1999) which after ligand binding heteromerizes with the signal transducer molecule gp130 that is also utilized by other cytokines of the same family, e.g., leukemia inhibitory factor (Taga et al. 1989; Rose-John and Heinrich 1994).

IL-6/sIL-6R complex or hyper-IL-6 (HIL-6), a fusion protein mimicking the effects of IL-6/sIL-6R (Fischer et al. 1997), increases nociceptor-specific release of CGRP and induces sensitization of heat-activated ionic currents (Opree and Kress 2000; Obreja et al. 2002b, 2005). The sensitization involved activation of the Janus tyrosine kinase (Jak) and protein kinase C (PKC) but no alteration of intracellular Ca^{2+}. Similar signaling pathways have been identified for IL-6 in promoting spinal axon regeneration (Cafferty et al. 2004; Qiu et al. 2005).

SIGNAL TRANSDUCTION PATHWAYS OF PROINFLAMMATORY CYTOKINES IN PAIN: ROLE OF P38 MAP KINASE

In some peripheral tissues, such as synovial fibroblasts, TNF-α as well as IL-1β are thought to act both up- and downstream of p38 MAP kinase (p38) activation (Chabaud-Riou and Firestein 2004). However, specifics of this signal transduction cascade differ among cell types and depend in part on unique characteristics of the tissue as well as of the initiating insult (Fig. 1). One of the variables is that cell type determines which isoforms of p38 are available; in the nervous system the options are limited to p38α and β. In some systems, activation of different p38 isoforms has opposing effects on cellular processes (Pramanik et al. 2003). Understanding the interface between TNF-α and p38, at the level of both the DRG and the spinal cord dorsal horn, is of interest because both cytokines have been proposed as therapeutic targets for various chronic pain states.

DORSAL ROOT GANGLIA

DRG neurons express extracellular signal regulated kinases (ERK), Jun N-terminal kinases (JNK), and p38 MAP kinases. Pollock et al. (2002) incubated DRG neuronal cultures with TNF-α and examined them for phosphorylation of all three families of MAP kinases. Exposure to TNF-α induced increases in phospho-p38 and phospho-JNK, but not phospho-ERK. All three MAP kinases in DRG neurons are phosphorylated subsequent to the spinal nerve ligation (SNL) type of nerve injury (Obata et al. 2004), which implies some selectivity of the action of pro-inflammatory cytokines, or at least of TNF-α, on the various MAP kinase targets.

Following nerve injury, TNF-α expression increases in the DRG of the injured nerves; at least some of this increased expression has been localized to neurons, primarily small nociceptive neurons (Shubayev and Myers 2001; Schäfers et al. 2003a). Other sources of TNF-α in the ganglia include activated macrophages and satellite cells. Following SNL (Schäfers et al. 2003c) and sciatic nerve crush (Ohtori et al. 2004), the number of TNF receptors is also reported to increase on DRG neurons. The phosphorylated (potentially activated) form of the MAP kinases also increases in DRG neurons following SNL (Schäfers et al. 2003a; Obata et al. 2004). The majority of this activation occurs in small, presumably nociceptive neurons that co-stain for the capsaicin receptor (TRPV1) (Jin et al. 2003) or isolectin B4 (Schäfers et al. 2003d), and many of these cells are also positive for TNF-α. Recent work indicates that both isoforms of p38 are present in DRG neurons (C. Sommer and L. Sorkin, unpublished data). There is disparity among the reports of time course for this phenomenon; our laboratory has reported an early, transient peak of phospho-p38 occurring within 5 hours after SNL (Schäfers et al. 2003d). However, others have reported the first peak at 3 days (Jin et al. 2003). Systemic pretreatment with the TNF-receptor antagonist etanercept (1 mg/kg i.p.) blocked this early SNL-induced increase in phospho-p38 in the DRG. Interestingly, systemic pretreatment with etanercept (1 mg/kg, i.p., once every 3 days) also reduced SNL-induced mechanical allodynia over a 3-week period, while identical treatment beginning 1 day post-injury was without effect. Taken together, these data support the idea that TNF-α is upstream of p38 activation in the DRG and that this early peak in DRG phospho-p38 helps to trigger SNL-induced allodynia. In animals that were given etanercept prior to injury, discontinuation of treatment resulted in full manifestation of the allodynia. Thus, maintained blockade of TNF-α in the DRG appears to merely delay the processes leading to allodynia.

SPINAL CORD

Nerve injuries result in fast activation of both microglia and astrocytes throughout the dorsal horn (Hashizume et al. 2000). Many of these activated glia cells produce proinflammatory cytokines, and nerve injury produces a parallel increase in spinal IL-1β and IL-6 as well as TNF-α (Raghavendra et al. 2003). Phosphorylation of p38 also occurs in the spinal cord following nerve injury; the vast majority of phospho-p38 is found in the activated microglia (Jin et al. 2003; Tsuda et al. 2004), with a small fraction being found in neurons. We have observed the onset of spinal phospho-p38 at 5 hours post-injury with expression peaking at day 1 (Schäfers et al. 2003d). Microglial inhibition with minocycline prior to spinal nerve transection dose-dependently reduces the resulting mechanical allodynia (Raghavendra et al. 2003). Importantly, this therapy only works as a pretreatment; when given after nerve injury, it is without effect. Interestingly, minocycline post-treatment is much more effective than pretreatment in reducing injury-induced increases in all three pro-inflammatory cytokines, implying that these increases are downstream of microglial and presumably p38 activation. We observe similar differences between pretreatment and post-treatment results with spinal administration of both the TNF-α antagonist etanercept and SB203580, a relatively specific p38 inhibitor (Schäfers et al. 2003d), again implying a triggering function for the phospho-p38. Intrathecal administration of etanercept, starting pre-injury, blocks phosphorylation of p38 in the spinal cord (Svensson et al. 2005). These data imply that TNF-α acts both up- and downstream of p38 in the spinal cord.

P38 ISOFORMS

A recent study indicates that p38β, but not p38α, is involved in spinal mediation of hyperalgesia after tissue injury (Svensson et al. 2005). Although similar studies have not been performed for nerve injury, SNL-induced allodynia is reduced in p38β knockout mice (Martin et al. 2005). In the dorsal horn of the spinal cord, p38α is found exclusively in neurons, while p38β is located in microglia (Svensson et al. 2005). These data, in combination with the strong association between microglial p38 activation and nerve-injury-induced allodynia, support the assertion that, as in tissue-injury-induced hyperalgesia, dorsal horn p38β mediates nerve-injury-induced allodynia. Given the known signal transduction pathway in peripheral tissue, this finding would implicate MAP kinase kinase (MKK) 6, rather than MKK3, as the upstream activator of phospho-p38 (Chabaud-Riou and Firestein 2004). Delineation of this pathway with respect to isoforms and upstream kinases may provide us with more specific and better therapeutic targets for pain control.

CYTOKINES IN PAINFUL DISEASES IN HUMANS

RHEUMATOID ARTHRITIS

Rheumatoid arthritis is the disease in which the role of cytokines in disease progression and pain generation has been best recognized so far (Dayer and Demczuk 1984; Ridderstad et al. 1991; Koch et al. 1995). TNF-α has mostly been regarded as the main player, and pain was markedly reduced in patients receiving TNF-α antagonists during clinical trials (Elliott et al. 1994; Rankin et al. 1995; Maini et al. 1999; Moreland et al. 1999; Weinblatt and al. 2003). The TNF-α antagonists etanercept and infliximab are now widely used in patients with rheumatoid arthritis refractory to other treatments. The IL-1 antagonist anakinra is also effective in combination with methotrexate in patients with rheumatoid arthritis (Cohen et al. 2004).

BACK PAIN

Experimental data indicate that cytokines, in particular TNF-α, mediate pain in disk herniation. In humans, cytokine production occurs in disk material (Takahashi et al. 1996; Burke et al. 2002). Higher levels of IL-8 correlated with pain (Ahn et al. 2002; Brisby et al. 2002), and patients with persisting pain after diskectomy had higher serum IL-6 levels than those without pain (Geiss et al. 1997). A functional IL-1α polymorphism that increases IL-1α synthesis was found to be associated with low back pain (Solovieva et al. 2004).

In the randomized controlled trial using etanercept in ankylosing spondylitis, etanercept was efficient in reducing back pain (Gorman et al. 2002). Only open-label studies using TNF-α inhibition in patients with chronic back pain of other etiologies have been reported. Case reports showed perispinal etanercept to be efficient in patients with chronic diskogenic pain (Tobinick and Britschgi-Davoodifar 2003), and an open-label study and further case reports found an improvement in patients with low back pain with intravenous infliximab (Karppinen et al. 2003; Atcheson and Dymeck 2004; Korhonen et al. 2004). Randomized controlled long term trials will have to prove the validity of this treatment approach.

NEUROPATHIC PAIN

Peripheral neuropathies may be painful or painless. It has been hypothesized that one factor determining the painfulness of a neuropathy may be the individual tendency to react with high or low production of pro-inflammatory cytokines upon nerve injury (Rutkowski et al. 1999; see Fig. 2). The classical example of a correlation between cytokine levels and neuropathic pain is leprosy, in which a subgroup of patients have elevated serum levels of TNF-α and IL-1β and suffer from excruciating pain (Sarno et al. 1991). Treatment with thalidomide reduces TNF-α secretion in peripheral blood mononuclear cells by more than 90% and significantly reduces pain in these patients (Barnes et al. 1992). In other neuropathies, preliminary data also point to a correlation between cytokine expression and pain. In two series of sural nerve biopsies, cytokine levels were increased more often in patients with painful neuropathies (Empl et al. 2001; Lindenlaub and Sommer 2003; see Fig. 3). In addition, our own preliminary data point to higher expression of mRNA for proinflammatory cytokines and lower expression of anti-inflammatory cytokines in blood cells from patients with painful neuropathies compared to those with painless neuropathies and to controls. Data for postherpetic neuralgia (PHN) are still controversial. One study with 30 patients could not identify a correlation between cytokine expression and the development of PHN (Zak-Prelich et al. 2003). In

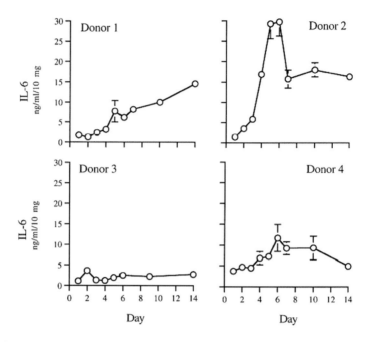

Fig. 2. Graphs depicting the release of cytokines by cultured human Schwann cells. Note the differences in temporal course and magnitude of cytokine release between donors. Reproduced from Rutkowski et al. (1999), with permission.

another study, however, an increase in serum IL-8 was identified as a predictor for the development of PHN (Kotani et al. 2004).

Complex regional pain syndrome (CRPS) is another condition in which the cytokine system has been suggested be involved. No differences in blood cytokine levels were found in a study comparing 26 patients with CRPS to controls (van de Beek et al. 2001). However, in a study using blister fluid and comparing cytokine levels from the affected and the unaffected side, an increase in IL-1β and TNF-α was found locally (Huygen et al. 2002, 2004). The same authors reported moderate improvement in two patients with CRPS treated with infliximab (Huygen et al. 2004a). One further case report describes remission of long-standing CRPS after treatment with thalidomide for Behçet's disease (Ching et al. 2003).

CHRONIC WIDESPREAD PAIN AND FIBROMYALGIA

In fibromyalgia, results of cytokine measurements are as yet conflicting, partly due to different methods used by the investigators and partly because of a variety of confounding factors such as concomitant diseases and medication.

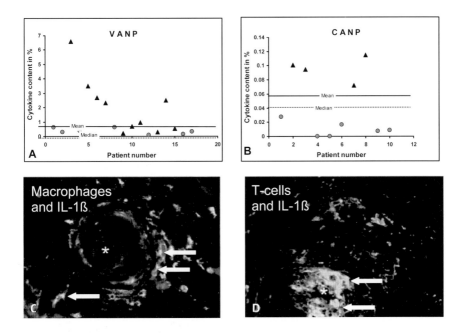

Fig. 3. Graphs showing quantification of cytokine immunoreactivity on sural nerve biopsy sections in patients with vasculitic neuropathy (VANP, A) and chronic axonal neuropathy (CANP, B). Black triangles represent patients with neuropathic pain, and gray circles patients without neuropathic pain. The solid line represents the mean value in each group, and the broken line the median in each group. Note that five patients with higher cytokine content than the mean and the median had neuropathic pain in VANP (A) and four in CANP (B). (C,D) Human sural nerve biopsy cryosections. Examples of immunostaining with double fluorescence (arrows) showing IL-1β immunoreactivity in macrophages (C) and T cells (D). Asterisks (*) denote endoneurial blood vessels. Adapted from Lindenlaub and Sommer (2003), with permission.

The published findings in fibromyalgia patients are a defect in IL-2 secretion (Hader et al. 1991); an increase in serum gp130, the common signal transducer protein of IL-6 and related cytokines, in soluble IL-6R and IL-1Ra (Maes et al. 1999); increases in IL-6, IL-8, and IL-1Ra (Wallace et al. 2001); an increase in IL-2 R and IL-8 (Gur et al. 2002); increased expression of IL-1β, IL-6, and TNF-α measured in skin biopsies from fibromyalgia patients (Salemi et al. 2003); and normal production of IL-1α, IL-6, TNF-α, and IL-10 by peripheral blood mononuclear cells from fibromyalgia patients (Amel Kashipaz et al. 2003). In our own series of 45 patients with chronic widespread pain, we found decreased levels of anti-inflammatory cytokines compared to controls (Üceyler et al. 2004).

TEMPOROMANDIBULAR JOINT DYSFUNCTION

Temporomandibular dysfunction (TMD) is another condition in which cytokines have been extensively studied (Lobbezoo et al. 2004). IL-1β, IL-6 and TNF-α were found in joint fluid (Fu et al. 1995a,b; Sandler et al. 1998; Kaneyama et al. 2002) and were associated with poor outcome, in particular IL-6 (Shafer et al. 1994; Alstergren et al. 1998). IL-1β was shown to induce IL-8 (Tobe et al. 2002) and CCL-5 (Ogura et al. 2004) in synovial cell fibroblasts. Other studies found a deficiency in the anti-inflammatory mediators IL-1Ra, IL-10, and transforming growth factor-β in TMD patients (Fang et al. 1999; Tominaga et al. 2004). Arthrocentesis has been used to reduce inflammatory mediators and IL-6 from the temporomandibular joint fluid as a therapeutic measure (Kaneyama et al. 2004).

CONCLUSIONS

Chronic pain states are modulated by a number of chemical mediators, among them pro- and anti-inflammatory cytokines. A large amount of pre-clinical data has been gathered over the last few years, elucidating the role of cytokines in different pain models and the molecular mechanisms by which cytokines may alter the function of nociceptive neurons. Clinical data on the function of cytokines in human pain states are also accumulating, supporting the relevance of these molecules for pain in clinical practice.

REFERENCES

Abe S, Mizusawa I, Kanno K, et al. Nitric oxide synthase expressions in rat dorsal root ganglion after a hind limb tourniquet. *Neuroreport* 2003; 14:2267–2270.

Ahn SH, Cho YW, Ahn MW, et al. mRNA expression of cytokines and chemokines in herniated lumbar intervertebral discs. *Spine* 2002; 27:911–917.

Alstergren P, Ernberg M, Kvarnstrom M, Kopp S. Interleukin-1 beta in synovial fluid from the arthritic temporomandibular joint and its relation to pain, mobility, and anterior open bite. *J Oral Maxillofac Surg* 1998; 56:1059–1065, discussion 1066.

Amel Kashipaz MR, Swinden D, Todd I, Powell RJ. Normal production of inflammatory cytokines in chronic fatigue and fibromyalgia syndromes determined by intracellular cytokine staining in short-term cultured blood mononuclear cells. *Clin Exp Immunol* 2003; 132:360–365.

Atcheson SG, Dymeck T. Rapid resolution of chronic sciatica with intravenous infliximab after failed epidural steroid injections. *Spine* 2004; 29:E248–250.

Barnes PF, Chatterjee D, Brennan PJ, et al. Tumor necrosis factor production in patients with leprosy. *Infect Immun* 1992; 60:1441–1446.

Brisby H, Olmarker K, Larsson K, et al. Proinflammatory cytokines in cerebrospinal fluid and serum in patients with disc herniation and sciatica. *Eur Spine J* 2002; 11:62–66.

Burke JG, Watson RW, McCormack D, et al. Spontaneous production of monocyte chemoat-tractant protein-1 and interleukin-8 by the human lumbar intervertebral disc. *Spine* 2002; 27:1402–1407.

Cafferty WB, Gardiner NJ, Das P, et al. Conditioning injury-induced spinal axon regeneration fails in interleukin-6 knock-out mice. *J Neurosci* 2004; 24:4432–4443.

Chabaud-Riou M, Firestein GS. Expression and activation of mitogen-activated protein kinase kinases-3 and -6 in rheumatoid arthritis. *Am J Pathol* 2004; 164:177–184.

Ching DWT, McClintock A, Beswick F. Successful treatment with low-dose thalidomide in a patient with both Behcet's disease and complex regional pain syndrome type I. *J Clin Rheumatology* 2003; 9:96–98.

Cohen SB, Moreland LW, Cush JJ, et al. A multicentre, double blind, randomised, placebo controlled trial of anakinra (Kineret), a recombinant interleukin 1 receptor antagonist, in patients with rheumatoid arthritis treated with background methotrexate. *Ann Rheum Dis* 2004; 63:1062–1068.

Copray JC, Mantingh I, Brouwer N, et al. Expression of interleukin-1 beta in rat dorsal root ganglia. *J Neuroimmunol* 2001; 118:203–211.

Cunha F, Poole S, Lorenzetti B, Ferreira S. The pivotal role of tumor necrosis factor alpha in the development of inflammatory hyperalgesia. *Br J Pharmacol* 1992; 107:660–664.

Cunha JM, Cunha FQ, Poole S, Ferreira SH. Cytokine-mediated inflammatory hyperalgesia limited by interleukin-1 receptor antagonist. *Br J Pharmacol* 2000; 130:1418–1424.

Dayer JM, Demczuk S. Cytokines and other mediators in rheumatoid arthritis. *Springer Semin Immunopathol* 1984; 7:387–413.

DeLeo JA, Colburn RW, Nichols M, Malhotra A. Interleukin-6-mediated hyperalgesia/allodynia and increased spinal IL-6 expression in a rat mononeuropathy model. *J Interferon Cytokine Res* 1996; 16:695–700.

Elliott MJ, Maini RN, Feldmann M, et al. Randomised double-blind comparison of chimeric monoclonal antibody to tumour necrosis factor alpha (cA2) versus placebo in rheumatoid arthritis. *Lancet* 1994; 344:1105–1110.

Empl M, Renaud S, Erne B, et al. TNF-alpha expression in painful and nonpainful neuropathies. *Neurology* 2001; 56:1371–1377.

Fang PK, Ma XC, Ma DL, Fu KY. Determination of interleukin-1 receptor antagonist, interleukin-10, and transforming growth factor-beta 1 in synovial fluid aspirates of patients with temporomandibular disorders. *J Oral Maxillofac Surg* 1999; 57:922–928; discussion 928–929.

Fehrenbacher JC, Burkey TH, Nicol GD, Vasko MR. Tumor necrosis factor alpha and interleukin-1 beta stimulate the expression of cyclooxygenase II but do not alter prostaglandin E_2 receptor mRNA levels in cultured dorsal root ganglia cells. *Pain* 2005; 113:113–122.

Ferreira S, Lorenzetti B, Bristow A, Poole S. Interleukin-1β as a potent hyperalgesic agent antagonized by a tripeptide analogue. *Nature* 1988; 334:698–700.

Ferreira S, Lorenzetti B, Poole S. Bradykinin initiates cytokine-mediated inflammatory hyperalgesia. *Br J Pharmacol* 1993; 110:1227–1231.

Fischer M, Goldschmitt J, Peschel C, et al. I. A bioactive designer cytokine for human hematopoietic progenitor cell expansion. *Nat Biotechnol* 1997; 15:142–145.

Freidin M, Bennett MV, Kessler JA. Cultured sympathetic neurons synthesize and release the cytokine interleukin 1 beta. *Proc Natl Acad Sci USA* 1992; 89:10440–10443.

Fu K, Ma X, Zhang Z, Chen W. Tumor necrosis factor in synovial fluid of patients with temporomandibular disorders. *J Oral Maxillofac Surg* 1995a; 53:424–426.

Fu K, Ma X, Zhang Z, et al. Interleukin-6 in synovial fluid and HLA-DR expression in synovium from patients with temporomandibular disorders. *J Orofac Pain* 1995b; 9:131–137.

Fu LW, Longhurst JC. Interleukin-1 beta sensitizes abdominal visceral afferents of cats to ischaemia and histamine. *J Physiol (Lond)* 1999; 521:249–260.

Fukuoka H, Kawatani M, Hisamitsu T, Takeshige C. Cutaneous hyperalgesia induced by peripheral injection of interleukin-1β in the rat. *Brain Res* 1994; 657:133–140.

Geiss A, Varadi E, Steinbach K, et al. Psychoneuroimmunological correlates of persisting sciatic pain in patients who underwent discectomy. *Neurosci Lett* 1997; 237:65–68.

Gorman JD, Sack KE, Davis JC, Jr. Treatment of ankylosing spondylitis by inhibition of tumor necrosis factor alpha. *N Engl J Med* 2002; 346:1349–1356.

Gur A, Karakoc M, Nas K, et al. Cytokines and depression in cases with fibromyalgia. *J Rheumatol* 2002; 29:358–361.

Hader N, Rimon D, Kinarty A, Lahat N. Altered interleukin-2 secretion in patients with primary fibromyalgia syndrome. *Arthritis Rheum* 1991; 34:866–872.

Hashizume H, DeLeo JA, Colburn RW, Weinstein JN. Spinal glial activation and cytokine expression after lumbar root injury in the rat. *Spine* 2000; 25:1206–1217.

Huygen FJ, De Bruijn AG, De Bruin MT, et al. Evidence for local inflammation in complex regional pain syndrome type 1. *Mediators Inflamm* 2002; 11:47–51.

Huygen FJ, Niehof S, Zijlstra FJ, et al. Successful treatment of CRPS 1 with anti-TNF. *J Pain Symptom Manage* 2004a; 27:101–103.

Huygen FJ, Ramdhani N, Van Toorenenbergen A, et al. Mast cells are involved in inflammatory reactions during complex regional pain syndrome type 1. *Immunol Lett* 2004b; 91:147–154.

Igwe OJ. c-Src kinase activation regulates preprotachykinin gene expression and substance P secretion in rat sensory ganglia. *Eur J Neurosci* 2003; 18:1719–1730.

Inoue A, Ikoma K, Morioka N, et al. Interleukin-1 beta induces substance P release from primary afferent neurons through the cyclooxygenase-2 system. *J Neurochem* 1999; 73:2206–2213.

Ji RR, Samad TA, Jin SX, et al. p38 MAPK activation by NGF in primary sensory neurons after inflammation increases TRPV1 levels and maintains heat hyperalgesia. *Neuron* 2002; 36:57–68.

Jin S-X, Zhuang Z-Y, Woolf C, Ji R. p38 mitogen-activated protein kinase is activated after a spinal nerve ligation in spinal cord microglia and dorsal root ganglion neurons and contributes to the generation of neuropathic pain. *J Neurosci* 2003; 23:4017–4022.

Junger H, Sorkin LS. Nociceptive and inflammatory effects of subcutaneous TNF alpha. *Pain* 2000; 85:145–151.

Kaneyama K, Segami N, Nishimura M, et al. Importance of proinflammatory cytokines in synovial fluid from 121 joints with temporomandibular disorders. *Br J Oral Maxillofac Surg* 2002; 40:418–423.

Kaneyama K, Segami N, Nishimura M, et al. The ideal lavage volume for removing bradykinin, interleukin-6, and protein from the temporomandibular joint by arthrocentesis. *J Oral Maxillofac Surg* 2004; 62:657–661.

Karppinen J, Korhonen T, Malmivaara A, et al. Tumor necrosis factor-alpha monoclonal antibody, infliximab, used to manage severe sciatica. *Spine* 2003; 28:750–753; discussion 753–754.

Koch AE, Kunkel SL, Strieter RM. Cytokines in rheumatoid arthritis. *J Investig Med* 1995; 43:28–38.

Korhonen T, Karppinen J, Malmivaara A, et al. Efficacy of infliximab for disc herniation-induced sciatica: one-year follow-up. *Spine* 2004; 29:2115–2119.

Kotani N, Kudo R, Sakurai Y, et al. Cerebrospinal fluid interleukin 8 concentrations and the subsequent development of postherpetic neuralgia. *Am J Med* 2004; 116:318–324.

Li Y, Ji A, Weihe E, Schafer MK. Cell-specific expression and lipopolysaccharide-induced regulation of tumor necrosis factor alpha (TNF alpha) and TNF receptors in rat dorsal root ganglion. *J Neurosci* 2004; 24:9623–9631.

Lindenlaub T, Sommer C. Cytokines in sural nerve biopsies from inflammatory and non-inflammatory neuropathies. *Acta Neuropathol* 2003; 105:593–602.

Lobbezoo F, Drangsholt M, Peck C, et al. Topical review: new insights into the pathology and diagnosis of disorders of the temporomandibular joint. *J Orofac Pain* 2004; 18:181–191.

Maes M, Libbrecht I, Van Hunsel F, et al. The immune-inflammatory pathophysiology of fibromyalgia: increased serum soluble gp130, the common signal transducer protein of various neurotrophic cytokines. *Psychoneuroendocrinology* 1999; 24:371–383.

Maini R, St Clair EW, Breedveld F, et al. Infliximab (chimeric anti-tumour necrosis factor alpha monoclonal antibody) versus placebo in rheumatoid arthritis patients receiving concomitant methotrexate: a randomised phase III trial. ATTRACT Study Group. *Lancet* 1999; 354:1932–1939.

Martin WM, BA M, J P, et al. p38b contributes to injury-induced nociceptive, but not inflammatory responses in mice. *Soc Neurosci Abstracts* 2005.

März P, Otten U, Rose-John S. Neural activities of IL-6-type cytokines often depend on soluble cytokine receptors. *Eur J Neurosci* 1999; 11:2995–3004.

Milligan ED, Twining C, Chacur M, et al. Spinal glia and proinflammatory cytokines mediate mirror-image neuropathic pain in rats. *J Neurosci* 2003; 23:1026–1040.

Moreland LW, Schiff MH, Baumgartner SW, et al. Etanercept therapy in rheumatoid arthritis. A randomized, controlled trial. *Ann Intern Med* 1999; 130:478–486.

Murphy PG, Ramer MS, Borthwick L, et al. Endogenous interleukin-6 contributes to hypersensitivity to cutaneous stimuli and changes in neuropeptides associated with chronic nerve constriction in mice. *Eur J Neurosci* 1999; 11:2243–2253.

Obata K, Yamanaka H, Kobayashi K, et al. Role of mitogen-activated protein kinase activation in injured and intact primary afferent neurons for mechanical and heat hypersensitivity after spinal nerve ligation. *J Neurosci* 2004; 24:10211–10222.

Obreja O, Rathee PK, Lips KS, et al. IL-1 beta potentiates heat-activated currents in rat sensory neurons: involvement of IL-1RI, tyrosine kinase, and protein kinase C. *Faseb J* 2002a; 16:1497–503.

Obreja O, Schmelz M, Poole S, Kress M. Interleukin-6 in combination with its soluble IL-6 receptor sensitises rat skin nociceptors to heat, in vivo. *Pain* 2002b; 96:57–62.

Obreja O, Biasio W, Andratsch M, et al. Fast modulation of heat-activated ionic current by proinflammatory interleukin 6 in rat sensory neurons. *Brain* 2005; 128:1634–1641.

Ogura N, Tobe M, Sakamaki H, et al. Interleukin-1 beta increases RANTES gene expression and production in synovial fibroblasts from human temporomandibular joint. *J Oral Pathol Med* 2004; 33:629–633.

Ohtori S, Takahashi K, Moriya H, Myers RR. TNF-alpha and TNF-alpha receptor type 1 upregulation in glia and neurons after peripheral nerve injury: studies in murine DRG and spinal cord. *Spine* 2004; 29:1082–1088.

Oka T, Oka K, Hosoi M, Hori T. Intracerebroventricular injection of interleukin-6 induces thermal hyperalgesia in rats. *Brain Res* 1995; 692:123–128.

Okamoto K, Martin DP, Schmelzer JD, et al. Pro- and anti-inflammatory cytokine gene expression in rat sciatic nerve chronic constriction injury model of neuropathic pain. *Exp Neurol* 2001; 169:386–391.

Opree A, Kress M. Involvement of the proinflammatory cytokines tumor necrosis factor-alpha, IL-1 beta, and IL-6 but not IL-8 in the development of heat hyperalgesia: effects on heat-evoked calcitonin gene-related peptide release from rat skin. *J Neurosci* 2000; 20:6289–6293.

Parada CA, Yeh JJ, Joseph EK, Levine JD. Tumor necrosis factor receptor type-1 in sensory neurons contributes to induction of chronic enhancement of inflammatory hyperalgesia in rat. *Eur J Neurosci* 2003; 17:1847–1852.

Perkins MN, Kelly D. Interleukin-1β-induced desArg⁹ bradykinin-mediated thermal hyperalgesia in the rat. *Neuropharmacology* 1994; 33:657–660.

Pollock J, McFarlane SM, Connell MC, et al. TNF-alpha receptors simultaneously activate Ca^{2+} mobilisation and stress kinases in cultured sensory neurones. *Neuropharmacology* 2002; 42:93–106.

Poole S, Cunha FQ, Selkirk S, et al. Cytokine-mediated inflammatory hyperalgesia limited by interleukin-10. *Br J Pharmacol* 1995; 115:684–688.

Pramanik R, Qi X, Borowicz S, et al. p38 isoforms have opposite effects on AP-1-dependent transcription through regulation of c-Jun. The determinant roles of the isoforms in the p38 MAPK signal specificity. *J Biol Chem* 2003; 278:4831–4839.

Qiu J, Cafferty WB, McMahon SB, Thompson SW. Conditioning injury-induced spinal axon regeneration requires signal transducer and activator of transcription 3 activation. *J Neurosci* 2005; 25:1645–1653.

Raghavendra V, Tanga F, DeLeo JA. Inhibition of microglial activation attenuates the development but not existing hypersensitivity in a rat model of neuropathy. *J Pharmacol Exp Ther* 2003; 306:624–630.

Rankin EC, Choy EH, Kassimos D, et al. The therapeutic effects of an engineered human anti-tumour necrosis factor alpha antibody (CDP571) in rheumatoid arthritis. *Br J Rheumatol* 1995; 34:334–342.

Ridderstad A, Abedi-Valugerdi M, Moller E. Cytokines in rheumatoid arthritis. *Ann Med* 1991; 23:219–223.

Rose-John S, Heinrich PC. Soluble receptors for cytokines and growth factors: generation and biological function. *Biochem J* 1994; 300(Pt 2):281–290.

Rutkowski JL, Tuite GF, Lincoln PM, et al. Signals for proinflammatory cytokine secretion by human Schwann cells. *J Neuroimmunol* 1999; 101:47–60.

Salemi S, Rethage J, Wollina U, et al. Detection of interleukin 1 beta (IL-1 beta), IL-6, and tumor necrosis factor-alpha in skin of patients with fibromyalgia. *J Rheumatol* 2003; 30:146–150.

Sandler NA, Buckley MJ, Cillo JE, Braun TW. Correlation of inflammatory cytokines with arthroscopic findings in patients with temporomandibular joint internal derangements. *J Oral Maxillofac Surg* 1998; 56:534-543; discussion 543–544.

Sarno EN, Grau GE, Vieira LM, Nery JA. Serum levels of tumour necrosis factor-alpha and interleukin-1 beta during leprosy reactional states. *Clin Exp Immunol* 1991; 84:103–108.

Schäfers M, Geis C, Svensson CI, et al. Selective increase of tumour necrosis factor-alpha in injured and spared myelinated primary afferents after chronic constrictive injury of rat sciatic nerve. *Eur J Neurosci* 2003a; 17:791–804.

Schäfers M, Lee DH, Brors D, et al. Increased sensitivity of injured and adjacent uninjured rat primary sensory neurons to exogenous tumor necrosis factor-alpha after spinal nerve ligation. *J Neurosci* 2003b; 23:3028–3038.

Schäfers M, Sorkin LS, Geis C, Shubayev VI. Spinal nerve ligation induces transient upregulation of tumor necrosis factor receptors 1 and 2 in injured and adjacent uninjured dorsal root ganglia in the rat. *Neurosci Lett* 2003c; 347:179–182.

Schäfers M, Svensson CI, Sommer C, Sorkin LS. Tumor necrosis factor-alpha induces mechanical allodynia after spinal nerve ligation by activation of p38 MAPK in primary sensory neurons. *J Neurosci* 2003d; 23:2517–2521.

Shafer DM, Assael L, White LB, Rossomando EF. Tumor necrosis factor-alpha as a biochemical marker of pain and outcome in temporomandibular joints with internal derangements. *J Oral Maxillofac Surg* 1994; 52:786–791; discussion 791–792.

Shubayev VI, Myers RR. Upregulation and interaction of TNF alpha and gelatinases A and B in painful peripheral nerve injury. *Brain Res* 2000; 855:83–89.

Shubayev VI, Myers RR. Axonal transport of TNF-alpha in painful neuropathy: distribution of ligand tracer and TNF receptors. *J Neuroimmunol* 2001; 114:48–56.

Solovieva S, Leino-Arjas P, Saarela J, et al. Possible association of interleukin 1 gene locus polymorphisms with low back pain. *Pain* 2004; 109:8–19.

Sommer C, Schäfers M. Painful mononeuropathy in C57BL/Wld mice with delayed Wallerian degeneration: differential effects of cytokine production and nerve regeneration on thermal and mechanical hypersensitivity. *Brain Res* 1998; 784:154–162.

Sommer C, Petrausch S, Lindenlaub T, Toyka KV. Neutralizing antibodies to interleukin 1-receptor reduce pain associated behavior in mice with experimental neuropathy. *Neurosci Lett* 1999; 270:25–28.

Sommer C, Lindenlaub T, Teuteberg P, et al. Anti-TNF-neutralizing antibodies reduce pain-related behavior in two different mouse models of painful mononeuropathy. *Brain Res* 2001; 913:86–89.

Svensson CI, Fitzsimmons B, Azizi S, et al. Spinal p38 beta isoform mediates tissue injury-induced hyperalgesia and spinal sensitization. *J Neurochem* 2005; 92:1508–1520.

Taga T, Hibi M, Hirata Y, et al. Interleukin-6 triggers the association of its receptor with a possible signal transducer, gp130. *Cell* 1989; 58:573–581.

Takahashi H, Suguro T, Okazima Y, et al. Inflammatory cytokines in the herniated disc of the lumbar spine. *Spine* 1996; 21:218–224.

Tobe M, Ogura N, Abiko Y, Nagura H. Interleukin-1 beta stimulates interleukin-8 production and gene expression in synovial cells from human temporomandibular joint. *J Oral Maxillofac Surg* 2002; 60:741–747.

Tobinick EL, Britschgi-Davoodifar S. Perispinal TNF-alpha inhibition for discogenic pain. *Swiss Med Wkly* 2003; 133:170–177.

Tominaga K, Habu M, Sukedai M, et al. IL-1 beta, IL-1 receptor antagonist and soluble type II IL-1 receptor in synovial fluid of patients with temporomandibular disorders. *Arch Oral Biol* 2004; 49:493–499.

Tsuda M, Mizokoshi A, Shigemoto-Mogami Y, et al. Activation of p38 mitogen-activated protein kinase in spinal hyperactive microglia contributes to pain hypersensitivity following peripheral nerve injury. *Glia* 2004; 45:89–95.

Üceyler N, Valenza R, Sprotte G, Sommer C. Fibromyalgia and cytokine expression under IVIG treatment. In: *Soc Neurosci Abstracts* 2004; Program No. 863.10.

van de Beek WJ, Remarque EJ, Westendorp RG, van Hilten JJ. Innate cytokine profile in patients with complex regional pain syndrome is normal. *Pain* 2001; 91:259–61.

Vogel C, Lindenlaub T, Tiegs G, et al. Pain related behavior in TNF-receptor deficient mice. In: Devor M, Rowbotham MC, Wiesenfeld-Hallin Z (Eds). *Proceedings of the 9th World Congress on Pain,* Progress in Pain Research and Management, Vol. 16. Seattle: IASP Press, 2000, pp 249–257.

Wagner R, Myers RR. Endoneurial injection of TNF-alpha produces neuropathic pain behaviors. *Neuroreport* 1996; 7:2897–901.

Wagner R, Janjigian M, Myers RR. Anti-inflammatory interleukin-10 therapy in CCI neuropathy decreases thermal hyperalgesia, macrophage recruitment, and endoneurial TNF-alpha expression. *Pain* 1998; 74:35–42.

Wallace DJ, Linker-Israeli M, Hallegua D, et al. Cytokines play an aetiopathogenetic role in fibromyalgia: a hypothesis and pilot study. *Rheumatology (Oxford)* 2001; 40:743–749.

Watkins LR, Maier SF. Implications of immune-to-brain communication for sickness and pain. *Proc Natl Acad Sci USA* 1999; 96:7710–7713.

Weinblatt ME, Keystone EC, Furst DE, et al. Adalimumab, a fully human anti-tumor necrosis factor alpha monoclonal antibody, for the treatment of rheumatoid arthritis in patients taking concomitant methotrexate: the ARMADA trial. *Arthritis Rheum* 2003; 48:35–45.

Woolf CJ, Allchorne A, Safieh-Garabedian B, Poole S. Cytokines, nerve growth factor and inflammatory hyperalgesia: the contribution of tumour necrosis factor alpha. *Br J Pharmacol* 1997; 121:417–424.

Xu XJ, Hao JX, Andell-Jonsson S, et al. Nociceptive responses in interleukin-6-deficient mice to peripheral inflammation and peripheral nerve section. *Cytokine* 1997; 9:1028–1033.

Zak-Prelich M, McKenzie RC, Sysa-Jedrzejowska A, Norval M. Local immune responses and systemic cytokine responses in zoster: relationship to the development of postherpetic neuralgia. *Clin Exp Immunol* 2003; 131:318–323.

Zhong J, Dietzel ID, Wahle P, et al. Sensory impairments and delayed regeneration of sensory axons in interleukin-6-deficient mice. *J Neurosci* 1999; 19:4305–4313.

Correspondence to: Prof. Dr. Claudia Sommer, Neurologische Klinik der Universität Josef-Schneider-Str. 11, D-97080 Würzburg, Germany. Fax: 49-931-201-23697; email: sommer@mail.uni-wuerzburg.de.

Proceedings of the 11th World Congress on Pain,
edited by Herta Flor, Eija Kalso, and Jonathan O.
Dostrovsky, IASP Press, Seattle, © 2006.

14

5-HT$_{1A}$ Receptors in Chronic Pain Processing and Control

Francis C. Colpaert,[a] Michel Hamon,[b] and Zsuzsanna Wiesenfeld-Hallin[c]

[a]Pierre Fabre Research Institute, Toulouse, France; [b]INSERM/UPMC, U677, Neuropsychopharmacology Department, Pierre and Marie Curie Faculty of Medicine, Paris, France; [c]Karolinska Institute, Department of Clinical Neuroscience, Section of Clinical Neurophysiology, Karolinska University Hospital, Huddinge, Stockholm, Sweden

Serotonin in the central nervous system (CNS) has long been considered to have an important role in the control of pain, for example through descending inhibition (Hamon and Bourgoin 1999). The serotonin (5-hydroxytryptamine [5-HT]) system is extremely complex, with a multitude of receptors mediating 5-HT's cellular effects (Barnes and Sharp 1999). However, the 5-HT$_{1A}$ subtype of serotonin receptors has never previously been considered as a molecular target for pain therapy (e.g., Dray and Rang 1998; Haegerstrand 1998; Kowaluk et al. 1998; Hunt and Mantyh 2001; Sah et al. 2003). This chapter presents evidence that the very high-efficacy activation of 5-HT$_{1A}$ receptors in the CNS may be more useful than opioid receptor activation for treating pain states. Previous studies of the mechanisms of opioid tolerance have paved the way for the present studies on 5-HT$_{1A}$-receptor actions.

SIGNAL TRANSDUCTION IN PAIN-PROCESSING SYSTEMS

We and our colleagues have proposed the theory that any input to pain-processing systems causes not a single effect, but dual effects that are bidirectional, or opposite in sign (Colpaert 1978, 1996; Colpaert and Frégnac 2001; Xu et al. 2003). Thus, morphine not only causes analgesia as a "first-order" effect, but also elicits a "second-order" hyperalgesia that outlasts opioid receptor activation for some period of time. The first-order analgesia results directly from the receptor activation; the second-order effect, however, is an indirect consequence of the analgesia that occurred and follows later in time. Upon chronic opioid exposure, the second-order pain, or sensitization to nociceptive input, grows and neutralizes the first-order analgesia. Thus, opioid tolerance may, paradoxically, be partly due to opioid-induced pain (Colpaert 1996; Mao 2002; Ossipov et al. 2003; Xu et al. 2003).

Furthermore, the same theory suggests that the stimulation of peripheral nociceptors should initially produce pain as a first-order effect, but also hypoalgesia as a second-order effect. In chronic pain states, the increase of the second-order hypoalgesia should progressively neutralize the first-order pain and develop into increasing analgesia (i.e., inverse tolerance). Equally important is the proposal that any noxious stimulus can, paradoxically, cooperate with another concomitant noxious stimulus, inducing second-order hypoalgesia (Colpaert 1978, 1996). Thus, finding the right agent should result in the relief of severe pain, even opioid-resistant chronic pains of neuropathic origin. A vast array of neuropharmacological tools have been tested in an attempt to identify a molecular action to verify this hypothesis. We now have identified very high-efficacy 5-HT$_{1A}$-receptor agonists that may permit us to achieve those neuroadaptive and therapeutic objectives (Colpaert et al. 2002).

F 13640: A HIGH-EFFICACY 5-HT$_{1A}$-RECEPTOR AGONIST

F 13640 is a newly discovered methylamino-pyridine with nanomolar affinity for both rat and human G-protein-coupled 5-HT$_{1A}$ receptors. This compound is highly selective, and even at a thousand-fold higher concentration it does not interact with any known neurotransmitter receptors, uptake sites, ion channels, or enzymes. Importantly, F 13640 causes activation of 5-HT$_{1A}$ receptors to a very large extent, stimulating the binding of the receptor to the G protein by a magnitude far greater than is observed with buspirone, 8-OH-DPAT, and other, more recently developed, selective 5-HT$_{1A}$-receptor agonists (Colpaert et al. 2002; Pauwels and Colpaert 2003; Wurch et al. 2003). This unique combination of potency, selectivity, and high efficacy is also observed in vivo. Following systemic administration, F 13640 readily penetrates the brain (Bardin et al. 2005), inhibits spinal cord wide dynamic neurons, and diminishes single motor unit responses to nociceptive electrical stimulation (You et al. 2005). It exerts analgesia from doses of 0.029 mg/kg onward (Bardin et al. 2003). Its effects are consistently antagonized by the selective 5-HT$_{1A}$ antagonist, WAY 100635 (Colpaert et al. 2002; Bardin et al. 2003; Buritova et al. 2003). In the amplitude of its 5-HT$_{1A}$-receptor-mediated actions, F 13640 is unrivaled by any other selective 5-HT$_{1A}$-receptor ligands (Colpaert et al. 2002; Bardin et al. 2003).

CO-OPERATION AND INVERSE TOLERANCE: ACUTE ACTIONS

Mechanical stimulation of the hindpaw sufficient to induce vocalization was used to test drug effects in rats (Colpaert et al. 2002). Whereas 5 mg/kg of morphine produced hypoalgesia followed by hyperalgesia, 0.63 mg/kg of F 13640 caused hyperalgesia followed by hypoalgesia. Thus, the data demonstrate bidirectional signal transduction and show that activation of 5-HT$_{1A}$ receptors results in effects that are the inverse of those following μ-opioid-receptor activation. Whereas repeated injection of morphine caused hyperalgesia and tolerance to its analgesic effect, repeated F 13640 injection caused hypoalgesia and tolerance to its proalgesic effect. Following a 14-day infusion of either 5 mg/kg/day of morphine or 0.63 mg/kg/day of F 13640, rats demonstrated normal sensitivity to mechanical stimulation. The opioid antagonist naloxone administered to morphine-infused animals caused hyperalgesia, whereas the 5-HT$_{1A}$ antagonist WAY 100635 in F 13640-infused animals caused powerful hypoalgesia (Colpaert et al. 2002), providing initial evidence that high-efficacy 5-HT$_{1A}$-receptor stimulation may exert a preemptive analgesic action on nociceptive pain.

F 13640 initially produces hyperalgesia in normal rats, but it produces antinociception in rats that have pain following an intraplantar formalin injection. Similar effects occur with other 5-HT$_{1A}$-receptor ligands (Bardin et al. 2001; Colpaert et al. 2002), but the magnitude of these effects depends on the efficacy of the ligands (Colpaert et al. 2002). Indeed, with the exception of morphine, none of the most commonly available analgesics rivals the magnitude of antinociception produced by F 13640 in this model (Bardin et al. 2003). The expression of c-Fos protein in spinal cord dorsal horn neurons following formalin injection was similarly suppressed by 20 mg/kg of intraperitoneal (i.p.) morphine and 0.63 mg/kg of i.p. F 13640 (Buritova et al. 2005).

The effect of F 13640 was also tested in a model of severe intra- and postoperative pain associated with orthopedic surgery in rats (Brennan et al. 1996; Houghton et al. 1997). Pre-operative i.p. injection of 0.63 mg/kg of the short-acting opioid remifentanil and the same dose of F 13640 lowered the requirement of intraoperative isoflurane anesthesia, indicating equivalent analgesic effect of the two drugs. F 13640 applied after surgery caused a long-lasting, powerful suppression of postoperative pain behaviors such as paw flexion and elevation, whereas remifentanil's analgesic effect was short-lived and was followed by a prolonged hyperalgesia (Kiss et al. 2005). Thus, high-efficacy 5-HT$_{1A}$ receptor agonists may be superior to opioids and also may eliminate the short- and long-term increases in postoperative pain induced by opioids.

LONG-TERM NEUROADAPTIVE ACTIONS

In the studies described in this section, drugs were infused by s.c. implanted osmotic pumps for 2 weeks or longer in rat models of chronic nociceptive or neuropathic pain.

CHRONIC NOCICEPTIVE PAIN

The elective drinking of a fentanyl solution is a measure of spontaneous, persistent, and severe chronic nociceptive pain associated with adjuvant arthritis in the rat (Colpaert 1987; Colpaert et al. 2001). In normal rats, F 13640 at 0.63 mg/kg/day causes hyperalgesia, whereas in arthritic rats it causes full antinociception that is at least equivalent to that reached with 5 mg/kg/day of morphine (Colpaert et al. 2002), a dose at which morphine produces dependence. Morphine infusion produces antinociception for 14 days in arthritic rats, a surprising observation given that the same treatment in normal rats can result in complete analgesic tolerance within 8 hours after pump implantation (Colpaert et al. 2002). These results suggest that nociceptive stimulation hampers the development of opioid tolerance (Colpaert 1996). Analgesics with other mechanisms of action (i.e., imipramine at 2.5 mg/kg/day, ketamine at 20 mg/kg/day, and gabapentin at 10 mg/kg/day) were inactive (Colpaert et al. 2002). As with tonic nociceptive pain, the data suggest that high-efficacy 5-HT_{1A}-receptor activation produces antinociception comparable to that obtained with morphine.

CHRONIC NEUROPATHIC PAIN

Unilateral chronic constriction injury of the common sciatic nerve is a model of peripheral neuropathic pain, and operated rats demonstrate a lowered threshold to mechanical stimulation (Bennett and Xie 1988). A 2-week infusion of morphine, ketamine, or imipramine produced no significant increase of the withdrawal threshold, while gabapentin had a significant effect. F 13640 produced a greater, highly significant increase, suggesting marked efficacy (Colpaert et al. 2002).

In a model of central neuropathic pain, ischemic injury to the spinal cord dorsal horn causes allodynic responses to cold and mechanical stimulations with von Frey filaments and brushing (Hao et al. 1998). Morphine, ketamine, imipramine, and gabapentin did not relieve the allodynia to any of the stimuli, whereas F 13640 robustly inhibited all three responses (Colpaert et al. 2002). In fact, the antinociceptive effects of F 13640 increased during the course of the 2-week treatment.

Acute administration of F 13640 and morphine counteracts allodynic responses to von Frey filament stimulation in rats with chronic constriction injury of the infra-orbital nerve (Deseure et al. 2002), a model of orofacial neuropathic pain (Vos et al. 1994). In this model, morphine initially produces robust, significant antinociception, but complete tolerance develops after 2 weeks. In another demonstration of inverse tolerance, the effects of F 13640 increased rather than diminished during the 2-week period (Deseure et al. 2003, 2004; see also Bruins Slot et al. 2003). These data suggest that high-efficacy 5-HT$_{1A}$-receptor activation may produce exceptionally powerful and sustained "symptomatic" analgesia in chronic neuropathic pains of peripheral or central origin.

PREEMPTIVE AND CURATIVE-LIKE ANALGESIA

Opioid-induced hyperalgesia and tolerance may outlast μ-opioid-receptor activation for a long time following the termination of opioid administration (Cochin and Kornetsky 1964; Colpaert 1996). The analgesic effect of F 13640 also outlasted its administration. Rats were infused with 0.63 mg/kg/day of F 13640 for 8 weeks starting 24 hours before the spinal cord injury. Reduction of cold and mechanical allodynia persisted unabated for 2 months following termination of treatment (Wu et al. 2003). These data suggest that high-efficacy 5-HT$_{1A}$-receptor activation may powerfully preempt pains ensuing from neuronal damage that may arise from ischemia, surgical nerve injury, or diabetes. Furthermore, rats with spinal cord injury that fully developed allodynia were infused with 0.63 mg/kg/day of F 13640 for 56 days. The treatment increasingly alleviated and eventually normalized the allodynic responses, further demonstrating inverse tolerance. More importantly, during the 70-day period that followed, the effects of F 13640 persisted, demonstrating an unprecedented curative-like action on neuropathic pain[1] (Colpaert et al. 2004). It remains to be shown whether these preemptive and curative-like actions are mediated by neuroprotective effects such as the inhibition of astroglial reactions by 5-HT$_{1A}$

---

[1] The terms "symptomatic," "preemptive," and "curative-like" distinguish three conditions in which the effects of analgesic drugs can be assessed. Traditionally, "symptomatic" analgesia is said to occur when a drug diminishes an established pain response by its molecular action. "Preemptive" analgesia refers to the observation that a drug, when administered prior to the development of a pain response, diminishes that response at a time when the drug action has ended. However, when F 13640 was administered, and then discontinued, at the time that a pain response had been well established, the drug effect persisted for a long, albeit finite, period of time during which the drug action was no longer ongoing; thus, in analogy to anticancer treatment effects assessed in similar conditions, we termed this effect "curative-like" (Colpaert et al. 2004).

agonists in ischemic brain tissue (Ramos et al. 2004). Another mechanism to be considered is the well-established regional difference in functional adaptation of 5-HT$_{1A}$ receptors upon long-term stimulation by agonists. Thus, chronic treatment with direct agonists or with indirect agonists (i.e., 5-HT reuptake inhibitors) produces a marked desensitization of 5-HT$_{1A}$ autoreceptors on 5-HT neurons in raphe nuclei, without altering the functional characteristics of postsynaptic 5-HT$_{1A}$ receptors in projection areas of these neurons (Lanfumey and Hamon 2004), such as the dorsal horn of the spinal cord (Hamon and Bourgoin 1999). As a result, the 5-HT$_{1A}$ autoreceptor-mediated inhibitory feedback control of 5-HT neurotransmission vanishes, which allows maximal 5-HT$_{1A}$ signaling at postsynaptic receptors (Lanfumey and Hamon 2004). Whether these differential adaptive receptor mechanisms contribute to the progressive increase of antiallodynic effects in the course of chronic F 13640 treatment should be investigated.

CONCLUSION

The evidence from animal studies suggests that high-efficacy 5-HT$_{1A}$-receptor stimulation presents a new approach for the treatment of a variety of pain states. Antinociception was achieved even in models that do not respond to high-efficacy opioids. As this approach has never before been studied in humans, clinical studies are now required to prove the concept.

ACKNOWLEDGMENTS

We gratefully acknowledge the participation in the studies summarized in this chapter by I. Kiss, L. Bardin, A. Degryse, I. Gomezde Segura, L. Arendt-Nielsen, J.P. Tarayre, W. Koek, P. Pauwels, T. Wurch, C. Cosi, E. Carilla, B. Vacher, M.B. Assié, J.P. Ribet, L. Bruins Slot, J. Buritova, J.M. Besson, K. Deseure, H. Adriaensen, H.J. You, S. Bourgoin, V. Kayser, J.-X. Hao, X.-J. Xu and W.-P. Wu.

REFERENCES

Bardin L, Tarayre JP, Koek W, Colpaert FC. In the formalin model of tonic nociceptive pain, 8-OH-DPAT produces 5-HT$_{1A}$ receptor-mediated, behaviorally specific analgesia. *Eur J Pharmacol* 2001; 421:109–114.

Bardin L, Tarayre JP, Malfetes N, Koek W, Colpaert FC. Profound, non-opioid analgesia produced by the high-efficacy 5-HT$_{1A}$ agonist F 13640 in the formalin model of tonic nociceptive pain. *Pharmacology* 2003; 67:182–194.

Bardin L, Assié MB, Pélissou M, et al. Dual, hyperalgesic and analgesic effects of the high-efficacy 5-hydroxytryptamine₁ₐ (5-HT₁ₐ) agonist F 13640 [(3-chloro-4-fluoro-phenyl)-[4-fluoro-4-{[(5-methyl-pyridin-2-ylmethyl)-amino]-methyl}piperidin-1-yl]methanone, fumaric acid salt]: relationship with 5-HT₁ₐ receptor occupancy and kinetic parameters. *J Pharmacol Exp Ther* 2005; 312:1034–1042.

Barnes NM, Sharp T. A review of central 5-HT receptors and their function. *Neuropharmacology* 1999; 38:1083–1152.

Bennett GJ, Xie YK. A peripheral mononeuropathy in rat that produces disorders of pain sensation like those seen in man. *Pain* 1988; 33:87–107.

Brennan TJ, Vandermeulen EP, Gebhart GF. Characterisation of a rat model of incisional pain. *Pain* 1996; 64:493–501.

Bruins Slot LA, Koek W, Tarayre JP, Colpaert FC. Tolerance and inverse tolerance to the hyperalgesic and analgesic actions, respectively, of the novel analgesic, F 13640. *Eur J Pharmacol* 2003; 466:271–279.

Buritova J, Tarayre JP, Besson JM, Colpaert F. The novel analgesic and high-efficacy 5-HT₁ₐ receptor agonist, F 13640, induces c-Fos protein expression in spinal cord dorsal horn neurons. *Brain Res* 2003; 974:212–221.

Buritova J, Larrue S, Aliaga M, Besson J-M, Colpaert F. Effects of the high-efficacy 5-HT₁ₐ receptor agonist, F 13640, in the formalin pain model: a c-Fos study. *Eur J Pharmacol* 2005; 514:121–130.

Cochin J, Kornetsky C. Development and loss of tolerance to morphine in the rat after single and multiple injections. *J Pharmacol Exp Ther* 1964; 145:1–10.

Colpaert FC. Narcotic cue, narcotic analgesia, and the tolerance problem: the regulation of sensitivity to drug cues and to pain by an internal cue processing model. In: Colpaert FC, Rosecrans JA (Eds). *Stimulus Properties of Drugs: Ten Years of Progress*. Amsterdam: Elsevier/North Holland Biomedical Press, 1978, pp 301–321.

Colpaert FC. Evidence that adjuvant arthritis in the rat is associated with chronic pain. *Pain* 1987; 28:201–222.

Colpaert FC. System theory of pain and of opiate analgesia: no tolerance to opiates. *Pharmacol Rev* 1996; 48:355–402.

Colpaert FC, Frégnac Y. Paradoxical signal transduction in neurobiological systems. *Mol Neurobiol* 2001; 24:145–168.

Colpaert FC, Tarayre JP, Alliaga M, et al. Opiate self-administration as a measure of chronic nociceptive pain in arthritic rats. *Pain* 2001; 91:33–45.

Colpaert FC, Tarayre JP, Koek W, et al. Large-amplitude 5-HT₁ₐ receptor activation: a new mechanism of profound central analgesia. *Neuropharmacology* 2002; 43:945–958.

Colpaert FC, Wu WP, Hao JX, et al. High-efficacy 5-HT₁ₐ receptor activation causes a curative-like action on allodynia in rats with spinal cord injury. *Eur J Pharmacol* 2004; 497:29–33.

Deseure K, Koek W, Colpaert FC, Adriaensen H. The 5-HT₁ₐ receptor agonist F 13640 attenuates mechanical allodynia in a rat model of trigeminal neuropathic pain. *Eur J Pharmacol* 2002; 456:51–57.

Deseure K, Koek W, Adriaensen H, Colpaert FC. Continuous administration of the 5-hydroxytryptamine₁ₐ agonist (3-chloro-4-fluoro-phenyl)-[4-fluoro-4-{[(5-methyl-pyridin-2-ylmethyl)-amino]-methyl}piperidin-1-yl]-methanone (F 13640) attenuates allodynia-like behavior in a rat model of trigeminal neuropathic pain. *J Pharmacol Exp Ther* 2003; 306:505–514.

Deseure KR, Adriaensen HF, Colpaert FC. Effects of the combined continuous administration of morphine and the high-efficacy 5-HT₁ₐ agonist, F 13640, in a rat model of trigeminal neuropathic pain. *Eur J Pain* 2004; 8:547–554.

Dray A, Rang H. The how and why of chronic pain states and the what of new analgesia therapies. *Trends Neurosci* 1998; 21:315–317.

Haegerstrand A. Trends and targets for treatment of pain, a pharmaceutical industry perspective. *Acta Anesthesiol Scand* 1998; 42(Suppl 113):31–33.

Hamon M, Bourgoin S. Serotonin and its receptors in pain control. In: Sawynok J, Cowan A (Eds). *Novel Aspects of Pain Management: Opioids and Beyond*. New York: Wiley, 1999, pp 203–228.

Hao JX, Wiesenfeld-Hallin Z, Xu XJ. Treatment of chronic allodynia in spinally injured rats: effects of intrathecal selective opioid receptor agonists. *Pain* 1998; 75:209–217.

Houghton AK, Hewitt E, Westlund K. Enhanced withdrawal responses to mechanical and thermal stimuli after bone injury. *Pain* 1997; 73:325–337.

Hunt SP, Mantyh PW. The molecular dynamics of pain control. *Nat Rev Neurosci* 2001; 2:83–91.

Kiss I, Degryse AD, Bardin L, Gomez De Segura IA. The novel analgesic, F 13640, produces intra- and postoperative analgesia in a rat model of surgical pain. *Eur J Pharmacol* 2005; 523:29–39.

Kowaluk EA, Arneric SP, Williams M. Opportunities in pain therapy: beyond the opioids and NSAIDS. *Expert Opin Emerg Drugs* 1998; 3:1–38.

Lanfumey L, Hamon M. 5-HT$_1$ receptors. *Curr Drug Targets CNS Neurol Disord* 2004; 3:1–10.

Mao J. Opioid-induced abnormal pain sensitivity: implications in clinical opioid therapy. *Pain* 2002; 100:213–217.

Ossipov MH, Lai J, Vanderah TW, Porreca F. Induction of pain facilitation by sustained opioid exposure: relationship to opioid nociceptive tolerance. *Life Sci* 2003; 73:783–800.

Pauwels PJ, Colpaert FC. Ca^{2+} responses in chinese hamster ovary-K1 cells demonstrate an atypical pattern of ligand-induced 5-HT$_{1A}$ receptor activation. *J Pharmacol Exp Ther* 2003; 307:608–614.

Ramos AJ, Rubio MD, Defagot C, et al. The 5-HT$_{1A}$ receptor agonist, 8-OH-DPAT, protects neurons and reduces astroglial reaction after ischemic damage caused by cortical devascularization. *Brain Res* 2004; 1030:201–220.

Sah DWY, Ossipov MH, Porreca F. Neurotrophic factors as novel therapeutics for neuropathic pain. *Nat Rev Drug Discov* 2003; 2:460–472.

Vos BP, Strassman AM, Maciewicz RJ. Behavioral evidence of trigeminal neuropathic pain following chronic constriction injury to the rat's infraorbital nerve. *J Neurosci* 1994; 14:2708–2723.

Wu WP, Hao JX, Xu XJ, et al. The very-high-efficacy 5-HT$_{1A}$ receptor agonist, F 13640, preempts the development of allodynia-like behaviors in rats with spinal cord injury. *Eur J Pharmacol* 2003; 478:131–137.

Wurch T, Colpaert FC, Pauwels PJ. Mutation in a protein kinase C phosphorylation site of the 5-HT$_{1A}$ receptor preferentially attenuates Ca^{2+} responses to partial as opposed to higher-efficacy 5-HT$_{1A}$ agonists. *Neuropharmacology* 2003; 44:873–881.

Xu XJ, Colpaert FC, Wiesenfeld-Hallin Z. Opioid hyperalgesia and tolerance versus 5-HT$_{1A}$ receptor-mediated inverse tolerance. *Trends Pharmacol Sci* 2003; 24:634–639.

You HJ, Colpaert FC, Arendt-Nielsen L. The novel analgesic and high-efficacy 5-HT$_{1A}$ receptor agonist F 13640 inhibits nociceptive responses, wind-up, and after-discharges in spinal neurons and withdrawal reflexes. *Exp Neurol* 2005; 191:174–183.

Correspondence to: Zsuzsanna Wiesenfeld-Hallin, PhD, Karolinska Institutet, Department of Clinical Neuroscience, Section of Clinical Neurophysiology, Karolinska University Hospital, Huddinge, 141 86 Stockholm, Sweden. Fax: 46-8-585-87050; email: zsuzsanna.wiesenfeld-hallin@ki.se.

Proceedings of the 11th World Congress on Pain,
edited by Herta Flor, Eija Kalso, and Jonathan O.
Dostrovsky, IASP Press, Seattle, © 2006.

15

Pathophysiology of Neurogenic Inflammation

Qing Lin,[a] Fernando Cervero,[b] and Martin Schmelz[c]

[a]Department of Neuroscience and Cell Biology, University of Texas Medical Branch, Galveston, Texas, USA; [b]Departments of Anesthesia and Dentistry and Centre for Research on Pain, McGill University, Montreal, Quebec, Canada; [c]Department of Anesthesiology, Faculty of Clinical Medicine, University of Heidelberg, Mannheim, Germany

Inflammation that is initiated by the release of inflammatory mediators from sensory nerve terminals (mainly nociceptors) is referred to as neurogenic inflammation (Richardson and Vasko 2002). Neurogenic inflammation has been implicated in the pathophysiology of various human diseases with uncertain etiology. Intradermal injection of capsaicin or mustard oil, or intra-articular injection of kaolin and carrageenan, have been experimentally established as effective means by which to induce neurogenic inflammation (Schaible and Schmidt 1985; Cervero and Laird 1996b; Lin et al. 1999; Garcia-Nicas et al. 2001). Peripherally, the released inflammatory substances would sensitize the terminals of primary afferents leading to enhanced pain sensation (primary hyperalgesia). Capsaicin is known to sensitize nociceptors selectively by activating the transient receptor potential vanilloid-1 (TRPV1) receptors on nociceptor terminals (Caterina et al. 1997; Szallasi and Blumberg 1999). Many primary afferent nociceptors (Aδ/C fibers) are peptidergic and have the capability to release inflammatory peptides, such as calcitonin gene-related peptide (CGRP) and substance P (Gibbins et al. 1985; Alvarez et al. 1988; Kruger et al. 1989). Thus, exposure of nociceptors to capsaicin or other chemical mediators not only sensitizes these nociceptive neurons, producing pain, but also induces the release of inflammatory peptides by several mechanisms, exacerbating pain (Kilo et al. 1997; Kessler et al. 1999). Centrally, neurogenic inflammation may lead to sensitization of nociceptive neurons of the spinal dorsal horn. Both mechanisms would contribute to the development of neurogenic inflammation and, in turn, exacerbate the perception of pain. Neurogenic inflammatory responses (vasodilation and edema) can be evoked experimentally by antidromic stimulation of either small myelinated or unmyelinated primary afferent axons (Szolcsanyi 1988; Jänig and Lisney 1989) through the release of CGRP and substance P (Habler et al. 1999; Kress et al. 1999; Peitl et al. 1999). This chapter updates the mechanisms of the pathophysiological process of neurogenic inflammation using animal and human models of somatosensory inflammatory pain in the light of results obtained by our different laboratory teams.

MECHANISMS BY WHICH DORSAL ROOT REFLEXES MEDIATE NEUROGENIC INFLAMMATION

PATHOGENIC MECHANISMS OF DORSAL ROOT REFLEXES

Dorsal root reflexes (DRRs) are triggered pathophysiologically by excessive primary afferent depolarization (PAD) of the central terminals in the spinal dorsal horn (Cervero and Laird 1996a; Willis 1999; Lin 2003). PAD is produced by the efflux of Cl⁻ ions from the synaptic terminals of primary afferents when $GABA_A$ receptors are activated by γ-aminobutyric acid (GABA) released from spinal GABAergic interneurons (Eccles et al. 1963; Alvarez et al. 1998; Rudomin and Schmidt 1999). Under normal conditions, PAD is evoked to produce presynaptic inhibition, reducing pain sensation (Cervero and Laird 1996a, Cervero et al. 2003). Following tissue injury or inflammation that sensitizes nociceptors, strong nociceptive barrages in turn sensitize GABAergic interneurons by activating *N*-methyl-D-aspartate (NMDA) and/or non-NMDA receptors on these interneurons. This event produces excessive PAD to generate DRRs that are then conducted antidromically in the primary afferents toward the periphery, causing neurogenic inflammation (Willis et al. 1998, Willis 1999; Lin 2003), and orthodromically, causing excitation of nociceptive neurons and hence pain (see the following section and Cervero and Laird 1996a; Cervero et al. 2003). Under these circumstances, PAD is no longer inhibitory but rather becomes an excitatory event.

RELEASE OF INFLAMMATORY PEPTIDES IS DRIVEN BY DORSAL ROOT REFLEXES AND CONTRIBUTES TO SENSITIZATION OF PRIMARY AFFERENT NOCICEPTORS

Studies by Lin et al. (1999, 2000) have shown that intradermal injection of capsaicin that is presumed to activate the TRPV1 receptors in primary afferent nociceptors can trigger and enhance DRRs, which accompany the spread of flare and edema in the paw (Lin et al. 1999). Obviously, there is a close relationship between the enhanced DRRs and centrally mediated inflammation evoked by capsaicin injection. Primary afferent fibers critically involved in triggering DRRs are capsaicin sensitive (C and some Aδ fibers) (Lin et al. 2000). Stimulation of capsaicin-sensitive afferent nociceptive fibers by capsaicin or other noxious stimuli can trigger the release of neuropeptides from their peripheral terminals to initiate neurogenic inflammation (Holzer 1991, 1993; Maggi 1993; Caterina and Julius 2001). Therefore, we propose that capsaicin-induced inflammation results from the release of inflammatory mediators from peptidergic primary afferent terminals. Lin et al.'s recent unpublished study shows that after DRRs were removed by dorsal rhizotomy, vasodilation and edema induced by capsaicin injection were almost completely blocked, but inflammation induced by CGRP and substance P was unchanged (Fig. 1). Also, the capsaicin-induced sensitization of primary afferent nociceptors (Aδ/C fibers) was attenuated after dorsal rhizotomy (Fig. 2). These data suggest that the release of neuropeptides in the periphery is relevant to the generation of DRRs, which contributes to the spread of cutaneous inflammation and to exacerbation of pain perception.

ACTIVITY OF GABAERGIC INTERNEURONS IS ENHANCED BY UPREGULATION OF GLUTAMATE RECEPTORS

Pharmacological studies have shown that the enhanced DRRs and inflammation after tissue injury are inhibited by spinally administering antagonists of NMDA, non-NMDA or $GABA_A$ receptors (Rees et al. 1995; Lin et al. 1999). Moreover, immunofluorescence double labeling and Western blots, which reveal the functional activation of GABAergic interneurons induced by strong noxious stimulation, indicate that Fos expression in GABAergic interneurons is increased following capsaicin injection; furthermore, this Fos expression can be inhibited after blockade of spinal NMDA or non-NMDA receptors (Zou et al. 2001). Thus, we propose that glutamate receptors are distributed in the GABAergic interneurons that are functionally activated following capsaicin injection to sensitize these interneurons, leading to triggering of DRRs. Our recent preliminary data support the view that the enhanced functional activity of dorsal horn GABAergic interneurons following capsaicin injection is closely associated with phosphorylation of NMDA-receptor NR1 subunits that are distributed in GABAergic interneurons following capsaicin injection (Zou et al. 2003). These anatomical findings support our hypothesis that excessive PAD is triggered to generate DRRs when GABAergic interneurons are hyperexcited in part by activation of NMDA receptors following capsaicin injection.

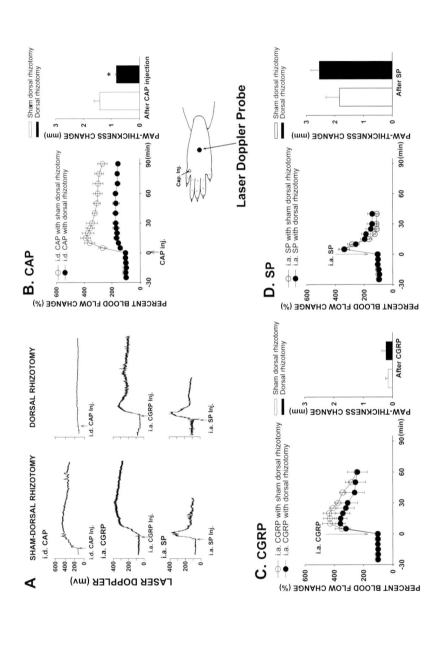

Laser Doppler Probe

A

SHAM-DORSAL RHIZOTOMY

i.d. CAP

i.a. CGRP

i.a. SP

DORSAL RHIZOTOMY

i.d. CAP Inj.

i.a. CGRP Inj.

i.a. SP Inj.

LASER DOPPLER (mv)

B. CAP

PERCENT BLOOD FLOW CHANGE (%)

i.d. CAP with sham dorsal rhizotomy
i.d. CAP with dorsal rhizotomy

CAP inj.

Sham dorsal rhizotomy
Dorsal rhizotomy

PAW-THICKNESS CHANGE (mm)

After CAP injection

*

C. CGRP

PERCENT BLOOD FLOW CHANGE (%)

i.a. CGRP with sham dorsal rhizotomy
i.a. CGRP with dorsal rhizotomy

i.a. CGRP

Sham dorsal rhizotomy
Dorsal rhizotomy

PAW-THICKNESS CHANGE (mm)

After CGRP

D. SP

PERCENT BLOOD FLOW CHANGE (%)

i.a. SP with sham dorsal rhizotomy
i.a. SP with dorsal rhizotomy

i.a. SP

Sham dorsal rhizotomy
Dorsal rhizotomy

PAW-THICKNESS CHANGE (mm)

After SP

Cap. Inj.

ROLE OF DORSAL ROOT REFLEXES IN TOUCH-EVOKED PAIN

TOUCH-EVOKED PAIN MEDIATED BY DORSAL ROOT REFLEXES

Persistent or intense noxious stimuli cause enhancement of pain sensitivity that can be described using the general term of hyperalgesia. These sensory alterations include the phenomenon known as touch-evoked pain (or tactile allodynia) detected in areas of injury and inflammation (primary hyperalgesia) and in zones outside an injury site (secondary hyperalgesia) (Treede et al. 1992; Cervero and Laird 2004). Tactile allodynia in areas of secondary hyperalgesia is thought to be caused by a state of central hyperexcitability known as central sensitization, generated in the central nervous system (CNS) by the originating injury or inflammatory focus (Woolf and Salter 2000). However, the mechanism by which central sensitization causes this sensory switch is not clear. Over the last decade, Cervero's group has developed the hypothesis that tactile allodynia is the result of altered processing at the level of the first synaptic relay in the CNS such that afferent Aβ fibers gain access to the nociceptive pathway through a presynaptic link with the terminals of Aδ and C afferent fibers (Cervero and Laird 1996a; Cervero et al. 2003). Under normal conditions, Aβ fibers activate spinal GABAergic interneurons to produce PAD, leading to presynaptic inhibition (Rudomin and Schmidt 1999; Willis 1999; see also the preceding section). Under conditions that generate tactile allodynia, the normal Aβ-fiber induction of PAD on the nociceptive terminals of fine afferent fibers is enhanced to the point that the depolarization can now generate spike activity in the afferent terminals, i.e., DRRs that orthodromically cause Aβ-fiber excitation of nociceptive neurons leading to pain (Cervero and Laird 1996a).

$NA^+/K^+/2Cl^-$ COTRANSPORTER AND TOUCH-EVOKED PAIN

A key element of the process leading to DRRs is PAD due to the GABA-mediated depolarizing currents (Rees et al. 1995; Sung et al. 2000) that result from the opening of Cl^- channels and efflux of Cl^- ions. The high gradient of Cl^- in primary sensory neurons is maintained by the activity of the $Na^+/K^+/2Cl^-$

← **Fig. 1.** (A) Laser Doppler flowmetry traces show changes in cutaneous blood flow of the rat hindpaw following ipsilateral intradermal (i.d.) injection of capsaicin (CAP) or intra-arterial (i.a.) injection of calcitonin gene-related peptide (CGRP) or substance P (SP) and the effects of dorsal rhizotomy. (B–D) Mean results of blood flow and paw-thickness recordings showing the effects of dorsal rhizotomy on the CGRP-, SP-, or CAP-evoked inflammation. Blood flow value of the predrug injection was expressed as 100%. Change in paw thickness following drug injection is presented as the difference in score before and after drug injection. Inset shows the sites where CAP was injected intradermally and blood flow was measured. $*P < 0.05$, compared to the value with sham dorsal rhizotomy. (Unpublished data from Q. Lin, Y. Ren, and X. Zou.)

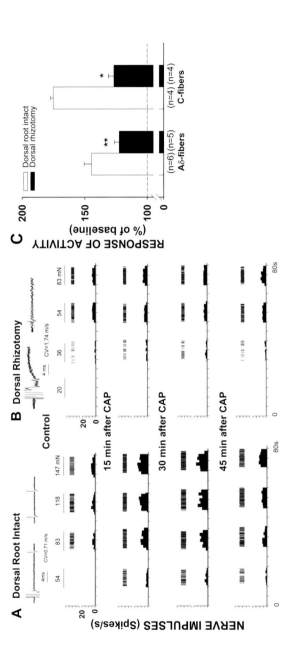

Fig. 2. Effects of dorsal rhizotomy on afferent responses of primary afferent nociceptive fibers to mechanical stimuli after intradermal injection of capsaicin (CAP). (A) Afferent response of a single C fiber in a rat with intact dorsal roots. (B) Afferent response of a single C fiber in a dorsal rhizotomized rat. Afferent activity was recorded from the distal end of the tibial or sural nerves. Inset shows the conduction velocity test and orthodromically evoked spikes. Spikes were evoked by orthodromically stimulating the receptive field with von Frey hairs. The upper trace of each panel shows recorded action potentials, and the lower trace of each panel shows a peristimulus time histogram converted from recorded action potentials. Horizontal lines above histograms indicate times of application of von Frey hairs. Bending forces are shown above the horizontal lines. (C) Grouped data of Aδ and C fibers. Baseline response before CAP injection is 100% (dashed line). * $P < 0.05$, ** $P < 0.01$, compared to the value of the intact dorsal root group. (Unpublished data from Q. Lin, Y. Ren, and X. Zou.)

cotransporter (NKCC1) (Sung et al. 2000). It has been proposed that persistent noxious stimulation can induce alterations in NKCC1 expression and activity in nociceptive afferents, producing a greater accumulation of intracellular Cl⁻ in their terminals and hence an increased GABA-mediated PAD when Aβ fibers are activated (Cervero et al. 2003). Multiple lines of evidence suggest that DRRs are generated in inflammatory conditions (Willis et al. 1998; Garcia-Nicas et al. 2001; Lin 2003). It has been demonstrated that DRRs conveyed in Aδ and C fibers are evoked by mechanical stimulation of the hindpaw following capsaicin injection (Lin et al. 2000). Aβ-fiber stimulation produces increases in blood flow following inflammation that were prevented by transection of the dorsal roots or of the sciatic nerve and blocked by peripheral CGRP-receptor antagonism (Garcia-Nicas et al. 2001). These findings are consistent with the hypothesis that Aβ-fiber stimulation can lead to DRR generation in Aδ and C fibers. DRRs also modulate the propagation of signaling of Aδ and C fibers onto ascending neurons of the superficial dorsal horn (Garcia-Nicas et al. 2003). Behavioral studies using NKCC1 knockout mice have further demonstrated that pain behavior in response to cotton-bud stroking following capsaicin injection is significantly attenuated in these mice when compared to their wild-type littermates (Laird et al. 2004). This finding supports the hypothesis that NKCC1 is involved in the development of touch-evoked allodynia following intense noxious stimulation.

A critical step in this interpretation is to show that NKCC1 can be up-regulated, or at least functionally enhanced, during inflammatory states. In a mouse model of visceral hyperalgesia and referred tactile allodynia (Laird et al. 2001), it has been shown that intense stimulation of capsaicin-sensitive colonic afferents leads to increases in spinal NKCC1 phosphorylation and trafficking (Fig. 3) that follow the time course of the behavioral development of referred tactile allodynia (Galan and Cervero 2005). These data provide evidence that alteration of spinal NKCC1 levels can be observed following intense activation of peripheral nociceptors, suggesting that a similar process could be started by more prolonged forms of noxious stimulation, such as inflammation or nerve lesions. A further study of whether NKCC1 is expressed in neurons involved in nociception was conducted using colocalization of NKCC1 mRNA and peripherin, a selective marker of small-diameter, unmyelinated and lightly myelinated neurons; CGRP, a marker of peptidergic unmyelinated afferents; and TRPV1, a marker of small nociceptive afferents. NKCC1 expression was found in about 50% of the peripherin-immunoreactive population and in similar populations of CGRP- and TRPV1-immunoreactive cells in both dorsal root ganglion and trigeminal ganglion cells (Fig. 4). Therefore, NKCC1 mRNA is expressed by a subpopulation of dorsal root and trigeminal ganglion neurons, most of which are of small and medium diameter and many of which are nociceptors because they also express TRPV1.

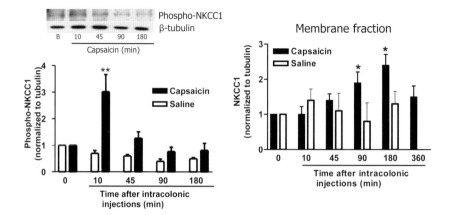

Fig. 3. Left graph: Intracolonic capsaicin induces NKCC1 co-transporter phosphorylation. Western blot (top) from membrane protein extracts showing the time course of NKCC1 phosphorylation. Lane marked "B" in the immunoblot contains control (basal) tissue. Membranes were re-incubated with β-tubulin as a loading control. The graph below shows the quantification of phospho-NKCC1 normalized to β-tubulin values after intracolonic capsaicin ($n = 6$ observations per time point). Asterisks indicate those groups that were significantly different from control levels (** $P < 0.01$). Right graph: Intracolonic capsaicin delivers NKCC1 into the plasma membrane of lumbosacral spinal cord cells. Time course ($n = 6$–8 observations per time point) of subcellular distribution of NKCC1 in the plasma membrane fraction of lumbosacral spinal cord at several times from intracolonic instillation of capsaicin or saline. Asterisks indicate those groups that were significantly different from control levels (* $P < 0.05$). (Data from Galan and Cervero 2005.)

NEUROGENIC INFLAMMATION IN HUMANS

NEURONAL BASIS OF NEUROGENIC INFLAMMATION IN HUMANS

Single nociceptive nerve fibers branch extensively in the periphery to form their receptive fields. Axonal branching is the structural basis for antidromic action potential propagation leading to neurogenic inflammation. The receptive field of primary afferent nociceptors is very small in rodents. However, in humans, skin innervation territories measuring up to 9 cm in diameter have been found (Schmelz et al. 1997).

In human skin, unmyelinated nociceptors fall into two basic classes: the majority of the fibers are mechano-heat-sensitive polymodal nociceptors, while about 20% are unresponsive to mechanical stimulation (Schmidt et al. 1995). These "silent" or "sleeping" nociceptors differ from conventional polymodal nociceptors in their receptive properties, their biophysical characteristics, and their functions. They have higher activation thresholds for heat but are not activated even by intense mechanical stimuli (Schmidt et al. 1995). Most interestingly, their high transcutaneous electrical thresholds and their activity-

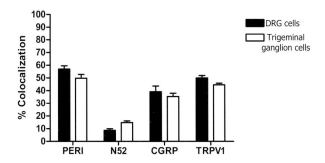

Fig. 4. Percentage colocalization of NKCC1 mRNA with sensory neuron population markers in rat dorsal root ganglia (DRG) and trigeminal ganglia. The percentage of neurons positive for NKCC1 mRNA is shown as a function of neurons that also expressed peripherin (PERI), N52, calcitonin gene-related peptide (CGRP), or TRPV1 in both the DRG and trigeminal ganglia ($n = 3$ for each marker). (Unpublished data from T.J. Price, K.M. Hargreaves, and F. Cervero.)

dependent hyperpolarization exceed by far the values observed in polymodal nociceptors. In rodents, antidromic activation of polymodal nociceptors was sufficient to cause neurogenic inflammation (Gee et al. 1997). In contrast, mechano-insensitive, but heat- and chemosensitive C nociceptors have been found to be responsible for the neurogenic vasodilation in pig skin (Lynn et al. 1996) and in humans (Sauerstein et al. 2000). The extent of the neurogenic erythema nicely matches the large cutaneous receptive fields of mechano-insensitive nociceptors, and their high electrical thresholds also match the strong currents required to provoke neurogenic flare. In healthy volunteers no neurogenic protein extravasation could be induced (Sauerstein et al 2000), but it may develop under pathophysiological conditions (Weber et al. 2001; Leis et al. 2003, 2004). Thus, neurogenic inflammation in humans differs from that in rodents, since in the latter it can be elicited by polymodal C nociceptors and consists of a combination of vasodilation and protein extravasation (Sauerstein et al. 2000; Weidner et al. 2000).

EPIDERMAL AXONAL BRANCHING IN HUMAN SKIN

Under physiological conditions, unmyelinated human nerve fibers entering the epidermis are found to be oriented straight up, and they reach the outermost layers of viable skin without pronounced branching (Hilliges et al. 1995). In some human skin diseases, extensive branching of epidermal nerve fibers has been described (Bohm-Starke et al. 1998). Increased intradermal nerve fiber density has been found in patients with chronic pruritus (Urashima and Mihara 1998). In addition, increased epidermal levels of neurotrophin 4 have been

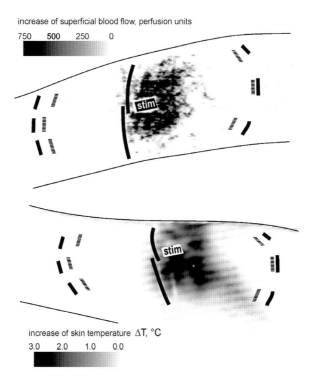

Fig. 5. Specimen of transcutaneous electrical stimulation (1 Hz, 50 mA, 0.5 ms; the stimulation site ["stim"] is marked by a rectangle) provoking an area of increased superficial blood flow, as assessed with a laser Doppler scanner (upper panel), and increased skin temperature, as measured by an infrared camera (lower panel). An anesthetic strip was induced by perfusing two intradermal microdialysis membranes (long black lines) with 2% lidocaine. The borders of hyperalgesia to punctate stimuli (short black lines) and to light stroking (dotted lines) are shown in the laser Doppler scan and the thermogram. Modified from Klede et al. (2003).

found in patients with atopic dermatitis, and massively increased serum levels of nerve growth factor (NGF) and substance P have been found to correlate with the severity of the disease in such patients (Toyoda et al. 2002). Increased fiber density and higher local NGF concentrations were also found in patients with contact dermatitis. Most interestingly, intra-epidermal axonal sprouting has also been found as a physiological response to circular skin incision (Rajan et al. 2003). Collateral sprouting from axons at the incision margins can lead to centripedal reconstitution of skin innervation, probably due to higher local NGF concentrations in the denervated skin (Rajan et al. 2003). It will be of interest in the future to assess the effects of this local sprouting on the sensory function of nociceptors. There is already evidence for increased epidermal nerve fiber sprouting in vulvodynia, as well as signs of nociceptor sensitization (Bohm-Starke et al. 2001).

NEUROGENIC INFLAMMATION AND SECONDARY HYPERALGESIA

The areas of vasodilation and warming around a noxious stimulation site are similar to the areas of secondary mechanical hyperalgesia (punctate hyperalgesia) (Serra et al. 1998). However, recent results suggest that by blocking axonal action potential propagation by a local anesthetic, only the spread of axon reflex vasodilation and warming can be blocked: in contrast, areas of punctate hyperalgesia developed symmetrically, even beyond a peripherally located "anesthetic strip" (Klede et al. 2003) (Fig. 5). This result speaks against a major role of DRRs in the generation of neurogenic inflammation in humans.

SUMMARY AND CONCLUSION

Studies in animal models reveal that DRRs produce an antidromic drive of primary afferent nociceptors, leading to the release of inflammatory peptides and the development of neurogenic inflammation and sensitization of nociceptors. The DRRs are thought to result from the enhancement of spinal GABAergic interneurons by upregulation of glutamate receptors and/or by upregulation of the NKCC1 transporter in primary afferents. Centrally, DRRs orthodromically cause Aβ-fiber excitation of nociceptive neurons, giving rise to touch-evoked pain. In humans, neurogenic inflammation involves the mechanically insensitive nociceptors in contrast to the C-polymodal nociceptors in the rat, and plasma extravasation does not appear to occur under normal conditions as is the case in the rat.

ACKNOWLEDGMENTS

The preparation of this chapter was supported by grants from the National Institutes of Health (NS 40723) to Q. Lin, from the Canadian Institutes of Health Research and Canadian Foundation for Innovation to F. Cervero, and from the German Research Foundation (DFG) grants SFB 353 and KFG 107 to M. Schmelz. Experimental protocols for the studies on animals were approved by the Animal Care and Use Committee of the University of Texas Medical Branch (Q. Lin) and by the McGill University Animal Care Committee (F. Cervero). The experimental protocol for the human study was approved by the ethics committee of the University of Erlangen, Germany.

REFERENCES

Alvarez FJ, Cervantes C, Blasco I, et al. Presence of calcitonin gene-related peptide (CGRP) and substance P (SP) immunoreactivity in intraepidermal free nerve endings of cat skin. *Brain Res* 1988; 442:391–395.

Alvarez FJ, Nani A, Marquez S. Chloride transport, osmotic balance, and presynaptic inhibition. In: Rudomin P, Romo R, Mendell LM (Eds). *Presynaptic Inhibition and Neuronal Control.* New York: Oxford University Press, 1998, pp 50–79.

Bohm-Starke N, Hilliges M, Falconer C, Rylander E. Increased intraepithelial innervation in women with vulvar vestibulitis syndrome. *Gynecol Obstet Invest* 1998; 46:256–260.

Bohm-Starke N, Hilliges M, Brodda-Jansen G, Rylander E, Torebjork E. Psychophysical evidence of nociceptor sensitization in vulvar vestibulitis syndrome. *Pain* 2001; 94:177–183.

Caterina MJ, Julius D. The vanilloid receptor: a molecular gateway to the pain pathway. *Ann Rev Neurosci* 2001; 24:487–517.

Caterina MJ, Schumacher MA, Tominaga M, et al. The capsaicin receptor: a heat-activated ion channel in the pain pathway. *Nature* 1997; 389:816–824.

Cervero F, Laird JM. Mechanisms of touch-evoked pain (allodynia): a new model. *Pain* 1996a; 68:13–23.

Cervero F, Laird JM. Mechanisms of allodynia: interactions between sensitive mechanoreceptors and nociceptors. *Neuroreport* 1996b; 7:526–528.

Cervero F, Laird, JMA. Referred visceral hyperalgesia: from sensations to molecular mechanisms. In: Brune K, Handwerker HO (Eds). *Hyperalgesia: Molecular Mechanisms and Clinical Implications,* Progress in Pain Research and Management, Vol. 30. Seattle: IASP Press, 2004, pp 229–250.

Cervero F, Laird JM, Garcia-Nicas E. Secondary hyperalgesia and presynaptic inhibition: an update. *Eur J Pain* 2003; 7:345–351.

Eccles JC, Schmidt RF, Willis WD. Pharmacological studies on presynaptic inhibition. *J Physiol* 1963; 168:500–530.

Galan A, Cervero F. Painful stimuli induce in vivo phosphorylation and membrane mobilization of mouse spinal cord NKCC1 co-transporter. *Neuroscience* 2005; 133:245–252.

Garcia-Nicas E, Laird J, Cervero F. Vasodilatation in hyperalgesic rat skin evoked by stimulation of afferent A beta-fibers: further evidence for a role of dorsal root reflexes in allodynia. *Pain* 2001; 94:283–291.

Garcia-Nicas E, Laird JM, Cervero F. Sensitization of nociceptor-specific neurons by capsaicin or mustard oil: effect of $GABA_A$-receptor blockade. In: Dostrovsky JO, Carr DB, Koltzenburg M (Eds). *Proceedings of the 10th World Congress on Pain,* Progress in Pain Research and Management, Vol. 24. Seattle: IASP Press, 2003, pp 327–335.

Gee MD, Lynn B, Cotsell B. The relationship between cutaneous C fibre type and antidromic vasodilatation in the rabbit and the rat. *J Physiol* 1997; 503:31–44.

Gibbins IL, Furness JB, Costa M, et al. Co-localization of calcitonin gene-related peptide-like immunoreactivity with substance P in cutaneous, vascular and visceral sensory neurons of guinea pig. *Neurosci Lett* 1985; 57:125–130.

Habler HJ, Timmermann L, Stegmann JU, et al. Involvement of neurokinins in antidromic vasodilatation in hairy and hairless skin of the rat hindlimb. *Neuroscience* 1999; 89:1259–1268.

Hilliges M, Wang L, Johansson O. Ultrastructural evidence for nerve fibers within all vital layers of the human epidermis. *J Invest Dermatol* 1995; 104:134–137.

Holzer P. Capsaicin: cellular targets, mechanisms of action, and selectivity for thin sensory neurons. *Pharmacol Rev* 1991; 43:143–201.

Holzer P. Capsaicin-sensitive nerves in the control of vascular effector mechanisms. In: Wood JN (Ed). *Capsaicin in the Study of Pain.* London: Academic Press, 1993, pp 191–218.

Jänig W, Lisney SJW. Small diameter myelinated afferents produce vasodilatation but not plasma extravasation in rat skin. *J Physiol* 1989; 415:477–486.

Kessler F, Habelt C, Averbeck B, et al. Heat-induced release of CGRP from isolated rat skin and effects of bradykinin and the protein kinase C activator PMA. *Pain* 1999; 83:289–295.

Kilo S, Harding-Rose C, Hargreaves KM, et al. Peripheral CGRP release as a marker for neurogenic inflammation: a model system for the study of neuropeptide secretion in rat paw skin. *Pain* 1997; 73:201–207.

Klede M, Handwerker HO, Schmelz M. Central origin of secondary mechanical hyperalgesia. *J Neurophysiol* 2003; 90:353–359.

Kress M, Guthmann C, Averbeck B, Reeh PW. Calcitonin gene-related peptide and prostaglandin E_2 but not substance P release induced by antidromic nerve stimulation from rat skin in vitro. *Neuroscience* 1999; 89:303–310.

Kruger L, Silverman JD, Mantyh PW, et al. Peripheral patterns of calcitonin-gene-related peptide general somatic sensory innervation: cutaneous and deep terminations. *J Comp Neurol* 1989; 280:291–302.

Laird JM, Martinez-Caro L, Garcia-Nicas E, et al. A new model of visceral pain and referred hyperalgesia in the mouse. *Pain* 2001; 92:335–342.

Laird JM, Garcia-Nicas E, Delpire EJ, et al. Presynaptic inhibition and spinal pain processing in mice: a possible role of the NKCC1 cation-chloride co-transporter in hyperalgesia. *Neurosci Lett* 2004; 361:200–203.

Leis S, Weber M, Isselmann A, et al. Substance-P-induced protein extravasation is bilaterally increased in complex regional pain syndrome. *Exp Neurol* 2003; 183:188–196.

Leis S, Weber M, Schmelz M, et al. Facilitated neurogenic inflammation in unaffected limbs of patients with complex regional pain syndrome. *Neurosci Lett* 2004; 359:163–166.

Lin Q. A contribution of dorsal root reflexes to neurogenic inflammation and pain. In: Chen J, Chen ACN, Han JS, et al (Eds). *Experimental Pathological Pain: From Molecules to Brain Functions*. Beijing: Science Press, 2003, pp 36–56.

Lin Q, Wu J, Willis WD. Dorsal root reflexes and cutaneous neurogenic inflammation following intradermal injection of capsaicin in rats. *J Neurophysiol* 1999; 82:2602–2611.

Lin Q, Zou X, Willis WD. Aδ and C primary afferents convey dorsal root reflexes after intradermal injection of capsaicin in rats. *J Neurophysiol* 2000; 84:2695–2698.

Lynn B, Schutterle S, Pierau FK. The vasodilator component of neurogenic inflammation is caused by a special subclass of heat-sensitive nociceptors in the skin of the pig. *J Physiol* 1996; 494:587–593.

Maggi CA. The pharmacological modulation of neurotransmitter release. In: Wood JN (Ed). *Capsaicin in the Study of Pain*. London: Academic Press, 1993, pp 161–189.

Peitl B, Petho G, Porszasz R, Nemeth J, Szolcsanyi J. Capsaicin-insensitive sensory-efferent meningeal vasodilatation evoked by electrical stimulation of trigeminal nerve fibres in the rat. *Br J Pharmacol* 1999; 127:457–467.

Rajan B, Polydefkis M, Hauer P, et al. Epidermal reinnervation after intracutaneous axotomy in man. *J Comp Neurol* 2003; 457:24–36.

Rees H, Sluka KA, Westlund KN, et al. The role of glutamate and GABA receptors in the generation of dorsal root reflexes by acute arthritis in the anaesthetised rat. *J Physiol* 1995; 484:437–445

Richardson JD, Vasko MR. Cellular mechanisms of neurogenic inflammation. *J Pharmacol Exp Ther* 2002; 302:839–845.

Rudomin P, Schmidt RF. Presynaptic inhibition in the vertebral spinal cord revisited. *Exp Brain Res* 1999; 129:1–37.

Sauerstein K, Klede M, Hilliges M, et al. Electrically evoked neuropeptide release and neurogenic inflammation differ between rat and human skin. *J Physiol* 2000; 529:803–810.

Schaible HG, Schmidt RF. Effects of an experimental arthritis on the sensory properties of fine articular afferent units. *J Neurophysiol* 1985; 54:1109–1126.

Schmidt R, Schmelz M, Forster C, et al. Novel classes of responsive and unresponsive C nociceptors in human skin. *J Neurosci* 1995; 15:333–341.

Schmelz M, Schmidt R, Bickel A, et al. Specific C-receptors for itch in human skin. *J Neurosci* 1997; 17:8003–8008.

Serra J, Campero M, Ochoa J. Flare and hyperalgesia after intradermal capsaicin injection in human skin. *J Neurophysiol* 1998; 80:2801–2810.

Sung KW, Kirby M, McDonald MP, et al. Abnormal GABAA receptor-mediated currents in dorsal root ganglion neurons isolated from Na-K-2Cl cotransporter null mice. *J Neurosci* 2000; 20:7531–7538.

Szallasi A, Blumberg PM. Vanilloid (capsaicin) receptors and mechanisms. *Pharmacol Rev* 1999; 51:159–211.

Szolcsanyi J. Antidromic vasodilatation and neurogenic inflammation. *Agents Actions* 1988; 23:4–11.

Toyoda M, Nakamura M, Makino T, et al. Nerve growth factor and substance P are useful plasma markers of disease activity in atopic dermatitis. *Br J Dermatol* 2002; 147:71–79.

Treede RD, Meyer RA, Raja SN, et al. Peripheral and central mechanisms of cutaneous hyperalgesia. *Prog Neurobiol* 1992; 38:397–421.

Urashima R, Mihara M. Cutaneous nerves in atopic dermatitis: a histological, immunohistochemical and electron microscopic study. *Virchows Arch Int J Pathol* 1998; 432:363–370.

Weber M, Birklein F, Neundorfer B, et al. Facilitated neurogenic inflammation in complex regional pain syndrome. *Pain* 2001; 91:251–257.

Weidner C, Klede M, Rukwied R, et al. Acute effects of substance P and calcitonin gene-related peptide in human skin—a microdialysis study. *J Invest Dermatol* 2000; 115:1015–1020.

Willis WD. Dorsal root potentials and dorsal root reflexes: a double-edged sword. *Exp Brain Res* 1999; 124:395–421.

Willis WD, Sluka KA, Rees H, et al. A contribution of dorsal root reflexes to peripheral inflammation. In: Rudomin P, Romo R, Mendell LM (Eds). *Presynaptic Inhibition and Neural Control*. New York: Oxford University Press, 1998, pp 407–423.

Woolf CJ, Salter MW. Neuronal plasticity: increasing the gain in pain. *Science* 2000; 288:1765–1769.

Zou X, Lin Q, Willis WD. NMDA and non-NMDA receptor antagonists attenuate increased Fos expression in spinal dorsal horn GABAergic neurons after intradermal injection of capsaicin in rats. *Neuroscience* 2001; 106:171–182.

Zou X, Lin Q, Willis WD. Phosphorylation of NMDA receptor NR1 subunit in spinal dorsal horn GABAergic neurons after intradermal injection of capsaicin in rats. *J Pain* 2003; 4(Suppl):42.

Correspondence to: Qing Lin, MD, PhD, Department of Neuroscience and Cell Biology, University of Texas Medical Branch, Galveston, TX 77555, USA. Tel: 409-772-2404; Fax: 409-772-2789; email: qilin@utmb.edu.

Proceedings of the 11th World Congress on Pain,
edited by Herta Flor, Eija Kalso, and Jonathan O.
Dostrovsky, IASP Press, Seattle, © 2006.

16

Substance P Enables C-Fiber-Mediated Nociceptive Responses in Naked Mole-Rats

Ying Lu,[a] Steven P. Wilson,[c] Charles E. Laurito,[a] Frank Rice,[d] and Thomas J. Park[b]

[a]Department of Anesthesiology and [b]Laboratory of Integrative Neuroscience, University of Illinois, Chicago, Illinois, USA; [c]Departments of Pharmacology, Physiology and Neuroscience, University of South Carolina School of Medicine, Columbia, South Carolina, USA; [d]Departments of Pharmacology and Neuroscience, Albany Medical College, Albany, New York, USA

Naked mole-rats have a distinct adaptation that makes their somatosensory system unique—they naturally lack the neuropeptides substance P and calcitonin gene-related peptide (CGRP) from the nerve fibers of their skin (Park et al. 2003); in contrast, the skin of naked mole-rats has an abundance of Aδ fibers. These neuropeptides are associated with nociceptors that express the TRPV1 (capsaicin) receptor, which are mostly expressed by unmyelinated C fibers and respond with a thermal activation threshold of ~43°C (Julius 2003). The neuropeptides substance P and CGRP coexist in unmyelinated C-fiber afferents (Gulbenkian 1986; Zachariou 1997) and are released from central terminals in the spinal cord in response to peripheral application of noxious thermal and mechanical stimuli or capsaicin application (Go and Yaksh 1987; Duggan et al. 1988, 1992; Collin 1991; Mantyh et al. 1995). In a previous study, we showed how the pain pathway responds in the absence of these transmitters in these unusual animals with their unique, natural knockout of gene expression.

Naked mole-rats also lack preprotachykinin (PPT) gene products in their cutaneous nociceptors. The use of recombinant herpes simplex viruses to modify gene expression in sensory neurons has proven of great use in elucidating the function of individual gene products and nociceptive mechanisms and in developing gene-based approaches to the treatment of chronic pain within complex systems (Wilson and Yeomans). Use of viral vectors makes it possible to overexpress missing gene products in naked mole-rats in order to test whether it is thus possible to restore capsaicin-dependent sensitization of thermal nociception.

This chapter summarizes experiments we conducted to investigate the effects of the natural absence of substance P and CGRP on nociceptive responses in naked mole-rats, to determine whether C-fiber and Aδ-fiber nociceptor activity is differentially affected by the absence of these neuropeptides, and to test the effects of introducing PPT cDNA into peripheral nerves of mole-rats using a recombinant herpes virus.

METHODS

Experimental animals. We used 24 naked mole-rats (35–45 g), together with 30 Swiss-Webster mice (20–30 g) as comparison animals. The mole-rats were housed under semi-natural conditions in an artificial burrow system within a colony room that was maintained under dim red lighting at 30°C with a relative humidity of 45–65% (Artwohl 2002). The University of Illinois at Chicago Institutional Animal Care and Use Committee approved the animal protocols.

A-delta vs C-fiber nociception test with capsaicin application. Naked mole-rats or mice were lightly anesthetized with 50 mg/kg pentobarbital, administered intraperitoneally. Foot-withdrawal responses were evoked by thermal activation of Aδ nociceptors (with a rapid heating rate of 6.5°C/second) and C nociceptors (with a low heating rate of 0.9°C/second) and were separately assessed. Baseline response latencies were measured in response to high or low rates of skin heating. Approximately 10 minutes after topical application of 2 mM capsaicin on the unilateral hindpaw skin and at 15-minute intervals thereafter, foot-withdrawal latencies were remeasured over approximately 1 hour to determine the nociceptive effects of tonic activation of C fibers.

A-delta vs. C-fiber nociception test with DMSO application. After naked mole-rats or mice were lightly anesthetized, baseline response latencies were measured in response to high or low rates of skin heating. Then we applied 100% dimethyl sulfoxide (DMSO) topically on one foot, and 10 minutes later we repeated the thermal pain test over 1 hour to measure the changes in foot-withdrawal latencies.

Recombinant herpes virus infection. The viral vectors have been designed either to overexpress transgenes or to knock down expression of endogenous genes. To induce production of PPT-derived peptides such as substance P within cutaneous C fibers, we employed gene transfer techniques, infecting one foot with a recombinant herpes virus containing the cDNA for PPT. The skin of a dorsal hindpaw was lightly abraded, and a recombinant herpes virus was topically applied. The recombinant viruses used contained an expression cassette composed of the human cytomegalovirus immediate-early enhancer-promoter, the desired cDNA, and a polyadenylation signal inserted into the indicated site of the viral gene. Viruses using the rat PPT cDNA inserted into the viral thymidine kinase gene included (1) PPPT, containing full-length cDNA inserted in sense orientation, and (2) PAPPT, containing the PPT cDNA inserted in antisense orientation relative to the promoter. A separate virus for knockdown of TRPV2, SATRPV2, was created by inserting the cassette containing the first 290 base pairs of the rat TRPV2 coding region in antisense orientation relative to the promoter into a site between the UL36 and UL37 genes of herpes simplex virus. In this procedure, the virus preferentially enters small fibers in the skin of the target foot and travels along the fibers to take residence in the cell bodies, where it will either overexpress PPT-derived peptides, including substance P, or produce antisense RNA for PPT or TRPV2. Two weeks after infection, the thermal pain behavior test was performed with topical capsaicin or DMSO application on the virus-infected foot. The uninfected foot served as a comparison.

RESULTS

The effects of capsaicin on withdrawal latencies to moderate noxious heat differed dramatically for mice and naked mole-rats. For mice, the withdrawal latencies of the foot treated with capsaicin were shortened by approximately 50%, indicative of thermal hyperalgesia (Fig. 1A, low heating rate curves). In contrast, naked mole-rats failed to develop thermal hyperalgesia from capsaicin (Fig. 1B, low heating rate curves). Note that baseline measures of withdrawal latencies prior to capsaicin application (the first three data points on each curve) did not differ for mice and naked mole-rats. Withdrawal to the high heating rate (associated with $A\delta$- fiber activity) was unaffected by capsaicin for both mice and naked mole-rats (Fig. 1A,B, high heating rate curves). The withdrawal latencies of mice infected with the PPT antisense virus resembled those of the naked mole-rats—the infected foot failed to show thermal hyperalgesia from capsaicin (Fig. 1C).

There were no differences in withdrawal latencies between mice and naked mole-rats after topical application of DMSO. Both mice (Fig. 2A) and naked mole-rats (Fig. 2B) show sensitization (shortened latencies) for the DMSO-treated foot with the high heating rate. Infection with the TRPV2 antisense virus affected both mice and naked mole-rats similarly—the infected foot in both species showed desensitization (increased latencies) after DMSO application (Fig. 2C,D).

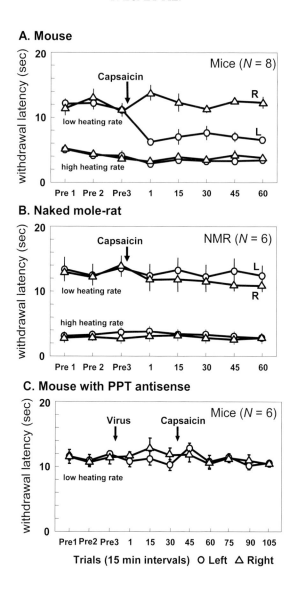

Fig. 1. Effects of topical capsaicin on foot-withdrawal latencies to low and high heating rates. Latencies were measured at 15-minute intervals for both the right (R) and left (L) foot. The first three data points on each curve reflect withdrawal latencies to acute noxious heat prior to capsaicin application (Pre 1–Pre 3). Capsaicin was then applied to the left foot only of (A) mice, (B) naked mole-rats, and (C) mice that were infected with PPT antisense virus (PAPPT).

Next we addressed the pivotal question of our study: Could we induce thermal hyperalgesia in naked mole-rats by infecting them with PPT sense virus? Two weeks after virus application, the infected naked mole-rat foot indeed

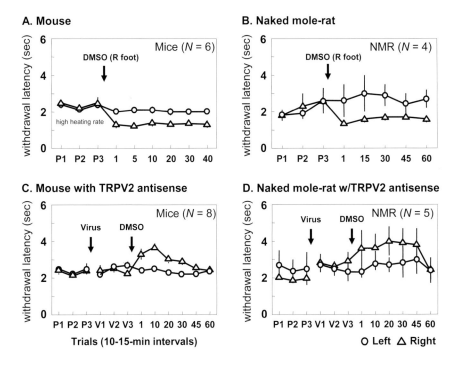

Fig. 2. Effects of topical dimethyl sulfoxide (DMSO) on foot-withdrawal latencies to the high heating rate. Latencies were measured at 10–15-minute intervals for both the right (R) and left (L) foot. The first three data points on each curve reflect withdrawal latencies prior to any manipulation (P1–P3). (A,B) DMSO was then applied to the right foot only in mice and naked mole-rats, respectively. (C,D) After collecting Pre data (P1–P3), mice and naked mole-rats were infected with TRPV2 antisense virus (SATRPV2). One week later, animals were tested again before (V1–V3) and after application of DMSO (trials 1–60).

showed sensitization from capsaicin that was comparable to that seen in mice (Fig. 3, low heating rate curves).

DISCUSSION

The main findings of this study are that naked mole-rats fail to show C-fiber-mediated sensitization from capsaicin, while they do show Aδ-fiber-mediated sensitization from DMSO comparable to that of mice. The experiments with TRPV2 antisense indicate normal (mouse-like) Aδ-fiber function for the naked mole-rats, suggesting that the lack of cutaneous neuropeptides specifically affects the C-fiber-mediated pathway. Introduction of PPT cDNA into naked mole-rat afferents via gene transfer techniques is sufficient to enable C-fiber-mediated sensitization from capsaicin. Taken together, these results are

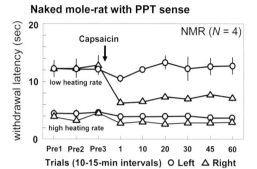

Fig. 3. Effects of infection with PPT sense virus (PPPT) on foot-withdrawal latencies of naked mole-rats. Virus was applied to the right (R) foot only. Testing was carried out 2 weeks later. The first three data points on each curve are withdrawal latencies after infection but prior to capsaicin application. Capsaicin was then applied to the right foot only.

consistent with the natural lack of substance P from cutaneous afferents in the naked mole-rat, and with the large body of evidence supporting a critical role for substance P in the development of thermal hyperalgesia (Cao et al. 1998; Furst 1999; Nichols et al. 1999; Woolf and Salter 2000; Hunt and Mantyh 2001; Willis 2001; Ikeda et al. 2003; Vierck 2003).

Several exciting animal models are currently being used to study the role of substance P in pain signaling, including PPT-A null mutant mice (Cao et al. 1998), neurokinin-1 knockout mice (De Felipe et al. 1998; Heikki et al. 1999; Laird et al. 2001), and rats treated with substance P-saporin conjugate (Mantyh et al. 1997; Nichols et al. 1999). In naked mole-rats, C fibers are present in the skin, as evidenced by the presence of small-diameter cell bodies in the dorsal root ganglia (Park et al. 2003), and they are easily identifiable in cross sections through the saphenous nerve (Y. Lu, personal observation, unpublished data). Thus, naked mole-rats should provide an additional valuable model for studying C-fiber-mediated function in the absence of substance P and after introduction of PPT via gene transfer techniques.

Peripheral application of capsaicin, the pungent ingredient in chili peppers that selectively activates receptors on C fibers, does not induce hypersensitivity to noxious heat (Lu 2002) and fails to elicit pain behavior responses in naked mole-rats (consistent with the apparent lack of acute sensitivity to capsaicin). These behavioral anomalies to painful stimuli could be explained simply by a lack of functional capsaicin-gated ion channels of the TRPV1 type expressed by sensory neurons. However, in electrophysiological recording of single cutaneous C fibers from naked mole-rats, we have observed C-fiber activation from capsaicin (G.R. Lewin and T.J. Park, unpublished data, 2004). Also, introduction of substance P alone into C fibers via infection with a transgenic herpes virus results in hypersensitivity from capsaicin that is comparable to that observed in other mammals to the low heating rate, which evokes C-fiber activation. Because the introduction of substance P alone is sufficient to enable C-fiber-mediated nociceptive responses in naked mole-rats, it seems that the lack of neuropeptides plays the main role in the lack of thermal hyperalgesia in this species.

Although C-fiber-mediated responses are affected dramatically, Aδ-fiber-mediated responses function normally, as seen in the experiments with the high heating rate where the response of naked mole-rats to DMSO was similar to that of mice. The animals showed no sensitization from DMSO when TRPV2-receptor activity was knocked down with the TRPV2 antisense virus. This finding indicates that Aδ and C nociceptors are affected differentially by the lack of neuropeptides in the peripheral nerves.

In summary, substance P and CGRP play a selective role in nociceptive responses mediated by C fibers. The activity of C and Aδ nociceptors is differentially affected by the absence of substance P, since Aδ-fiber activation remains unchanged. The introduction of PPT-derived peptides appears sufficient to enable a pathway that presumably was inactivated millions of years ago through evolutionary adaptation.

ACKNOWLEDGMENTS

The experimental work of the author and her colleagues was supported by the Departments of Anesthesiology and Biological Sciences at the University of Illinois at Chicago.

REFERENCES

Artwohl J, Hill T, Comer C, Park T. Naked mole-rats: unique opportunities and husbandry challenges. *Lab Anim (NY)* 2002; 31:32–36.

Cao YQ, Mantyh PW, Carlson EJ, et al. Primary afferent tachykinins are required to experience moderate to intense pain. *Nature* 1998; 392:390–394.

Collin E, Mauborgne A, Bourgoin S, et al. In vivo tonic inhibition of spinal substance P (-like material) release by endogenous opioid(s) acting at delta receptors. *Neuroscience* 1991; 44:725–731.

Collin E, Mantelet S, Frechilla D, et al. Increased in vivo release of calcitonin gene-related peptide-like material from the spinal cord in arthritic rats. *Pain* 1993; 54:203–211.

De Felipe C, Herrero JF, O'Brien JA, et al. Altered nociception, analgesia and aggression in mice lacking the receptor for substance P. *Nature* 1998; 392:394–397.

Duggan AW. Neuropharmacology of pain. *Curr Opin Neurol Neurosurg* 1992; 5:503–507.

Duggan AW, Hendry IA, Morton CR, Hutchison WD, Zhao ZQ. Cutaneous stimuli releasing immunoreactive substance P in the dorsal horn of the cat. *Brain Res* 1988; 451:261–273.

Go VL, Yaksh T. Release of substance P from the cat spinal cord. *J Physiol* 1987; 391:141–167.

Furst S. Transmitters involved in antinociception in the spinal cord. *Brain Res Bull* 1999;48:129–141.

Gulbenkian S, Merighi A, Wharton J, Varndell IM, Polak JM. Ultrastructural evidence for the co-existence of calcitonin gene-related peptide and substance P in secretory vesicles of peripheral nerves in the guinea pig. *J Neurocytol* 1986; 15:535–542.

Hamamoto DT, Ortiz-Gonzalez XR, Honda JM, Kajander KC. Intraplantar injection of hyaluronic acid at low pH into the rat hindpaw produces tissue acidosis and enhances withdrawal responses to mechanical stimuli. *Pain* 1998; 74:225–234.

Hunt SP, Mantyh PW. The molecular dynamics of pain control. *Nat Rev Neurosci* 2001; 2:83–91.

Ikeda H, Kusudo K, Ryu PD, Murase K. Effects of corticotropin-releasing factor on plasticity of optically recorded neuronal activity in the substantia gelatinosa of rat spinal cord slices. *Pain* 2003;106:197–207.

Julius D: The molecular biology of thermosensation. In: Dostrovsky JO, Carr DB, Koltzenburg M (Eds). *Proceedings of the 10th World Congress on Pain,* Progress in Pain Research and Management, Vol. 24. Seattle: IASP Press, 2002, pp 63–70.

Laird JM, Roza C, De Felipe C, Hunt SP, Cervero F. Role of central and peripheral tachykinin NK1 receptors in capsaicin-induced pain and hyperalgesia in mice. *Pain* 2001; 90:97–103.

LaMotte RH, Lundberg LE, Torebjork HE. Pain, hyperalgesia and activity in nociceptive C units in humans after intradermal injection of capsaicin. *J Physiol* 1992; 448:749–764.

Lindahl O. Pain: a chemical explanation. *Acta Rheumatol Scand* 1962; 8:161–169.

Lu Y, Park T, Rice F, Laurito C. The absence of substance P and CGRP in the dorsal root ganglia of naked mole rats correlates with an absence of hyperalgesia to heat. In: Dostrovsky JO, Carr DB, Koltzenburg M (Eds). *Proceedings of the 10th World Congress on Pain,* Progress in Pain Research and Management, Vol. 24. Seattle: IASP Press, 2002, pp 235–243.

Mantyh PW, Allen CJ, Ghilardi JR, et al. Rapid endocytosis of a G protein-coupled receptor: substance P evoked internalization of its receptor in the rat striatum in vivo. *Proc Natl Acad Sci USA* 1995;92:2622–2626.

Mantyh PW, Rogers SD, Honore P, et al. Inhibition of hyperalgesia by ablation of lamina I spinal neurons expressing the substance P receptor. *Science* 1997; 278:275–279.

Park TJ, Comer C, Carol A, et al. Somatosensory organization and behavior in naked mole-rats: II. Peripheral structures, innervation, and selective lack of neuropeptides associated with thermoregulation and pain. *J Comp Neurol* 2003; 465:104–120.

Nichols ML, Allen BJ, Rogers SD, et al. Transmission of chronic nociception by spinal neurons expressing the substance P receptor. *Science* 1999; 286:1558–1561.

Sakurada T, Katsumata K, Tan-No K, Sakurada S, Kisara K. The capsaicin test in mice for evaluating tachykinin antagonists in the spinal cord. *Neuropharmacology* 1992; 31:1279–1285.

Simone DA. Inhibition of hyperalgesia by ablation of lamina I spinal neurons expressing the substance P receptor. *Science* 1997; 278:275–279.

Tzabazis A, Klyukinov M, Manering N, et al. Differential activation of trigeminal C or A-delta noci-ceptors by infrared diode laser in rats: behavioral evidence. *Brain Res* 2005;1037:148–156.

Vierck CJ Jr, Kline RH, Wiley RG. Intrathecal substance p-saporin attenuates operant escape from nociceptive thermal stimuli. *Neuroscience* 2003; 119:223–232.

Willis WD. Role of neurotransmitters in sensitization of pain responses. *Ann N Y Acad Sci* 2001; 933:142–156.

Wilson SP, Yeomans DC. Genetic therapy for pain management. *Curr Rev Pain* 2000; 4:445–450.

Wilson SP, Yeomans DC. Virally mediated delivery of enkephalin and other neuropeptide transgenes in experimental pain models. *Ann N Y Acad Sci* 2002; 971:515–521.

Woolf CJ, Salter MW. Neuronal plasticity: increasing the gain in pain. *Science* 2000;288:1765–1769.

Wright C, Goudas LC, Bentch A, et al. Hyperalgesia in outpatients with dermal injury: quantitative sensory testing versus a novel simple technique. *Pain Med* 2004; 5:162–167.

Yaksh T, Go VL. Survey of distribution of substance P, vasoactive intestinal polypeptide, cholecystokinin, neurotensin, Met-enkephalin, bombesin and PHI in the spinal cord of cat, dog, sloth and monkey. *Peptides* 1988; 9:357–372.

Yeomans D, Proudfit H. Nociceptive responses to high and low rates of noxious cutaneous heating are mediated by different nociceptors in the rat: electrophysiological evidence. *Pain* 1996; 68:141–150.

Yeomans D, Pirec V, Proudfit H. Nociceptive responses to high and low rates of noxious cutaneous heating are mediated by different nociceptors in the rat: behavioral evidence. *Pain* 1996; 68:133–140.

Zachariou V, Goldstein BD, Yeomans DC. Low but not high rate noxious radiant skin heating evokes a capsaicin-sensitive increase in spinal cord dorsal horn release of substance P. *Brain Res* 1997; 752:143–150.

Correspondence to: Ying Lu, MD, Department of Anesthesiology, University of Illinois at Chicago, 1740 West Taylor Street, Suite 3200 West, Chicago, IL 60612-7239, USA. Fax: 425-643-0481; email: yinglu@uic.edu.

Proceedings of the 11th World Congress on Pain,
edited by Herta Flor, Eija Kalso, and Jonathan O.
Dostrovsky, IASP Press, Seattle, © 2006.

17

Different Effects of Spinally Applied COX-1, COX-2, and Nonselective Cyclooxygenase Inhibitors on Inflammation-Evoked Spinal Hyperexcitability

Alejandro Telleria-Diaz,[a] Anne-Kathrin Neubert,[a]
Florian Schache,[a] Enrique Vazquez,[a,b]
Andrea Ebersberger,[a] Horacio Vanegas,[a,b]
and Hans-Georg Schaible[a]

[a]*Department of Physiology, Friedrich Schiller University of Jena, Jena, Germany;*
[b]*Venezuelan Institute for Scientific Research, Caracas, Venezuela*

Hyperexcitability of spinal cord neurons (central sensitization) is regarded as a fundamental mechanism in persistent pain conditions. Current evidence indicates that spinal prostaglandins contribute to central sensitization caused by peripheral inflammation. Indeed, peripheral inflammation induces upregulation of cyclooxygenase-2 (COX-2) in dorsal root ganglia and the spinal cord and increases spinal prostaglandin release (Vanegas and Schaible 2001). Spinally applied prostaglandin E_2 (PGE_2) receptor agonists evoke responses in nociceptive spinal cord neurons similar to those evoked by inflammation in the knee (Bär et al. 2004), and spinal pretreatment with COX inhibitors attenuates the generation of inflammation-induced central sensitization (Vanegas and Schaible 2001; Svensson and Yaksh 2002).

However, studies of spinal pretreatment with COX inhibitors do not clarify the roles of spinal prostaglandins, COX, and COX inhibitors in the maintenance of neuronal hyperexcitability (Vanegas and Schaible 2001). In some studies, spinally applied nonselective COX inhibitors have failed to reverse inflammation-induced behavioral hyperalgesia (Dirig et al. 1998) or hyperexcitability of spinal nociceptive neurons (Vasquez et al. 2001), once inflammation was established, whereas in other studies selective COX-2 inhibitors did reduce behavioral hyperalgesia (Yamamoto and Nozaki-Taguchi 1996; Samad et al. 2001). This chapter describes a study in which we compared the action of spinally applied COX-1, COX-2, and nonselective COX inhibitors on inflammation-evoked activity of nociceptive spinal cord neurons with knee joint input. COX inhibitors were applied either before or during established inflammation. In the latter situation we also measured the release of spinal prostaglandins. Because COX-2 in the brain is also involved in the metabolic breakdown of endocannabinoids (Kim and Alger 2004; Kozak et al. 2004), which have analgesic properties (Lichtman and Martin 1991; Richardson et al. 1998), we also tested whether an endocannabinoid-dependent pathway (see Gühring et al. 2002) might be involved in the putative effects of COX-2 inhibitors.

METHODS

Male Wistar rats (315–396 g) were anesthetized with thiopentone. Spinal cord segments L1–L4 were exposed by laminectomy, and a trough over the recording region was built with a rubber ring (about 3×5 mm). Injection of kaolin and carrageenan into the knee joint cavity produced acute inflammation. Action potentials were recorded extracellularly from dorsal horn neurons that responded to pressure onto the ipsilateral knee but not to brushing or squeezing of the skin over the knee. The knee joint was compressed in the mediolateral axis at innocuous (1.9 N/40 mm^2 holding pressure) and noxious intensity (5.9 or 7.8 N/40 mm^2). Innocuous and noxious pressure was applied with clips to the ankle and paw. Each stimulus lasted for 15 seconds. Test responses to each stimulus type were averaged within successive blocks of either 25 or 60 minutes.

Compounds pipetted into the spinal trough were: (1) indomethacin (8 mM, see Vasquez et al. 2001), (2) diclofenac (3 mM, dissolved in Tyrode and 0.07% ethanol), (3) SC-560 (3 mM, dissolved in dimethylformamide and distilled water 1:1), (4) L-745,337 (Boyce et al. 1994) (0.3 and 3 mM, dissolved in 5% glucose), (5) NS-398 (1.3 mM, dissolved in dimethylformamide and distilled water 1:1), and (6) the cannabinoid receptor 1 (CB1) antagonist AM-251 (1 μM, dissolved in 0.07% dimethylsulfoxide and 0.07% ethanol). COX inhibitors or their vehicles were given either before induction of inflammation or when inflammation was fully established (7–12 hours after kaolin), in order to test their effects on the responses of neurons to pressure onto the knee and ankle. During inflammation, we also tested the influence of AM-251 on the effects of COX inhibitors.

We assessed effects of COX inhibitors on prostaglandin release in samples from the spinal trough, beginning 7 hours after kaolin injection. First, vehicle was applied into the trough for 15 minutes and then aspirated for PGE_2 determination. After three such samples, the COX inhibitor was applied spinally. After 60 minutes three 15-minute sampling runs were carried out with the COX inhibitor solution. Samples were frozen immediately, and immunoreactive PGE_2 ($iPGE_2$) was determined by enzyme immunoassay (detection level 15 pg/mL).

RESULTS

All sampled neurons were located in the deep dorsal horn of L1–L4 at depths of 700–1200 µm (mean $\pm$ SD = 924 $\pm$ 205 µm). In addition to the knee, the receptive field usually included deep tissues of the thigh and lower leg. Some neurons had cutaneous receptive fields, but not over the knee.

EFFECT OF COX INHIBITORS ON THE GENERATION OF SPINAL HYPEREXCITABILITY

With vehicle on the cord, dorsal horn neurons developed hyperexcitability after induction of inflammation. They showed enhanced responses to noxious pressure upon the injected knee (Fig. 1 top, open squares) and, as an indicator of central sensitization, novel or enhanced responses to pressure of the non-inflamed ankle (Fig. 1 bottom, open squares) and paw. When the selective COX-1 inhibitor SC-560 was applied, the development of neuronal hyperexcitability was attenuated in the first 2 hours after kaolin, but not later (filled circles). By contrast, the spinally applied selective COX-2 inhibitor L-745,337 fully prevented increases of the responses to the inflamed knee and the non-inflamed ankle (filled squares). The increase in knee circumference was similar in these experimental groups and the vehicle-treated controls, indicating similar peripheral inflammation.

SPINAL APPLICATION OF COX INHIBITORS DURING INFLAMMATION

COX inhibitors were spinally applied once inflammation-evoked spinal hyperexcitability was established. SC-560 did not change responses to noxious pressure (7 neurons, see example in Fig. 2A). By contrast, L-745,337 reduced responses to noxious pressure (see neuron displayed in Fig. 2B). On average, responses to noxious pressure were significantly reduced to 58% after 75–100 minutes by 3 mM (11 neurons), and to 67% after 75–100 minutes by 0.3 mM L-745,337 (7 neurons). The vehicle had no effect (10 neurons). In the absence of inflammation, L-745,337 had no effect on the responses (5 neurons). The selective COX-2 inhibitor NS-398 also reduced inflammation-evoked neuronal

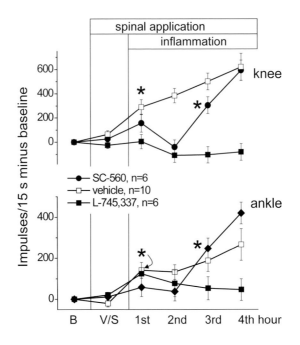

Fig. 1. Effects of spinally applied COX inhibitors on the generation of inflammation-evoked spinal hyperexcitability. The graph shows changes of responses to noxious pressure onto the knee joint (top graph) and onto the non-inflamed ankle (bottom graph) after induction of knee inflammation. The initial baseline (B) was set to zero, and the other values (mean ± SEM) show changes from baseline. Inflammation was induced 30 minutes after spinal drug administration. V/S, either vehicle or substance; COX-1 inhibitor SC-560, 3 mM; COX-2 inhibitor L-745,337, 3 mM. Asterisks show the first values that were different from baseline (Wilcoxon matched-pairs signed-rank test, $P < 0.05$).

responses. Nonselective COX inhibitors diclofenac and indomethacin had no effect. Fig. 2C shows a neuron whose responses were not changed by diclofenac but were reduced by subsequent L-745,337 application.

Since the difference between various COX inhibitors might result from different degrees of COX inhibition, release of iPGE$_2$ into the spinal trough during inflammation was measured when the trough contained either Tyrode (a neutral control solution), indomethacin (8 mM), L-745,377 (3 mM), or SC-560 (3 mM). Mechanical stimulation was continuously performed as in experiments with recordings from neurons. Compared to their vehicles, all COX inhibitors depressed iPGE$_2$ release significantly by about 60% (Fig. 2D) in samples taken 60–105 minutes after application. Therefore, there was no correlation between inhibition of prostaglandin synthesis and inhibition of responses to mechanical stimulation during inflammation.

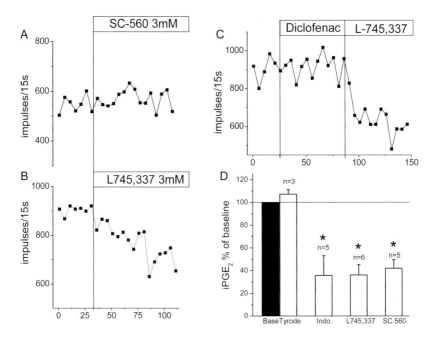

Fig. 2. Effects of spinally applied COX inhibitors on the enhanced responses of spinal cord neurons to noxious pressure onto the inflamed knee (at least 7 hours after induction of knee inflammation). (A–C) Responses of single neurons before and during drug application. (A) No change in a neuron under 3 mM SC-560. (B) Reduction of responses in a neuron by L-745,337. (C) No effect of diclofenac and effect of L-745,337 on a neuron. (D) Reduced release of iPGE$_2$ from the spinal cord into the solution in the trough during knee inflammation, before (Base) and 60–105 minutes after application of Tyrode, indomethacin (8 mM), L-745,337 (3 mM), or SC-560 (3 mM). Asterisks (*) denote significant reductions ($P < 0.05$, Wilcoxon matched-pairs signed-rank test).

ENDOCANNABINOIDS AND ANTINOCICEPTION BY COX-2 INHIBITORS

We tested whether the antinociceptive effect of L-745,337 during inflammation is influenced by AM-251, an antagonist of the cannabinoid-1 (CB1) receptor. Spinal application of AM-251 (1 µM) alone for 2 hours did not change neuronal responses (6 neurons, example in Fig. 3A). When L-745,337 (3 mM) was coadministered to the spinal cord with AM-251 (1 µM) during inflammation, responses to noxious and innocuous pressure onto the inflamed knee were not significantly reduced (8 neurons, example in Fig. 3B). Furthermore, AM-251 reversed the reduction of the responses by L-745,337 when added to the COX-2 inhibitor after 100 minutes (8 neurons, example in Fig. 3C). By contrast, the negative effect of indomethacin on neuronal responses was not modified by coadministration of AM-251 (6 neurons).

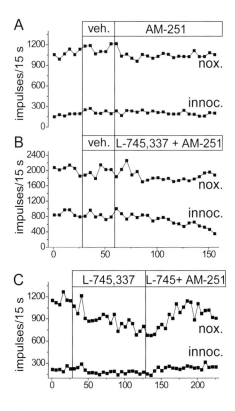

Fig. 3. Influence of AM-251, antagonist at cannabinoid-1 receptors, on neuronal responses to innocuous (innoc.) and noxious (nox.) pressure onto the inflamed knee joint, as well as on the effects of L-745,337. (A) No reduction of responses by AM-251. (B) No reduction of responses to noxious pressure upon coadministration of L-745,337 (3 mM) and AM-251 (1 μM). (C) Reduction of responses to noxious pressure during application of L-745,337 (3 mM) alone, and reversal of this effect upon coadministration of L-745,337 (3 mM) and AM-251 (1 μM).

DISCUSSION

Spinal pretreatment with COX-1 inhibitors hindered the initiation of central sensitization, which suggests a role for constitutive COX-1 at this stage. But this effect was transient, probably because induction of COX-2 eventually elevates spinal prostaglandin levels. Inhibiting COX-2 indeed had a profound and long-lasting effect upon the responses of nociceptive neurons, consistent with results from behavioral experiments in which spinal pretreatment with selective COX-2 inhibitors prevented the sensitization of nociceptive motor responses caused by subsequent inflammation (Yamamoto and Nozaki-Taguchi 1996; Dirig et al. 1998).

During established inflammation, only the spinal application of the COX-2 inhibitors—not COX-1 or nonselective COX inhibitors—reduced responses to mechanical stimulation. Interestingly, however, all COX inhibitors reduced the spinal release of PGE_2, which shows a clear discrepancy between reduction of prostaglandin release and reduction of neuronal activity. It was therefore necessary to reconsider the mechanism of action of these compounds, at least in the spinal cord. In fact, an antagonist to the CB1 receptor prevented and reversed the attenuation of neuronal hyperexcitability caused by L-745,337, a selective COX-2 inhibitor, during inflammation. We assume therefore that, independent from its effects on prostaglandin synthesis, L-745,337 fosters endogenous cannabinoid activity. This assumption is based on the fact that spinal application of the CB1 antagonist had no effect unless L-745,337 was acting. The most likely explanation is that COX-2 inhibition by L-745,337 decreased endocannabinoid breakdown so that endocannabinoids such as 2-arachidonylglycerol and anandamide reached a sufficiently high concentration to act on CB1 receptors.

Further studies have to test whether this interaction with endocannabinoids applies to all COX-2 inhibitors. Furthermore, it needs to be clarified why indomethacin, which inhibits both COX-1 and COX-2, neither had an effect upon neuronal responses nor was influenced by AM-251 during inflammation. Nevertheless, after oral administration, several selective COX-2 inhibitors reach concentrations well above their IC_{50} (the concentration that inhibits activity by 50%) in the cerebrospinal fluid and the spinal cord (Dembo et al. 2005). The results described in this chapter clearly show that COX-2 inhibitors might be superior to nonselective COX inhibitors concerning spinal effects during inflammation.

ACKNOWLEDGMENTS

We thank Merck Frosst, Kirkland, Quebec, Canada, for providing L-745,337.

REFERENCES

Bär KJ, Natura G, Telleria-Diaz A, et al. Changes in the effect of spinal prostaglandin E2 during inflammation: prostaglandin E (EP1-EP4) receptors in spinal nociceptive processing of input from the normal or inflamed knee joint. *J Neurosci* 2004; 24:642–651.

Boyce S, Chan CC, Gordon R, et al. L-745,337: a selective inhibitor of cyclooxygenase-2 elicits antinociception but not gastric ulceration in rats. *Neuropharmacology* 1994; 33:1609–1611.

Dembo G, Park SB, Kharasch ED. Central nervous system concentrations of cyclooxygenase-2 inhibitors in humans. *Anesthesiology* 2005; 102:409–415.

Dirig DM, Isakson PC, Yaksh TL. Effect of COX-1 and COX-2 inhibition on induction and maintenance of carrageenan-evoked thermal hyperalgesia in rats. *J Pharmacol Exp Ther* 1998; 285:1031–1038.

Gühring H, Hamza M, Sergejeva M, et al. A role for endocannabinoids in indomethacin-induced spinal antinociception. *Eur J Pharmacol* 2002; 454:153–163.

Kim J, Alger BE. Inhibition of cyclooxygenase-2 potentiates retrograde endocannabinoid effects in hippocampus. *Nature Neurosci* 2004; 7:697–698.

Kozak KR, Prusakiewicz JJ, Marnett LJ. Oxidative metabolism of endocannabinoids by COX-2. *Curr Pharm Des* 2004; 10:659–667.

Lichtman AH, Martin BR. Spinal and supraspinal components of cannabinoid-induced antinociception. *J Pharmacol Exp Ther* 1991; 258:517–523.

Richardson JD, Aanonsen L, Hargreaves KM. Antihyperalgesic effects of spinal cannabinoids. *Eur J Pharmacol* 1998; 345:145–153.

Samad TA, Moore KA, Sapirstein A, et al. Interleukin-1β-mediated induction of COX-2 in the CNS contributes to inflammatory pain hypersensitivity. *Nature* 2001; 410:471–475.

Svensson CI, Yaksh TL. The spinal phospholipase-prostanoid cascade in nociceptive processing. *Annu Rev Pharmacol Toxicol* 2002; 42:553–583.

Vanegas H, Schaible H-G. Prostaglandins and cyclooxygenases in the spinal cord. *Prog Neurobiol* 2001; 64:327–363.

Vasquez E, Bär K-J, Ebersberger A, et al. Spinal prostaglandins are involved in the development but not the maintenance of inflammation-induced spinal hyperexcitability. *J Neurosci* 2001; 21:9001–9008.

Yamamoto T, Nozaki-Taguchi N. Analysis of the effects of cyclooxygenase (COX)-1 and COX-2 spinal nociceptive transmission using indomethacin, a non-selective COX inhibitor, and NS-398, a COX-2 selective inhibitor. *Brain Res* 1996; 739:104–110.

Correspondence to: Professor Dr. Hans-Georg Schaible, Department of Physiology, University of Jena, Teichgraben 8, D-07740 Jena, Germany Tel: 49-3641-938810; Fax: 49-3641-938812; email: hans-georg.schaible@mti.uni-jena.de.

Proceedings of the 11th World Congress on Pain,
edited by Herta Flor, Eija Kalso, and Jonathan O.
Dostrovsky, IASP Press, Seattle, © 2006.

18

Paclitaxel-Induced Mechanical Allodynia in Rats Is Inhibited by Spinal Delivery of Plasmid DNA Encoding Interleukin-10

Annemarie Ledeboer,[a] Evan M. Sloane,[a]
Erin D. Milligan,[a] Stephen J. Langer,[b] Steven F.
Maier,[a] Kirk W. Johnson,[c] Leslie A. Leinwand,[b]
Raymond A. Chavez,[c] and Linda R. Watkins[a]

[a]Department of Psychology and the Center for Neuroscience, and [b]Department
of Molecular, Cellular and Developmental Biology, University of Colorado
at Boulder, Boulder, Colorado, USA; [c]Avigen Inc., Alameda, California, USA

Paclitaxel is a chemotherapeutic drug that is frequently associated with the development of painful peripheral neuropathy (Dougherty et al. 2004). Little is known about the mechanisms underlying this dose-limiting adverse effect. Recent data strongly support the concept that activated glial cells in the spinal cord critically contribute to the facilitation of other neuropathic pain states, in particular through the release of proinflammatory cytokines, such as interleukin-1 (IL-1) (Watkins et al. 2001; Watkins and Maier 2003; DeLeo et al. 2004). These findings raise the question of whether paclitaxel activates spinal cord glia and, if so, whether this chemotherapy-induced neuropathic pain state may be mediated by spinal release of proinflammatory cytokines.

This chapter describes a study using a rat model of paclitaxel-induced neuropathic pain, in which repeated intraperitoneal injections of paclitaxel induce stable changes in pain behavior that last for several months (Polomano et al. 2001; Flatters and Bennett 2004). In order to examine whether proinflammatory cytokines mediate paclitaxel-induced pain changes, we explored whether paclitaxel-induced mechanical allodynia could be reversed by intrathecal (i.t.) interleukin-1 receptor antagonist (IL-1ra) and/or by a novel i.t. interleukin-10 (IL-10) gene therapy. These two complementary approaches were chosen for two reasons. First, spinal IL-1 has been repeatedly implicated as a mediator of diverse enhanced pain states (Watkins and Maier 2003), indicating that IL-1ra may be effective for paclitaxel-induced neuropathic pain as well. Second, the anti-inflammatory cytokine IL-10 suppresses the production and activity of several proinflammatory cytokines, including IL-1 (Moore et al. 2001). We have previously shown that i.t. administration of either IL-10 protein or IL-10 gene therapy with viral vectors prevents or reverses mechanical allodynia induced by traumatic neuropathy such as chronic constriction injury (CCI) and sciatic inflammatory neuropathy (Milligan et al. 2005a,c). More recently, we have been pursuing a novel nonviral approach, which utilizes i.t. delivery of "naked" plasmid DNA encoding IL-10 (pDNA-IL-10). In studies to date, i.t. pDNA-IL-10 has been reported to produce prolonged reversal of CCI-induced mechanical allodynia (Milligan et al. 2005b; Sloane et al. 2005). Thus, we used this improved i.t. gene therapy approach for the present study.

METHODS

Drugs. Paclitaxel (6 mg/mL in vehicle consisting of surfactant/ethanol 1:1) was diluted in 0.9% sterile saline to a concentration of 1 or 2 mg/mL prior to injection. Endotoxin-free solutions of recombinant human interleukin-1 receptor antagonist (IL-1ra; 100 µg/µL) were used. Plasmid DNA encoding for rat IL-10 (pDNA-IL-10) was identical to the expression cassette used in our previous studies with adeno-associated virus, encoding rat IL-10 under the control of a hybrid cytomegalovirus (CMV) enhancer/chicken β-actin promoter (Milligan et al. 2005c). Here it was used in the absence of the viral vector; that is, as naked DNA. The control plasmid (pDNA-control) was identical to the pDNA-IL-10 plasmid but without the IL-10 gene. Plasmids were purified using an endotoxin-free purification kit. Plasmid DNA was suspended in sterile phosphate-buffered saline (pH 7.2) with 3% sucrose.

Intrathecal (i.t.) drug delivery. Acute i.t. injections were performed under brief isoflurane anaesthesia using an 18-gauge sterile needle temporarily inserted between lumbar vertebrae L5 and L6. This needle served as a guide cannula for drug and pDNA delivery via a polyethylene (PE-10) injection catheter, as described previously (Ledeboer et al. 2005).

Experimental procedures. All experiments were approved by the Institutional Animal Care and Use Committee at the University of Colorado at Boulder. In all experiments, adult male Sprague Dawley rats (n = 5–7/group) received four intraperitoneal (i.p.) injections of vehicle or paclitaxel (1 or 2 mg/kg; cumulative dose: 4 or 8 mg/kg) on four alternate days, as described in Polomano et al. (2001). In experiment 1, rats received a single i.t. injection of IL-1ra (150 µg) or vehicle, 3 weeks after the first i.p. injection of paclitaxel (4 mg/kg). In experiments 2 and 3, rats were tested for the efficacy of pDNA-

IL10, beginning 5 weeks after the first i.p. injection of paclitaxel (4 mg/kg in experiment 2 and 8 mg/kg in experiment 3) or vehicle. The dosing regimen for pDNA-IL10 was based on our prior studies, demonstrating that a 100-μg dose of pDNA-IL10, followed 3 days later by a second pDNA-IL10 dose of 25 μg, results in a prolonged reversal of CCI-induced mechanical allodynia (Sloane et al. 2005). The effects of pDNA-IL10 were compared to those of equal doses of pDNA-control and phosphate-buffered saline delivered identically to pDNA-IL10.

Behavioral testing. Rats were tested for mechanical allodynia by assessing their touch/pressure thresholds within the sciatic innervation area of the hindpaws using the von Frey test (Chaplan et al. 1994), as previously described (Milligan et al. 2000). Thresholds were assessed prior to i.p. injections (baseline), and weekly thereafter. After i.t. injections, responses to the von Frey test were reassessed throughout the remainder of the time course as indicated in the figures. As paclitaxel induces bilateral allodynia, and response thresholds did not differ between left and right hindpaws, values represent average thresholds from both hindpaws.

Statistical analysis. Data were analyzed by one-way analysis of variance (ANOVA) for baseline measures, and by repeated-measures ANOVA for time-course measures, followed by Fisher's protected least significant difference post-hoc comparisons, where appropriate.

RESULTS

Paclitaxel-treated rats developed a pronounced bilateral mechanical allodynia, as assessed by the von Frey test, with onset of allodynia between 2–3 weeks after the first i.p. injection (Figs. 1–3), whereas vehicle-treated rats did not exhibit significant allodynia.

In experiment 1, we first assessed whether spinal IL-1 is involved in paclitaxel-induced mechanical allodynia by using the specific IL-1 antagonist, IL-1ra. Fig. 1 shows that baseline assessments on the von Frey test revealed no differences between groups prior to drug treatment, and that repeated paclitaxel injections induced reliable allodynia by day 18 after the first i.p. injection. A single i.t. injection of IL-1ra given on this day transiently reversed allodynia in both hindpaws, with maximal effect 2 hours after IL-1ra injection.

We next investigated whether IL-10 gene therapy would be effective in reversing paclitaxel-induced allodynia. In experiment 2, baseline responses to the von Frey test showed no differences between groups prior to drug treatment, and repeated paclitaxel injections (cumulative dose 4 mg/kg) induced mechanical allodynia by 3 weeks after the first i.p. injection (Fig. 2). pDNA-IL-10 resulted in a partial reversal of allodynia, which lasted for at least 4 weeks.

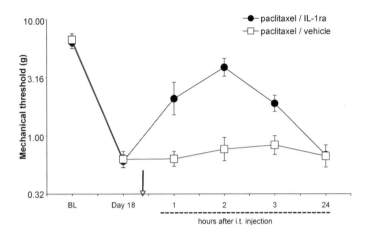

Fig. 1. A single intrathecal injection of IL-1ra transiently reverses paclitaxel-induced mechanical allodynia. Rats received four intraperitoneal injections of paclitaxel (4 × 1 mg/kg) on alternate days, and IL-1ra (150 μg) or vehicle was administered intrathecally 18 days after the first paclitaxel injection (indicated by the arrow). Low-threshold mechanical sensitivity was assessed by the von Frey test, at baseline (BL), on day 18, and 1, 2, 3, and 24 hours after injection.

In experiment 3, baseline mechanical thresholds again did not differ between groups, and repeated paclitaxel injections (cumulative dose 8 mg/kg) induced mechanical allodynia by 3 weeks after the first i.p. injection, as compared to vehicle-injected controls (Fig. 3). pDNA-IL-10 partially reversed allodynia, an effect that lasted for approximately 5 weeks. Basal response thresholds of vehicle-injected animals were not affected by treatment with pDNA-IL-10. Interestingly, paclitaxel-treated rats that were injected with the control plasmid (pDNA-control) also showed a partial reversal of allodynia, but this lasted for approximately 1 week only (Fig. 3). This transient effect of non-encoding pDNA is in accordance with our previous studies (Sloane et al. 2005).

DISCUSSION

The present study shows that intrathecal IL-1ra and IL-10 gene therapy both attenuate paclitaxel-induced pain behavior. These results demonstrate that spinal cord proinflammatory cytokines are importantly involved in neuropathic pain induced by this widely used chemotherapeutic agent. Consistent with previous observations (Polomano et al. 2001), the 4 mg/kg and 8 mg/kg paclitaxel doses induced comparable magnitudes of mechanical allodynia. Similarly, pDNA-IL-10 was equally effective in reversing allodynia induced by a cumulative dose of 4 or 8 mg/kg paclitaxel.

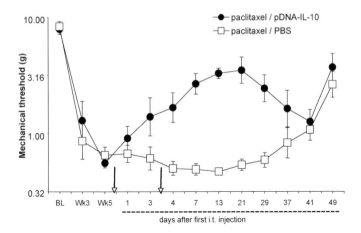

Fig. 2. Intrathecal IL-10 gene therapy partially reverses mechanical allodynia induced by paclitaxel (4 mg/kg). Rats received four intraperitoneal injections of paclitaxel (4 × 1 mg/kg) on alternate days. Two intrathecal injections of pDNA-IL-10 (100 and 25 μg, respectively) or vehicle (phosphate-buffered saline) were given 5 weeks after the first paclitaxel injection, 3 days apart (indicated by the arrows). Low-threshold mechanical sensitivity was assessed by the von Frey test, at baseline (BL), at 3 weeks and 5 weeks after the first paclitaxel injection, and up to 49 days after the first intrathecal injection.

The fact that i.t. IL-1ra was able to affect paclitaxel-induced pain changes suggests that at least IL-1 is involved in mediating paclitaxel-induced allodynia in the spinal cord. It is noteworthy that the efficacy of IL-1ra does not preclude the involvement of other proinflammatory cytokines, such as tumor necrosis factor or interleukin-6. Spinal proinflammatory cytokines are often released as part of a cascade, such that blockade of one proinflammatory cytokine can decrease the production of others (Milligan et al. 2001). Thus, given the specificity of IL-1ra for IL-1 receptors, the effect of IL-1ra clearly indicates paclitaxel-induced release of IL-1, but does not negate the involvement of other spinal proinflammatory cytokines.

While i.t. IL-1ra and i.t. IL-10 can each reverse neuropathic pain (Milligan et al. 2005a), the effects of both are short-lived, due to their rapid degradation and/or clearance. This transient duration of effect limits their therapeutic potential. Therefore, we have been pursuing i.t. IL-10 gene therapy in order to attain prolonged spinal release of IL-10. Intrathecal delivery of nonviral "naked" plasmid DNA has proven especially effective in this regard. Previously, we reported that an initial i.t. injection of pDNA-IL-10 reversed mechanical allodynia induced by CCI for a short period (4–5 days) (Milligan et al. 2005b). Remarkably, repeated i.t. pDNA-IL10 injections yielded reversal of allodynia for a prolonged period (more than 3 months) (Milligan et al. 2005b; Sloane et

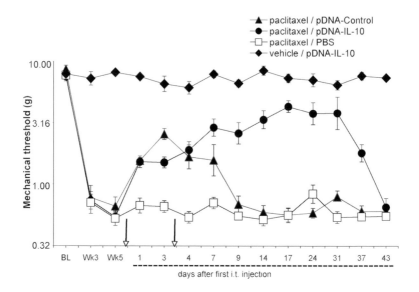

Fig. 3. Intrathecal IL-10 gene therapy partially reverses mechanical allodynia induced by paclitaxel (8 mg/kg). Rats received four intraperitoneal injections of paclitaxel (4×2 mg/kg) on alternate days. Two intrathecal injections of pDNA-IL-10 or pDNA-control (100 and 25 µg, respectively) or vehicle (phosphate-buffered saline) were given 5 weeks after the first paclitaxel injection, 3 days apart (indicated by the arrows). Low-threshold mechanical sensitivity was assessed by the von Frey test, at baseline (BL), 3 weeks, and 5 weeks after the first paclitaxel or vehicle injection, and up to 43 days after the first intrathecal injection.

al. 2005). In accordance with these prior studies, prolonged reversal of pacli-taxel-induced allodynia was observed in response to two sequential i.t. injec-tions of pDNA-IL-10 administered 3 days apart. From the data published so far, it appears that the first i.t. injection of pDNA "primes" cells surrounding the lumbosacral cerebrospinal fluid space, thereby rendering the second i.t. injection more effective (Milligan et al. 2005b; Sloane et al. 2005). Studies investigating the mechanisms of this "priming" effect are currently in progress.

It is also notable that pDNA was able to transiently reverse paclitaxel-induced allodynia, in the absence of the IL-10 transgene (pDNA-control). These findings replicate our prior observation that pDNA-control produces a transient reversal of CCI-induced allodynia (Sloane et al. 2005). While these findings were initially surprising, recent studies document that pDNA-control induces a transient anti-inflammatory response when administered to the intra-thecal compartment. This work is supported by the finding that IL-10 protein levels in lumbosacral cerebrospinal fluid are increased 3 days after intrathecal pDNA-control injections, relative to vehicle-injected controls (Sloane et al. 2005). This finding suggests that pDNA-control elicits an endogenous IL-10 response, which may account for the observed short-term reversal of allodynia.

Ongoing studies demonstrate, however, that inclusion of the IL-10 transgene in the plasmid DNA construct is required for prolonged (more than 3 months) reversal of allodynia attained by a subsequent plasmid injection. That this prolonged behavioral reversal is indeed due to prolonged spinal release of IL-10 is supported by the fact that, even a month after CCI-induced allodynia was reversed by pDNA-IL10 therapy, anti-IL10 (but not control antibody) abolished the anti-allodynic effects of pDNA-IL10. That is, anti-IL10 treatment returned pDNA-IL10-treated CCI rats to a fully allodynic state (Sloane et al. 2005).

Lastly, the present data would suggest that paclitaxel-induced allodynia is associated with glial activation in the spinal cord. Indeed, preliminary observations indicate that paclitaxel induces microglial activation, as reflected by increases in OX-6 (labeling MHC class II) and OX-42 (labeling CD11b) immunoreactivity, in the spinal cord. Studies defining which proinflammatory cytokines are upregulated by paclitaxel are in progress.

Taken together, the data presented in this chapter suggest that paclitaxel-induced painful neuropathies are mediated by spinal proinflammatory cytokines such as IL-1. Our findings indicate that spinal IL-10 gene therapy may be a promising strategy for controlling paclitaxel-induced neuropathic pain.

ACKNOWLEDGMENTS

We thank Amgen (Thousand Oaks, California) for kindly providing the IL-1ra and its vehicle. Supported by Avigen and by NIH grants DA015642, NS40696, NS38020, DA015656, AI51093, and DA018156.

REFERENCES

Chaplan SR, Bach FW, Pogrel JW, Chung JM, Yaksh TL. Quantitative assessment of tactile allodynia in the rat paw. *J Neurosci Methods* 1994; 53:55–63.

DeLeo JA, Tanga FY, Tawfik VL. Neuroimmune activation and neuroinflammation in chronic pain and opioid tolerance/hyperalgesia. *Neuroscientist* 2004; 10:40–52.

Dougherty PM, Cata JP, Cordella JV, Burton A, Weng HR. Taxol-induced sensory disturbance is characterized by preferential impairment of myelinated fiber function in cancer patients. *Pain* 2004; 109:132–142.

Flatters SJ, Bennett GJ. Ethosuximide reverses paclitaxel- and vincristine-induced painful peripheral neuropathy. *Pain* 2004; 109:150–161.

Ledeboer A, Sloane EM, Milligan ED, et al. Minocycline attenuates mechanical allodynia and proinflammatory cytokine expression in rat models of pain facilitation. *Pain* 2005; 115:71–83.

Milligan ED, Mehmert KK, Hinde JL, et al. Thermal hyperalgesia and mechanical allodynia produced by intrathecal administration of the human immunodeficiency virus-1 (HIV-1) envelope glycoprotein, gp120. *Brain Res* 2000; 861:105–116.

Milligan ED, O'Connor KA, Nguyen KT, et al. Intrathecal HIV-1 envelope glycoprotein gp120 induces enhanced pain states mediated by spinal cord proinflammatory cytokines. *J Neurosci* 2001; 21:2808–2819.

Milligan ED, Langer SJ, Sloane EM, et al. Controlling pathological pain by adenovirally driven spinal production of the anti-inflammatory cytokine, interleukin-10. *Eur J Neurosci* 2005a; 21:2136–2148.

Milligan ED, Sloane EM, Hughes T, et al. Neuropathic pain control in rats by intrathecal (IT) plasmid DNA vectors encoding the anti-inflammatory cytokine, interleukin-10 (IL10). *Abstracts: 11th World Congress on Pain.* Seattle: IASP Press, 2005b.

Milligan ED, Sloane EM, Langer SJ, et al. Controlling neuropathic pain by adeno-associated virus driven production of the anti-inflammatory cytokine, interleukin-10. *Mol Pain* 2005c; 1:9.

Moore KW, de Waal Malefyt R, Coffman RL, O'Garra A. Interleukin-10 and the interleukin-10 receptor. *Annu Rev Immunol* 2001; 19:683–765.

Polomano RC, Mannes AJ, Clark US, Bennett GJ. A painful peripheral neuropathy in the rat produced by the chemotherapeutic drug, paclitaxel. *Pain* 2001; 94:293–304.

Sloane EM, Langer S, Milligan ED, et al. Resolution of neuropathic pain by intrathecal (IT) gene therapy to induce interleukin-10 (IL10): initial exploration of mechanisms. *Abstracts: 11th World Congress on Pain.* Seattle: IASP Press, 2005.

Watkins LR, Maier SF. Glia: a novel drug discovery target for clinical pain. *Nat Rev Drug Discov* 2003; 2:973–985.

Watkins LR, Milligan ED, Maier SF. Glial activation: a driving force for pathological pain. *Trends Neurosci* 2001; 24:450–455.

Correspondence to: Annemarie Ledeboer, PhD, Avigen, Inc., 1301 Harbor Bay Parkway, Alameda, CA 94502, USA. Email: aledeboer@avigen.com.

Proceedings of the 11th World Congress on Pain,
edited by Herta Flor, Eija Kalso, and Jonathan O.
Dostrovsky, IASP Press, Seattle, © 2006.

19

The Thalamic Amplifier after Spinal Cord Injury: Upregulation of the Na$_V$1.3 Sodium Channel and Autonomous Hyperexcitability

Bryan C. Hains and Stephen G. Waxman

Department of Neurology and Center for Neuroscience and Regeneration Research, Yale University School of Medicine, New Haven, Connecticut, USA, and Rehabilitation Research Center, VA Connecticut Healthcare System, West Haven, Connecticut, USA

Spinal cord injury (SCI) triggers electrophysiological changes in the discharge properties of dorsal horn somatosensory neurons (Yezierski and Park 1993; Drew et al. 2001; Hains et al. 2003a,b; Hao et al. 2004). These changes contribute to pain-like behaviors in animals and humans (Widerstrom-Noga 2003). Both nociceptive and non-nociceptive neurons of the dorsal horn project directly and indirectly to relay neurons of the thalamus (Jones 1998; Willis and Coggeshall 2004). Specifically, ventroposterior lateral (VPL) thalamic neurons relay tactile and nociceptive impulses to the cortex for interpretation. Thalamic changes have been associated with pain following SCI in humans (Lenz et al. 1989; Pattany et al. 2002), in primates (Weng et al. 2000), and in rodent models (Koyama et al. 1993; Gerke et al. 2003), but the underlying molecular mechanisms are still not well understood.

Na$_V$1.3 sodium channels display rapid recovery from inactivation, and thus support neuronal firing at higher-than-normal frequencies (Cummins and Waxman 1997; Cummins et al. 2001). We have recently shown that after thoracic contusive SCI, expression of Na$_V$1.3 is upregulated in neurokinin-1-positive (and thus presumably nociceptive) dorsal horn neurons and that it contributes to hyperexcitability of these second-order neurons. However, no prior studies have focused on the potential role of Na$_V$1.3 and on changes in excitability at higher levels along the neuraxis after SCI, especially in the thalamus.

This chapter summarizes a study in which we examined whether SCI can trigger supraspinal changes in sodium channel expression within thalamic neurons, and considered whether it can contribute to functional changes. In this study we demonstrated that following SCI, thalamic neurons develop altered electrophysiological properties that persist after afferent barrage from the injured spinal cord is eliminated. We showed that these changes are accompanied by upregulated expression of $Na_V1.3$ (Hains et al. 2005). We also showed that these changes are reversed following intrathecal administration of $Na_V1.3$ antisense and that they persist after elimination of ascending activity from the dorsal horn by spinal cord transection. These results suggest a link between altered nociceptive processing and misexpression of $Na_V1.3$ within thalamic neurons following SCI.

MATERIALS AND METHODS

Spinal contusion injury was produced in 24 rats at spinal segment T9 using an impact injury device (Gruner 1992; Hains et al. 2001). A 10-g, 2.0-mm diameter rod was released from a 25-mm height onto the exposed spinal cord. For sham surgery, we performed a laminectomy in 20 control (intact) rats and placed the rats into the vertebral clips of the impactor without impact injury.

Antisense (AS) oligodeoxynucleotide sequences corresponding to the translation initiation site of $Na_V1.3$ (SCI + AS, $n = 12$ rats), or its mismatch (SCI + MM, $n = 12$ rats), were produced as previously described (see Hains et al. 2003b, 2004). Twenty-eight days after SCI, under anesthesia with ketamine/ xylazine (80/5 mg/kg administered intraperitoneally), a sterile, premeasured 32-gauge intrathecal (i.t.) catheter was threaded down to the lumbar enlargement. Three days after catheter placement (day 31 after SCI), under brief (<1 minute) halothane sedation (3% by facial mask), i.t. administration of antisense or mismatch was initiated. For 4 days, 45 µg/5 µL twice daily of either antisense or mismatch in artificial cerebrospinal fluid (CSF) was injected followed by a 10-µL flush of artificial CSF.

At day 35, coronal sections were collected from the brain, corresponding to the ventrobasal complex of the thalamus (bregma –3.14 mm) of animals from the following groups: intact ($n = 5$), SCI ($n = 5$), SCI + MM ($n = 6$), and SCI + AS ($n = 6$). Thin (12-µm) cryosections ($n = 4–7$ sections/animal/group) were processed simultaneously for detection of $Na_V1.3$ protein using a subtype-specific primary antibody raised in rabbits against $Na_V1.3$ (Hains et al. 2002, 2003b, 2004). A neuronal marker, mouse anti-NeuN, was used to identify neurons.

Also at day 35, animals from intact ($n = 7$), SCI ($n = 5$), SCI + MM ($n = 7$), and SCI + AS ($n = 6$) groups underwent extracellular single unit recording according to established methods (Hains et al. 2003b, 2004). The activity of 3–7 units per animal were recorded, yielding 12–36 cells per group. Neuronal units were isolated from the ventroposterior lateral (VPL) and ventroposterior medial (VPM) nuclei of the thalamus (respective stereotactic coordinates in millimeters: bregma [–3.30, –2.12], lateral [2.6, 3.5], vertical [4.8, 6.8]). Once a cell was identified by gentle probing of body surface, its receptive field was mapped and stimulated by an experimenter blinded to the treatment of the animal. Background activity was measured followed by cutaneous receptive field mapping and stimulation with: (1) a cotton brush; (2) von Frey filaments of increasing force (0.39 g, 1.01 g, and 20.8 g); (3) pressure, by attaching a large arterial clip with a weak grip to a fold of the skin (144 g/mm^2); and (4) pinch, by applying a small arterial clip with a strong grip to a fold of skin (583 g/mm^2). Multireceptive units were identified by their responsiveness to brush, pressure, and pinch, and with increasing responsiveness to von Frey stimuli of increasing intensity. Low-threshold or high-threshold phenotype units were classified as such based on their rate of response to brush, von Frey stimulation, or pinch. Evoked responses were calculated by subtracting the pre-stimulus baseline activity to yield the net number of spikes per response.

To ascertain whether high rates of spontaneous firing were due to increased afferent barrage from neurons close to the SCI lesion, we also recorded from VPL neurons before and after application of 2% lidocaine and subsequent cord transection.

RESULTS

NA$_V$1.3 IMMUNOCYTOCHEMISTRY

Levels of Na$_V$1.3 signal are very low within the thalamus of intact animals (Fig. 1A). In contrast, 28 days following T9 SCI, the Na$_V$1.3 signal was increased within both the ventral posterior medial (VPM) nucleus and the ventral posterior lateral (VPL) nucleus of the thalamus (Fig. 1B). Na$_V$1.3 signal was higher in the VPL than the VPM in all cases, but some neurons within the VPM were positive. No other regions of the thalamus were Na$_V$1.3-positive. Na$_V$1.3-positive neuronal cell bodies were approximately 20–25 μm in diameter and displayed characteristic neuronal morphologies. Na$_V$1.3 signal was colocalized with NeuN, indicating that the expression of Na$_V$1.3 occurred primarily in neurons.

Forty-seven percent of NeuN-positive cells were Na$_V$1.3-positive. Four days after initiation of oligodeoxynucleotide administration, levels of Na$_V$1.3

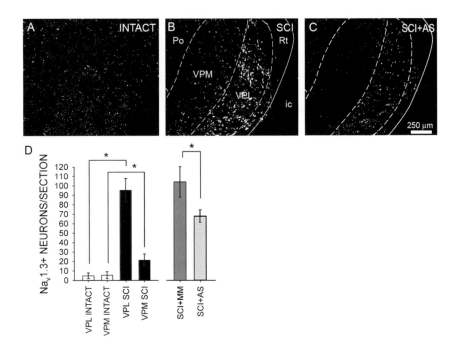

Fig. 1. $Na_V1.3$ immunostaining revealed very low levels of expression in the thalamus in intact animals (A). In contrast, 28 days after T9 spinal cord injury (SCI), $Na_V1.3$ was increased within the ventral posterior lateral (VPL) nucleus and, to a smaller extent, the ventral posterior medial (VPM) nucleus of the thalamus (B). After $Na_V1.3$ antisense (AS) delivery, levels of $Na_V1.3$ expression were reduced (C). Quantification of the mean number of $Na_V1.3$-positive neurons per section (D) revealed that following SCI, significantly upregulation of $Na_V1.3$ occurred in the VPL and VPM nuclei (*$P < 0.05$). $Na_V1.3$ AS, but not mismatch (MM), administration resulted in a significant (*$P < 0.05$) reduction in the number of $Na_V1.3$ profiles within the VPL after SCI.

expression in the VPL were unaffected in the SCI + MM group. In contrast, in the SCI + AS group there was a reduction in the level of $Na_V1.3$ expression within the VPL (Fig. 1C).

Quantification showed that intact animals demonstrated very limited expression of $Na_V1.3$-positive neurons (4.1 ± 2.3 per section); in contrast, following SCI, VPL neurons demonstrated significant ($P < 0.05$) upregulation of $Na_V1.3$-positive neurons (95.7 ± 12.6 per section) (Fig. 1D). Mismatch administration resulted in no change in the number of $Na_V1.3$-immunopositive neuronal profiles (101.5 ± 15.8) compared to SCI (95.7 ± 12.6). In contrast, antisense administration significantly ($P < 0.05$) reduced the number of $Na_V1.3$-immunopositive neuronal profiles within the VPL (66.4 ± 6.3) (Fig. 1D).

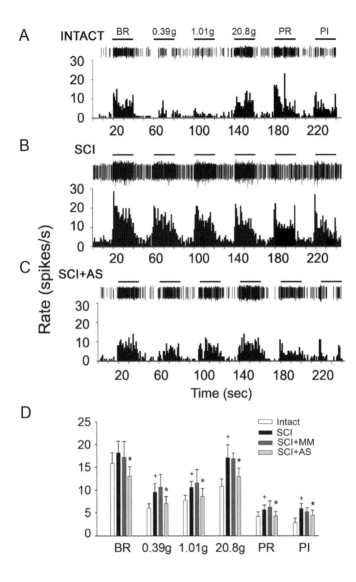

Fig. 2. Evoked activity from VPL units of intact and SCI animals and animals receiving $Na_V 1.3$ antisense (AS). In each record, the upper panel shows individual spikes and time of application of natural stimuli, each applied for 20 seconds. BR = brush, PR = pressure from von Frey filaments of increasing intensities, and PI = pinch. Spike activity is also plotted as peristimulus time histograms (1 bin/second). Compared to intact animals (A), increases were observed in spontaneous background firing and evoked discharges to peripheral stimulation after SCI (B). In SCI animals receiving $Na_V 1.3$ AS, there was reduced evoked activity (C). Bar histograms represent data from intact animals, animals with SCI, and SCI animals receiving $Na_V 1.3$ AS (D). Significant increases ($+ P < 0.05$) were observed in response to all stimuli (except for BR stimulus) after SCI, compared to intact animals, which were significantly ($* P < 0.05$) reduced by administration of $Na_V 1.3$ AS.

EVOKED ACTIVITY

Compared to the activity of a unit from an intact animal (Fig. 2A), the response rate of units to natural stimuli was increased after SCI (Fig. 2B). Quantification revealed that this increase was statistically significant for all stimuli except for brush after SCI (Fig. 2D). Increases on the order of 200–300% were observed (ranging up to 21.6 ± 3.1 spikes/second in SCI animals).

Evoked responsiveness after $Na_V1.3$ mismatch administration was not significantly different from SCI animals. However, administration of $Na_V1.3$ antisense significantly ($P < 0.05$) reversed increases in evoked activity to natural stimuli (Fig. 2C), suggesting a reversal of neuronal hyperresponsiveness after SCI. Evoked discharge rates were not significantly different from discharge rates from intact animals in response to von Frey filaments, press, or pinch. In response to brush, however, evoked rates after antisense administration (11.6 ± 2.3 spikes/second) were below those for intact animals (16.3 ± 1.9 spikes/second) (Fig. 2D).

AUTONOMOUS ACTIVITY

Recordings from VPL neurons 28 days after SCI demonstrated a high rate of spontaneous firing in neurons with hindlimb receptive fields (Fig. 3A). T1 blockade of ascending spinal barrage via 2% lidocaine and spinal cord transection reduced evoked responses to brush (and pinch, not shown), but it did not attenuate the high level of spontaneous firing in thalamic neurons (Fig. 3A).

BACKGROUND ACTIVITY

After SCI, although SCI and intact groups showed some overlap (Fig. 3B), the mean spontaneous background activity of the entire population of units studied was significantly increased in SCI animals (6.7 ± 1.2 spikes/second) when compared to that in intact animals (3.1 ± 0.9 spikes/second). When separated according to the receptive field and functional phenotype, this increase manifested mostly in multireceptive units (6.9 ± 1.6 spikes/second in SCI animals compared to 2.7 ± 0.9 in intact animals, $P < 0.05$) and in those with lower-body receptive fields (7.4 ± 1.2 spikes/second in SCI animals compared to 1.7 ± 0.6 in intact animals, $P < 0.01$).

Administration of $Na_V1.3$ antisense significantly reduced the average rate of background activity in all units (3.2 ± 0.2 spikes/second compared to 6.7 ± 1.2 in SCI, $P < 0.05$, and 6.1 ± 0.6 in SCI + MM animals), multireceptive units (2.9 ± 0.7 spikes/second compared to 6.9 ± 1.6 in SCI, $P < 0.05$, and 6.4 ± 0.6 in SCI + MM animals), and lower-body receptive field units (4.5 ± 0.2 spikes/second compared to 7.4 ± 1.2 in SCI and 7.0 ± 1.5 in SCI + MM animals, $P < 0.05$).

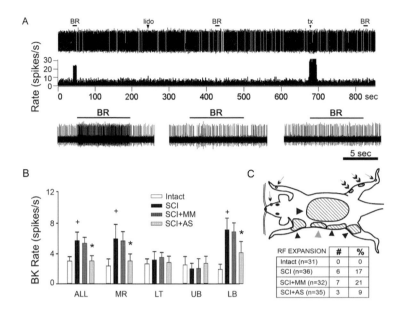

Fig. 3. Spontaneous and evoked activity of a VPL neuron with a hindlimb receptive field before and after T1 application of lidocaine (lido) and cord transection (tx). (A) Spontaneous activity persisted after cord interruption, but evoked responses to brush (BR) did not. (B) Spontaneous background (BK) activity (spikes/second) of VPL units from intact, SCI, and SCI animals receiving $Na_v1.3$ mismatch (MM) or antisense (AS). Mean BK activities are plotted for all units and for multireceptive (MR), low-threshold (LT), upper-body (UB), and lower-body (LB) units. Significant increases (+ $P < 0.05$) were observed in BK activity in SCI animals, compared to intact animals in all units, MR, and LB units. SCI + AS animals demonstrated significant (*$P < 0.05$) decreases in BK activity compared to SCI and SCI + MM animals. (C) Schematic illustration showing comparative receptive field sizes in intact (arrow), SCI (black arrowhead), SCI + MM (gray arrowhead), and SCI + AS animals (double arrow). Receptive field expansion shows number (#) and percentage (%) of neurons with expanded receptive field sizes in intact, SCI, and SCI animals receiving $Na_v1.3$ MM or AS. In SCI + AS animals, receptive field sizes were reduced compared to SCI or SCI + MM.

RECEPTIVE FIELD EXPANSION

Most receptive fields mapped to the body of intact animals were clearly identified and restricted in dimensions (typically 1–2 mm² surface area). Representative mapped receptive field areas are shown in Fig. 3C. Receptive fields of 10 neurons, out of a total population of 36 units mapped (17%), were dramatically expanded in SCI rats compared to intact animals (0 out of 31 units, $P < 0.05$) (Fig. 3C). Expansion of peripheral receptive fields was observed in only 3 neurons out of a population of 35 units mapped (9%) in SCI + AS animals, in contrast to results shown for untreated animals with SCI (6/36, 17%). In SCI + MM animals, there was no effect on receptive field size, a result that was comparable to SCI (7/32, 21%).

DISCUSSION

Spinal cord injury can alter somatosensory circuitry within the spinal dorsal horn, which can contribute to chronic neuropathic pain both in humans and in animal models. We have previously documented development of hyperresponsiveness of lumbar dorsal horn nociceptive neurons associated with pain-related behavior after thoracic contusion SCI in rats. We have reported a contribution of upregulated $Na_V1.3$ expression within second-order nociceptive neurons to this hyperresponsiveness (Hains et al. 2003b). Dorsal horn nociceptive neurons project rostrally to the thalamic VPL nucleus. In the study described in this chapter, we hypothesized that in addition to triggering pain-associated modifications of spinal nociceptive circuitry, SCI would also induce supraspinal changes within thalamic neurons that contribute to the processing of ascending signals.

This chapter has described recent results that show both $Na_V1.3$ upregulation and an increase in the spontaneous activity and responses to natural stimuli in thalamic VPL neurons following SCI (Hains et al. 2005). These were not pure nociceptive units, however, since they responded to both noxious and non-noxious stimuli. Upregulated $Na_V1.3$ within VPL neurons following SCI may be functionally important because $Na_V1.3$ recovers from inactivation rapidly and produces a depolarizing response to small stimuli close to resting potential, increasing excitability in cells that express $Na_V1.3$ (Cummins and Waxman 1997; Cummins et al. 2001). Lumbar intrathecal administration of $Na_V1.3$ antisense in SCI animals reduced the number of neurons displaying $Na_V1.3$ upregulation within the VPL, and reversed thalamic electrophysiological abnormalities caused by SCI. We cannot exclude the possibility that factors other than $Na_V1.3$ also contribute to the reconfiguration of the firing properties of thalamic units following SCI because the magnitudes of change of $Na_V1.3$ expression levels did not perfectly match the magnitude of the electrophysiological changes. Our results demonstrate for the first time, nevertheless, changes in ion channel expression within the thalamus that are associated with abnormal sensory processing. Reversal of $Na_V1.3$ expression with antisense functionally influenced the thalamus, suggesting a contribution of $Na_V1.3$ to an increase in the intrinsic excitability of thalamic neurons following SCI. Our experiments, however, could not definitively confirm a direct action of antisense on VPL neurons (as opposed to a direct effect on dorsal horn neurons, with a secondary effect on their thalamic targets), because we have shown (Hains et al. 2003b, 2004) that intrathecal administration of $Na_V1.3$ antisense has a direct effect on dorsal horn neurons. Thus, we can not exclude the possibility that an increased barrage to thalamic neurons from dorsal horn neurons and/or the nucleus gracilis (which could relay abnormal sensory information from the damaged dorsal column pathway) contributes to increased activity or other changes in these neurons after SCI. Importantly, however, we observed that the increased level of activity in VPL neurons after SCI persists after spinal cord transection that disconnects the site of SCI and ascending projections from the lumbar enlargement from the thalamus, indicating a degree of autonomous hyperexcitability of the thalamus.

In summary, our findings demonstrate changes in excitability and expression of $Na_V1.3$ within VPL neurons following SCI. We also report that hyperexcitability of thalamic neurons following SCI is to at least some degree autonomous, since it persists following spinal cord transection that abolishes ascending barrages from spinal cord neurons near or below the injury site. Together with our earlier results on dorsal root ganglion and dorsal horn neurons (Hains et al. 2003b), these results provide evidence suggesting that dysregulation of sodium channel $Na_V1.3$ expression at both supraspinal and spinal levels contributes to altered processing of somatosensory information and may contribute to dysesthesias after SCI.

ACKNOWLEDGMENTS

This work was supported in part by grants from the Medical Research Service and Rehabilitation Research Service, Department of Veterans Affairs, the National Multiple Sclerosis Society, and by generous gifts from J. Pelkey and K. and R. Kimball. The Center for Neuroscience and Regeneration Research is a Collaboration of the Paralyzed Veterans of America and the United Spinal Association. B.C. Hains was funded by The Christopher Reeve Paralysis Foundation (HB1-0304-2), the NIH/NINDS (1 F32 NS046919-01), and Pfizer (Scholar's Grant in Pain Medicine).

REFERENCES

Cummins TR, Waxman SG. Down-regulation of tetrodotoxin-resistant sodium currents and up-regulation of a rapidly repriming tetrodotoxin-sensitive sodium current in small spinal sensory neurons following nerve injury. *J Neurosci* 1997; 17:3503–3514.

Cummins TR, Aglieco F, Renganathan M, et al. $Na_V1.3$ sodium channels: rapid repriming and slow closed-state inactivation display quantitative differences after expression in a mammalian cell line and in spinal sensory neurons. *J Neurosci* 2001; 21:5952–5961.

Drew GM, Siddall PJ, Duggan AW. Responses of spinal neurones to cutaneous and dorsal root stimuli in rats with mechanical allodynia after contusive spinal cord injury. *Brain Res* 2001; 893:59–69.

Gerke MB, Duggan AW, Xu L, Siddall PJ. Thalamic neuronal activity in rats with mechanical allodynia following contusive spinal cord injury. *Neuroscience* 2003; 117:715–722.

Gruner JA. A monitored contusion model of spinal cord injury in the rat. *J Neurotrauma* 1992; 9:123–126.

Hains BC, Yucra JA, Hulsebosch CE. Selective COX-2 inhibition with NS-398 preserves spinal parenchyma and attenuates behavioral deficits following spinal contusion injury. *J Neurotrauma* 2001; 18:409–423.

Hains BC, Black JA, Waxman SG. Primary motor neurons fail to up-regulate voltage-gated sodium channel Na(v)1.3/brain type III following axotomy resulting from spinal cord injury. *J Neurosci Res* 2002; 70:546–552.

Hains BC, Johnson KM, Eaton MJ, Willis WD, Hulsebosch CE. Serotonergic neural precursor cell grafts attenuate bilateral hyperexcitability of dorsal horn neurons after spinal hemisection in rat. *Neuroscience* 2003a; 116:1097–1110.

Hains BC, Klein JP, Saab CY, et al. Upregulation of sodium channel $Na_V1.3$ and functional involvement in neuronal hyperexcitability associated with central neuropathic pain after spinal cord injury. *J Neurosci* 2003b; 23:8881–8892.

Hains BC, Saab CY, Klein JP, Craner MJ, Waxman SG. Altered sodium channel expression in second-order spinal sensory neurons contributes to pain after peripheral nerve injury. *J Neurosci* 2004; 24:4832–4839.

Hains BC, Saab CY, Waxman SG. Changes in electrophysiologic properties and sodium channel $Na_V1.3$ expression in thalamic neurons after spinal cord injury. *Brain* 2005; 128:2359–2371.

Hao JX, Kupers RC, Xu XJ. Response characteristics of spinal cord dorsal horn neurons in chronic allodynic rats after spinal cord injury. *J Neurophysiol* 2004; 92:1391–1399.

Jones EG. Viewpoint: the core and matrix of thalamic organization. *Neuroscience* 1998; 85:331–345.

Koyama S, Katayama Y, Maejima S, et al. Thalamic neuronal hyperactivity following transection of the spinothalamic tract in the cat: involvement of N-methyl-D-aspartate receptor. *Brain Res* 1993; 612:345–350.

Lenz FA, Kwan HC, Dostrovsky JO, Tasker RR. Characteristics of the bursting pattern of action potentials that occurs in the thalamus of patients with central pain. *Brain Res* 1989; 496:357–360.

Pattany PM, Yezierski RP, Widerstrom-Noga EG, et al. Proton magnetic resonance spectroscopy of the thalamus in patients with chronic neuropathic pain after spinal cord injury. *Am J Neuroradiol* 2002; 23:901–905.

Weng HR, Lee JI, Lenz FA, Schwartz A, et al. Functional plasticity in primate somatosensory thalamus following chronic lesion of the ventral lateral spinal cord. *Neuroscience* 2000; 101:393–401.

Widerstrom-Noga E. Chronic pain and nonpainful sensations after spinal cord injury: is there a relation? *Clin J Pain* 2003; 19:39–47.

Willis WD, Coggeshall RE. *Sensory Mechanisms of the Spinal Cord,* 3rd ed. New York: Plenum Press, 2004.

Yezierski RP, Park SH. The mechanosensitivity of spinal sensory neurons following intraspinal injections of quisqualic acid in the rat. *Neurosci Lett* 1993; 157:115–119.

Correspondence to: Bryan C. Hains, PhD, Center for Neuroscience and Regeneration Research, Department of Neurology, Yale School of Medicine, 950 Campbell Avenue, West Haven, CT 06511, USA. Tel: 203-937-3802; Fax: 203-937-3801; email: bryan.hains@yale.edu.

Part III

Nociceptive Pathways and Central Processing

Proceedings of the 11th World Congress on Pain,
edited by Herta Flor, Eija Kalso, and Jonathan O.
Dostrovsky, IASP Press, Seattle, © 2006.

20

Emerging Role of Spinal Microglia in Neuropathic Pain Plasticity

Michael W. Salter

University of Toronto Centre for the Study of Pain, Toronto, Ontario, Canada

Pain has three mechanistically distinct types—nociceptive, inflammatory, and neuropathic. Nociceptive pain is a critical mechanism that warns an individual of recent or imminent damage to the body; it is the physiological consequence of the normal functioning of the peripheral and central nervous systems. Inflammatory or neuropathic pains, by contrast, reflect aberrant functioning of the peripheral or central nervous system (Woolf and Salter 2000, 2006). Typically, these persistent pains are not directly related to tissue damage, and they may be maintained long after any tissue damage that may have initiated nociceptive pain has subsided. Pathological alterations underlying and amplifying chronic pain occur in the peripheral nervous system or in numerous sites within the central nervous system (CNS), leading to the concept that chronic pain is a nervous system disorder. Given the diversity of chronic pain, it should be considered a group of mechanistically separable nervous system disorders produced and maintained by one or more abnormal cellular signaling processes.

The dorsal horn of the spinal cord contains a complex nociceptive processing network through which inputs from the periphery are transduced and modulated (Fig. 1). This network includes local, as well as descending, inhibitory control mechanisms, and its output is transmitted to other areas of the CNS involved in sensory, emotional, autonomic, and motor processing. Normally, this network reliably transduces inputs from nociceptive primary afferents such that its output, which of course serves as the input to these brain areas, is well-matched to the degree of peripheral tissue damage. The result is nociceptive pain (Fig. 1a). By contrast, a prominent feature of persistent pain is aberrant activation of intracellular signaling pathways, the ultimate effect of which is alteration of the normally finely tuned balance of excitation and inhibition in the dorsal horn nociceptive processing network. As a result, the output of this network, for a given input, is increased (Fig. 1b). This increased output may

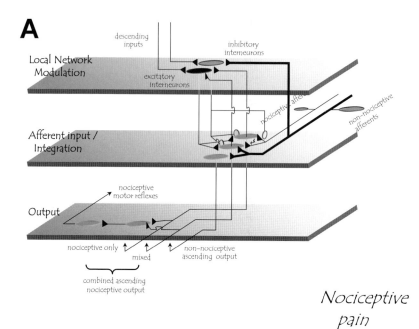

*Nociceptive
pain*

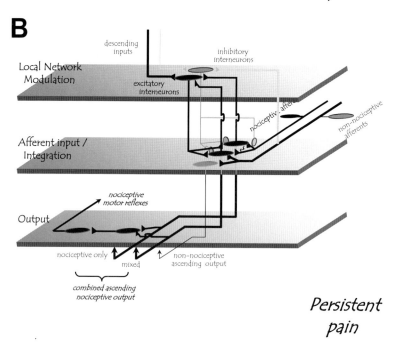

*Persistent
pain*

arise from alteration of the intrinsic voltage-dependent or voltage-independent currents in dorsal horn neurons, from enhancement of excitatory inputs or depression of inhibitory control mechanisms, or from a combination of these events. These diverse neuronal mechanisms have been the subject of several recent reviews (Ji et al. 2003; Ji and Strichartz 2004; Lewin et al. 2004; Salter 2005; Woolf and Salter 2006). Therefore, I will focus here on the emerging role of glial cells, and of neuronal-glial-neuronal signaling, in nerve-injury-induced pain.

In the CNS, glial cells outnumber neurons by approximately 10:1, but these cells have traditionally been considered to play mainly housekeeping or supportive roles. This view has, however, changed dramatically over the past decade. Glial cells are known to play key roles in regulating synaptic transmission and participating in synaptic plasticity (Fields and Stevens-Graham 2002; Auld and Robitaille 2003; Pascual and Haydon 2003; Zhang and Haydon 2005). For pain resulting from peripheral nerve injury, a growing body of evidence indicates that hyperalgesia, allodynia, and ongoing pain involve active participation of glia in the spinal dorsal horn (Wieseler-Frank et al. 2004; Tsuda et al. 2005). The CNS contains three types of glia—astrocytes, oligodendrocytes, and microglia. Microglia comprise 5–10% of the total glial population in the CNS and are roughly equal in number to neurons (Kreutzberg 1996; Stoll and Jander 1999). These cells have emerged as a critical glial cell type in pain hypersensitivity after peripheral nerve injury (Tsuda et al. 2003, 2005).

In the unperturbed CNS, microglia are in a so-called "resting" state, which is now known to be an active surveillance mode in which these cells continuously and vigorously monitor the local environment (Davalos et al. 2005; Nimmerjahn et al. 2005). Even in the "resting" state, microglia show responses within minutes to neural damage (Nimmerjahn et al. 2005). In addition, a wide variety of stimuli that threaten physiological homeostasis evoke a program of changes in morphology, gene expression, function, and number of microglia (Perry 1994). The four cardinal signs of microglial activation, based on responses to neuroinflammatory stimulation, are: (1) hypertrophy and shape

---

← **Fig. 1.** Schematic representation of the organization of the nociceptive network in the dorsal horn showing input, output, and local modulatory connections, and changes occurring during persistent pain. (A) Nociceptive and non-nociceptive inputs, and motor and ascending outputs, with layered local excitatory and inhibitory modulatory control, which can be accessed by supraspinal, local, or primary afferent inputs. (B) Mechanisms for enhancing the output of the nociceptive processing network, underlying some forms of persistent pain, are indicated by thicker lines and boldface type. These mechanisms include increased activity of primary afferent nociceptors and enhancement of transmission onto nociceptive output neurons; enhanced activity or transmission of excitatory interneurons; depressed number, activity, or transmission of inhibitory interneurons; and alteration of the intrinsic membrane properties of the nociceptive output neurons. The net result is increased output of the network.

change, (2) proliferation, (3) immunophenotypic change, and (4) a change in the secretory molecules produced (Streit et al. 1999). Activated microglia change their morphology from a resting, ramified shape, progressively retracting small secondary and tertiary processes. The main processes become engorged, and ultimately the activated microglia take on an ameboid shape (Kreutzberg 1996; Stoll and Jander 1999; Streit et al. 1999; Nakajima and Kohsaka 2001). Such fully activated microglia are capable of performing phagocytosis, giving rise to the view that these cells are resident macrophages of the CNS. Not only do microglia undergo dramatic morphological changes, but they also proliferate, generating new cells capable of local action. Indeed microglia are the only non-stem cells in the mature CNS that are capable of division. In addition to shape changes and proliferation, during activation these cells dramatically alter the repertoire of molecules expressed on the cell surface. These molecules include the CR3 (CD11b/CD18) receptor, composed of integrin subunits α_M (CD11b) and β_2 (CD18) (Ehlers 2000). Activated microglia also show enhanced expression of immune system molecules such as major histocompatibility complex (MHC) class II (Kreutzberg 1996; Stoll and Jander 1999; Streit et al. 1999), which play a role in antigen presentation to T lymphocytes. Activated microglia produce and release various chemical mediators, including proinflammatory cytokines, which can produce immunological actions and can also act on neurons to alter their function (Stoll and Jander 1999; Nakajima and Kohsaka 2001; Hanisch 2002).

Activation is not uniform, however; different responses are evoked by different types of stimulation, and responses to the same stimulation differ in various regions of the CNS (Carson et al. 2004). Therefore, the response state of microglia needs to be investigated based on the CNS region and on the stimulus producing activation. Within the spinal cord dorsal horn, the four cardinal signs of microglial activation develop in a stereotyped fashion following injury to a peripheral nerve. Evidence for microglial activation after injury to sensory nerves goes back more than 25 years (Ling 1979). The state of microglia in the spinal cord has been examined in a variety of models: compression, ligation, or transection of the sciatic nerve (Bennett and Xie 1988), of the spinal nerves (Kim and Chung 1992), and of peripheral branches of the sciatic nerve (Decosterd and Woolf 2000). A common feature of these models, and one that is often considered to be clinically relevant, is that after nerve injury, withdrawal behaviors are evoked by stimuli that are innocuous, such as gentle mechanical stimulation (Beggs and Salter 2006). The potential clinical relevance of this behavior change is that it reflects allodynia, which is a common, and often severe, component of neuropathic pain in humans (Zimmermann 2001; Jensen and Baron 2003; Woolf 2004).

Following peripheral nerve injury, a series of changes occur in microglia within the spinal dorsal horn (Eriksson et al. 1993; Liu et al. 1995; Coyle 1998; Tanga et al. 2004), although there may be some variability among the models in terms of the extent and time course of the changes (Colburn et al. 1997, 1999). Within hours after peripheral nerve injury, signs of microglial activation are observed, with the small soma becoming hypertrophic and the long and thin processes withdrawing (Eriksson et al. 1993). A subsequent proliferation of microglia occurs, which peaks about 3 days after nerve injury (Gehrmann and Banati 1995). After peripheral nerve injury, the microglia in the dorsal horn show an increased level of several activation "marker" proteins including CR3 (CD11b/CD18) (Eriksson et al. 1993; Liu et al. 1995; Coyle 1998; Tsuda et al. 2003), toll-like receptor 4 (TLR4) (Tanga et al. 2004), cluster determinant 14 (CD14) (Tanga et al. 2004), CD4 (Sweitzer et al. 2002), and MHC class II protein (Sweitzer and DeLeo 2002; Sweitzer et al. 2002). While many reports have shown a positive correlation between activation of microglia and signs of pain hypersensitivity, only recently was it established that microglia have a causal role in these nerve-injury-evoked pain behaviors in studies implicating $P2X_4$ receptors (Tsuda et al. 2003) and p38 mitogen-activated protein (MAP) kinase (Jin et al. 2003; Tsuda et al. 2004).

$P2X_4$ receptors are a subtype of the P2X family of ligand-gated ion channels, i.e., ionotropic purinoceptors, that are activated by adenosine triphosphate (ATP) (North 2002). Mechanical allodynia following spinal nerve ligation is acutely reversed by intrathecal administration of a $P2X_4$ antagonist. $P2X_4$ receptors are undetectable in either neurons or astrocytes (Tsuda et al. 2003) in the dorsal horn, but they are expressed in microglia. Their expression is low in the naive spinal cord, but it increases progressively in the days following nerve injury, paralleling the development of mechanical allodynia. Inhibiting the rise in $P2X_4$ expression prevents the development of allodynia. Thus, microglial $P2X_4$ receptors are required for mechanical allodynia after nerve injury. Moreover, in otherwise naive animals, mechanical allodynia develops after administration of microglia in which $P2X_4$ receptors have been stimulated in vitro. By contrast, unstimulated microglia do not cause allodynia (Tsuda et al. 2003). Thus, stimulation of $P2X_4$ receptors in activated microglia appears to be sufficient as well as necessary for causing mechanical allodynia.

Like blockade of $P2X_4$ receptors, pharmacological inhibition of p38 MAP kinase by means of an intrathecally administered inhibitor reverses mechanical allodynia following spinal nerve ligation (Jin et al. 2003). Infusing the p38 inhibitor beginning prior to the nerve injury prevented allodynia from developing. The nerve lesion leads to persistent activation of p38 MAP kinase, as judged by labeling for a phosphorylated form of p38 MAP kinase, which is restricted to microglia. Thus, these two proteins, $P2X_4$ receptors and p38 MAP kinase, and by inference activated microglia themselves, are critical for maintaining mechanical allodynia after peripheral nerve injury. These findings have opened the question of whether agents that inhibit the function or expression of these proteins might alleviate neuropathic pain in humans. One potential strategy is inhibition of microglial activation with agents such as minocycline, which, by an unknown mechanism, suppresses signs of microglial activation and has other effects including inhibition of matrix metalloproteinases (Zemke and Majid 2004). Minocycline is unable to reverse pain hypersensitivity after peripheral nerve injury, although it can suppress its development (Raghavendra et al. 2003; Ledeboer et al. 2005). Such a dissociation between microglial "activation" and maintenance of pain behaviors is not surprising, given that suppression of $P2X_4$-receptor expression with antisense prevented the development of pain hypersensitivity but did not affect enhanced "activation" in a study that used OX-42 labeling to determine CR3 expression (Tsuda et al. 2003). Together, these findings suggest that the pathways inhibited by minocycline, the identity of which remains to be determined, are not required for maintaining pain hypersensitivity, whereas those involving $P2X_4$ receptors and p38 MAP kinase *are* necessary. By inference, these latter two pathways are not expected to be inhibited by minocycline.

One key mechanistic issue is to determine how microglia in the spinal cord become activated after nerve injury in the periphery. A large number of molecules are known to be capable of activating microglia, and thus there are many candidates for the signaling molecules most proximal to these cells. Recently it was reported that mice lacking TLR4, a member of the interleukin-1/toll-like receptor superfamily (Cook et al. 2004), show markedly reduced mechanical allodynia following peripheral nerve injury compared to wild-type controls (Tanga et al. 2005). Moreover, suppression of TLR4 expression in the spinal cord by antisense oligonucleotides administered daily prevented the development of allodynia. Not only was allodynia suppressed, but the activation of the microglia, as judged by expression of CR3 and other molecular markers, was also markedly blunted. Thus, TLR4 in spinal microglia appears to be a key mediator of microglial activation after peripheral nerve injury. One minor caveat is that intrathecally administered antisense oligonucleotides may be able to reach the dorsal root ganglia, and therefore it is possible that depressed expression of TLR4 there is involved. Nevertheless, this report opens up important questions: What is the identity of the endogenous ligand for TLR4, and which cells are producing it? Also, because neither the allodynia nor the microglia activation was completely prevented, either in the knockouts or by the antisense oligonucleotides, there must be additional molecules and signaling pathways that participate in the response to peripheral nerve injury. Identifying these additional pathways is a crucial goal for the future.

Another key issue is to determine how microglia signal to neurons in the dorsal horn nociceptive network in order to effect an increase in network output. There are a number of possibilities to consider because microglia could conceivably interact with neurons through direct contact factors, through release of diffusible chemical mediators, or even by phagocytosis of neuroactive molecules in the local environment (Tsuda et al. 2005). Moreover, the effect of the microglia signaling on the dorsal horn neurons could be mediated by facilitation of excitatory synaptic transmission or of the activity of local excitatory neurons, by suppression of inhibition or inhibitory neuron activity, by alteration of the intrinsic membrane properties of the dorsal horn nociceptive output neurons, or by a combination of these mechanisms.

The effect of microglia on spinal neurons in lamina I of the dorsal horn has recently been investigated in the rat. These neurons were studied because they are one of the major outputs of the dorsal horn nociceptive network (Craig 2000, 2003) and because a rise in their intracellular chloride concentration, which causes disinhibition, is a key mechanism for mechanical allodynia following peripheral nerve injury (Coull et al. 2003). The key new findings are that administering ATP-stimulated microglia intrathecally in naive rats causes intracellular accumulation of the anion chloride in lamina I neurons (Coull et al. 2005). Moreover, acute pharmacological blockade of $P2X_4$ receptors in the dorsal horn reverses the increase in chloride in lamina I neurons observed following peripheral nerve injury. In addition, it was discovered that microglia produce this increased chloride by releasing brain-derived neurotrophic factor (BDNF), which acts on its cognate receptor, trkB, on lamina I neurons. These findings define a cellular signaling pathway from microglia to neurons that has a major role in producing mechanical allodynia following experimental nerve injury. The extent to which this pathway is activated in humans with neuropathic pain, and the extent to which it contributes to such pain, are open questions for investigation.

In conclusion, it is now apparent that damage to a peripheral nerve stimulates a program of changes in the dorsal horn that evokes neuroplasticity, leading to neuropathic pain. Importantly, recent evidence demonstrates that critical molecular mechanisms are not restricted to neurons but also involve glial cells and glial-neuronal signaling in the spinal cord, with the preponderance of evidence to date implicating microglia. Undoubtedly, further elucidation of the roles of microglia may lead to strategies for diagnosing and managing neuropathic pain that have not previously been considered by investigators viewing this type of pain as solely as a disorder of neurons.

ACKNOWLEDGMENTS

The work of the author is supported by grants from the Canadian Institutes of Health Research and from Brain Repair Program of Neuroscience Canada. The author holds a Canada Research Chair (Tier I), in Neuroplasticity and Pain.

REFERENCES

Auld DS, Robitaille R. Glial cells and neurotransmission: an inclusive view of synaptic function. *Neuron* 2003; 40:389–400.
Beggs S, Salter MW. Neuropathic pain: symptoms, models and mechanisms. *Drug Dev Res* 2006; in press.
Bennett GJ, Xie YK. A peripheral mononeuropathy in rat that produces disorders of pain sensation like those seen in man. *Pain* 1988; 33:87–107.
Carson MJ, Thrash JC, Lo D. Analysis of microglial gene expression: identifying targets for CNS neurodegenerative and autoimmune disease. *Am J Pharmacogenomics* 2004; 4:321–330.
Colburn RW, DeLeo JA, Rickman AJ, et al. Dissociation of microglial activation and neuropathic pain behaviors following peripheral nerve injury in the rat. *J Neuroimmunol* 1997; 79:163–175.
Colburn RW, Rickman AJ, DeLeo JA. The effect of site and type of nerve injury on spinal glial activation and neuropathic pain behavior. *Exp Neurol* 1999; 157:289–304.
Cook DN, Pisetsky DS, Schwartz DA. Toll-like receptors in the pathogenesis of human disease. *Nat Immunol* 2004; 5:975–979.
Coull JA, Boudreau D, Bachand K, et al. Trans-synaptic shift in anion gradient in spinal lamina I neurons as a mechanism of neuropathic pain. *Nature* 2003; 424:938–942.
Coull JA, Beggs S, Boudreau D, et al. BDNF from microglia mediates the shift in neuronal anion gradient that underlies neuropathic pain. *Nature* 2005; 438:1017–1021.
Coyle DE. Partial peripheral nerve injury leads to activation of astroglia and microglia which parallels the development of allodynic behavior. *Glia* 1998; 23:75–83.
Craig AD. The functional anatomy of lamina I and its role in post-stroke central pain. *Prog Brain Res* 2000; 129:137–151.
Craig AD. A new view of pain as a homeostatic emotion. *Trends Neurosci* 2003; 26:303–307.
Davalos D, Grutzendler J, Yang G, et al. ATP mediates rapid microglial response to local brain injury in vivo. *Nat Neurosci* 2005; 8:752–758.
Decosterd I, Woolf CJ. Spared nerve injury: an animal model of persistent peripheral neuropathic pain. *Pain* 2000; 87:149–158.
Ehlers MR. CR3: a general purpose adhesion-recognition receptor essential for innate immunity. *Microbes Infect* 2000; 2:289–294.
Eriksson NP, Persson JK, Svensson M, et al. A quantitative analysis of the microglial cell reaction in central primary sensory projection territories following peripheral nerve injury in the adult rat. *Exp Brain Res* 1993; 96:19–27.
Fields RD, Stevens-Graham B. New insights into neuron-glia communication. *Science* 2002; 298:556–562.
Gehrmann J, Banati RB. Microglial turnover in the injured CNS: activated microglia undergo delayed DNA fragmentation following peripheral nerve injury. *J Neuropathol Exp Neurol* 1995; 54:680–688.
Hanisch UK. Microglia as a source and target of cytokines. *Glia* 2002; 40:140–155.
Jensen TS, Baron R. Translation of symptoms and signs into mechanisms in neuropathic pain. *Pain* 2003; 102:1–8.
Ji RR, Strichartz G. Cell signaling and the genesis of neuropathic pain. *Sci STKE* 2004; 252: reE14.

Ji RR, Kohno T, Moore KA, Woolf CJ. Central sensitization and LTP: do pain and memory share similar mechanisms? *Trends Neurosci* 2003; 26:696–705.

Jin SX, Zhuang ZY, Woolf CJ, Ji RR. p38 mitogen-activated protein kinase is activated after a spinal nerve ligation in spinal cord microglia and dorsal root ganglion neurons and contributes to the generation of neuropathic pain. *J Neurosci* 2003; 23:4017–4022.

Kim SH, Chung JM. An experimental model for peripheral neuropathy produced by segmental spinal nerve ligation in the rat. *Pain* 1992; 50:355–363.

Kreutzberg GW. Microglia: a sensor for pathological events in the CNS. *Trends Neurosci* 1996; 19:312–318.

Ledeboer A, Sloane EM, Milligan ED, et al. Minocycline attenuates mechanical allodynia and pro-inflammatory cytokine expression in rat models of pain facilitation. *Pain* 2005; 115:71–83.

Lewin GR, Lu Y, Park TJ. A plethora of painful molecules. *Curr Opin Neurobiol* 2004; 14:443–449.

Ling EA. Evidence for a haematogenous origin of some of the macrophages appearing in the spinal cord of the rat after dorsal rhizotomy. *J Anat* 1979; 128:143–154.

Liu L, Tornqvist E, Mattsson P, et al. Complement and clusterin in the spinal cord dorsal horn and gracile nucleus following sciatic nerve injury in the adult rat. *Neuroscience* 1995; 68:167–179.

Nakajima K, Kohsaka S. Microglia: activation and their significance in the central nervous system. *J Biochem (Tokyo)* 2001; 130:169–175.

Nimmerjahn A, Kirchhoff F, Helmchen F. Resting microglial cells are highly dynamic surveillants of brain parenchyma in vivo. *Science* 2005; 308:1314–1318.

North RA. Molecular physiology of P2X receptors. *Physiol Rev* 2002; 82:1013–1067.

Pascual O, Haydon PG. Synaptic inhibition mediated by glia. *Neuron* 2003; 40:873–875.

Perry VH. Modulation of microglia phenotype. *Neuropathol Appl Neurobiol* 1994; 20:177.

Raghavendra V, Tanga F, DeLeo JA. Inhibition of microglial activation attenuates the development but not existing hypersensitivity in a rat model of neuropathy. *J Pharmacol Exp Ther* 2003; 306:624–630.

Salter MW. Cellular signalling pathways of spinal pain neuroplasticity as targets for analgesic development. *Curr Top Med Chem* 2005; 5:557–567.

Stoll G, Jander S. The role of microglia and macrophages in the pathophysiology of the CNS. *Prog Neurobiol* 1999; 58:233–247.

Streit WJ, Walter SA, Pennell NA. Reactive microgliosis. *Prog Neurobiol* 1999; 57:563–581.

Sweitzer SM, DeLeo JA. The active metabolite of leflunomide, an immunosuppressive agent, reduces mechanical sensitivity in a rat mononeuropathy model. *J Pain* 2002; 3:360–368.

Sweitzer SM, White KA, Dutta C, DeLeo JA. The differential role of spinal MHC class II and cellular adhesion molecules in peripheral inflammatory versus neuropathic pain in rodents. *J Neuroimmunol* 2002; 125:82–93.

Tanga FY, Raghavendra V, DeLeo JA. Quantitative real-time RT-PCR assessment of spinal microglial and astrocytic activation markers in a rat model of neuropathic pain. *Neurochem Int* 2004; 45:397–407.

Tanga FY, Nutile-McMenemy N, DeLeo JA. The CNS role of Toll-like receptor 4 in innate neuro-immunity and painful neuropathy. *Proc Natl Acad Sci USA* 2005; 102:5856–5861.

Tsuda M, Shigemoto-Mogami Y, Koizumi S, et al. P2X4 receptors induced in spinal microglia gate tactile allodynia after nerve injury. *Nature* 2003; 424:778–783.

Tsuda M, Mizokoshi A, Shigemoto-Mogami Y, Koizumi S, Inoue K. Activation of p38 mitogen-activated protein kinase in spinal hyperactive microglia contributes to pain hypersensitivity following peripheral nerve injury. *Glia* 2004; 45:89–95.

Tsuda M, Inoue K, Salter MW. Neuropathic pain and spinal microglia: a big problem from molecules in 'small' glia. *Trends Neurosci* 2005; 28:101–107.

Wieseler-Frank J, Maier SF, Watkins LR. Glial activation and pathological pain. *Neurochem Int* 2004; 45:389–395.

Woolf CJ. Dissecting out mechanisms responsible for peripheral neuropathic pain: implications for diagnosis and therapy. *Life Sci* 2004; 74:2605–2610.

Woolf CJ, Salter MW. Neuronal plasticity: increasing the gain in pain. *Science* 2000; 288:1765–1769.

Woolf CJ, Salter MW. Plasticity and pain: role of the dorsal horn. In: McMahon SB, Koltzenberg M (Eds). *Melzack and Wall's Textbook of Pain,* 5th ed. London: Elsevier, 2006, pp 91–106.

Zemke D, Majid A. The potential of minocycline for neuroprotection in human neurologic disease. *Clin Neuropharmacol* 2004; 27:293–298.

Zhang Q, Haydon PG. Roles for gliotransmission in the nervous system. *J Neural Transm* 2005; 112:121–125.

Zimmermann M. Pathobiology of neuropathic pain. *Eur J Pharmacol* 2001; 429:23–37.

Correspondence to: Michael W. Salter, MD, PhD, The Hospital for Sick Children, 555 University Avenue, Toronto, Ontario, Canada M5G 1X8. Tel: 416-813-6272; Fax: 416-813-7921; email: mike.salter@utoronto.ca.

Proceedings of the 11th World Congress on Pain, edited by Herta Flor, Eija Kalso, and Jonathan O. Dostrovsky, IASP Press, Seattle, © 2006.

21

Central Sensitization, Referred Pain, and Deep Tissue Hyperalgesia in Musculoskeletal Pain

Thomas Graven-Nielsen,[a] Michele Curatolo,[b] and Siegfried Mense[c]

[a]Center for Sensory-Motor Interaction (SMI), Laboratory for Experimental Pain Research, Aalborg University, Denmark; [b]Department of Anesthesiology, Division of Pain Therapy, Inselspital, Berne, Switzerland; [c]Institute of Anatomy and Cell Biology, University of Heidelberg, Heidelberg, Germany

It is generally accepted that pain from deep tissues constitutes a special diagnostic and therapeutic challenge. Further insights into the peripheral and central neurobiological mechanisms are thus necessary to improve diagnosis and management strategies. This chapter considers the possible mechanisms underlying muscle pain, discussing basic animal studies on muscle pain, with a focus on afferent sensitization and neuroplastic changes related to muscle nociception, as well as human experimental muscle pain in terms of referred pain and muscle hyperalgesia. Finally, we will also discuss clinical studies that have investigated temporal summation and enlarged areas of referred pain.

In contrast to the sharp, localized characteristics of cutaneous pain, muscle pain is described as aching and cramping, with diffuse localization. Kellgren (1938), one of the pioneers of experimental studies of the diffuse characteristics of muscle pain, determined the locations of referred pain triggered by selective activation of specific muscle groups. The sensation of acute muscle pain is the result of activation of group III and group IV polymodal muscle nociceptors. Sensitization of muscle nociceptors may eventually lead to central hyperexcitability of dorsal horn neurons, which is manifested as prolonged neuronal discharges, increased responses to noxious stimuli, responses to non-noxious stimuli, and expansion of the receptive field. Therefore, in muscle pain disorders, the plasticity of dorsal horn neurons is likely to manifest as deep tissue hyperalgesia, an enlarged area of referred pain, and facilitated temporal summation.

DORSAL HORN NEURON PLASTICITY
AND MUSCLE NOCICEPTION

An important metabolic factor for the development of muscle pain is the nitric oxide–cyclic guanosine monophosphate (NO-cGMP) pathway. The role of NO and cGMP in nociception is controversial (Callsen-Cencic et al. 1999). Many of the discrepancies in the literature appear to be due to the fact that some studies investigated the effects of NO with systemic administration of drugs that interfere with the NO-cGMP pathway, whereas others used spinal (intrathecal) administration of these compounds.

A recent study addressed the question whether the spinal and supraspinal effects of NO and cGMP are different (Hoheisel et al. 2005b). The levels of NO and cGMP were manipulated in rats by either spinal or supraspinal application of inhibitors of the pathway. Spinal administration consisted of spinal superfusion of the lumbar segments 4 and 5, and supraspinal administration was accomplished by injection into the third cerebral ventricle. Nociceptive neurons were recorded with microelectrodes in the L4 and L5 segments. The inhibitors used were N-nitro-L-arginine methyl ester (L-NAME), an inhibitor of all isoforms of NO synthase; ODQ, a blocker of the cGMP-synthesizing enzyme guanylyl cyclase; and sildenafil, an inhibitor of phosphodiesterase 5, the enzyme that degrades cGMP to 5'-GMP. Recently, sildenafil has attracted interest because some patients taking the drug have complained of myalgias or low back pain (Lim et al. 2002).

A local spinal lack of NO or cGMP (induced by superfusing L4/L5 with L-NAME or ODQ, respectively) was highly effective in exciting predominantly nociceptive neurons (Fig. 1). Chronic experimental myositis is associated with a reduction of NO synthesis in the spinal cord, and a therapeutic increase in spinal NO or cGMP synthesis thus may be an interesting approach to the alleviation of chronic muscle pain. Increasing the local cGMP level by superfusing the spinal cord with sildenafil or 8-bromo-cGMP (a membrane-permeable cGMP analogue) slightly reduced the activity of nociceptive dorsal horn neurons (Hoheisel et al. 2005b).

In contrast to the data obtained at the spinal level, lowering NO or cGMP levels in supraspinal centers by injecting L-NAME and ODQ into the third ventricle had no effect on the activity of nociceptive horn neurons. On the other hand, injection of sildenafil and 8-bromo-cGMP into the third ventricle caused a strong activation of lumbar nociceptive dorsal horn neurons (Fig. 1). Apparently, the myalgias of patients treated with sildenafil are due to the fact that the drug acts primarily at the supraspinal level, where it increases the activity of nociceptive spinal neurons through pain-modulating descending pathways.

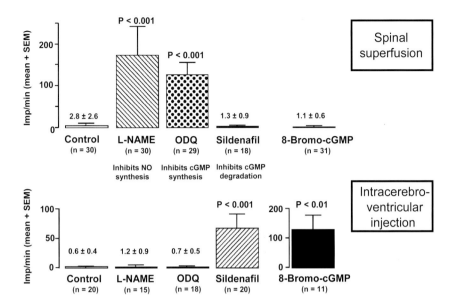

Fig. 1. Discharge frequency of rat dorsal horn neurons after spinal and supraspinal administration of drugs that change the CNS concentration of NO and cGMP, respectively. Spinal administration was performed by superfusing the lumbar segments 4 and 5, supraspinal administration by intracerebroventricular injection into the third cerebral ventricle. Superfusion of the lumbar spinal cord (upper panel) with drugs that increased the NO or cGMP level (sildenafil and 8-bromo-cGMP, respectively) caused a very slight reduction in neuronal activity compared with control, whereas a decrease of NO or cGMP (by L-NAME or ODQ, respectively) induced a marked excitation. Injection into the third cerebral ventricle (lower panel) had the opposite effect: increasing the local NO or cGMP level (by sildenafil or 8-bromo-cGMP, respectively) excited the lumbar neurons, whereas a decreased NO or cGMP concentration did not affect the neurons. The data show that at the spinal level, a decrease in NO and cGMP is excitatory for nociceptive neurons, whereas at the supraspinal level an increase has this action. Based on data from Hoheisel and Mense (2005b).

The muscle hyperalgesia of patients with muscle pain can largely be explained by sensitization of peripheral muscle nociceptors in addition to the sensitization of central neurons. The input from muscle nociceptors that is responsible for central sensitization reaches the spinal cord mainly via unmyelinated (group IV) afferent fibers equipped with tetrodotoxin (TTX)-resistant sodium channels. Interestingly, the cord dorsum potential caused by electrical stimulation of group IV fibers in the nerve of the gastrocnemius soleus muscle increased in amplitude when the TTX-sensitive fibers were blocked with TTX. This finding indicates that normally the synaptic efficacy of muscle group IV afferents in the spinal cord is inhibited by activity in TTX-sensitive (largely myelinated) afferent fibers. The input from cutaneous C fibers did not show this effect. These findings are a strong indication of a differential synaptic connectivity of muscle group IV fibers compared to cutaneous C fibers (Steffens et al. 2003).

A highly interesting substance for the induction of muscle pain is nerve growth factor (NGF). When injected intramuscularly (i.m.) in healthy subjects, NGF does not cause immediate pain, but after about a day, the injected muscle becomes hyperalgesic to mechanical stimuli (Svensson et al. 2003a). Perhaps the lack of pain upon injection could be due to the possibility that NGF may not excite muscle nociceptors, although rat nociceptors were strongly excited by the growth factor (Hoheisel et al. 2005a). Compared to other stimulating substances, NGF is unique in that it excites only those unmyelinated afferent units that have a high mechanical threshold in the noxious range (putative nociceptors). Another study has shown that these high-threshold, mechano-sensitive muscle receptors have TTX-resistant afferent fibers (Steffens et al. 2003). Therefore, the NGF-induced input most likely reaches the spinal cord via TTX-resistant fibers.

A possible reason for the lack of pain upon i.m. injection of NGF is that the growth factor does not elicit action potentials in dorsal horn neurons. Instead, it mainly elicits subthreshold excitatory postsynaptic potentials (EPSPs). To test this assumption, Hoheisel and Mense performed intracellular recordings from rat dorsal horn neurons in vivo. The results, previously unpublished, show that most of the nociceptive dorsal horn neurons that reacted to i.m. NGF exhibit only EPSPs (Fig. 2). Moreover, the few dorsal horn neurons that responded to NGF with action potentials in addition to EPSPs showed a very short-lasting excitation that apparently was not effectively transmitted to higher centers, given that blood pressure recordings showed almost no reaction. In contrast, an injection of hypertonic saline into the same muscle—which always causes pain in humans—elicited a strong activation of the same dorsal horn neuron and a marked increase in blood pressure. The finding that the main action of NGF at the spinal level is subthreshold may explain the lack of pain during and directly after i.m. injection. The question to address in the future is whether the NGF-induced subthreshold EPSPs are sufficient to cause long-lasting muscle hyperalgesia.

DEEP-TISSUE HYPERALGESIA

Algesic substances such as capsaicin, bradykinin, serotonin, and hypertonic saline are known to induce muscle pain in humans, as are ischemia or strong mechanical or electrical stimuli (Graven-Nielsen and Arendt-Nielsen 2003). The sensitization of muscle nociceptors is the best-established peripheral mechanism

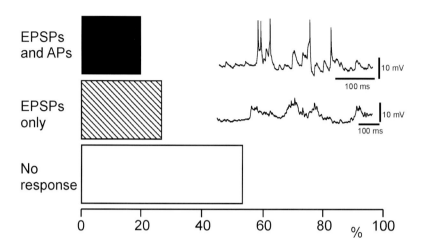

Fig. 2. Reactions of rat dorsal horn neurons to injection of nerve growth factor (0.8 μM, 25 μL) into the gastrocnemius soleus muscle. The neurons were recorded intracellularly in anesthetized animals. The open bar represents neurons without any response. The hatched bar represents neurons that reacted only with subthreshold excitatory postsynaptic potentials (EPSPs). The solid bar represents neurons responding with action potentials (APs) in addition to EPSPs. The original registrations show examples of the behavior of single cells. Some of the action potentials are truncated. Note that of those neurons that reacted to NGF, the majority showed subthreshold potentials (U. Hoheisel and S. Mense, unpublished data).

for the subjective tenderness and the pain felt during movement after muscle damage. Pain increases over time during a sequence of brief mechanical stimuli repeated every 10 or 30 seconds at the threshold for pressure pain, most likely reflecting sensitization of the muscle nociceptors (Nie et al. 2005a). Pressure pain thresholds decrease after i.m. injections of capsaicin (Witting et al. 2000; Polianskis et al. 2002; Qerama et al. 2004). Intra-arterial injections of serotonin, bradykinin, and prostaglandin have been found effective in sensitizing animal nociceptors (Mense 1993). Moreover, in humans, single or combined injections of endogenous substances such as bradykinin, serotonin, substance P, prostaglandin E_2, adenosine triphosphate, and histamine induce deep-tissue hyperalgesia at the injection site (Jensen and Norup 1992; Babenko et al. 1999; Mørk et al. 2003).

An interesting model of deep-tissue hyperalgesia is the delayed-onset muscle soreness arising 24–48 hours after eccentric (contraction during muscle lengthening) muscle exercise. A detailed evaluation of the pressure-pain sensitivity along the musculoskeletal unit (from the proximal to the distal tendon) did not find general hyperalgesia, but rather an increased sensitivity to pressure at various sites (Fig. 3; Andersen et al. 2005). These sites of reversible muscle hyperalgesia might involve mechanisms similar to those underlying the initial development of trigger points seen in myofascial pain patients (Simons et al. 1999) and further studies should explore this in details. Microdialysis reveals an increased intramuscular level of glutamate during delayed-onset muscle soreness (Tegeder et al. 2002), suggesting that glutamate could be involved in the sensitizing process. A similar mechanism might be involved in myalgia of the trapezius muscle, given that a study in patients with this condition was able to correlate the extracellular level of glutamate to the degree of hyperalgesia to pressure (Rosendal et al. 2004). In human studies, i.m. injections of glutamate produce local hyperalgesia to pressure stimuli that outlasts the muscle pain (Svensson et al. 2003b; Ge et al. 2005). Similarly, in rat studies, i.m. gluta-mate sensitizes muscle afferents (Cairns et al. 2002). The glutamate-induced muscle pain is attenuated in humans by i.m. injection of glutamate together with ketamine, an N-methyl-D-aspartate (NMDA) receptor antagonist (Cairns et al. 2003). Ketamine injection also decreases the afferent activity recorded in animals (Cairns et al. 2003). These findings indicate that activation of periph-eral NMDA receptors may contribute to muscle pain and that these receptors might be a valuable target for new analgesics. Facilitated central mechanisms may also be involved in models of delayed hyperalgesia. For example, temporal summation of muscle pain was facilitated during delayed-onset muscle soreness (Bajaj et al. 2000; Nie et al. 2005b).

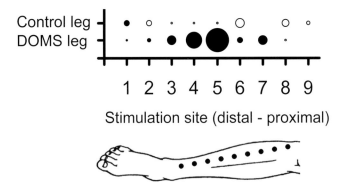

Fig. 3. Sites of hyperalgesia to pressure stimulation after induction of delayed onset muscle soreness (DOMS) induced by eccentric exercise in one subject. Each circle represents the change of pressure pain thresholds for the DOMS leg and the control leg. The width of the circles represents the amount of either hyperalgesia (filled circles) or hypoalgesia (open circles) compared to pre-exercise recordings taken 2 days previously. Interestingly, one site with extensive hyperalgesia is located close to a site with no or very little change in the deep tissue sensitivity. Based on data from Andersen et al. (2005).

REFERRED PAIN

Referred pain is a specific characteristic of muscle pain. Previous studies have focused on referred pain elicited from muscle and joint structures. A recent study in healthy volunteers reported that hypertonic saline injection in tendons evokes referred pain with a comparable frequency to pain induced by injection into the muscle belly (Gibson et al. 2005). Typically, referred pain is described as a sensation from deep structures (Graven-Nielsen et al. 2002) in contrast to visceral referred pain, which is both superficially and deeply located. Referred pain is probably a combination of central processing and peripheral input, given that it is possible to induce referred pain to limbs with complete sensory loss due to an anesthetic block (Kellgren 1938).

Data from animal experiments show that the input from muscle nociceptors causes marked neuroplastic changes in sensory neurons of the dorsal horn (Hoheisel et al. 1994). These changes include the opening of ineffective (silent) synapses, changes in gene expression and neuronal metabolism, and hyperexcitability of nociceptive neurons, i.e., central sensitization, which in this case is mainly due to activation of NMDA channels and neurokinin-1 receptors (Hoheisel et al. 1997). The sensitization of dorsal horn neurons by input from muscle nociceptors is likely to be responsible for the referral of muscle pain. There is a complex network of extensive collateral synaptic connections for each muscle afferent fiber onto multiple dorsal horn neurons (Mense and Simons 2001). Under normal conditions, afferent fibers have fully functional synaptic connections with dorsal horn neurons as well as latent synaptic connections to other neurons within the same region of the spinal cord. Following ongoing strong noxious input, latent synaptic connections become operational, thereby allowing for convergence of input from more than one source. Recordings from a dorsal horn neuron with a receptive field located in the biceps femoris muscle show new receptive fields in the anterior tibial muscle and at the foot after i.m. injection of bradykinin into the anterior tibial muscle (Hoheisel et al. 1993). In the context of referred pain, the unmasking of new receptive fields due to central sensitization could mediate referred pain. The appearance of referred pain is delayed by 20–40 seconds compared to local muscle pain (Graven-Nielsen et al. 1997; Laursen et al. 1997), indicating that a time-dependent process, perhaps the unmasking of new synaptic connections, is involved in the neural mediation of referred pain. The frequency of referred pain from prolonged mechanical stimulation on the anterior tibial muscle is significantly higher than for brief stimulation, again indicating the time dependency of referred pain (Gibson et al. 2005). Moreover, saline-induced referred pain occurred less frequently in healthy subjects treated with ketamine compared to a placebo treatment (Schulte et al. 2003), indicating the involvement of central sensitization.

REFERRED PAIN, HYPERALGESIA, AND TEMPORAL SUMMATION IN CHRONIC MUSCULOSKELETAL PAIN

Clinical knowledge is substantial on the patterns of referred muscle pain from various skeletal muscles and after activation of trigger points in myofascial pain patients (Simons et al. 1999). The pattern and size of referral seem to be changed in chronic musculoskeletal pain conditions. For example, fibromyalgia patients experience more severe pain and larger referred areas after experimental muscle pain (induced by hypertonic saline injection) compared to matched controls (Sörensen et al. 1998). Pain from the anterior tibial muscle is normally projected distally to the ankle; only rarely is it projected proximally. Enlarged areas of referred pain in patients with chronic pain suggest an increase in the efficacy of central processing (central sensitization). Moreover, the expanded area of referred pain in fibromyalgia patients was partly inhibited by ketamine, a finding that also implicates central sensitization (Graven-Nielsen et al. 2000). Extended areas of referred pain from the anterior tibial muscle have also been shown in patients suffering from chronic whiplash pain; extended areas of referred pain were also found in the neck and shoulder region after saline injection into the infraspinatus muscle (Johansen et al. 1999). Similarly, patients with lateral epicondylitis (tennis elbow) pain mapped larger pain areas (Fig. 4) and reported a higher frequency of pain referral compared to controls after experimental pain was induced in a wrist extensor muscle (Slater et al. 2005). Patients suffering from chronic osteoarthritic knee pain reported extended areas of saline-induced referred pain (Bajaj et al. 2001). Such findings show that noxious input from the joints to the central nervous system facilitates the mechanisms of referred pain from muscles, possibly due to central sensitization.

Repeated stimuli of constant intensity may evoke an increase in the intensity of perception until they are eventually perceived as painful (Price 1972; Arendt-Nielsen et al. 1994). This phenomenon reflects neuronal integration processes and is called temporal summation. Assessment of temporal summation provides information on central integrative mechanisms of sensory processing. To elicit temporal summation, a stimulus is repeated at constant intervals, e.g., five times with a frequency of 2 Hz, at constant intensity. The intensity of the five constant stimuli is increased gradually until the subject feels an increase in pain perception during the repeated stimulation. As an example, repeated pressure stimulation on muscle tissue with a 1-second interstimulus interval evokes a progressive increase in pain intensity (Nie et al. 2005a). Pain thresholds to intramuscular electrical stimulation were assessed in patients with fibromyalgia (Sörensen et al. 1998). The stimulation was applied to muscles that were not spontaneously painful. While there was no difference in cutaneous pain thresholds to single stimulations between patients and healthy controls, temporal summation

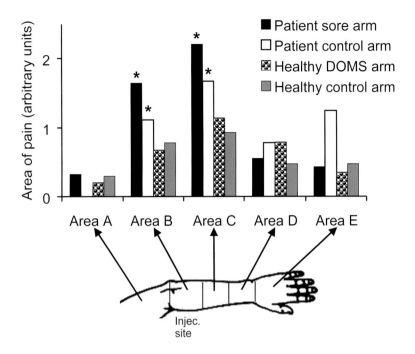

Fig. 4. Mean areas of pain after injections of hypertonic saline (1 mL, 5.8%) into the extensor carpi radialis brevis muscle of the sore arm in patients with lateral epicondylitis pain and their contralateral control arm (pain free). The controls were a group of healthy subjects in whom delayed-onset muscle soreness (DOMS) was induced in one arm (injections were made in both arms). The arm was divided into five areas for assessment of local and referred pain. In patients, both the injected area and the distal areas showed significantly (*$P < 0.05$) larger areas of pain in both the sore and pain-free arms compared to both DOMS and pain-free arms in controls. The effects of expanded pain areas on the contralateral arm in patients might indicate involvement of central sensitization. Based on data from Slater et al. (2005).

after intramuscular stimulation was facilitated in fibromyalgia patients. Later, temporal summation was studied in fibromyalgia patients and healthy controls by delivering repeated mechanical stimuli. Temporal summation was greatly exaggerated in fibromyalgia patients (Staud et al. 2003). These findings indicate generalized central sensitization in fibromyalgia.

A study on chronic whiplash patients measured pain thresholds to electrical stimulation applied both on the skin and in the muscles of the neck and lower limb (Curatolo et al. 2001). Patients displayed lower pain thresholds than healthy controls for both cutaneous and muscular electrical stimulation (Fig. 5). Lower stimulus intensity was sufficient to induce the increase in pain sensation during repeated stimulation (temporal summation) in patients, compared with controls, suggesting facilitated temporal summation. This phenomenon can also

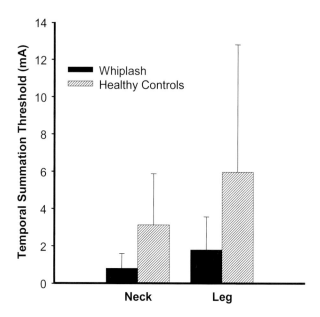

Fig. 5. Temporal summation thresholds for intramuscular electrical stimulation in whiplash patients and healthy controls in the neck and leg muscles. The differences between the two groups were statistically significant in both the neck and leg. Note that no spontaneous pain was reported in the leg. Based on data from Curatolo et al. (2001).

be investigated using the nociceptive withdrawal reflex, an electrophysiological method in which an increase in the electromyographic response is observed during repeated transcutaneous electrical stimulation (Arendt-Nielsen et al. 1994). The threshold for the withdrawal reflex during repeated stimulation was significantly lower in fibromyalgia and whiplash patients compared to healthy controls, indicating spinal cord hyperexcitability in these patients (Banic et al. 2004). Facilitated temporal summation might explain the pain after minimal ongoing nociceptive input arising from minimally damaged tissues or even after innocuous stimulation, an attractive explanation for those cases in which there is pain without clear evidence for tissue damage. Interestingly, infiltration of a local anesthetic into the painful and tender muscles (not at the threshold assessment site) did not reduce either neck pain or pain thresholds (Curatolo et al. 2001). This finding suggests that the source of pain was not located in the muscles and indicates that the muscle hypersensitivity may be due to central mechanisms rather than to primary muscle pathology. However, it is uncertain whether infiltration with local anesthetics is a valid model for investigation of muscle pathology as a primary source of pain.

While muscle hyperalgesia and enhanced temporal summation occur in various musculoskeletal pain conditions, their clinical significance is not fully understood. It is important to distinguish whether these phenomena are the result of primary muscle pathology, or rather the result of central sensitization, with the primary nociceptive focus being located within another anatomical structure. Regardless of the primary origin of pain, muscle hyperalgesia and facilitated temporal summation have high clinical relevance because they contribute substantially to pain and disability. Therefore, a relevant question is whether attenuating these mechanisms may reduce suffering and disability in those patients in which it is impossible to treat the primary cause of pain.

Because hyperalgesia and enhanced temporal summation probably result from central sensitization, treatments aiming at attenuating central plasticity changes may be useful. The extensive literature on basic research and the great improvement in knowledge gained in the last two decades have only minimally been translated into effective treatments. Preventing nociceptive input from arriving at the spinal cord is expected to prevent central plasticity changes. However, with few exceptions (Lord et al. 1996), there is no way of implementing this concept in most clinical musculoskeletal pain conditions. Different drugs act at spinal and supraspinal mechanisms involved in central sensitization. A review of the possible pharmacological approaches is beyond the scope of this chapter. Worth mentioning are opioids, NMDA antagonists (Staud et al. 2005), anticonvulsants acting at the calcium channel $\alpha_2\delta_1$ subunit (Gottrup et al. 2004), cyclooxygenase inhibitors (Yamamoto and Sakashita 1998), $5HT_3$-receptor inhibitors (Farber et al. 2001), and antidepressants (Bendtsen and Jensen 2000). Even nonpharmacological approaches, including physical and psychological treatments, may play a role. Unfortunately, the sparse published evidence and clinical experience show, at best, only modest efficacy for currently available treatment modalities.

CONCLUSION

It has become increasingly evident that the neural plasticity in muscle nociception is significant and that such changes might be important for the muscle hyperalgesia, referred pain, referred hyperalgesia, and widespread hyperalgesia seen in chronic musculoskeletal pain. Quantitative sensory assessments of deep-tissue sensitivity and referred pain from muscles have revealed new and important knowledge for diagnosis and therapy. For example, experimentally induced referred pain may be used to assess a potential involvement of central sensitization in musculoskeletal pain conditions. Attenuating these mechanisms is likely to reduce suffering and disability. Existing treatment modalities have only modest efficacy, so new treatment modalities incorporating evidence on sensitization mechanisms are needed.

ACKNOWLEDGMENT

Dr. Graven-Nielsen was supported by the Danish Research Council. Dr. Curatolo was supported by the scientific funds of the Department of Anesthesiology. Dr. Mense was supported by the Deutsche Forschungsgemeinschaft, project KFG 107.

REFERENCES

Andersen H, Arendt-Nielsen L, Danneskiold-Samsøe B, et al. Muscle hardness and spatial pressure sensitivity in delayed onset muscle soreness. *Abstracts: 11th World Congress on Pain.* Seattle: IASP Press, 2005, p 174.

Arendt-Nielsen L, Brennum J, Sindrup S, et al. Electrophysiological and psychophysical quantification of temporal summation in the human nociceptive system. *Eur J Appl Physiol* 1994; 68:266–273.

Babenko V, Graven-Nielsen T, Svensson P, et al. Experimental human muscle pain and muscular hyperalgesia induced by combinations of serotonin and bradykinin. *Pain* 1999; 82:1–8.

Bajaj P, Graven-Nielsen T, Wright A, et al. Muscle hyperalgesia in postexercise muscle soreness assessed by single and repetitive ultrasound stimuli. *J Pain* 2000; 1:111–121.

Bajaj P, Bajaj P, Graven-Nielsen T, et al. Osteoarthritis and its association with muscle hyperalgesia: an experimental controlled study. *Pain* 2001; 93:107–114.

Banic B, Petersen-Felix S, Andersen OK, et al. Evidence for spinal cord hypersensitivity in chronic pain after whiplash injury and in fibromyalgia. *Pain* 2004; 107:7–15.

Bendtsen L, Jensen R. Amitriptyline reduces myofascial tenderness in patients with chronic tension-type headache. *Cephalalgia* 2000; 20:603–610.

Cairns BE, Gambarota G, Svensson P, et al. Glutamate-induced sensitization of rat masseter muscle fibers. *Neuroscience* 2002; 109:389–399.

Cairns BE, Svensson P, Wang K, et al. Activation of peripheral NMDA receptors contributes to human pain and rat afferent discharges evoked by injection of glutamate into the masseter muscle. *J Neurophysiol* 2003; 90:2098–2105.

Callsen-Cencic P, Hoheisel U, Kaske A, et al. The controversy about spinal neuronal nitric oxide synthase: under which conditions is it up—or downregulated? *Cell Tissue Res* 1999; 295:183–194.

Curatolo M, Petersen-Felix S, Arendt-Nielsen L, et al. Central hypersensitivity in chronic pain after whiplash injury. *Clin J Pain* 2001; 17:306–315.

Farber L, Stratz TH, Bruckle W, et al. Short-term treatment of primary fibromyalgia with the 5-HT3-receptor antagonist tropisetron. Results of a randomized, double-blind, placebo-controlled multicenter trial in 418 patients. *Int J Clin Pharmacol Res* 2001; 21:1–13.

Ge H-Y, Madeleine P, Arendt-Nielsen L. Gender differences in pain modulation evoked by repeated injections of glutamate into the human trapezius muscle. *Pain* 2005; 113:134–140.

Gibson W, Arendt-Nielsen L, Graven-Nielsen T. Experimentally induced saline pain from human tendon and muscle: a comparison of pain characteristics and referred pain areas. *Abstracts: 11th World Congress on Pain.* Seattle: IASP Press, 2005, p 172.

Gottrup H, Juhl G, Kristensen AD, et al. Chronic oral gabapentin reduces elements of central sensitization in human experimental hyperalgesia. *Anesthesiology* 2004; 101:1400–1408.

Graven-Nielsen T, Arendt-Nielsen L. Induction and assessment of muscle pain, referred pain, and muscular hyperalgesia. *Curr Pain Headache Rep* 2003; 7:443–451.

Graven-Nielsen T, Arendt-Nielsen L, Svensson P, et al. Stimulus-response functions in areas with experimentally induced referred muscle pain—a psychophysical study. *Brain Res* 1997; 744:121–128.

Graven-Nielsen T, Kendall SA, Henriksson KG, et al. Ketamine reduces muscle pain, temporal summation, and referred pain in fibromyalgia patients. *Pain* 2000; 85:483–491.

Graven-Nielsen T, Gibson SJ, Laursen RJ, et al. Opioid-insensitive hypoalgesia to mechanical stimuli at sites ipsilateral and contralateral to experimental muscle pain in human volunteers. *Exp Brain Res* 2002; 146:213–222.

Hoheisel U, Mense S, Simons DG, et al. Appearance of new receptive fields in rat dorsal horn neurons following noxious stimulation of skeletal muscle: a model for referral of muscle pain? *Neurosci Lett* 1993; 153:9–12.

Hoheisel U, Koch K, Mense S. Functional reorganization in the rat dorsal horn during an experimental myositis. *Pain* 1994; 59:111–118.

Hoheisel U, Sander B, Mense S. Myositis-induced functional reorganisation of the rat dorsal horn: effects of spinal superfusion with antagonists to neurokinin and glutamate receptors. *Pain* 1997; 69:219–230.

Hoheisel U, Unger T, Mense S. Excitatory and modulatory effects of inflammatory cytokines and neurotrophins on mechanosensitive group IV muscle afferents in the rat. *Pain* 2005a; 114:168–176.

Hoheisel U, Unger T, Mense S. The possible role of the NO-cGMP pathway in nociception: different spinal and supraspinal action of enzyme blockers on rat dorsal horn neurones. *Pain* 2005b;117:358–367.

Jensen K, Norup M. Experimental pain in human temporal muscle induced by hypertonic saline, potassium and acidity. *Cephalalgia* 1992; 12:101–106.

Johansen MK, Graven-Nielsen T, Olesen AS, et al. Generalised muscular hyperalgesia in chronic whiplash syndrome. *Pain* 1999; 83:229–234.

Kellgren JH. Observations on referred pain arising from muscle. *Clin Sci* 1938; 3:175–190.

Laursen RJ, Graven-Nielsen T, Jensen TS, et al. Quantification of local and referred pain in humans induced by intramuscular electrical stimulation. *Eur J Pain* 1997; 1:105–113.

Lim PH, Ng FC, Cheng CW, et al. Clinical safety profile of sildenafil in Singaporean men with erectile dysfunction: pre-marketing experience (ASSESS-I evaluation). *J Int Med Res* 2002; 30:137–143.

Lord SM, Barnsley L, Wallis BJ, et al. Percutaneous radio-frequency neurotomy for chronic cervical zygapophyseal-joint pain. *N Engl J Med* 1996; 335:1721–1726.

Mense S. Nociception from skeletal muscle in relation to clinical muscle pain. *Pain* 1993; 54:241–289.

Mense S, Simons DG. *Muscle Pain. Understanding its Nature, Diagnosis, and Treatment.* Philadelphia: Lippincott Williams & Wilkins, 2001.

Mørk H, Ashina M, Bendtsen L, et al. Experimental muscle pain and tenderness following infusion of endogenous substances in humans. *Eur J Pain* 2003; 7:145–153.

Nie H, Arendt-Nielsen L, Andersen H, et al. Temporal summation of pain evoked by mechanical stimulation in deep and superficial tissue. *J Pain* 2005a; 6:348–355.

Nie H, Arendt-Nielsen L, Madeleine P, et al. Enhanced temporal summation of pressure pain in the trapezius muscle after delayed onset muscle soreness. *Exp Brain Res* 2005b; 23:1–9.

Polianskis R, Graven-Nielsen T, Arendt-Nielsen L. Pressure-pain function in desensitized and hypersensitized muscle and skin assessed by cuff algometry. *J Pain* 2002; 3:28–37.

Price DD. Characteristics of second pain and flexion reflexes indicative of prolonged central summation. *Exp Neurol* 1972; 37:371–387.

Qerama E, Fuglsang-Frederiksen A, Kasch H, et al. Evoked pain in the motor endplate region of the brachial biceps muscle: an experimental study. *Muscle Nerve* 2004; 29:393–400.

Rosendal L, Larsson B, Kristiansen J, et al. Increase in muscle nociceptive substances and anaerobic metabolism in patients with trapezius myalgia: microdialysis in rest and during exercise. *Pain* 2004; 112:324–334.

Schulte H, Graven-Nielsen T, Sollevi A, et al. Pharmacological modulation of experimental phasic and tonic muscle pain by morphine, alfentanil and ketamine in healthy volunteers. *Acta Anaesthesiol Scand* 2003; 47:1020–1030.

Simons DG, Travell JG, Simons L. *Myofascial Pain and Dysfunction: The Trigger Point Manual.* Philadelphia: Lippincott Williams & Wilkins, 1999.

Slater H, Arendt-Nielsen L, Wright A, et al. Sensory and motor effects of experimental muscle pain in patients with lateral epicondylalgia and controls with delayed onset muscle soreness. *Pain* 2005; 114:118–130.

Sörensen J, Graven-Nielsen T, Henriksson KG, et al. Hyperexcitability in fibromyalgia. *J Rheumatol* 1998; 25:152–155.

Staud R, Cannon RC, Mauderli AP, et al. Temporal summation of pain from mechanical stimulation of muscle tissue in normal controls and subjects with fibromyalgia syndrome. *Pain* 2003; 102:87–95.

Staud R, Vierck CJ, Robinson ME, et al. Effects of the N-methyl-D-aspartate receptor antagonist dextromethorphan on temporal summation of pain are similar in fibromyalgia patients and normal control subjects. *J Pain* 2005; 6:323–332.

Steffens H, Eek B, Trudrung P, et al. Tetrodotoxin block of A-fibre afferents from skin and muscle—a tool to study pure C-fibre effects in the spinal cord. *Pflugers Arch* 2003; 445:607–613.

Svensson P, Cairns BE, Wang K, et al. Injection of nerve growth factor into human masseter muscle evokes long-lasting mechanical allodynia and hyperalgesia. *Pain* 2003a; 104:241–247.

Svensson P, Cairns BE, Wang K, et al. Glutamate-evoked pain and mechanical allodynia in the human masseter muscle. *Pain* 2003b; 101:221–227.

Tegeder I, Zimmermann J, Meller ST, et al. Release of algesic substances in human experimental muscle pain. *Inflamm Res* 2002; 51:393–402.

Witting N, Svensson P, Gottrup H, et al. Intramuscular and intradermal injection of capsaicin: a comparison of local and referred pain. *Pain* 2000; 84:407–412.

Yamamoto T, Sakashita Y. COX-2 inhibitor prevents the development of hyperalgesia induced by intrathecal NMDA or AMPA. *Neuroreport* 1998; 9:3869–3873.

Correspondence to: Thomas Graven-Nielsen, PhD, Center for Sensory-Motor Interaction (SMI), Laboratory for Experimental Pain Research, Aalborg University, Fredrik Bajers Vej 7D-3, DK-9220 Aalborg E, Denmark. Tel: 45-96359832; Fax: 45-98154008; email: tgn@hst.aau.dk.

Proceedings of the 11th World Congress on Pain,
edited by Herta Flor, Eija Kalso, and Jonathan O.
Dostrovsky, IASP Press, Seattle, © 2006.

22

Role of Central Sensitization in Chronic Pain: Osteoarthritis and Rheumatoid Arthritis Compared to Neuropathic Pain

Michael C. Rowbotham[a], Bruce L. Kidd,[b] and Frank Porreca[c]

[a]Department of Neurology and Pain Clinical Research Center, University of California at San Francisco, California, USA; [b]Royal London Hospital, London, United Kingdom; [c]Department of Pharmacology, University of Arizona, Tucson, Arizona, USA

Osteoarthritis (OA) affects 13% of people aged >55 years. The total number affected is expected to double by 2020, due to increases in life expectancy and obesity (Melton 2003). Rheumatoid arthritis (RA) affects approximately 0.5–1% of the population (Silman and Pearson 2002). In the United States alone, the prevalence of OA and RA is estimated to be 21 million and 2.5 million, respectively (Lawrence et al. 1998). Together, OA and RA comprise the most common cause of adult disability (Mili et al. 2002).

Although pain is not an inevitable consequence of joint disease, it is its most common symptom (Kidd et al. 2004). Pain in OA and RA is characterized by hyperalgesia and spontaneous pain (Schaible et al. 2002). Patients have lowered pain thresholds as well as increased sensitivity to pressure and temperature. Verbal descriptions are unable to discriminate between pain in OA and RA (Helliwell 1995). In both, pain is described by patients as "aching" and "throbbing," interspersed by activity-related episodes of "sharp" and "stabbing" pain (Wagstaff et al. 1985). Although symptoms are mostly experienced in or near the affected joint, referred pain and tenderness may also occur (Kidd 2003).

The "cause" of pain in OA has been attributed to a number of peripheral factors, including increased synovial activity (McCrae et al. 1992), synovial thickening (Hill et al. 2001), and bone marrow edema (Felson et al. 2001). However, these factors alone are unlikely to produce pain symptoms (Kellgren and Samuel 1950; Schaible and Grubb 1993; Kidd 2003). Whereas RA is an autoimmune disorder in which inflammation is the primary pathophysiological mechanism, OA results from the degeneration of hyaline articular cartilage, which secondarily results in local inflammation and pain (Niissalo et al. 2002). Although acute inflammation is essential to the body's defense, chronic inflammation can result in tissue injury and pain (D'Agostino et al. 2005).

PLASTICITY AND PERIPHERAL SENSITIZATION

The nervous system is able to modify its function according to different conditions, an attribute termed "plasticity" (Coderre et al. 1993). Plasticity is pivotal to the generation of the hypersensitivity underlying inflammatory pain (Kidd and Urban 2001). Nociceptors are highly sensitive to changes within their microenvironment, which can reduce their threshold for activation (Kidd 2003). Following tissue injury, inflammatory mediators are released from damaged cells, including ions (K^+, H^+), bradykinin, histamine, serotonin (5-hydroxytryptamine), adenosine triphosphate, and nitric oxide. Activation of the arachidonic acid pathway leads to the production of prostanoids and leukotrienes; immune cells are recruited to the site of injury and release further inflammatory mediators, including cytokines and growth factors (Kidd and Urban 2001). During inflammation, primary afferent neurons in the joint become sensitized. The response to pressure and movement of low-threshold, non-nociceptive mechanoreceptors (Aβ fibers) becomes enhanced. High-threshold nociceptors (Aδ and C fibers) start to respond to light pressure and movement, and "silent nociceptors" (mechanoinsensitive fibers) become responsive to mechanical stimulation (Schaible et al. 2002). The net result is that the nociceptive system is activated by normally innocuous and nonpainful stimuli, a condition known as "peripheral sensitization" (Schaible and Grubb 1993).

INDICATIONS OF CENTRAL INVOLVEMENT
IN INFLAMMATORY PAIN

The observation that patients with OA may suffer abnormal, generalized pain sensitivity only in response to stimulation of deep muscle tissue, together with findings that pain sensitivity and modulation are normalized following osteotomy or joint replacement, strongly suggest that a central mechanism contributes to OA pain (Bradley et al. 2004). This suggestion has been supported by studies of hyperalgesia in OA patients (Farrell et al. 2000; Bajaj et al. 2001) and by the finding that unilateral administration of local anesthetic in the knee of an OA patient can have bilateral effects (Creamer et al. 1996). Similarly, studies of capsaicin-induced hyperalgesia in RA patients (Jolliffe et al. 1995; Morris et al. 1997), as well as a comparison of the response to pain induced by intranasal stimulation with gaseous carbon dioxide between RA patients and controls (Hummel et al. 2000), have indicated that joint symptoms in RA arise from central factors, in addition to peripheral ones.

MECHANISMS AND MEDIATORS OF CENTRAL SENSITIZATION

In chronic inflammatory conditions, such as OA and RA, sustained or repetitive activation of primary afferent fibers results in changes to the function and activity of central neurogenic pathways (Kidd and Urban 2001). Such changes manifest as enhanced responses to pressure in areas adjacent to the inflamed tissue and even in remote, non-inflamed "normal" tissue; often, the total receptive field of neurons is increased (Schaible et al. 2002). The induction of "wind-up," whereby repeated nerve stimulations result in increased electrical activity in spinal dorsal horn neurons, and the ensuing long-lasting changes in spinal excitability are known collectively as "central sensitization." The generation and maintenance of central sensitization are dependent on the action of transmitter/receptor systems in the spinal cord. Peripheral sensitization increases the evoked release of transmitters from the spinal terminals of afferent neurons, representing the presynaptic component of central sensitization. Activation of receptors and secondary messenger systems lead to changes in receptor sensitivity, thereby increasing the excitability of spinal cord neurons, representing the postsynaptic component of central sensitization (Schaible et al. 2002) (Fig. 1).

Glutamate is the key neurotransmitter responsible for communication between the periphery and spinal dorsal horn. When innocuous pressure is applied to a non-inflamed joint, glutamate is released from low-threshold non-nociceptive Aβ fibers onto spinal cord neurons, where it opens ligand-gated cation channels on α-amino-3-hydroxy-5-methyl-isoxazole-4-propionic acid (AMPA) receptors (Schaible et al. 2002). Under such circumstances, N-methyl-D-aspartate (NMDA) receptors are not opened, since they are blocked by Mg^{2+} ions. When noxious pressure is applied, non-nociceptive Aβ fibers and nociceptive Aδ and C fibers are activated, resulting in enhanced glutamate release and strong depolarization, which expels Mg^{2+} ions and opens NMDA- and AMPA-receptor channels (Schaible et al. 2002). Likewise, when an inflamed joint is stimulated, both NMDA and AMPA receptors are opened. NMDA receptors play an essential role in the development and maintenance of central sensitization (Neugebauer et al. 1993).

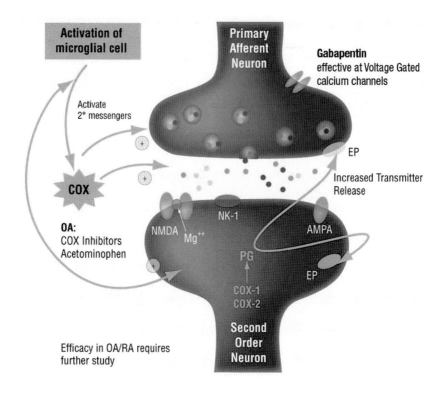

Fig. 1. Mechanisms of central sensitization common to chronic inflammatory pain and neuropathic pain. AMPA = α-amino-3-hydroxy-5-methyl-isoxazole-4-propionic acid; COX-1 = cyclooxygenase-1; COX-2 = cyclooxygenase-2; EP = PGE$_2$ family of prostanoid receptors; Mg^{++} = magnesium ions; NK-1 = neurokinin-1; OA = osteoarthritis; PG = prostaglandin; RA = rheumatoid arthritis.

A number of neuromodulators augment central sensitization. During inflammation, neuropeptides such as substance P, neurokinin A, and calcitonin gene-related peptide (Sluka and Westlund 1993; Niissalo et al. 2002; Schaible 2004) and neurotrophic peptides such as brain-derived neurotrophic factor (Pezet et al. 2002) are released from the central terminals of primary afferent neurons, where they act as co-transmitters (Woolf 1983), probably by enhancing glutamatergic synaptic transmission (Ebersberger et al. 2000). The antinociceptive effect of neuropeptide receptor antagonists is much weaker than that of glutamate receptor antagonists, but neuropeptide receptors may be involved in long-term changes in pain sensitivity during inflammation (Schaible et al. 2002).

Prostaglandins are important mediators of inflammation, fever, and pain and are synthesized by cyclooxygenase-1 (COX-1) and its isoform enzyme COX-2, which is induced in peripheral tissues by cytokines, growth factors, and other inflammatory mediators (Ballou et al. 2000). Prostaglandins can directly activate nociceptors, but they are generally considered to be sensitizing agents, increasing levels of cellular cyclic adenosine monophosphate (cAMP) and enhancing nociceptor sensitivity by lowering the activation threshold for tetrodotoxin-resistant sodium channels via a protein kinase A pathway (England et al. 1996). Prostaglandins sensitize primary afferents to bradykinin and other mediators (Neugebauer et al. 1989) and are thought to be involved at multiple sites along the nociceptive pathway (Rueff and Dray 1993). COX-1 and COX-2 synthesize prostaglandins in dorsal root ganglion (DRG) and spinal cord neurons (Schaible et al. 2002). Prostaglandin receptors are located not only on primary afferent neurons, but also on spinal cord neurons, indicating that prostaglandins act both pre- and postsynaptically (Vanegas and Schaible 2001). Animal models have demonstrated that COX-2 products contribute to increased spinal excitability during persistent peripheral inflammation (Seybold et al. 2003). Animal studies have also shown that there is a tonic release of immunoreactive prostaglandin E_2 from the spinal cord following the induction of arthritis, which is accompanied by enhanced expression of COX-2 protein in the spinal cord, indicating that intraspinal prostaglandins may play a role in inflammation-evoked central sensitization (Ebersberger et al. 1999).

The proinflammatory cytokine interleukin-1β (IL-1β) is a major inducer of central COX-2 upregulation, thereby contributing to central sensitization (Samad et al. 2001). Interleukin-1 plays an important role in the pathogenesis of both RA (Kay and Calabrese 2004) and OA (Chevalier et al. 2005). Tumor necrosis factor-α (TNF-α) is a pleiotropic cytokine that is overproduced in rheumatoid joints, triggering a cascade of secondary mediators involved in the recruitment of inflammatory cells (Camussi and Lupia 1998). Studies in rat models have demonstrated that TNF-α mediates carrageenin-induced inflammatory knee-joint incapacitation (Tonussi and Ferreira 1999) and that it plays a key role in Freund's adjuvant-induced inflammatory hyperalgesia, directly acting on neurons via TNF-receptor 1 and facilitating the accumulation of macrophages in the DRG via a pathway mediated by TNF-receptor 2 (Inglis et al. 2005). A recent study indicates that the autocrine/paracrine activities of TNF-α and IL-1 in articular cartilage may play important roles in cartilage matrix degradation in some OA patients (Kobayashi et al. 2005). Nitric oxide facilitates spinal excitability (Wu et al. 1998), possibly by enhancing the phosphorylation of cAMP-responsive element-binding protein (CREB) in the spinal cord (Wu et al. 2002).

Under normal circumstances, enhanced spinal excitability is counteracted by descending inhibitory systems, mediated by opioids, cannabinoids, norepinephrine, adenosine, and other substances (Kidd 2003; Strangman and Walker 1999). Endogenous opioids and α_2-adrenergic agonists decrease spinal excitability by inhibiting presynaptic C-fiber neurotransmitter release and postsynaptic hyperpolarization of second-order neurons (Besson 1999). Dysfunction in in-hibitory systems has been shown to play a role in a number of musculoskeletal disorders, including OA (Kosek and Ordeberg 2000a). Once central sensitiza-tion is initiated, spinal glial cells are activated by a variety of the mediators responsible for hyperplasia, including prostaglandins, substance P, and nitric oxide (Watkins et al. 2001). This activation causes the glial cells themselves to release proinflammatory cytokines (TNF-α, IL-1, IL-6), substance P, nitric ox-ide, prostaglandins, adenosine triphosphate, and excitatory amino acids, which in turn further increase the release of excitatory amino acids and substance P from Aδ and C afferents synapsing in the dorsal horn, thus enhancing the hy-perexcitability of the dorsal horn neurons (Watkins et al. 2001; Milligan et al. 2003; Bradley et al. 2004).

DIFFERENTIATING NEUROPATHIC FROM INFLAMMATORY PAIN

Whereas inflammatory pain is related to tissue damage, neuropathic pain is caused by neural damage (Romanelli and Esposito 2004). Experimental models of arthritis and neuropathic pain, involving the injection of proinflammatory agents into joints (e.g., Freund's adjuvant; Julkunen and Rokkanen 1970) or near nerves (e.g., formalin; Puig and Sorkin 1996), have demonstrated that, at the peripheral level, inflammatory pain and neuropathic pain have elements in common, because nerve damage induces inflammatory events that play a crucial role in the pathogenesis of neuropathic pain (Tal 1999). Furthermore, OA-associated degenerative changes may result in mechanical compression of nerves, and leakage of cytokines into nerve roots may result in nerve inflam-mation ("neuritis"), introducing a neuropathic component to OA and RA pain (Tal 1999; Ordeberg 2004).

Similar to tissue damage, neural damage results in the release of neu-rotransmitters and neuropeptides that can induce peripheral sensitization and lead to central sensitization (Romanelli and Esposito 2004). The mechanisms leading to central sensitization in neuropathic pain may differ from those in-volved in arthritis. A characteristic feature of neuropathic pain is allodynia to gentle dynamic mechanical stimulation of the skin, a condition that can result from central sensitization (Romanelli and Esposito 2004). It is uncertain what arthritis symptom(s) would be analogous to neuropathic allodynia. Whereas prostaglandins are the primary mediators of inflammatory pain, nerve damage enhances the expression of sodium channels at the lesion site and induces the expression of adrenergic receptors, eliciting ectopic discharges in nociceptive afferents (Jänig et al. 1996; Eglen et al. 1999; Tal 1999; Schaible and Vanegas

2000). Such differences may have important implications for the efficacy of different types of therapy in arthritis and neuropathic pain, as evidenced by the fact that many elements of neuropathic pain are unresponsive to current analgesics (Garry and Fleetwood-Walker 2004). However, some of the mechanisms leading to central sensitization are likely to be common to neuropathic and inflammatory pain (Fig. 1). For example, murine studies have demonstrated that following sciatic nerve injury, the expression of TNF-α and TNF-α receptor 1 are upregulated in dorsal horn glial cells and spinal neurons, respectively, indicating that the TNF-signaling pathway may be involved in the pathogenesis of neuropathic pain, as well as inflammatory pain (Ohtori et al. 2004).

Studies of experimental neuropathic pain have shown that although enhanced discharge following nerve injury may be responsible for the initiation of neuropathic pain, its maintenance involves other systems. Neuroplastic changes in the rostral ventromedial medulla (RVM) enhance central descending pain facilitation, with an associated increase in the release of the hormone cholecystokinin (Kovelowski et al. 2000; Porreca et al. 2002), and elevate spinal levels of the endogenous opioid peptide dynorphin (Burgess et al. 2002). These findings are supported by experiments showing that lidocaine administered to the RVM blocks neuropathic pain without altering acute nociception (Kovelowski et al. 2000; Burgess et al. 2002). Similarly, enhanced descending facilitation has been demonstrated in experimental models of inflammatory hyperalgesia, involving a time-dependent increase in RVM neurotransmission by excitatory amino acids, via modulation of NMDA and AMPA receptors (Guan et al. 2002, 2003). However, whereas the maintenance of inflammatory hyperalgesia appears to depend primarily on a peripheral driver—as evidenced by the finding that, in the majority of OA patients, hyperalgesia stops following joint replacement surgery (Kosek and Ordeberg 2000b)—the maintenance of neuropathic pain appears to require both the enhanced descending facilitation arising in the brainstem as well as increased or abnormal peripheral input (Porreca et al. 2002).

Neuropathic pain is resistant to centrally acting analgesics, to which inflammatory pain responds well (Garry and Fleetwood-Walker 2004). This contrast may in part be due to subtle differences in neuroreceptors involved in inflammatory and neuropathic pain. For example, the NMDA receptor has two main types of subunit, NR1 and NR2, which determine specific channel characteristics (Chen et al. 1999). The intracellular C terminus of the NR2 subunit mediates interactions with membrane-associated guanylate kinase (MAGUK) proteins, thought to play key roles in neuronal plasticity (Garry and Fleetwood-Walker 2004). Recent research has demonstrated that different MAGUKs are associated with inflammatory and neuropathic pain (Garry and Fleetwood-Walker 2004), which might help explain differences in response to current treatment and point the way to more targeted forms of future therapy (Tao and Raja 2004).

TARGETING CENTRAL SENSITIZATION:
IMPLICATIONS FOR TREATMENT OF PAIN

An understanding of the importance of central sensitization in inflammatory pain not only helps to explain the variability in efficacy of current treatment options, but also informs the development of future therapies, with many of the mediators of central sensitization providing useful targets for drug development.

At present, pain and inflammation associated with RA and OA are treated with nonsteroidal anti-inflammatory drugs (NSAIDs), often in conjunction with analgesics and steroids. NSAIDs are typically classed as selective or nonselective, dependent on their interaction with COX enzymes. Patients with RA may also receive disease-modifying antirheumatic drugs or biological response modifiers such as anti-TNF-α fusion protein or interleukin-1 receptor antagonists.

Recent data suggest that some peripherally acting NSAIDs, such as ketoprofen, may have the ability to penetrate the brain and spinal cord to directly affect pain mediated by 5-hydroxytryptamine (5-HT) receptors, specifically 5-HT$_{1-3}$ and 5-HT$_7$ receptors (Diaz-Reval et al. 2004). Similarly, emerging evidence from animal models suggests that the use of a selective NSAID may prevent the perpetuation of central pain sensitization (You et al. 2003; Ghilardi et al. 2004; Veiga et al. 2004). In one study, intrathecal infusion of a COX-2 inhibitor prior to tissue injury prevented the development of significant tactile allodynia, whereas infusion of a COX-1 inhibitor did not (Ghilardi et al. 2004). In another study, formalin-induced secondary hyperalgesia was prevented by pretreatment with a locally applied COX-2 inhibitor, which was not effective when applied after formalin stimulation. However, hyperalgesia was prevented by spinal administration of the drug, whether given before or after formalin stimulation (Veiga et al. 2004).

NMDA-receptor antagonists not only prevent the hypersensitivity of dorsal horn neurons during the development of arthritis in the rat knee joint (Neugebauer et al. 1993), but also reduce central sensitization once it is established (Neugebauer et al. 1994). They appear to be more affective in ameliorating the effects of mechanical than thermal hyperalgesia (Hama et al. 2003). However, the potential therapeutic use of NMDA-receptor antagonists is hampered by the fact that NMDA receptors are present in most of the brain, affecting many neuronal systems (Schaible and Vanegas 2000). With some NMDA antagonists injected intrathecally, doses near the antihyperalgesic range impair motor coordination (Hama et al. 2003).

Immunomodulatory and disease-modifying drugs have demonstrated efficacy in the treatment of inflammatory pain, particularly in RA. For example, several TNF-α blockers (such as etanercept, infliximab, and adalimumab) are approved for treatment of RA. These drugs are effective for short- and long-term therapy, although, given the pleiotropic nature of TNF-α, careful monitoring is required in order to avoid secondary infections (Hochberg et al. 2005). Similarly, an IL-1-receptor antagonist has been developed specifically to block the activity of IL-1 in synovial joints; it has shown efficacy in reducing inflammatory and joint destructive processes in adults with RA (Waugh and Perry 2005). A study demonstrating a role for TNF-α and IL-1 in the matrix metalloprotease degradation of cartilage in OA patients suggests that therapeutic inhibition of IL-1 and TNF-α may also be beneficial in some patients (Kobayashi et al. 2005). A recent study of intra-articular administration of IL-1-receptor antagonist in OA patients demonstrated a significant improvement in pain, together with good tolerability (Chevalier et al. 2005). Disease-modifying drugs may have the potential to prevent the process of central sensitization from developing or to reverse existing processes.

TREATMENTS FOR NEUROPATHIC PAIN AND THEIR ROLE IN THE TREATMENT OF INFLAMMATORY PAIN

Whereas inflammatory mediators, such as prostaglandins, provide effective therapeutic targets for inflammatory pain, no distinct targets have as yet been identified for central sensitization (Garry and Fleetwood-Walker 2004), although antidepressants, anticonvulsants, topical therapies, and opioids have all been shown to be effective in the treatment of neuropathic pain (Backonja 2004; Spina and Perugi 2004; Hempenstall et al. 2005). Some neuropathic pain therapies have also been used to treat arthritis pain.

Antidepressants. Tricyclic antidepressants and the newer serotonin-norepinephrine reuptake inhibitors are highly effective in the treatment of neuropathic pain disorders (Mattia et al. 2002; Iyengar et al. 2004; Saarto and Wiffen 2005). The efficacy of tricyclic antidepressants may be further enhanced by their ability to block voltage-gated sodium channels (Wang et al. 2004). Tricyclic antidepressants have also shown efficacy in the treatment of arthritis pain, independent of their antidepressive effects (Ash et al. 1999).

Anticonvulsants. Antiepileptic drugs are increasingly used for the treatment of chronic pain, especially neuropathic pain (Spina and Perugi 2004). Phenytoin, a sodium-channel-blocking antiepileptic drug, has shown efficacy as a disease-modifying agent for RA (Naidu et al. 1991; Rao et al. 1995). Gabapentin and pregabalin are approved for the treatment of neuropathic pain, such as postherpetic neuralgia (Rowbotham et al. 1998) and painful diabetic neuropathy (Backonja et al. 1998). These drugs target the $\alpha_2\delta$ subunit on neuronal calcium channels, selectively inhibiting neuronal calcium influx and thereby reducing the activation of AMPA heteroreceptors on noradrenergic nerve terminals (Fink et al. 2002).

Pregabalin has also shown efficacy in reducing pain and fatigue and improving sleep quality in patients with fibromyalgia (Crofford et al. 2005). Fibromyalgia is a syndrome characterized by widespread musculoskeletal pain, fatigue, and sleep abnormalities. Recently gathered evidence of hyperalgesia to mechanical, thermal, chemical, and electrical stimuli has led to the hypothesis that central sensitization plays a key role in the syndrome (Staud and Smitherman 2002; Marcus 2003), and it is likely that the efficacy of pregabalin in treating fibromyalgic pain is a result of its central action on calcium channels. Fibromyalgia is reported in approximately 6% of patients with painful neuropathic disorders (Berger et al. 2004) and 17% of RA patients (Wolfe and Michaud 2004); it may represent a final common phenotype in a number of different chronic pain disorders.

Although there are currently no published trials of the use of gabapentin or pregabalin for OA or RA pain, a randomized controlled trial of pregabalin for OA that enrolled nearly 300 subjects was described in detail in 2001, but remains unpublished (Farrar et al. 2001). Animal experimental models using intra-articular injection of proinflammatory agents have demonstrated that gabapentin can reverse allodynia when administered orally (Fernihough et al. 2004). In animal studies, gabapentin reduced nociception when administered either centrally against thermal hyperalgesia (Lu and Westlund 1999) or peripherally against mechanical hyperalgesia (Hanesch et al. 2003). Other studies of experimental arthritis in animals have invoked actions of pregabalin not clearly related to the $\alpha_2\delta$ subunit (Boileau et al. 2005). Similarly, human models of heat- and capsaicin-induced cutaneous secondary hyperalgesia have demonstrated efficacy of gabapentin; these models have elements similar to inflammatory pain and neuropathic pain (Dirks et al. 2002; Gottrup et al. 2004).

Topicals. Topical therapies with demonstrated efficacy for neuropathic pain include the 5% lidocaine patch (Rowbotham et al. 1996; Galer et al. 1999; Meier et al. 2003; Hempenstall et al. 2005) and capsaicin (Hempenstall et al. 2005). The 5% lidocaine patch has also shown efficacy in the treatment of peripheral pain in OA patients (Burch et al. 2004; Gammaitoni et al. 2004). The mode of action of lidocaine in these pain scenarios is to block voltage-gated sodium channels (Wood et al. 2004). The neurotoxin capsaicin selectively activates C-nociceptors, inducing the release of substance P. In addition, there is a specific blockade of transport and de novo synthesis of substance P, such that repeated applications of topical capsaicin result in long-lasting (but reversible) desensitization to pain, by increasing the pain threshold (Yoshimura et al. 2000; Keitel et al. 2001). Topically applied nonselective NSAIDs overcome the major gastrointestinal adverse effects associated with oral NSAIDs (McQuay et al. 1997) and are widely used to treat inflammatory pain in OA and RA.

Opioids. Opioids act both in the peripheral nervous system and in multiple CNS locations. Controlled trials of intravenous and oral opioids have all shown efficacy in the treatment of neuropathic pain, but randomized controlled trials have all been of less than 2–3 months' duration, and conclusions regarding the risks of tolerance and addiction remain controversial (Kalso et al. 2004; Eisenberg et al. 2005). Some evidence from animal models indicates that the administration of an opioid may itself contribute to the maintenance of neuropathic pain, by increasing the level of spinal dynorphin (Lai et al. 2001), by upregulating cholecystokinin production in the RVM (Ossipov et al. 2004), or by inducing IL-1 production (Shavit et al. 2005), thereby enhancing descending pain facilitation.

Oral morphine has shown efficacy in patients with chronic regional pain of soft-tissue or musculoskeletal origin, who have previously not responded to treatment with codeine, anti-inflammatory agents, or antidepressants (Moulin et al. 1996). Intra-articular morphine has also demonstrated efficacy in the treatment of chronic pain in OA (Likar et al. 1997) and RA (Stein et al. 1999). Weak to moderate potency opioids, with or without acetaminophen (paracetamol), have had mixed results in clinical trials for OA (Kjaersgaard-Andersen et al. 1990; Caldwell et al. 1999; Peloso et al. 2000). For example, in a study comparing the use of codeine plus acetaminophen with acetaminophen alone for the treatment of pain associated with OA of the hip, codeine plus acetaminophen significantly reduced pain over the first 7 days of treatment; however, this combination was associated with a high rate of treatment-related adverse events, which resulted in early study termination (Kjaersgaard-Andersen et al. 1990).

Cannabinoids. The endocannabinoid system forms part of the descending nociceptive inhibitory system. It involves two G-protein-coupled receptors, CB1 and CB2, which are localized primarily to the nervous system and the immune system, respectively (Cravatt and Lichtman 2004). Synthetic cannabinoids have shown efficacy in the treatment of neuropathic pain (Karst et al. 2003), although their use has been associated with psychotropic side effects (Fox and Bevan 2005), and their potential clinical benefit is currently uncertain (Campbell et al. 2001; Attal et al. 2004). However, animal models continue to elucidate the mechanisms of action involved in the endocannabinoid system. For example, CB1 stimulation alters calcium influx and substance P release in rat DRG cells, modulating the activities of transient receptor potential vanilloid 1 (TRPV1), a cloned capsaicin receptor (Oshita et al. 2005). Activation of CB2 receptors attenuates the response of wide-dynamic-range neurons to mechanical stimulation in models of neuropathic and inflammatory pain (Elmes et al. 2004). Cannabinoids have shown anti-inflammatory and immunosuppressive effects in models of arthritis (Malfait et al. 2000; Sumariwalla et al. 2004). Direct application of a cannabinoid to the spinal cord can prevent central sensitization (Johanek and Simone 2005).

TNF-alpha-blockers. Although preclinical data demonstrating the potential efficacy of TNF-α blockade in the treatment of neuropathic pain (Sommer et al. 1998), no clinical trials have as yet been conducted. TNF-α may be involved in the dissipation of neuropathic pain (Ignatowski et al. 2005). As previously mentioned, TNF-α-blockers are now widely used for the treatment of RA (Sharma et al. 2004; Hochberg et al. 2005).

Current treatment practices for inflammatory pain associated with arthritis and neuropathic pain have only small areas of overlap. Both types of disorders involve an element of inflammation that may vary from mild to marked, and evidence is steadily accruing that pro-inflammatory cytokines play an important role in both types of pain (Sommer and Kress 2004). Treatments that are effective in both chronic inflammatory and neuropathic pain appear to be those that are able to affect central mechanisms.

Combination therapy. Concomitant treatment with different classes of drugs can result in beneficial synergistic interactions and may allow lower doses of individual drugs to be administered. Moreover, where associated adverse effects discourage the use of a drug that might otherwise be effective, the co-administration of another drug, capable of blocking these adverse effects, may prove advantageous. Another approach might be to use drugs with different routes of administration, such as an intra-articular opioid combined with an oral NSAID. Generally, the most successful therapies are likely to be those that target multiple sites at both the peripheral and central level and thus provide an opportunity for synergistic interactions with other compounds.

CONCLUSIONS

Evidence is growing that central sensitization plays a role in both chronic inflammatory and neuropathic pain. Central sensitization in OA and RA, and in many patients with neuropathic pain, appears to be maintained by sustained or repetitive activation of primary afferent fibers, by changes in the release of spinal cord neurotransmitters, and by enduring changes in neuronal excitability. Treatments for neuropathic pain, particularly those affecting central mechanisms, have been tested in only a limited way for treatment of chronic inflammatory pain; a more systematic examination of these medications for arthritis pain is warranted because the mechanisms underlying central sensitization in neuropathic pain overlap with those involved in inflammatory pain. Central sensitization due to chronic inflammation may be mitigated by selective NSAIDs as well as traditional neuropathic pain medications, such as tricyclic antidepressants. As the understanding of the mechanisms underlying central sensitization increases, targeted therapies are likely to emerge that are more effective than traditional analgesics. These mechanisms include not only those associated with the central "wind-up" of pain, but also those involved in descending inhibitory pathways.

ACKNOWLEDGMENTS

Dr. Kidd acknowledges the support of the Arthritis Research Campaign of the United Kingdom.

REFERENCES

Ash G, Dickens CM, Creed FH, et al. The effects of dothiepin on subjects with rheumatoid arthritis and depression. *Rheumatology (Oxford)* 1999; 38:959–967.

Attal N, Brasseur L, Guirimand D, et al. Are oral cannabinoids safe and effective in refractory neuropathic pain? *Eur J Pain* 2004; 8:173–177.

Backonja M. Neuromodulating drugs for the symptomatic treatment of neuropathic pain. *Curr Pain Headache Rep* 2004; 8:212–216.

Backonja M, Beydoun A, Edwards KR, et al. Gabapentin for the symptomatic treatment of painful neuropathy in patients with diabetes mellitus: a randomized controlled trial. *JAMA* 1998; 280:1831–1836.

Bajaj P, Bajaj P, Graven-Nielsen T, Arendt-Nielsen L. Osteoarthritis and its association with muscle hyperalgesia: an experimental controlled study. *Pain* 2001; 93:107–114.

Ballou LR, Botting RM, Goorha S, et al. Nociception in cyclooxygenase isozyme-deficient mice. *Proc Natl Acad Sci USA* 2000; 97:10272–10276.

Berger A, Dukes EM, Oster G. Clinical characteristics and economic costs of patients with painful neuropathic disorders. *J Pain* 2004; 5:143–149.

Besson JM. The neurobiology of pain. *Lancet* 1999; 353:1610–1615.

Boileau C, Martel-Pelletier J, Brunet J, et al. Oral treatment with PD-0200347, an alpha-2-delta ligand, reduces the development of experimental osteoarthritis by inhibiting metalloproteinases and inducible nitric oxide synthase gene expression and synthesis in cartilage chondrocytes. *Arthritis Rheum* 2005; 52:488–500.

Bradley LA, Kersh BC, DeBerry JJ, et al. Lessons from fibromyalgia: abnormal pain sensitivity in knee osteoarthritis. *Novartis Found Symp* 2004; 260:258–270.

Burch F, Codding C, Patel N, Sheldon E. Lidocaine patch 5% improves pain, stiffness, and physical function in osteoarthritis pain patients. A prospective, multicenter, open-label effectiveness trial. *Osteoarthritis Cartilage* 2004; 12:253–255.

Burgess SE, Gardell LR, Ossipov MH, et al. Time-dependent descending facilitation from the rostral ventromedial medulla maintains, but does not initiate, neuropathic pain. *J Neurosci* 2002; 22:5129–5136.

Caldwell JR, Hale ME, Boyd RE, et al. Treatment of osteoarthritis pain with controlled release oxycodone or fixed combination oxycodone plus acetaminophen added to nonsteroidal antiinflammatory drugs: a double blind, randomized, multicenter, placebo controlled trial. *J Rheumatol* 1999; 26:862–869.

Campbell FA, Tramer MR, Carroll D, et al. Are cannabinoids an effective and safe treatment option in the management of pain? A qualitative systematic review. *BMJ* 2001; 323:13–16.

Camussi G, Lupia E. The future role of anti-tumour necrosis factor (TNF) products in the treatment of rheumatoid arthritis. *Drugs* 1998; 55:613–620.

Chen N, Luo T, Raymond LA. Subtype-dependence of NMDA receptor channel open probability. *J Neurosci* 1999; 19:6844–6854.

Chevalier X, Giraudeau B, Conrozier T, et al. Safety study of intraarticular injection of interleukin 1 receptor antagonist in patients with painful knee osteoarthritis: a multicenter study. *J Rheumatol* 2005; 32:1317–1323.

Coderre TJ, Katz J, Vaccarino AL, Melzack R. Contribution of central neuroplasticity to pathological pain: review of clinical and experimental evidence. *Pain* 1993; 52:259–285.

Cravatt BF, Lichtman AH. The endogenous cannabinoid system and its role in nociceptive behavior. *J Neurobiol* 2004; 61:149–160.

Creamer P, Hunt M, Dieppe P. Pain mechanisms in osteoarthritis of the knee: effect of intraarticular anesthetic. *J Rheumatol* 1996; 23:1031–1036.

Crofford LJ, Rowbotham MC, Mease PJ, et al. Pregabalin for the treatment of fibromyalgia syndrome: results of a randomized, double-blind, placebo-controlled trial. *Arthritis Rheum* 2005; 52:1264–1273.

D'Agostino MA, Conaghan P, Le Bars M, et al. EULAR report on the use of ultrasonography in painful knee osteoarthritis. Part 1: prevalence of inflammation in osteoarthritis. *Ann Rheum Dis* 2005; 64:1703–1709.

Diaz-Reval MI, Ventura-Martinez R, Deciga-Campos M, et al. Evidence for a central mechanism of action of S+-ketoprofen. *Eur J Pharmacol* 2004; 483:241–248.

Dirks J, Petersen KL, Rowbotham MC, Dahl JB. Gabapentin suppresses cutaneous hyperalgesia following heat-capsaicin sensitization. *Anesthesiology* 2002; 97:102–107.

Ebersberger A, Grubb BD, Willingale HL, et al. The intraspinal release of prostaglandin E2 in a model of acute arthritis is accompanied by an up-regulation of cyclo-oxygenase-2 in the spinal cord. *Neuroscience* 1999; 93:775–781.

Ebersberger A, Charbel Issa P, Vanegas H, Schaible HG. Differential effects of calcitonin gene-related peptide and calcitonin gene-related peptide 8-37 upon responses to N-methyl-D-aspartate or (R, S)-alpha-amino-3-hydroxy-5-methylisoxazole-4-propionate in spinal nociceptive neurons with knee joint input in the rat. *Neuroscience* 2000; 99:171–178.

Eglen RM, Hunter JC, Dray A. Ions in the fire: recent ion-channel research and approaches to pain therapy. *Trends Pharmacol Sci* 1999; 20:337–342.

Eisenberg E, McNicol ED, Carr DB. Efficacy and safety of opioid agonists in the treatment of neuropathic pain of nonmalignant origin: systematic review and meta-analysis of randomized controlled trials. *JAMA* 2005; 293:3043–3052.

Elmes SJ, Jhaveri MD, Smart D, et al. Cannabinoid CB2 receptor activation inhibits mechanically evoked responses of wide dynamic range dorsal horn neurons in naive rats and in rat models of inflammatory and neuropathic pain. *Eur J Neurosci* 2004; 20:2311–2320.

England S, Bevan S, Docherty RJ. PGE_2 modulates the tetrodotoxin-resistant sodium current in neonatal rat dorsal root ganglion neurones via the cyclic AMP-protein kinase A cascade. *J Physiol* 1996; 495:429–440.

Farrar JT, Young JP Jr, LaMoreaux L, Werth JL, Poole RM. Clinical importance of changes in chronic pain intensity measured on an 11-point numerical pain rating scale. *Pain* 2001; 94:149–158.

Farrell M, Gibson S, McMeeken J, Helme R. Pain and hyperalgesia in osteoarthritis of the hands. *J Rheumatol* 2000; 27:441–447.

Felson DT, Chaisson CE, Hill CL, et al. The association of bone marrow lesions with pain in knee osteoarthritis. *Ann Intern Med* 2001; 134:541–549.

Fernihough J, Gentry C, Malcangio M, et al. Pain related behaviour in two models of osteoarthritis in the rat knee. *Pain* 2004; 112:83–93.

Fink K, Dooley DJ, Meder WP, et al. Inhibition of neuronal Ca^{2+} influx by gabapentin and pregabalin in the human neocortex. *Neuropharmacology* 2002; 42:229–236.

Fox A, Bevan S. Therapeutic potential of cannabinoid receptor agonists as analgesic agents. *Expert Opin Investig Drugs* 2005; 14:695–703.

Galer BS, Rowbotham MC, Perander J, Friedman E. Topical lidocaine patch relieves postherpetic neuralgia more effectively than a vehicle topical patch: results of an enriched enrollment study. *Pain* 1999; 80:533–538.

Gammaitoni AR, Galer BS, Onawola R, et al. Lidocaine patch 5% and its positive impact on pain qualities in osteoarthritis: results of a pilot 2-week, open-label study using the Neuropathic Pain Scale. *Curr Med Res Opin* 2004; 20(Suppl 2):S13–S19.

Garry EM, Fleetwood-Walker SM. Organizing pains. *Trends Neurosci* 2004; 27:292–294.

Ghilardi JR, Svensson CI, Rogers SD, et al. Constitutive spinal cyclooxygenase-2 participates in the initiation of tissue injury-induced hyperalgesia. *J Neurosci* 2004; 24:2727–2732.

Gottrup H, Juhl G, Kristensen AD, et al. Chronic oral gabapentin reduces elements of central sensitization in human experimental hyperalgesia. *Anesthesiology* 2004; 101:1400–1408.

Guan Y, Terayama R, Dubner R, Ren K. Plasticity in excitatory amino acid receptor-mediated descending pain modulation after inflammation. *J Pharmacol Exp Ther* 2002; 300:513–520.

Guan Y, Guo W, Zou SP, et al. Inflammation-induced upregulation of AMPA receptor subunit expression in brain stem pain modulatory circuitry. *Pain* 2003; 104:401–413.

Hama A, Woon Lee J, Sagen J. Differential efficacy of intrathecal NMDA receptor antagonists on inflammatory mechanical and thermal hyperalgesia in rats. *Eur J Pharmacol* 2003; 459:49–58.

Hanesch U, Pawlak M, McDougall JJ. Gabapentin reduces the mechanosensitivity of fine afferent nerve fibres in normal and inflamed rat knee joints. *Pain* 2003; 104:363–366.

Helliwell PS. The semeiology of arthritis: discriminating between patients on the basis of their symptoms. *Ann Rheum Dis* 1995; 54:924–926.

Hempenstall K, Nurmikko TJ, Johnson RW, et al. Analgesic therapy in postherpetic neuralgia: a quantitative systematic review. *PLoS Med* 2005; 2:e164.

Hill CL, Gale DG, Chaisson CE, et al. Knee effusions, popliteal cysts, and synovial thickening: association with knee pain in osteoarthritis. *J Rheumatol* 2001; 28:1330–1337.

Hochberg MC, Lebwohl MG, Plevy SE, et al. The benefit/risk profile of TNF-blocking agents: findings of a consensus panel. *Semin Arthritis Rheum* 2005; 34:819–836.

Hummel T, Schiessl C, Wendler J, Kobal G. Peripheral and central nervous changes in patients with rheumatoid arthritis in response to repetitive painful stimulation. *Int J Psychophysiol* 2000; 37:177–183.

Ignatowski TA, Sud R, Reynolds JL, et al. The dissipation of neuropathic pain paradoxically involves the presence of tumor necrosis factor-alpha (TNF). *Neuropharmacology* 2005; 48:448–460.

Inglis JJ, Nissim A, Lees DM, et al. The differential contribution of tumour necrosis factor to thermal and mechanical hyperalgesia during chronic inflammation. *Arthritis Res Ther* 2005; 7:R807–816.

Iyengar S, Webster AA, Hemrick-Luecke SK, et al. Efficacy of duloxetine, a potent and balanced serotonin-norepinephrine reuptake inhibitor in persistent pain models in rats. *J Pharmacol Exp Ther* 2004; 311:576–584.

Jänig W, Levine JD, Michaelis M. Interactions of sympathetic and primary afferent neurons following nerve injury and tissue trauma. *Prog Brain Res* 1996; 113:161–184.

Johanek LM, Simone DA. Cannabinoid agonist, CP 55,940, prevents capsaicin-induced sensitization of spinal cord dorsal horn neurons. *J Neurophysiol* 2005; 93:989–997.

Jolliffe VA, Anand P, Kidd BL. Assessment of cutaneous sensory and autonomic axon reflexes in rheumatoid arthritis. *Ann Rheum Dis* 1995; 54:251–255.

Julkunen H, Rokkanen P. Arthritis induced with Freund's adjuvant and its relationship to changes in the stomach, small intestine and thymus. A histological and tritiated thymidine study on rats. *Acta Rheumatol Scand* 1970; 16:22–29.

Kalso E, Edwards JE, Moore RA, McQuay HJ. Opioids in chronic non-cancer pain: systematic review of efficacy and safety. *Pain* 2004; 112:372–380.

Karst M, Salim K, Burstein S, et al. Analgesic effect of the synthetic cannabinoid CT-3 on chronic neuropathic pain: a randomized controlled trial. *JAMA* 2003; 290:1757–1762.

Kay J, Calabrese L. The role of interleukin-1 in the pathogenesis of rheumatoid arthritis. *Rheumatology (Oxford)* 2004; 43(Suppl 3):2–9.

Keitel W, Frerick H, Kuhn U, et al. Capsicum pain plaster in chronic non-specific low back pain. *Arzneimittelforschung* 2001; 51:896–903.

Kellgren J, Samuel E. The sensitivity and innervation of the articular capsule. *J Bone Joint Surg* 1950; 32:84–91.

Kidd B. Peripheral and central pain mechanisms in osteoarthritis. In: Brandt KD, Doherty M, Lohmander S (Eds). *Osteoarthritis*. Oxford University Press, 2003, pp 185–89.

Kidd BL, Urban LA. Mechanisms of inflammatory pain. *Br J Anaesth* 2001; 87:3–11.

Kidd BL, Photiou A, Inglis JJ. The role of inflammatory mediators on nociception and pain in arthritis. *Novartis Found Symp* 2004; 260:122–133.

Kjaersgaard-Andersen P, Nafei A, Skov O, et al. Codeine plus paracetamol versus paracetamol in longer-term treatment of chronic pain due to osteoarthritis of the hip. A randomised, double-blind, multi-centre study. *Pain* 1990; 43:309–318.

Kobayashi M, Squires GR, Mousa A, et al. Role of interleukin-1 and tumor necrosis factor alpha in matrix degradation of human osteoarthritic cartilage. *Arthritis Rheum* 2005; 52:128–135.

Kosek E, Ordeberg G. Lack of pressure pain modulation by heterotopic noxious conditioning stimulation in patients with painful osteoarthritis before, but not following, surgical pain relief. *Pain* 2000a; 88:69–78.

Kosek E, Ordeberg G. Abnormalities of somatosensory perception in patients with painful osteoarthritis normalize following successful treatment. *Eur J Pain* 2000b; 4:229–238.

Kovelowski CJ, Ossipov MH, Sun H, et al. Supraspinal cholecystokinin may drive tonic descending facilitation mechanisms to maintain neuropathic pain in the rat. *Pain* 2000; 87:265–273.

Lai J, Ossipov MH, Vanderah TW, et al. Neuropathic pain: the paradox of dynorphin. *Mol Interv* 2001; 1:160–167.

Lawrence RC, Helmick CG, Arnett FC, et al. Estimates of the prevalence of arthritis and selected musculoskeletal disorders in the United States. *Arthritis Rheum* 1998; 41:778–799.

Likar R, Schafer M, Paulak F, et al. Intraarticular morphine analgesia in chronic pain patients with osteoarthritis. *Anesth Analg* 1997; 84:1313–1317.

Lu Y, Westlund KN. Gabapentin attenuates nociceptive behaviors in an acute arthritis model in rats. *J Pharmacol Exp Ther* 1999; 290:214–219.

Malfait AM, Gallily R, Sumariwalla PF, et al. The nonpsychoactive cannabis constituent cannabidiol is an oral anti-arthritic therapeutic in murine collagen-induced arthritis. *Proc Natl Acad Sci USA* 2000; 97:9561–9566.

Marcus DA. Current trends in fibromyalgia research. *Expert Opin Pharmacother* 2003; 4:1687–1695.

Mattia C, Paoletti F, Coluzzi F, Boanelli A. New antidepressants in the treatment of neuropathic pain. A review. *Minerva Anestesiol* 2002; 68:105–114.

McCrae F, Shouls J, Dieppe P, Watt I. Scintigraphic assessment of osteoarthritis of the knee joint. *Ann Rheum Dis* 1992; 51:938–942.

McQuay HJ, Moore RA, Eccleston C, et al. Systematic review of outpatient services for chronic pain control. *Health Technol Assess* 1997; 1:i–iv, 1–135.

Meier T, Wasner G, Faust M, et al. Efficacy of lidocaine patch 5% in the treatment of focal peripheral neuropathic pain syndromes: a randomized, double-blind, placebo-controlled study. *Pain* 2003; 106:151–158.

Melton L. Osteoarthritis pain goes central. *Lancet Neurol* 2003; 2:524.

Mili F, Helmick CG, Zack MM. Prevalence of arthritis: analysis of data from the US Behavioral Risk Factor Surveillance System 1996–99. *J Rheumatol* 2002; 29:1981–1988.

Milligan ED, Twining C, Chacur M, et al. Spinal glia and proinflammatory cytokines mediate mirror-image neuropathic pain in rats. *J Neurosci* 2003; 23:1026–1040.

Morris VH, Cruwys SC, Kidd BL. Characterisation of capsaicin-induced mechanical hyperalgesia as a marker for altered nociceptive processing in patients with rheumatoid arthritis. *Pain* 1997; 71:179–186.

Moulin DE, Iezzi A, Amireh R, et al. Randomised trial of oral morphine for chronic non-cancer pain. *Lancet* 1996; 347:143–147.

Naidu MU, Ramesh Kumar T, Anuradha RT, Rao UR. Evaluation of phenytoin in rheumatoid arthritis—an open study. *Drugs Exp Clin Res* 1991; 17:271–275.

Neugebauer V, Schaible HG, Schmidt RF. Sensitization of articular afferents to mechanical stimuli by bradykinin. *Pflugers Arch* 1989; 415:330–335.

Neugebauer V, Lucke T, Schaible HG. N-methyl-D-aspartate (NMDA) and non-NMDA receptor antagonists block the hyperexcitability of dorsal horn neurons during development of acute arthritis in rat's knee joint. *J Neurophysiol* 1993; 70:1365–1377.

Neugebauer V, Lucke T, Grubb B, Schaible HG. The involvement of N-methyl-D-aspartate (NMDA) and non-NMDA receptors in the responsiveness of rat spinal neurons with input from the chronically inflamed ankle. *Neurosci Lett* 1994; 170:237–240.

Nicholson B. Responsible prescribing of opioids for the management of chronic pain. *Drugs* 2003; 63:17–32.

Niissalo S, Hukkanen M, Imai S, et al. Neuropeptides in experimental and degenerative arthritis. *Ann N Y Acad Sci* 2002; 966:384–399

Ohtori S, Takahashi K, Moriya H, Myers RR. TNF-alpha and TNF-alpha receptor type 1 upregulation in glia and neurons after peripheral nerve injury: studies in murine DRG and spinal cord. *Spine* 2004; 29:1082–1088.

Ordeberg G. Characterization of joint pain in human OA. *Novartis Found Symp* 2004; 260:105–115.

Oshita K, Inoue A, Tang HB, et al. CB(1) cannabinoid receptor stimulation modulates transient receptor potential vanilloid receptor 1 activities in calcium influx and substance P release in cultured rat dorsal root ganglion cells. *J Pharmacol Sci* 2005; 97:377–385.

Ossipov MH, Lai J, King T, et al. Antinociceptive and nociceptive actions of opioids. *J Neurobiol* 2004; 61:126–148.

Peloso PM, Bellamy N, Bensen W, et al. Double blind randomized placebo control trial of controlled release codeine in the treatment of osteoarthritis of the hip or knee. *J Rheumatol* 2000; 27:764–771.

Pezet S, Malcangio M, McMahon SB. BDNF: a neuromodulator in nociceptive pathways? *Brain Res Brain Res Rev* 2002; 40:240–249.

Porreca F, Ossipov MH, Gebhart GF. Chronic pain and medullary descending facilitation. *Trends Neurosci* 2002; 25:319–325.

Puig S, Sorkin LS. Formalin-evoked activity in identified primary afferent fibers: systemic lidocaine suppresses phase-2 activity. *Pain* 1996; 64:345–355.

Rao UR, Naidu MU, Kumar TR, et al. Comparison of phenytoin with auranofin and chloroquine in rheumatoid arthritis—a double blind study. *J Rheumatol* 1995; 22:1235–1240.

Romanelli P, Esposito V. The functional anatomy of neuropathic pain. *Neurosurg Clin N Am* 2004; 15:257–268.

Rowbotham MC, Davies PS, Verkempinck C, Galer BS. Lidocaine patch: double-blind controlled study of a new treatment method for post-herpetic neuralgia. *Pain* 1996; 65:39–44.

Rowbotham M, Harden N, Stacey B, et al. Gabapentin for the treatment of postherpetic neuralgia: a randomized controlled trial. *JAMA* 1998; 280:1837–1842.

Rueff A, Dray A. Sensitization of peripheral afferent fibres in the in vitro neonatal rat spinal cord-tail by bradykinin and prostaglandins. *Neuroscience* 1993; 54:527–535.

Samad TA, Moore KA, Sapirstein A, et al. Interleukin-1-beta-mediated induction of Cox-2 in the CNS contributes to inflammatory pain hypersensitivity. *Nature* 2001; 410:471–475.

Saarto T, Wiffen P. Antidepressants for neuropathic pain. *Cochrane Database Syst Rev* 2005; 3: CD005454.

Schaible HG. Spinal mechanisms contributing to joint pain. *Novartis Found Symp* 2004; 260:4–22.

Schaible HG, Grubb BD. Afferent and spinal mechanisms of joint pain. *Pain* 1993; 55:5–54.

Schaible HG, Vanegas H. How do we manage chronic pain? *Baillieres Best Pract Res Clin Rheumatol* 2000; 14:797–811.

Schaible HG, Ebersberger A, Von Banchet GS. Mechanisms of pain in arthritis. *Ann N Y Acad Sci* 2002; 966:343–354.

Seybold VS, Jia YP, Abrahams LG. Cyclo-oxygenase-2 contributes to central sensitization in rats with peripheral inflammation. *Pain* 2003; 105:47–55.

Sharma PK, Hota D, Pandhi P. Biologics in rheumatoid arthritis. *J Assoc Physicians India* 2004; 52:231–236.

Shavit Y, Wolf G, Goshen I, Livshits D, Yirmiya R. Interleukin-1 antagonizes morphine analgesia and underlies morphine tolerance. *Pain* 2005; 115:50–59.

Silman AJ, Pearson JE. Epidemiology and genetics of rheumatoid arthritis. *Arthritis Res* 2002; 4(Suppl 3):S265–S272.

Sluka KA, Westlund KN. Spinal cord amino acid release and content in an arthritis model: the effects of pretreatment with non-NMDA, NMDA, and NK1 receptor antagonists. *Brain Res* 1993; 627:89–103.

Sommer C, Marziniak M, Myers RR. The effect of thalidomide treatment on vascular pathology and hyperalgesia caused by chronic constriction injury of rat nerve. *Pain* 1998; 74:83–91.

Sommer C, Kress M. Recent findings on how proinflammatory cytokines cause pain: peripheral mechanisms in inflammatory and neuropathic hyperalgesia. *Neurosci Lett* 2004; 361:184–187.

Spina E, Perugi G. Antiepileptic drugs: indications other than epilepsy. *Epileptic Disord* 2004; 6:57–75.

Staud R, Smitherman ML. Peripheral and central sensitization in fibromyalgia: pathogenetic role. *Curr Pain Headache Rep* 2002; 6:259–266.

Strangman NM, Walker JM. Cannabinoid WIN 55,212-2 inhibits the activity-dependent facilitation of spinal nociceptive responses. *J Neurophysiol* 1999; 82:472–477.

Stein A, Yassouridis A, Szopko C, et al. Intraarticular morphine versus dexamethasone in chronic arthritis. *Pain* 1999; 83:525–532.

Sumariwalla PF, Gallily R, Tchilibon S, et al. A novel synthetic, nonpsychoactive cannabinoid acid (HU-320) with antiinflammatory properties in murine collagen-induced arthritis. *Arthritis Rheum* 2004; 50:985–998.

Tal M. A role for inflammation in chronic pain. *Curr Rev Pain* 1999; 3:440–446.

Tao YX, Raja SN. Are synaptic MAGUK proteins involved in chronic pain? *Trends Pharmacol Sci* 2004; 25:397–400.

Tonussi CR, Ferreira SH. Tumour necrosis factor-alpha mediates carrageenin-induced knee-joint incapacitation and also triggers overt nociception in previously inflamed rat knee-joints. *Pain* 1999; 82:81–87.

Vanegas H, Schaible HG. Prostaglandins and cyclooxygenases in the spinal cord. *Prog Neurobiol* 2001; 64:327–363.

Veiga AP, Duarte IP, Avila MN, et al. Prevention by celecoxib of secondary hyperalgesia induced by formalin in rats. *Life Sci* 2004; 75:2807–2817.

Wagstaff S, Smith OV, Wood PH. Verbal pain descriptors used by patients with arthritis. *Ann Rheum Dis* 1985; 44:262–265.

Wang GK, Russell C, Wang SY. State-dependent block of voltage-gated Na+ channels by amitriptyline via the local anesthetic receptor and its implication for neuropathic pain. *Pain* 2004; 110:166–174.

Watkins LR, Milligan ED, Maier SF. Glial activation: a driving force for pathological pain. *Trends Neurosci* 2001; 24:450–455.

Waugh J, Perry CM. Anakinra: a review of its use in the management of rheumatoid arthritis. *BioDrugs* 2005; 19:189–202.

Wolfe F, Michaud K. Severe rheumatoid arthritis (RA), worse outcomes, comorbid illness, and sociodemographic disadvantage characterize RA patients with fibromyalgia. *J Rheumatol* 2004; 31:695–700.

Wood JN, Boorman JP, Okuse K, Baker MD. Voltage-gated sodium channels and pain pathways. *J Neurobiol* 2004; 61:55–71.

Woolf CJ. Evidence for a central component of post-injury pain hypersensitivity. *Nature* 1983; 306:686–688.

Wu J, Lin Q, McAdoo DJ, Willis WD. Nitric oxide contributes to central sensitization following intradermal injection of capsaicin. *Neuroreport* 1998; 9:589–592.

Wu J, Fang L, Lin Q, Willis WD. The role of nitric oxide in the phosphorylation of cyclic adenosine monophosphate-responsive element-binding protein in the spinal cord after intradermal injection of capsaicin. *J Pain* 2002; 3:190–198.

Yoshimura M, Yonehara N, Ito T, et al. Effects of topically applied capsaicin cream on neurogenic inflammation and thermal sensitivity in rats. *Jpn J Pharmacol* 2000; 82:116–121.

You HJ, Morch CD, Chen J, Arendt-Nielsen L. Differential antinociceptive effects induced by a selective cyclooxygenase-2 inhibitor (SC-236) on dorsal horn neurons and spinal withdrawal reflexes in anesthetized spinal rats. *Neuroscience* 2003; 121:459–472.

Correspondence to: Michael C. Rowbotham, MD, UCSF Pain Clinical Research Center, 1701 Divisadero Street, Suite 480, San Francisco, CA 94115, USA. Fax: 415-885-7855; email: michael.rowbotham@ucsf.edu.

Proceedings of the 11th World Congress on Pain,
edited by Herta Flor, Eija Kalso, and Jonathan O.
Dostrovsky, IASP Press, Seattle, © 2006.

23

Pain Memory and Central Sensitization in Humans

Rolf-Detlef Treede, Thomas Klein, and Walter Magerl

Institute of Physiology and Pathophysiology, Johannes Gutenberg University, Mainz, Germany

Central sensitization in nociceptive pathways may be defined as increased responsiveness of nociceptive neurons in the central nervous system (CNS) to their normal afferent input. It has been studied most extensively in the spinal cord, but may also occur in the thalamus, cortex, or other nociceptive regions in the CNS (Willis 2001; Ji et al. 2003). Its mechanisms may be pre- or post-synaptic and may include an enhancement of excitatory synaptic efficacy or a decrease of inhibitory controls. Central sensitization may or may not lead to increased pain sensitivity (hyperalgesia, including dynamic tactile allodynia), depending on whether it involves projection neurons of the spinothalamocortical pathways leading to pain perception, reflex interneurons, or even inhibitory interneurons (J. Sandkühler et al., unpublished manuscript).

The term "pain memory" may have several different connotations, depending on which subtype of learning and memory it is referring to. Memory processes can be divided into explicit and implicit types. Explicit memory is also called declarative memory, because its contents can be told verbally, and the learning process is usually conscious. Explicit memory consists of semantic memory about facts (e.g., we know that injury hurts) and episodic memory about events (e.g., we may or may not remember the pain of a past injury). This type of pain memory is tapped in the patient whenever a medical history is being taken (Erskine et al. 1990).

Implicit memory is also called non-declarative memory, because its contents consist of behavior and cannot be told verbally, and we are usually not consciously aware of the learning process. Contents of implicit memory range from simple reflexes to complex behaviors (Kandel et al. 2000). There are two types of implicit learning and memory, associative and non-associative, both of which are highly relevant in pain research and therapy. Associative implicit memory includes classical conditioning (as demonstrated by Pavlov using paired stimuli) and operant conditioning (as demonstrated by Skinner using stimulus-reward pairing). Associative implicit memory is thought to contribute to the development of chronic low back pain (Flor 2000). Its extinction by relearning is a core concept of behavioral therapy (Vlaeyen and Linton 2000). Non-associative implicit memory includes habituation and sensitization to repetitive stimulation (Prescott 1998). Thus, the word "sensitization" is used in both pain research and memory research to describe increases in neural or behavioral responses, which raises the question as to what extent this term has the same connotations in these two areas of the neurosciences.

In this chapter, we will compare neural mechanisms of non-associative implicit memory and central sensitization of nociceptive pathways. In order to provide a link from basic pain research at the cellular and molecular level to clinical pain research, we will show how evidence for central sensitization can be obtained in humans, both in experimental surrogate models and in clinical assessment of individual patients. Finally, we will review the clinical evidence for the potential roles of central sensitization in acute and chronic pain, including both nociceptive and neuropathic pain states.

SENSITIZATION AND HABITUATION: TWO ELEMENTARY MECHANISMS OF IMPLICIT MEMORY

Sensitization is listed in neuroscience textbooks as one of the elementary mechanisms of non-associative implicit memory, along with its counterpart, habituation (Kandel et al. 2000). The neurobiological mechanisms of habituation and sensitization have been elaborated in much detail in reduced animal models such as the gill withdrawal reflex in *Aplysia californica* (Prescott 1998). Whereas repetition of harmless stimuli such as touching the animal's syphon with a gentle water jet leads to progressively smaller motor responses (habituation; Pinsker et al. 1970), noxious stimuli such as pinching the tail increase the motor response (intrinsic sensitization; Illich and Walters 1997). As shown in Fig. 1, a single noxious stimulus can sensitize the system for several minutes even to the harmless tactile stimulus (extrinsic sensitization). Repeating the noxious stimulus or pairing both types of stimuli in a classical conditioning paradigm can consolidate intrinsic or extrinsic sensitization into a long-term form (Kandel 2001). Whereas short-term and long-term habituation are homosynaptic processes, short-term and long-term sensitization require the heterosynaptic interaction of two input pathways, wherein one pathway modulates the sensitivity of the other (Prescott 1998; Bailey et al. 2000).

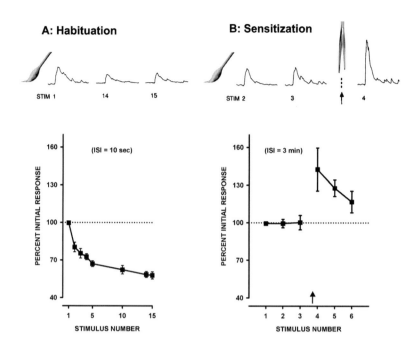

Fig. 1. Non-associative mechanisms of implicit memory in an invertebrate animal model (gill withdrawal reflex in *Aplysia californica*). (A) Habituation occurs when harmless stimuli (e.g., touching the syphon with a gentle water jet) are repeated at a relatively fast rate (every 10 seconds). Habituation is a homosynaptic process. (B) Sensitization occurs when a harmful stimulus (e.g., tail pinch) is applied. In this experiment, the harmless test stimuli were given at a low, non-habituating rate (once every 3 minutes). Sensitization is a heterosynaptic process involving two input pathways. (Data from Nolen and Carew 1988: excitatory postsynaptic potentials in motoneuron R2).

According to the dual process theory of plasticity, repeated stimulation simultaneously activates the mechanisms of habituation and sensitization in all sensory systems (Prescott 1998). However, in most sensory systems, habituation predominates to such an extent that the presence of sensitization can only be deduced indirectly from a reduction in habituation. In the nociceptive system, on the other hand, each injury as an adequate stimulus is regularly followed by pronounced increases in pain sensitivity above the pre-injury level (Raja et al. 1988; Treede et al. 1992b). Moreover, extrinsic sensitization as a learning process in non-nociceptive pathways is usually achieved by an intervening noxious stimulus. Thus, sensitization as a mechanism of implicit, non-associative memory is typical for noxious or other aversive stimuli.

As illustrated in Fig. 2, sensitization of the nociceptive system can occur at synapses within the CNS (central sensitization) and at the primary afferent nerve terminals (peripheral sensitization). While central sensitization bears a close resemblance to the mechanisms of synaptic plasticity that are relevant for

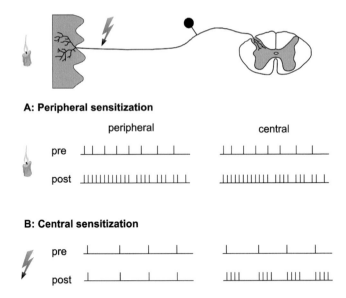

Fig. 2. Peripheral and central sensitization of the vertebrate nociceptive system. (A) Peripheral sensitization. Noxious heat stimuli activate free nerve endings of primary nociceptive afferents, and the resulting action potentials are transmitted to the spinal cord. Strong heat stimuli and other types of injury sensitize nociceptive nerve terminals to subsequent heat stimulation. Note that peripheral sensitization also increases the output of central neurons, since it enhances the afferent input to those neurons. (B) Central sensitization. Electrical stimuli circumvent the transduction process at peripheral nerve terminals and can ensure a reproducible input to central nociceptive neurons. Electrical stimuli can also mimic the injury discharge and induce central sensitization, i.e., an increased responsiveness of nociceptive neurons in the central nervous system to their normal afferent input. Each vertical dash represents one action potential, as would be recorded from the peripheral nerve (left) or spinal cord (right).

memory (Treede and Magerl 1995; Sandkühler 2000; Ji et al. 2003), peripheral sensitization evokes its own specific set of neural mechanisms (McCleskey and Gold 1999; Julius and Basbaum 2001). Injury leads to both peripheral sensitization (via release of inflammatory mediators by tissue damage) and central sensitization (via centripetally conducted action potentials and retrograde axonal transport). In the 1960s and 1970s, pain researchers were mainly focusing on peripheral sensitization and had little interaction with memory researchers. With the new focus on central sensitization (Woolf 1983), it became evident that pain research and memory research study closely related phenomena, sometimes even in the same experimental models, such as withdrawal reflexes (Woolf and Walters 1991).

USE-DEPENDENT SYNAPTIC PLASTICITY
IN THE NOCICEPTIVE SYSTEM

As a primitive mechanism of non-associative learning, sensitization is a form of use-dependent synaptic plasticity. From the perspective of memory research, sensitization means that the nervous system learns that a frequently activated synapse is important. From the perspective of pain research, central sensitization is induced by the high-frequency neural discharges of nociceptive afferents induced by an injury, i.e., the central nociceptive synapses increase their strength as a function of being activated frequently (LaMotte et al. 1991).

Use-dependent synaptic plasticity in the vertebrate nervous system has been studied most extensively in the hippocampus and neocortex (Kandel 2001). Reduced electrophysiological models consist of the electrical stimulation of defined synaptic input pathways and recordings from individual postsynaptic neurons or population signals from functionally homogenous groups of neurons. In both the hippocampus and neocortex, use-dependent synaptic plasticity depends on the frequency of the conditioning electrical pulse trains: whereas high-frequency stimulation (100 Hz) leads to long-term potentiation (LTP), low-frequency stimulation (1 Hz) induces long-term depression (LTD) of synaptic strength (Malenka and Bear 2004). Low-frequency stimulation can also reverse a previously established LTP. This process, known as depotentiation, may be considered as an active mechanism of forgetting. Long-term potentiation, long-term depression, and depotentiation can probably occur at all glutamatergic synapses throughout the CNS.

Studies in isolated spinal cord slices have shown that the conditioning high-frequency stimulus protocols that induce LTP in the hippocampus and neocortex also induce LTP at the first synapse of the nociceptive pathways (Randic et al. 1993; Liu and Sandkühler 1995). In turn, the conditioning low-frequency stimulus protocols that induce LTD in the hippocampus and neocortex also depress synaptic strength in spinal cord slices (Randic et al. 1993; Liu et al. 1998). Thus, the first synaptic relay of the nociceptive pathways in the superficial dorsal horn exhibits the same patterns of use-dependent plasticity known from other glutamatergic synapses (Fig. 3A). Some of these findings have been reproduced in intact animals and in the deep dorsal horn (Sandkühler and Liu 1998; Svendsen et al. 1999).

The behavioral consequences of nociceptive LTP and LTD have not yet been studied in animal models, but we have recently established corresponding experimental human surrogate models (Klein et al. 2004). Synaptic strength in the dorsal horn is not accessible in humans. Therefore, as indirect evidence we have obtained pain ratings to weak electrical test stimuli through a specially designed surface electrode that preferentially activates superficial nociceptive

A: Dorsal horn electrophysiology in rats

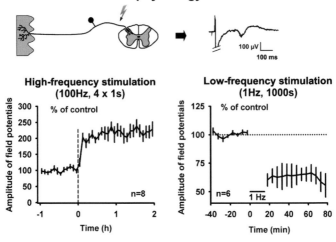

B: Pain perception in humans

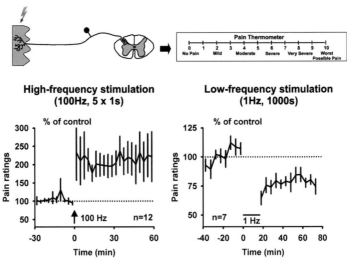

Fig. 3. Use-dependent synaptic plasticity in the nociceptive system. (A) Rat spinal cord slice preparation, showing C-fiber evoked field potentials in lamina I. High-frequency conditioning stimulation leads to long-term potentiation (LTP) of synaptic strength, whereas low-frequency conditioning stimulation leads to long-term depression (LTD) of synaptic strength in the spinal cord dorsal horn. (Data from Liu and Sandkühler 1997 and Liu et al. 1998). (B) Human psychophysics, showing pain ratings to single electrical test pulses. High-frequency conditioning stimulation leads to long-term enhancement (perceptual LTP), whereas low-frequency conditioning stimulation leads to long-term decrease (perceptual LTD) of pain elicited by electrical test stimuli. (Data from Lang et al. 2005 and Klein et al. 2004.)

nerve terminals. Conditioning electrical stimulus trains through the same electrode at high frequency (100 Hz) induced a long-term enhancement of pain
perception for several hours, whereas low-frequency stimulation (1 Hz) led to
a long-term decrease (Fig. 3B). Using a different low-frequency stimulation
protocol, we could also reverse a previously induced long-term potentiation of
human pain perception (Hansen et al. 2005). Thus, use-dependent plasticity of
human pain perception encompasses behavioral correlates of LTP, LTD, and
depotentiation.

CENTRAL SENSITIZATION AND LONG-TERM POTENTIATION OF THE NOCICEPTIVE SYSTEM

Animal studies on nociceptive LTP in the spinal cord have revealed the
following characteristics. Spinal LTP is dependent on the N-methyl-D-aspartate
(NMDA) receptor in both the superficial (Liu and Sandkühler 1995) and deep
dorsal horn (Svendsen et al. 1999). Spinal LTP is dependent on activation of
neurokinin-1 (NK1) receptors (Liu and Sandkühler 1997), and in particular on
activation of a NK1-receptor-expressing population of lamina I neurons that
project to the parabrachial nucleus (Mantyh et al. 1997; Ikeda et al. 2003).
Thus, the induction of nociceptive LTP requires activation of peptidergic C-fiber nociceptors. Spinal LTP is specific to the conditioned input (homosynaptic
LTP), because responses of wide dynamic range neurons in deep dorsal horn
to Aβ-fiber input are not facilitated (Svendsen et al. 1998).

Human studies on nociceptive LTP have shown that use-dependent
plasticity of pain perception is frequency dependent, related to activation of
peptidergic C fibers and to the activation of NMDA-type glutamate receptors
(Klein et al. 2000, 2003, 2004). However, its behavioral consequences are not
restricted to the conditioning input pathway; quantitative sensory testing with
a comprehensive battery covering all somatosensory submodalities (Rolke et
al. 2006) revealed that C-fiber-mediated percepts (innocuous warmth, noxious
heat, and noxious cold) were unchanged, whereas some A-fiber mediated percepts (pinprick-evoked pain) were significantly enhanced (Lang et al. 2005).
Moreover, high-frequency stimulation also induced static mechanical hyperalgesia to pinpricks and dynamic tactile allodynia to light touch surrounding
the conditioning electrode, i.e., in parts of the skin that had not received any
conditioning stimulation (Klein et al. 2004). This dual lack of input specificity (modality, spatial extent) sets perceptual LTP apart from the homosynaptic
phenomena observed in both the spinal cord and hippocampus. However, the
observed pattern of sensory changes is identical to that of secondary hyperalgesia surrounding a site of injury (Raja et al. 1984), which has previously been
attributed to central sensitization.

PERCEPTUAL CORRELATES OF PERIPHERAL
AND CENTRAL SENSITIZATION

Injury induces two types of hyperalgesia: primary hyperalgesia of the injured tissue itself and secondary hyperalgesia in surrounding uninjured tissue. Primary hyperalgesia is the perceptual correlate of peripheral sensitization. Peripheral sensitization is strictly localized to the injury site without any significant spread into uninjured tissue (Thalhammer and LaMotte 1982; Schmelz et al. 1996). It increases sensitivity to heat stimuli but not mechanical stimuli (Treede et al. 1992b) and probably reflects functional alterations of the heat-sensitive ion channel TRPV1 (Julius and Basbaum 2001).

Secondary hyperalgesia is the perceptual correlate of central sensitization, which is characterized by increased sensitivity to mechanical stimuli but not heat stimuli, both in skin surrounding a real injury (Raja et al. 1984) and in skin surrounding injury simulated by capsaicin injection, which induces strong nociceptor discharges but no tissue damage (Ali et al. 1996). Using the capsaicin injection model for induction of secondary hyperalgesia, the laboratories of Robert H. LaMotte and William D. Willis have shown that both wide-dynamic-range and high-threshold spinal neurons increase their responsiveness to punctate mechanical stimuli and to light touch (Simone et al. 1991), whereas responses of both A- and C-fiber peripheral nociceptors remain unchanged (Baumann et al. 1991).

The human surrogate model of spinal LTP also simulates nociceptor discharges associated with injury, but without any tissue damage. As in the capsaicin injection model, we observed static mechanical hyperalgesia and dynamic tactile allodynia without any heat hyperalgesia. The fact that the pattern of sensory changes at the conditioned site was the same as in the surrounding secondary zone suggests that mechanical hyperalgesia and allodynia may be due to central sensitization, even within the primary hyperalgesia zone. Given that primary afferents are not sensitized to mechanical stimuli even at the injury site itself, with the exception of pain to blunt pressure after freeze injury (Kilo et al. 1994), central sensitization may even be a necessary condition for punctate mechanical hyperalgesia and dynamic tactile allodynia in the zone of primary hyperalgesia.

IMPLICATIONS FOR THE MECHANISMS OF CENTRAL
SENSITIZATION FROM HUMAN SURROGATE MODELS

Since secondary hyperalgesia is due to central sensitization, it can be used as a surrogate model to reveal further details about mechanisms of central sensitization in humans. Studies on secondary hyperalgesia following real injury (burns) or simulated injury (capsaicin injection, high-frequency electrical stimulation) have shown that central sensitization is induced by the activation of a specific class of nociceptive afferents: these afferents are unmyelinated C fibers, are chemosensitive (e.g., to capsaicin), have relatively large receptive fields, and exhibit little mechanical sensitivity (Meyer et al. 1992; Schmidt et al. 2002). The resulting hypersensitivity, however, is mediated by a different class of afferents: these afferents are myelinated A fibers, are insensitive to the blocking action of capsaicin cream, and exhibit little if any heat sensitivity, but are sensitive to mechanical stimuli (Ziegler et al. 1999; Fuchs et al. 2000; Magerl et al. 2001).

According to these functional properties, the following histological markers are predicted to characterize the conditioning pathway: positive for the vanilloid receptor TRPV1 (because these afferents are capsaicin sensitive) and negative for the plant lectin IB4 (because these afferents express substance P and calcitonin gene-related peptide). These characteristics identify a well-known subclass of C-fiber nociceptors. In contrast, little is known about the facilitated pathway, except that these afferents should express myelin markers but no TRPV1. The neuropharmacological characterization of this class of A-fiber nociceptors is a challenging task for future basic research that may lead to new drug targets for treating mechanical hyperalgesia.

These findings suggest that secondary hyperalgesia requires heterosynaptic interactions, wherein one pathway sensitizes another (Fig. 4A). Although the induction of central sensitization depends on capsaicin-sensitive C fibers, the resulting hypersensitivity is mediated by two classes of capsaicin-insensitive A fibers, namely Aδ-fiber high-threshold mechanoreceptors for punctate hyperalgesia and Aβ-fiber low-threshold mechanoreceptors for dynamic tactile allodynia. In memory research, this type of mechanism is called extrinsic sensitization (Prescott 1998). It has been proposed that consolidation of LTP into behaviorally relevant phenomena requires heterosynaptic facilitation (Bailey et al. 2000). Mechanisms of secondary hyperalgesia may be more similar to heterosynaptic reflex sensitization in *Aplysia* than to homosynaptic hippocampal LTP in rats. Heterosynaptic interactions in secondary hyperalgesia may also involve descending facilitation, which appears to be specific for mechanosensitive inputs and is spatially more restricted than descending inhibition (Suzuki et al. 2004).

SIGNS OF CENTRAL SENSITIZATION IN PATIENTS: ASSESSMENT AND TAXONOMY

Synaptic strength in the dorsal horn is not accessible for testing in humans, so indirect evidence needs to be obtained. For this purpose, either electrical or mechanical test stimuli are used, because in contrast to heat, these test stimuli

A: Gain control model of central sensitization

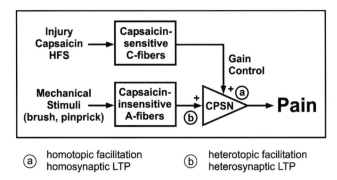

(a) homotopic facilitation
    homosynaptic LTP

(b) heterotopic facilitation
    heterosynaptic LTP

B: Clinical assessment of central sensitization

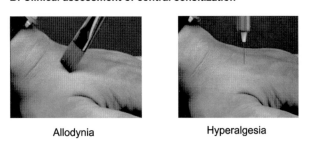

Allodynia   Hyperalgesia

Fig. 4. (A) Gain control model of central sensitization. Central sensitization involves heterosynaptic interaction of two nociceptive inputs. Conditioning stimulation of peptidergic, capsaicin-sensitive (TRPV1-positive) C fibers leads to enhanced pain mediated by the conditioned pathway (homotopic facilitation as a perceptual correlate of homosynaptic long-term potentiation [LTP]). The same conditioning stimulation also leads to enhanced pain mediated by another input pathway: capsaicin-insensitive (TRPV1-negative) A fibers (Aβ-fiber tactile receptors and Aδ-fiber nociceptors). The perceptual correlate of this heterosynaptic LTP is heterotopic facilitation of pain, i.e., secondary hyperalgesia to light touch (dynamic tactile allodynia) and to pinprick (static mechanical hyperalgesia). CPSN = central pain-signaling neuron. (Modified from Magerl et al. 2001). (B) Clinical assessment of central sensitization in humans. Left: Allodynia: pain due to a stimulus that does not normally provoke pain. Test: gentle stroking of the skin (dynamic tactile allodynia). Right: Hyperalgesia: an increased response to a stimulus which is normally painful. Test: pinprick stimuli (static mechanical hyperalgesia, characterized by both reduced thresholds and increased suprathreshold responses). Both phenomena are induced by central sensitization.

cause little or no peripheral sensitization. The sensory pattern of central sensitization comprises hyperalgesia to pinpricks and allodynia to moving tactile stimuli. Fig. 4B illustrates how these two positive sensory signs may be assessed in clinical practice using quantitative sensory testing (Koltzenburg et al. 1992; Baumgärtner et al. 2002; Treede et al. 2004; Rolke et al. 2006).

Dynamic tactile allodynia is assessed by gently stroking the skin with light tactile stimuli that do not activate nociceptive afferents. It is mediated by central sensitization to A-fiber tactile receptor input. This is the clinical phenomenon for which the taxonomy task force of IASP coined the term "allodynia" in 1979 at the request of one of its members, Noordenbos, who asked for a term to describe pain arising from non-noxious stimuli to otherwise normal tissue (Merskey 2005, p. 331). Dynamic tactile allodynia needs to be distinguished from static mechanical hyperalgesia (Koltzenburg et al. 1992; Ochoa and Yarnitsky 1993), which is assessed by applying pressure to the skin via small-diameter probes (LaMotte et al. 1991; Treede et al. 2002), preferably with a cylindrical tip or a blunt needle (Greenspan and McGillis 1991; Chan et al. 1992; Ziegler et al. 1999). Static mechanical hyperalgesia to pinprick is due to central sensitization to A-fiber nociceptor input. Either of these two positive sensory signs may occur alone, or they may occur in combination (Treede and Cole 1993; Baumgärtner et al. 2002), and either of them is sufficient to provide evidence for central sensitization in a given patient or healthy volunteer.

CLINICAL RELEVANCE OF CENTRAL SENSITIZATION

Evidence for central sensitization has been provided in a number of acute and chronic pain states. The vicinity of the surgical wound becomes hyperalgesic to punctate mechanical stimuli and electrical stimuli during acute postoperative pain (Richmond et al. 1993; Wilder-Smith et al. 1996). In delayed-onset muscle soreness following eccentric exercise, vibration increases pain instead of relieving it (Weerakkody et al. 2003), and muscle tenderness can be reduced by an A-fiber block (Barlas et al. 2000). These observations suggest that central sensitization to muscle spindle input ("proprioceptive allodynia") contributes to acute post-exercise muscle pain. Muscle spindle afferents exhibit a dynamic response to changes in muscle length and are large-diameter non-nociceptive A fibers, thus sharing several properties with the cutaneous afferents that mediate dynamic tactile allodynia.

Several acute and chronic visceral pain states are associated with tenderness to electrical stimulation, which also suggests a mechanism of central sensitization (Arendt-Nielsen et al. 2000; Giamberardino et al. 2005). Behavioral signs of central sensitization are a constant feature in recent animal models of cancer pain, but there is surprisingly little clinical information on the incidence and severity of hyperalgesia in cancer pain patients (Gottrup et al. 2000). A large body of literature has described signs of central sensitization in subgroups of patients suffering from chronic neuropathic pain conditions (Fields et al. 1998; Baumgärtner 2002). This list of examples illustrates that mechanical hyperalgesia and allodynia as signs of central sensitization do not indicate that pain has become chronic, as they can also occur with acute pain conditions. Even long-lasting hyperalgesia in chronic neuropathic pain may sometimes be relieved rapidly with appropriate nerve blocks (Gracely et al. 1992; Treede et al. 1992a), emphasizing that the nociceptive system is highly plastic and may change its sensitivity within minutes.

COMPARISON OF ACUTE AND CHRONIC PAIN WITH SHORT-TERM AND LONG-TERM MEMORY

Human memory processes may be divided into short-term and long-term storage systems consisting of four stages (Werner 1980). Short-term memory comprises sensory memory (lasting fractions of a second for all sensory inputs) and primary memory (lasting many seconds after verbal labels have been attached to some of the sensory inputs). Some of the contents of sensory or primary memory are transferred to long-term storage in secondary memory that lasts from minutes to years. Forgetting in secondary memory appears to require "unlearning" and interference with either previously (proactive inhibition) or subsequently (retroactive inhibition) learned material. Some memory contents such as one's own name are extremely durable and readily accessible; for this stage the term "tertiary memory" has been introduced.

Comparing the time scales of nociceptive processing with those of memory suggests that wind-up may be conceived as the equivalent of sensory memory, maintaining the neural representation of nociceptive stimulation within the first nociceptive relay nucleus for a few seconds at most (Fig. 5). This process of temporal summation of slow excitatory postsynaptic potentials is part of the normal transient activation of the nociceptive system by its adequate stimuli. When low-frequency stimulation is continued over minutes, wind-up turns into long-term depression, i.e., it is not maintained with prolonged stimulation (Klein et al. 2004). Hence, wind-up is involved in the processing of phasic painful stimuli, but its clinical relevance is questionable.

In nociceptive processing there is no obvious equivalent to what is called primary memory in the usual explicit memory processes. Nociceptive LTP in the spinal cord and its behavioral correlates in humans last for more than an hour (see Fig. 3A,B) and thus fall into the time window of secondary memory—the classical long-term memory. Secondary hyperalgesia and the underlying central sensitization are also measured in terms of hours up to one day (Simone et al. 1989; LaMotte et al. 1991). The underlying processes are part of the normal repertoire of the nociceptive system and its modulation; they cover the time range of acute pain (Fig. 5) and are usually reversible. Thus, mechanisms of

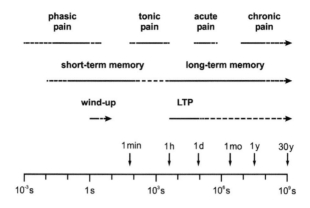

Fig. 5. Pain memory and central sensitization: comparison of time scales. Experimental pain models use phasic or tonic stimuli. Clinical pain may be acute or chronic. The duration of these four phenomena covers more than nine orders of magnitude. Short-term memory lasts from fractions of a second to a few minutes, approximately equivalent to the duration of phasic experimental pain models. Long-term memory processes cover the time from several minutes up to a lifetime, equivalent to the duration of tonic experimental pain models, as well as acute and chronic clinical pain. Of the mechanisms of enhanced synaptic efficacy in the spinal cord, wind-up is restricted to the same time range as short-term memory, whereas long-term potentiation extends into the duration of acute pain and may also be relevant for chronic pain. Note the logarithmic time scale, ranging from milliseconds to a lifetime. (Modified from Treede 1995.)

long-term memory are already relevant for acute pain; they do not necessarily imply chronic pain.

Long-term memory spans many orders of magnitude of different durations, eventually extending into the time range of chronic pain (Fig. 5). In discussing the relationship of LTP persistence and memory retention, several subtypes of LTP can be distinguished (for review see Abraham 2003): early LTP (LTP1) decays with time constants of 2–3 hours, whereas late LTP decays with time constants of 4 days (LTP2) or 3 weeks (LTP3). In that sense, nociceptive LTP as studied so far is equivalent to LTP1, and does not yet explain the transition of pain from acute to chronic. In the fear-conditioning model of associative implicit learning, persistence of memory over several weeks requires consolidation by repeated paired stimulation, and this process is paralleled by a transition from early to late LTP in the amygdala and hippocampus (Frey et al. 2001). Central sensitization in chronic pain may be retained by similar neural mechanisms, including altered gene transcription and de novo protein biosynthesis (Woolf and Salter 2000). Whereas altered gene transcription in chronic pain would suggest that central sensitization has become independent of the initiating event, there is some clinical evidence that it may still be dynamically maintained by peripheral nociceptive input. For peripheral neuropathic pain, several authors have shown examples of reversibility of hyperalgesia as a sign of central sensitization even after years of chronic pain (Gracely et al. 1992; Treede et al. 1992a). How often pain memory may be irreversibly fixed needs to be addressed by appropriate treatment trials.

SUMMARY AND CONCLUSIONS

Central sensitization plays a role in both acute and chronic pain. Evidence for central sensitization has been provided in postoperative pain, visceral pain, delayed-onset muscle soreness, cancer pain, and neuropathic pain. When comparing neural mechanisms of pain with those of memory, it is important to note that short-term memory lasts only for a few minutes. Thus, mechanisms of long-term memory such as LTP are already relevant for acute clinical pain and even in tonic experimental pain models; they do not apply to chronic pain exclusively. In the nociceptive system, as has been proposed for consolidation of other types of memory, consolidation of LTP into behaviorally relevant phenomena appears to require heterosynaptic facilitation. Two correlates of heterosynaptic facilitation can be assessed clinically: dynamic tactile allodynia to light touch and static mechanical hyperalgesia to pinpricks. Although it has not yet been fully tested, the pharmacology of homosynaptic and heterosynaptic facilitation appears to be different, suggesting the need to develop new treatment strategies including pharmacotherapy as well as neurostimulation.

ACKNOWLEDGMENTS

Supported by the Deutsche Forschungsgemeinschaft (DFG grant Tr 236/16-2) and by the Bundesministerium für Bildung und Forschung (BMBF grant 01EM0506).

REFERENCES

Abraham WC. How long will long-term potentiation last? *Philos Trans R Soc London Biol Sci* 2003; 358:735–744.

Ali Z, Meyer RA, Campbell JN. Secondary hyperalgesia to mechanical but not heat stimuli following a capsaicin injection in hairy skin. *Pain* 1996; 68:401–411.

Arendt-Nielsen L, Laursen RJ, Drewes AM. Referred pain as an indicator for neural plasticity. In: Sandkühler J, Bromm B, Gebhart GF (Eds). *Nervous System Plasticity and Chronic Pain, Progress in Brain Research*. Amsterdam: Elsevier, 2000, pp 343–356.

Bailey CH, Giustetto M, Huang Y-Y, Hawkins RD, Kandel ER. Is heterosynaptic modulation essential for stabilizing Hebbian plasticity and memory? *Nat Rev Neurosci* 2000; 1:11–20.

Barlas P, Walsh DM, Baxter GD, Allen JM. Delayed onset muscle soreness: effect of an ischaemic block upon mechanical allodynia in humans. *Pain* 2000; 87:221–225.

Baumann TK, Simone DA, Shain CN, LaMotte RH. Neurogenic hyperalgesia: the search for the primary cutaneous afferent fibers that contribute to capsaicin-induced pain and hyperalgesia. *J Neurophysiol* 1991; 66:212–227.

Baumgärtner U, Magerl W, Klein T, Hopf HC, Treede RD. Neurogenic hyperalgesia versus painful hypoalgesia: two distinct mechanisms of neuropathic pain. *Pain* 2002; 96:141–151.

Chan AW, MacFarlane IA, Bowsher D, Campbell JA. Weighted needle pinprick sensory thresholds: a simple test of sensory function in diabetic peripheral neuropathy. *J Neurol Neurosurg Psychiatry* 1992; 55:56–59.

Erskine A, Morley S, Pearce S. Memory for pain: a review. *Pain* 1990; 41:255–265.

Fields HL, Rowbotham M, Baron R. Postherpetic neuralgia: irritable nociceptors and deafferentation. *Neurobiol Dis* 1998; 5:209–227.

Flor H. The functional organization of the brain in chronic pain. In: Sandkühler J, Bromm B, Gebhart GF (Eds). *Nervous System Plasticity and Chronic Pain,* Progress in Brain Research. Amsterdam: Elsevier, 2000, pp 313–322.

Frey S, Bergado-Rosado J, Seidenbecher T, Pape HC, Frey JU. Reinforcement of early long-term potentiation (early-LTP) in dentate gyrus by stimulation of the basolateral amygdala: heterosynaptic induction mechanisms of late-LTP. *J Neurosci* 2001; 21:3697–3703.

Fuchs PN, Campbell JN, Meyer RA. Secondary hyperalgesia persists in capsaicin desensitized skin. *Pain* 2000; 84:141–149.

Giamberardino MA, Affaitati G, Lerza R, et al. Relationship between pain symptoms and referred sensory and trophic changes in patients with gallbladder pathology. *Pain* 2005; 114:239–249.

Gottrup H, Andersen J, Arendt-Nielsen L, Jensen TS. Psychophysical examination in patients with post- mastectomy pain. *Pain* 2000; 87:275–284.

Gracely RH, Lynch SA, Bennett GJ. Painful neuropathy: altered central processing, maintained dynamically by peripheral input. *Pain* 1992; 51:175–194.

Greenspan JD, McGillis SLB. Stimulus features relevant to the perception of sharpness and mechanically evoked cutaneous pain. *Somatosens Motor Res* 1991; 8:137–147.

Hansen N, Klein T, Magerl W, Treede RD. Metaplasticity and homeostatic plasticity of nociceptive long-term potentiation (LTP) in humans. *Abstracts: 11th World Congress on Pain,* Seattle: IASP Press, 2005, pp 445–446.

Ikeda H, Heinke B, Ruscheweyh R, Sandkühler J. Synaptic plasticity in spinal lamina I projection neurons that mediate hyperalgesia. *Science* 2003; 299:1237–1240.

Illich PA, Walters ET. Mechanosensory neurons innervating *Aplysia* siphon encode noxious stimuli and display nociceptive sensitization. *J Neurosci* 1997; 17:459–469.

Ji RR, Kohno T, Moore KA, Woolf CJ. Central sensitization and LTP: do pain and memory share similar mechanisms? *Trends Neurosci* 2003; 26:696–705.

Julius D, Basbaum AI. Molecular mechanisms of nociception. *Nature* 2001; 413:203–210.

Kandel ER. The molecular biology of memory storage: a dialogue between genes and synapses. *Science* 2001; 294:1030–1038.

Kandel ER, Schwartz JH, Jessell TM. *Principles of Neural Science,* 4th ed. New York: McGraw-Hill, 2000, pp 1227–1279.

Kilo S, Schmelz M, Koltzenburg M, Handwerker HO. Different patterns of hyperalgesia induced by experimental inflammation in human skin. *Brain* 1994; 117:385–396.

Klein T, Magerl W, Hopf HC, et al. Electrical stimulation of peptidergic afferents in human skin: Functional evidence from laser Doppler imaging. *Pflugers Arch Suppl* 2000; 439(6):R340.

Klein T, Magerl W, Mantzke U, et al. Perceptual correlates of long-term potentiation in the spinal cord. In: Dostrovsky J, Carr D, Koltzenburg M (Eds). *Proceedings of the 10th World Congress on Pain,* Progress in Pain Research and Management, Vol. 24. Seattle: IASP Press, 2003, pp 407–415.

Klein T, Magerl W, Hopf HC, Sandkühler J, Treede RD. Perceptual correlates of nociceptive long-term potentiation and long-term depression in humans. *J Neurosci* 2004; 24:964–971.

Koltzenburg M, Lundberg LER, Torebjörk HE. Dynamic and static components of mechanical hyperalgesia in human hairy skin. *Pain* 1992; 51:207–219.

LaMotte RH, Shain CN, Simone DA, Tsai E-FP. Neurogenic hyperalgesia: psychophysical studies of underlying mechanisms. *J Neurophysiol* 1991; 66:190–211.

Lang S, Klein T, Magerl W, Treede RD. Human nociceptive long-term potentiation (LTP) elicits modality-specific changes in somatosensory perception. *Abstracts: 11th World Congress on Pain*. Seattle: IASP Press, 2005, p 61.

Liu XG, Sandkühler J. Long-term potentiation of C-fiber-evoked potentials in the rat spinal dorsal horn is prevented by spinal N-methyl-D- aspartic acid receptor blockage. *Neurosci Lett* 1995; 191:43–46.

Liu XG, Sandkühler J. Characterization of long-term potentiation of C-fiber- evoked potentials in spinal dorsal horn of adult rat: essential role of NK1 and NK2 receptors. *J Neurophysiol* 1997; 78:1973–1982.

Liu XG, Morton CR, Azkue JJ, Zimmermann M, Sandkühler J. Long-term depression of C-fibre-evoked spinal field potentials by stimulation of primary afferent A delta-fibres in the adult rat. *Eur J Neurosci* 1998; 10:3069–3075.

Magerl W, Fuchs PN, Meyer RA, Treede RD. Roles of capsaicin-insensitive nociceptors in pain and secondary hyperalgesia. *Brain* 2001; 124:1754–1764.

Malenka RC, Bear MF. LTP and LTD: an embarrassment of riches. *Neuron* 2004; 44:5–21.

Mantyh PW, Rogers SD, Honore P, et al. Inhibition of hyperalgesia by ablation of lamina I spinal neurons expressing the substance P receptor. *Science* 1997; 278:275–279.

McCleskey EW, Gold MS. Ion channels of nociception. *Annu Rev Physiol* 1999; 61:835–856.

Merskey H. Terms and taxonomy: paper tools at the cutting edge of study. In: Merskey H, Loeser JD, Dubner R (Eds). *The Paths of Pain 1975–2005*. Seattle: IASP Press, 2005, pp 329–337.

Meyer RA, Treede RD, Raja SN, Campbell JN. Peripheral versus central mechanisms for secondary hyperalgesia. Is the controversy resolved? *Am Pain Soc J* 1992; 1:127–131.

Nolen TG, Carew TJ. The cellular analog of sensitization in *Aplysia* emerges at the same time in development as behavioral sensitization. *J Neurosci* 1988; 8:212–222.

Ochoa JL, Yarnitsky D. Mechanical hyperalgesias in neuropathic pain patients: dynamic and static subtypes. *Ann Neurol* 1993; 33:465–472.

Pinsker H, Kipfermann I, Castellucci V, Kandel E. Habituation and dishabituation of the gill-withdrawal reflex in *Aplysia*. *Science* 1970; 167:1740–1742.

Prescott SA. Interactions between depression and facilitation within neural networks: updating the dual-process theory of plasticity. *Learn Mem* 1998; 5:446–466.

Raja SN, Campbell JN, Meyer RA. Evidence for different mechanisms of primary and secondary hyperalgesia following heat injury to the glabrous skin. *Brain* 1984; 107:1179–1188.

Raja SN, Meyer RA, Campbell JN. Peripheral mechanisms of somatic pain. *Anesthesiology* 1988; 68:571–590.

Randic M, Jiang MC, Cerne R. Long-term potentiation and long-term depression of primary afferent neurotransmission in the rat spinal cord. *J Neurosci* 1993; 13:5228–5241.

Richmond CE, Bromley LM, Woolf CJ. Preoperative morphine pre-empts postoperative pain. *Lancet* 1993; 342:73–75.

Rolke R, Magerl W, Andrews-Campbell K, et al. Quantitative sensory testing: a comprehensive protocol for clinical trials. *Eur J Pain* 2006; 10:77–88.

Sandkühler J. Learning and memory in pain pathways. *Pain* 2000; 88:113–118.

Sandkühler J, Liu X. Induction of long-term potentiation at spinal synapses by noxious stimulation or nerve injury. *Eur J Neurosci* 1998; 10:2476–2480.

Schmelz M, Schmidt R, Ringkamp M, et al. Limitation of sensitization to injured parts of receptive fields in human skin C-nociceptors. *Exp Brain Res* 1996; 109:141–147.

Schmidt R, Schmelz M, Weidner C, Handwerker HO, Torebjörk HE. Innervation territories of mechano-insensitive C nociceptors in human skin. *J Neurophysiol* 2002; 88:1859–1866.

Simone DA, Baumann TK, LaMotte RH. Dose-dependent pain and mechanical hyperalgesia in humans after intradermal injection of capsaicin. *Pain* 1989; 38:99–107.

Simone DA, Sorkin LS, Oh U, et al. Neurogenic hyperalgesia: Central neural correlates in responses of spinothalamic tract neurons. *J Neurophysiol* 1991; 66:228–246.

Suzuki R, Rahman W, Hunt SP, Dickenson AH. Descending facilitatory control of mechanically evoked responses is enhanced in deep dorsal horn neurones following peripheral nerve injury. *Brain Res* 2004; 1019:68–76.

Svendsen F, Tjolsen A, Hole K. AMPA and NMDA receptor-dependent spinal LTP after nociceptive tetanic stimulation. *Neuroreport* 1998; 9:1185–1190.

Svendsen F, Tjolsen A, Rygh LJ, Hole K. Expression of long-term potentiation in single wide dynamic range neurons in the rat is sensitive to blockade of glutamate receptors. *Neurosci Lett* 1999; 259:25–28.

Thalhammer JG, LaMotte RH. Spatial properties of nociceptor sensitization following heat injury of the skin. *Brain Res* 1982; 231:257–265.

Treede RD. Peripheral acute pain mechanisms. *Ann Med* 1995; 27:213–216.

Treede RD, Cole JD. Dissociated secondary hyperalgesia in a subject with a large-fibre sensory neuropathy. *Pain* 1993; 53:169–174.

Treede RD, Magerl W. Modern concepts of pain and hyperalgesia: beyond the polymodal C-nociceptor. *News Physiol Sci* 1995; 10:216–228.

Treede RD, Davis KD, Campbell JN, Raja SN. The plasticity of cutaneous hyperalgesia during sympathetic ganglion blockade in patients with neuropathic pain. *Brain* 1992a; 115:607–621.

Treede RD, Meyer RA, Raja SN, Campbell JN. Peripheral and central mechanisms of cutaneous hyperalgesia. *Prog Neurobiol* 1992b; 38:397–421.

Treede RD, Rolke R, Andrews K, Magerl W. Pain elicited by blunt pressure: neurobiological basis and clinical relevance. *Pain* 2002; 98:235–240.

Treede RD, Handwerker HO, Baumgärtner U, Meyer RA, Magerl W. Hyperalgesia and allodynia: taxonomy, assessment, and mechanisms. In: Brune K, Handwerker HO (Eds). *Hyperalgesia: Molecular Mechanisms and Clinical Implications*, Progress in Pain Research and Management, Vol. 30. Seattle: IASP Press, 2004, pp 1–15.

Vlaeyen JWS, Linton SJ. Fear-avoidance and its consequences in chronic musculoskeletal pain: a state of the art. *Pain* 2000; 85:317–332.

Weerakkody NS, Percival P, Hickey MW, et al. Effects of local pressure and vibration on muscle pain from eccentric exercise and hypertonic saline. *Pain* 2003; 105:425–435.

Werner G. Higher functions of the nervous system. In: Mountcastle VB (Ed). *Medical Physiology,* 14th ed. St. Louis: C.V. Mosby, 1980, pp 629–646.

Wilder-Smith OHG, Tassonyi E, Senly C, Otten P, Arendt-Nielsen L. Surgical pain is followed not only by spinal sensitization but also by supraspinal antinociception. *Br J Anaesth* 1996; 76:816–821.

Willis WD. Role of neurotransmitters in sensitization of pain responses. *Ann NY Acad Sci* 2001; 933:142–156.

Woolf CJ. Evidence for a central component of post-injury pain hypersensitivity. *Nature* 1983; 306:686–688.

Woolf CJ, Salter MW. Neuronal plasticity: increasing the gain in pain. *Science* 2000; 288:1765–1769.

Woolf CJ, Walters ET. Common patterns of plasticity contributing to nociceptive sensitization in mammals and *Aplysia*. *Trends Neurosci* 1991; 14:74–78.

Ziegler EA, Magerl W, Meyer RA, Treede RD. Secondary hyperalgesia to punctate mechanical stimuli: central sensitization to A-fibre nociceptor input. *Brain* 1999; 122:2245–2257.

Correspondence to: Prof. Dr. Rolf-Detlef Treede, Institute of Physiology and Pathophysiology, Johannes Gutenberg University, Saarstr. 21, D-55099 Mainz, Germany. Fax: 49-6131-392 5902; email: treede@uni-mainz.de.

Proceedings of the 11th World Congress on Pain,
edited by Herta Flor, Eija Kalso, and Jonathan O.
Dostrovsky, IASP Press, Seattle, © 2006.

24

Spinal Cord Nociceptive Pathways

William D. Willis

*Department of Neuroscience and Cell Biology, University of Texas
Medical Branch, Galveston, Texas, USA*

SPINAL CORD ASCENDING NOCICEPTIVE PATHWAYS

Several pathways that originate from neurons in the spinal cord and project to the brain have nociceptive components. These pathways include the spinothalamic tract (STT), which has traditionally been regarded as the most important pathway for sensory discrimination of painful and thermal stimuli (Gybels and Sweet 1989; Willis and Coggeshall 2004). The STT is also thought to contribute to the motivational-affective aspects of pain. However, nociceptive signals are also transmitted by at least some neurons belonging to the postsynaptic dorsal column, spinocervical, spinoreticular, spinomesencephalic, spinohypothalamic, spinoparabrachial, and spinolimbic pathways (Willis and Coggeshall 2004; Willis and Westlund 2004).

Many nociceptive projection neurons respond to both somatic and visceral stimuli. This characteristic is often suggested to help account for the clinical observation that pain that originates in visceral structures is often referred to the body wall (e.g., Cervero 1995). Ways to distinguish which pathways are more important for visceral or somatic pain include behavioral or electrophysiological experiments in animals before and after transecting a candidate pathway. Even more convincing are demonstrations of changes in pain perception in human patients as the result of lesions of ascending spinal cord pathways.

THE SPINOTHALAMIC TRACT AND THE POSTSYNAPTIC
DORSAL COLUMN PATHWAY SIGNAL PAIN IN HUMANS

Evidence for a role of the STT in somatic and visceral pain and the postsynaptic dorsal column (PSDC) pathway in visceral pain comes from both clinical observations and animal experiments.

Anterolateral cordotomy.   It has been known for many years that an anterolateral cordotomy can reduce both somatic and visceral pain in patients (see
review by Gybels and Sweet 1989). The somatic analgesia is contralateral to
and below the level of the lesion and is generally attributed to the interruption
of the STT and associated pathways that ascend in the anterolateral white matter
of the spinal cord. There is also a loss of thermal sense that overlaps the analgesic region on the side opposite the lesion. The optimum lesion for pain relief
interrupts much of the anterolateral white matter and extends to just dorsal to
the denticulate ligament (Fig. 1A; Nathan et al. 2001). Anterolateral cordotomy
can also relieve visceral pain (Gybels and Sweet 1989), especially if the cordotomy is made bilaterally (since many visceral organs are innervated bilaterally). Unfortunately, a bilateral cordotomy can result in a number of unwanted
side effects, such as respiratory failure in the case of high cervical cordotomies
and urinary bladder and bowel incontinence. Rather than performing bilateral
cordotomies, the neurosurgeon can interrupt the axons of STT cells located on
both sides of the spinal cord as they cross the midline by a procedure known as
a commissural myelotomy (Gybels and Sweet 1989). However, this procedure
generally must be carried out over several segments. When Dargent et al. (1963)
reviewed the cases reported by Wertheimer and Lecuire (1953), they concluded
that commissural myelotomy was effective in relieving only vaginal and visceral
pain. This result can be explained if the effect of commissural myelotomy is

A

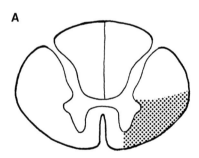

B

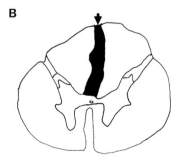

Fig. 1. (A) Area occupied by the spinothalamic tract and associated ascending nociceptive pathways at a thoracic level of the
human spinal cord, as shown by the results
of anterolateral cordotomies for pain relief.
Complete analgesia and thermoanesthesia
requires interruption of the entire dotted
area. (From Nathan et al. 2001.) (B) Drawing
showing the distribution of a limited midline
myelotomy in the posterior columns at T10
in a patient whose colon cancer pain was
completely alleviated by the lesion. (From
Hirshberg et al. 1996.)

the result of the interruption of the pelvic visceral pain pathway that is found near the midline of the posterior columns, rather than from cutting the crossing axons of STT cells (Nauta et al. 1997).

Midline myelotomy. Neurosurgical lesions have been made in the posterior midline of the spinal cord at a midthoracic level to relieve pelvic cancer pain (Gildenberg and Hirshberg 1984; Hirshberg et al. 1996). Examination of a postmortem specimen from a patient whose colon cancer pain was completely relieved by such a limited midline myelotomy at T10 revealed that the lesion was restricted to the gracile fasciculi (Fig. 1B; Hirshberg et al. 1996). This operation is a modification of the "stereotactic C1 central myelotomy" reported earlier (Hitchcock 1970, 1974, 1977; Schvarcz 1984; see Gybels and Sweet 1989). The beneficial effects of limited midline myelotomy have been confirmed by several groups (Nauta et al. 1997, 2000; Becker et al. 1999; Kim and Kwon 2000).

EFFECTS OF SPINAL CORD LESIONS ON CHANGES IN EXPLORATORY ACTIVITY INDUCED BY NOXIOUS SOMATIC OR VISCERAL STIMULI

One type of behavioral analysis of nociceptive responses in animals depends on an evaluation of exploratory activity. To measure exploratory activity, a rat is placed in a plastic box through which several infrared light beams are passed to test for movements of the rat from one place to another within the box. Interruptions of the beams are recorded automatically by a computer. Typically, a normal animal explores the box actively when it is first placed in it. As the rat becomes familiar with its new environment, the exploratory activity declines, and by 45 minutes the activity reaches a low level (Fig. 2A, open symbols). However, if the animal's movements result in pain, the rat will avoid exploratory activity. Consequently, the number of entries of the animal into a different area of the box will be reduced, and the time that the rat spends quietly "resting" will increase.

For instance, assuming that animals respond like humans to an intradermal injection of capsaicin, mechanical allodynia and hyperalgesia will develop in the area surrounding the injection site (Simone et al. 1989; LaMotte et al. 1991). Hence, movements are likely to be painful. During a period of 45 minutes after an intradermal injection of capsaicin, the exploratory activity of rats is much less than normal (Fig. 2A, filled circles; Palecek et al. 2002). A capsaicin injection has no effect on exploratory activity if made on the side of dorsal rhizotomies that denervate the skin in the area to be injected (Fig. 2B, RHIZ-I) or if a lesion of the lateral funiculus is made that interrupts the STT and accompanying

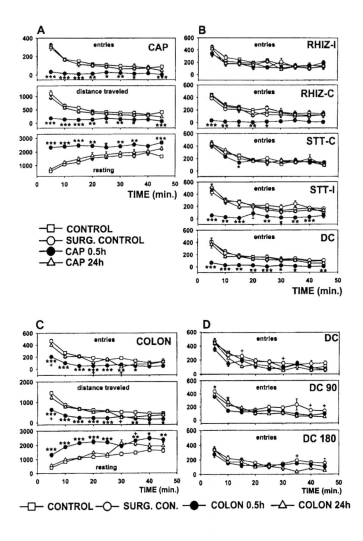

Fig. 2. The effect of pain on exploratory activity. (A) Under control conditions (open squares and open circles), rats showed a gradually declining level of activity, measured in terms of entries, distance traveled, and resting time. Half an hour after injection of capsaicin (filled circles) into one foot, the exploratory activity was greatly reduced. Twenty-four hours later, the activity had returned to the control level (open triangles). (B) The effect of a capsaicin injection in reducing exploratory activity was prevented by rhizotomy (RHIZ-I) of the lumbosacral dorsal roots ipsilateral to the injection or by interruption of the spinothalamic tract contralateral to the injection (STT-C), However, contralateral dorsal rhizotomies (RHIZ-C), ipsilateral interruption of the STT (STT-I), or bilateral interruption of the dorsal columns (DC) had no effect. (C) The effect of colon inflammation with mustard oil, plus mild distension of the colon, significantly reduced exploratory activity (filled circles). (D) Bilateral interruption of the dorsal columns at an upper cervical level nearly eliminated the effect of colon inflammation and distension (DC). This action was still apparent at 90 days (DC 90) and at 180 days (DC 180) after the DC lesion. (From Palecek et al. 2002.)

tracts on the side contralateral to the injection (Fig. 2B, STT-C). By contrast, a lesion of the ipsilateral STT (Fig. 2B, STT-I) or a bilateral lesion of the dorsal columns (Fig. 2B, DC) does not prevent the capsaicin injection from reducing the exploratory activity. The implication is that the nociceptive input to the brain that follows a capsaicin injection reduces exploratory activity and this input requires intact dorsal roots on the side ipsilateral to the injection and an intact STT on the side contralateral to the injection. The ineffectiveness of bilateral interruption of the dorsal column indicates that the dorsal column has little or no role in the response to injection of capsaicin into the skin.

Exploratory activity was also reduced during slight colorectal distension following inflammation of the colon (Fig. 2C, COLON). A bilateral lesion of the dorsal columns prevented this effect of colon inflammation and distension, and the lesion remained effective for at least 180 days (Fig. 2D, DC, DC 90, and DC 180; Palecek et al. 2002). This finding suggests that intact dorsal columns are required for this behavioral response to colon inflammation and distension. Similarly, a dorsal column lesion in rats with pancreatitis reversed the reduction in exploratory activity observed in this condition (Houghton et al. 1997).

ORGANIZATION OF THE PRIMATE SPINOTHALAMIC TRACT

Locations and response properties of STT cells. The locations of the cells of origin of the primate STT have been mapped following retrograde labeling (Willis et al. 1979; Apkarian and Hodge 1989a) and also by antidromic microstimulation in the thalamus (Applebaum et al. 1979; Zhang et al. 2000a,b). Primate STT cells are distributed in three major regions of the spinal cord gray matter: laminae I, IV–V, and VI–VIII. These three populations of STT cells have distinctive response properties and projection targets.

The receptive fields of lamina I STT cells tend to be smaller than those of STT cells in deeper layers (Fig. 3C, D; Willis 1989). This finding suggests that lamina I STT cells would be more suited for localizing painful stimuli than are STT cells in deeper laminae. Furthermore, the receptive fields of lamina I STT cells are clearly somatotopically organized in a fashion similar to other dorsal horn neurons with cutaneous input, whereas deeper STT cells are not (Willis et al. 1974; Brown and Fuchs 1975). This finding suggests that the receptive fields of lamina I STT cells are organized in a fashion that would contribute to spatial discrimination of painful stimuli. By contrast, STT cells in the intermediate region and ventral horn typically have very large receptive fields that often extend over the entire body and face (Giesler et al. 1981). These STT cells are unlikely to provide information about stimulus localization but instead would be suited to evoke arousal, activate attentional mechanisms, or provoke motivational-affective responses.

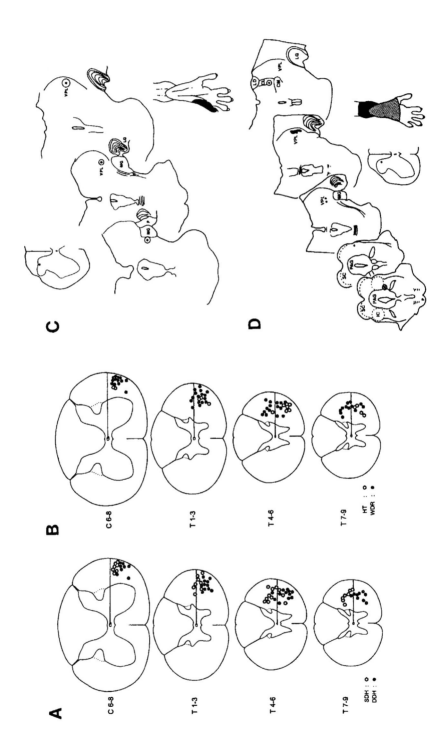

STT cells generally respond to mechanical, thermal, and chemical stimuli applied to restricted receptive fields in the skin. However, responses to innocuous thermal stimuli appear to be confined to STT cells located in lamina I (Christensen and Perl 1970; Ferrington et al. 1987; Dostrovsky and Craig 1996; Craig and Andrew 2002). In primates, most STT cells in lamina I, as in the deep layers of the dorsal horn, respond to both innocuous and noxious mechanical stimuli, although their best responses are to noxious intensities (see Fig. 5B, right panel; Owens et al. 1992). These are often called "wide-dynamic-range" responses (Mendell 1966). Very few STT cells respond primarily to tactile stimuli. Some "high-threshold" STT cells in the superficial and deep layers of the dorsal horn and in lamina VII are activated chiefly by noxious intensities of mechanical stimuli (Giesler et al. 1981; Owens et al. 1992; see Fig. 5B). Besides the STT cells in the superficial dorsal horn that can be activated by innocuous warm and cool thermal stimuli, many STT cells in both the superficial and deep dorsal horn discharge in response to noxious heat or cold (Kenshalo et al. 1979; Surmeier et al. 1986a,b; Ferrington et al. 1987). Many STT cells can be excited by intradermal injection of capsaicin (Simone et al. 1991; Dougherty and Willis 1992) or by injection of kaolin and carrageenan into the knee joint (Dougherty et al. 1992). STT cells in the deep dorsal horn of the lumbar enlargement have been shown to respond to mechanical and chemical stimulation of muscle nociceptors (Foreman et al. 1979).

STT cells often respond to visceral as well as to somatic stimuli. STT cells in the upper thoracic spinal cord can be activated by injection of bradykinin into a coronary artery (Foreman 1999). Recordings have been made from STT cells that are activated by both electrical and chemical stimulation of cardiopulmonary afferents (see Foreman 1989, 1999); by mechanical stimulation of the urinary bladder and testicle (Milne et al. 1981); by colorectal distension (Al-Chaer et al. 1999); and by stimulation of renal (Ammons 1987), ureteral (Ammons 1989), and gallbladder afferents (Ammons et al. 1984).

←— **Fig. 3.** Identification of primate STT cells or their axons by microstimulation. (A) Locations of the axons of primate STT cells ascending through thoracic and cervical segments of the spinal cord. Axons originating from lamina I STT cells of the superficial dorsal horn (SDH) are shown by open circles and those from STT cells of the deep dorsal horn (DDH) by filled circles. (B) The same axons are classified as belonging to wide-dynamic-range (WDR) or high-threshold (HT) STT cells. (From Zhang et al. 2000b.) (C) Low-threshold points found very close to the terminations of the axon of a primate lamina I STT cell. The location of the recording site near the neuron, low-threshold points in the posterior complex and ventral posterior lateral (VPL) nucleus, and the receptive field of the neuron are shown. (D) Sites for antidromic activation of a primate STT cell located in lamina IV of the deep dorsal horn. Low-threshold points are shown in the midbrain, the VPL nucleus, and the central lateral (CL) nucleus. The neuron was therefore an STT cell that projected to both the lateral and medial thalamus. The location of the recording site in lamina IV and the receptive field are also shown. (From Applebaum et al. 1979.)

Projections to the thalamus. The axons of STT cells in lamina I project to the brain by way of the contralateral lateral funiculus (Fig. 3A; Craig 2000; Zhang et al. 2000a,b). These axons tend to be concentrated in the middle of the lateral funiculus in an area occupied by the pathway for thermal sensation (Fig. 3A; Norrsell 1989a,b). The axons of STT cells in the deep dorsal horn also cross and ascend in the lateral funiculus. However, they tend to be located more ventrally than are the axons of lamina I STT cells (Fig. 3A; Zhang et al. 2000a,b).

Target nuclei in the thalamus. The spinothalamic tract of primates, including humans, terminates in a number of thalamic nuclei, including the ventral posterior lateral (VPL) nucleus, the ventral posterior inferior (VPI) nucleus, the posterior complex in the lateral thalamus, and the central lateral nucleus in the medial thalamus (Mehler et al. 1960; Applebaum et al. 1979; Boivie 1979; Kenshalo et al. 1980; Giesler et al. 1981; Apkarian and Hodge 1989b; Apkarian and Shi 1994; Zhang et al. 2000a,b). Apparently, some lamina I STT cells also project to the posterior ventromedial nucleus in the lateral thalamus (Craig et al. 1994; Craig 2004; see Graziano and Jones 2004). However, many other lamina I STT cells project to the VPL and adjacent nuclei, such as the VPI and the posterior complex (Fig. 3C; Graziano and Jones 2004). STT cells in the deep layers of the dorsal horn project chiefly to the lateral thalamus, including the VPL nucleus, or to both the lateral and medial thalamus (the VPL and the central lateral nucleus; Fig. 3D; Applebaum et al. 1979; Giesler et al. 1981; Zhang et al. 2000a,b). STT cells in laminae VI–VIII project to the central lateral nucleus (Giesler et al. 1981).

The diverse spinothalamic inputs to the VPL nucleus account for the recordings of neurons in this thalamic nucleus that respond chiefly to strong noxious stimuli, as well as neurons that respond to both innocuous and noxious stimuli (Kenshalo et al. 1980). Presumably, such inputs also account for recordings from both of these types of neurons in the somatosensory cortex of monkeys (Kenshalo and Isensee 1983; Kenshalo et al. 1988). Similar recordings have been made in the trigeminal system from the magnocellular part of the ventral posterior medial (VPM) nucleus from neurons that respond either to noxious stimulation or to both innocuous and noxious stimulation applied sequentially to the face (Bushnell et al. 1993; Duncan et al. 1993).

ORGANIZATION OF THE POSTSYNAPTIC
DORSAL COLUMN PATHWAY

Locations and response properties of postsynaptic dorsal column neurons. Most PSDC neurons are concentrated in laminae III and IV of the spinal cord dorsal horn (see review by Willis and Coggeshall 2004). There are also PSDC cells in the central part of the spinal gray matter, including lamina X. Although the initial recordings from visceral nociceptive PSDC neurons suggested that these neurons were concentrated in lamina X and adjacent laminae in the central region of the spinal cord (Al-Chaer et al. 1996b), a later study demonstrated Fos expression following distension of the ureter in a substantial fraction of PSDC neurons in the dorsal horn, as well as in those in the central part of the cord (Palecek et al. 2003a). Many STT cells in the same animals also expressed Fos.

Recordings from PSDC neurons identified by antidromic activation from the dorsal column nuclei or from the dorsal column near the dorsal column nuclei (Fig. 4A,B) have also demonstrated responses to several types of visceral stimuli, including colorectal distension (Fig. 4D) and colon inflammation with mustard oil (Fig. 4F; Al-Chaer et al. 1996b, 1999). The same neurons also respond to innocuous and noxious stimulation of somatic receptive fields (Fig. 4C,E).

Interruption of the dorsal columns prevents responses of VPL neurons to innocuous mechanical stimulation of the skin, but not those to noxious mechanical stimulation of the skin. The latter responses are blocked by interruption of the STT. In one study, about 10% of the neurons in the dorsal column nuclei from which recordings were made could be excited following noxious chemical stimulation of the pancreas with bradykinin (Wang and Westlund 2001).

Projection. The axons of PSDC neurons in the sacral spinal cord that respond to visceral stimuli can be activated by antidromic stimulation of the dorsal columns near the level of the dorsal column nuclei (Hirshberg et al. 1996). Injection of the anterograde tracer, *Phaseolus* leukoagglutinin (PHA-L), into the central gray region of the sacral spinal cord labels axons that ascend in the midline of the spinal cord and terminate in the medial part of the gracile nuclei (Wang et al. 1999). This finding offers an explanation of why midline myelotomy can block pelvic visceral pain, assuming that a comparable pathway exists in humans. On the other hand, injection of PHA-L into the central gray matter of the spinal cord at a mid-thoracic level labels axons that ascend in the dorsal column lateral to the midline near the dorsal intermediate septum (Wang et al. 1999). Experiments show that nociceptive responses to distension of the duodenum in rats are not blocked by midline lesions but are blocked by bilateral lesions of the dorsal columns in the area of the dorsal intermediate septa (Feng et al. 1998).

Projection targets. The visceral nociceptive pathway that ascends in the dorsal columns originates from PSDC neurons (Al Chaer et al. 1996b) and forms synapses on neurons of the dorsal column nuclei (Wang et al. 1999). Neurons of the dorsal column nuclei in turn project to the contralateral ventrobasal thalamus, as well as to sites in the brainstem (Al-Chaer et al. 1996b; see review by Willis et al. 1999; Willis and Coggeshall 2004).

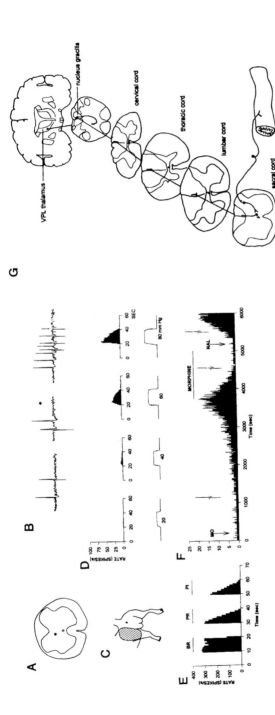

Fig. 4. (A–F) Responses of a rat postsynaptic dorsal column (PSDC) neuron to visceral and somatic stimulation. (A) Site of recording from a PSDC neuron. (B) Antidromic activation of the PSDC cell from stimulation of the dorsal column at an upper cervical level. Collision of the antidromic action potential with orthodromic activity and high frequency following are demonstrated. (C) The somatic receptive field is shown. (D) Graded responses to colorectal distension of 20, 40, 60, and 80 mm Hg. (E) Responses to brush (BR), pressure (PR), and pinch (PI) stimuli applied to the receptive field. (F) Response to inflammation of the colon with mustard oil (MO) applied at the time indicated by the first arrow. The enhanced spontaneous activity was greatly diminished by microdialysis administration of morphine into the sacral spinal cord. The morphine action was reversed by an intravenous injection of naloxone. (From Al-Chaer et al. 1996b.) (G) The course of the dorsal column visceral pain pathway from pelvic viscera, such as the lower colon. Visceral afferents synapse in the dorsal horn on interneurons that activate PSDC neurons. The PSDC neurons at a sacral level project their axons near the midline to the nucleus gracilis. The nucleus gracilis then relays nociceptive information to the contralateral ventral posterior lateral (VPL) nucleus. (From Willis and Westlund 1997.)

PLASTIC CHANGES IN SPINOTHALAMIC TRACT CELLS IN RESPONSE TO SEVERE NOXIOUS STIMULATION

As mentioned, the majority of the STT cells from which my colleagues and I have recorded are activated to some extent by innocuous mechanical stimuli applied to the skin, although they respond best to noxious stimuli (Owens et al. 1992). My colleagues and I speculate that the sensory role of these wide-dynamic-range neurons (Mendell 1966) is to signal pain. It is our view that the minor responses to tactile stimuli seen under ordinary experimental conditions are disregarded by higher centers in the pain system. Conditions that would produce severe pain in humans, such as intradermal injection of capsaicin, repeated damage to the skin, or peripheral nerve lesions that produce neuropathic pain result in greatly enhanced responses of primate STT cells to tactile stimuli (e.g., see Simone et al. 1991; Dougherty and Willis 1992; Owens et al. 1992; Palecek et al. 1992). We propose that such responses would result in mechanical allodynia, since the responses are often as large as or larger than the responses of the same STT cells to noxious stimuli under normal conditions (Fig. 5A,B, right panels). A similar enhancement of the responses of STT cells to innocuous thermal stimuli can be observed in monkeys with peripheral neuropathy. Following the same reasoning, increased response to innocuous thermal stimuli would result in thermal allodynia.

The plastic changes in the responses of STT cells following intradermal capsaicin injection or peripheral neuropathy have been investigated extensively and are termed "central sensitization." Similarities of central sensitization to long-term potentiation (LTP) in such brain structures as the hippocampus have been noted, and my colleagues and I have proposed that central sensitization is a spinal cord form of LTP (see Willis 2002; Willis and Coggeshall 2004).

NEUROTRANSMITTERS AND PROJECTION NEURONS

Immunostaining of synaptic contacts with identified STT cells has demonstrated the presence of a variety of neurotransmitters, including glutamate, γ-aminobutyric acid (GABA), substance P, calcitonin gene-related peptide (CGRP), serotonin (5HT), and norepinephrine (Willis and Coggeshall 2004). Receptors for these neurotransmitters and a variety of pharmacological agents have been investigated by iontophoretic release or by microdialysis administration of drugs in the vicinity of recorded STT cells (Willis and Coggeshall 2004). The effective agents include both excitatory neurotransmitters (glutamate, aspartate, substance P, CGRP) and inhibitory ones (GABA, glycine, 5HT, norepinephrine, opioids).

Little is known about the neurotransmitters that act on PSDC neurons. These cells normally lack neurokinin-1 (NK1) receptors, although some PSDC neurons upregulate NK1 receptors after colon inflammation by mustard oil (Palecek et al. 2003b). Microdialysis administration of the glutamate receptor antagonist CNQX or of morphine into the sacral spinal cord blocks the excitation of VPL neurons following colorectal distension, presumably by interfering

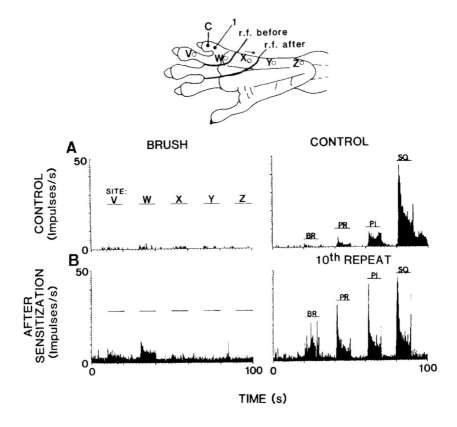

Fig. 5. The skin of the foot of an anesthetized monkey was stimulated repeatedly at several intensities, including very strong squeezing using serrated forceps. Responses were recorded from an STT cell. A drawing of the foot is shown at the top. The entire series of mechanical brush (BR), pressure (PR), pinch (PI), and squeezing (SQ) stimuli was applied at C and at 1 (shown in the drawing at top). Brush stimuli were applied at sites designated V, W, X, Y, and Z. The receptive field was mapped using a von Frey filament. The receptive field increased in size after repeated stimulation. A, left: Responses to BR at sites V–Z before repeated application of the stimulus series. A, right: The responses to the initial control series of BR, PR, PI, and SQ stimuli applied to point C. B, left: The increased background discharges and enhanced responses to BR stimuli applied at V–Z after repeated applications of the entire mechanical stimulus series to point C. B, right: The responses are shown to the 10th repetition of the entire series of graded mechanical stimuli applied at point C. Note that the response to BR is now larger than the original response to PI. (From Owens et al. 1992.)

with the excitation of PSDC neurons in the sacral cord (Fig. 4F; Al-Chaer et al. 1996b). However, it is unclear whether the site of action was directly on the PSDC neurons or on interneurons interposed between the primary afferents and the PSDC neurons.

DESCENDING CONTROL OF PROJECTION NEURONS

STT cells are under the inhibitory influence of a number of brain structures and mediated by pathways that descend from the brain into the spinal cord (reviewed in Willis and Coggeshall 2004). For example, primate STT cells can be inhibited by stimulation in the periaqueductal gray, nucleus raphe magnus, medullary reticular formation, anterior pretectal nucleus, ventrobasal thalamus, and postcentral gyrus. By contrast, stimulation in the pontomedullary reticular formation or the primary motor cortex can excite STT cells. Much less is known about the descending controls of PSDC neurons.

In summary, several sensory pathways that ascend from the spinal cord to the brain convey signals that lead to visceral pain. This chapter has emphasized the spinothalamic tract and the postsynaptic dorsal column pathway, since visceral pain in human patients can be alleviated when the spinothalamic tract is interrupted bilaterally by anterolateral cordotomy or commissural myelotomy or when the postsynaptic dorsal column pathway is interrupted by midline myelotomy. Experimental work using behavioral, electrophysiological, and pharmacological techniques confirms that a visceral pain pathway is also present in the dorsal columns of animals.

ACKNOWLEDGMENTS

The author thanks Kelli Gondesen and Griselda Gonzales for their expert technical assistance. The work was supported by NIH grants NS 09743 and NS 11255.

REFERENCES

Al-Chaer ED, Lawand NB, Westlund KN, Willis WD. Visceral nociceptive input into the ventral posterolateral nucleus of the thalamus: a new function for the dorsal column pathway. *J Neurophysiol* 1996a; 76:2661–2674.

Al-Chaer, ED, Lawand NB, Westlund, KN, Willis WD. Pelvic visceral input into the nucleus gracilis is largely mediated by the postsynaptic dorsal column pathway. *J Neurophysiol* 1996b; 76:2675–2690.

Al-Chaer ED, Feng Y, Willis WD. Comparative study of viscerosomatic input onto postsynaptic dorsal column and spinothalamic tract neurons in the primate. *J Neurophysiol* 1999; 82:1876–1882.

Ammons WS. Characteristics of spinoreticular and spinothalamic neurons with renal input. *J Neurophysiol* 1987; 50:480–495.

Ammons WS. Primate spinothalamic cell responses to ureteral occlusion. *Brain Res* 1989; 496:124–130.

Ammons WS, Blair RW, Foreman RD. Responses of primate T1-T5 spinothalamic neurons to gallbladder distension. *Am J Physiol* 1984; 247:R995–R1002.

Apkarian AV, Hodge CJ. The primate spinothalamic pathways. I. A quantitative study of the cells of origin of the spinothalamic pathway. *J Comp Neurol* 1989a; 288:447–473.

Apkarian AV, Hodge CJ. The primate spinothalamic pathways. III. Thalamic terminations of the dorsolateral and ventral spinothalamic pathways. *J Comp Neurol* 1989b; 288:493–511.

Apkarian VA, Shi T. Squirrel monkey lateral thalamus. I. Somatic nociresponsive neurons and their relation to spinothalamic terminals. *J Neurosci* 1994; 14:6779–6795.

Applebaum AE, Leonard RB, Kenshalo DR, Martin RF, Willis WD. Nuclei in which functionally identified spinothalamic tract neurons terminate. *J Comp Neurol* 1979; 188:575–586.

Becker R, Sure U, Bertalanffy H. Punctate midline myelotomy. A new approach in the management of visceral pain. *Acta Neurochir (Wien)* 1999; 141:881–883.

Boivie J. An anatomical reinvestigation of the termination of the spinothalamic tract in the monkey. *J Comp Neurol* 1979; 186:343—370.

Brown PB, Fuchs JL. Somatotopic representation of hindlimb skin in cat dorsal horn. *J Neurophysiol* 1975; 38:1–9.

Bushnell MC, Duncan GH, Tremblay N. Thalamic VPM nucleus in the behaving monkey. I. Multimodal and discriminative properties of thermosensitive neurons. *J Neurophysiol* 1993; 69:739–752.

Cervero F. Mechanisms of visceral pain: past and present. In: Gebhart GF (Ed). *Visceral Pain, Progress in Pain Research and Management*, Vol. 5. Seattle: IASP Press, 1995, pp 25–40.

Christensen BN, Perl ER. Spinal neurons specifically excited by noxious or thermal stimuli: marginal zone of the dorsal horn. *J Neurophysiol* 1970; 33:293–307.

Craig AD. Spinal location of ascending lamina I axons in the macaque monkey. *J Pain* 2000; 1:33–45.

Craig AD. Distribution of trigeminothalamic and spinothalamic lamina I terminations in the macaque monkey. *J Comp Neurol* 2004; 477:119–148.

Craig AD, Andrew D. Responses of spinothalamic lamina I neurons to repeated brief contact heat stimulation in the cat. *J Neurophysiol* 2002; 87:1902–1914.

Craig AD, Bushnell MC, Zhang ET, Blomqvist A. A thalamic nucleus specific for pain and temperature sensation. *Nature* 1994; 372:770–771.

Dargent M, Mansuy L, Cohen J, De Rougemont J. Les problémes posées par la douleur dans l'évolution des cancers gynécologiques. *Lyon Chir* 1963; 59:62–83.

Dostrovsky JO, Craig AD. Cooling-specific spinothalamic neurons in the monkey. *J Neurophysiol* 1996; 76:3656–3665.

Dougherty PM, Willis WD. Enhanced responses of spinothalamic tract neurons to excitatory amino acids accompany capsaicin-induced sensitization in the monkey. *J Neurosci* 1992; 12:883–894.

Dougherty PM, Sluka KA, Sorkin LS, Westlund KN, Willis WD. Neural changes in acute arthritis in monkeys. I. Parallel enhancement of responses of spinothalamic tract neurons to mechanical stimulation and excitatory amino acids. *Brain Res Rev* 1992; 17:1–13.

Duncan GH, Bushnell MC, Oliveras JL, et al. Thalamic VPM nucleus in the behaving monkey. III. Effects of reversible inactivation by lidocaine on thermal and mechanical discrimination. *J Neurophysiol* 1993; 70:2086–2096.

Feng Y, Cui M, Al-Chaer ED, Willis WD. Epigastric antinociception by cervical dorsal column lesions in rats. *Anesthesiology* 1998; 89:411–420.

Ferrington DG, Sorkin LS, Willis WD. Responses of spinothalamic tract cells in the superficial dorsal horn of the primate lumbar spinal cord. *J Physiol* 1987; 388:277–291.

Foreman RD. Organization of the spinothalamic tract as a relay for cardiopulmonary sympathetic afferent fiber activity. In: Ottoson D (Ed). *Progress in Sensory Physiology*, Vol. 9. New York: Springer-Verlag, 1989, pp 1–51.

Foreman RD. Mechanisms of cardiac pain. *Annu Rev Physiol* 1999; 61:143–167.

Foreman RD, Schmidt RF, Willis WD. Effects of mechanical and chemical stimulation of fine muscle afferents upon primate spinothalamic tract cells. *J Physiol* 1979; 286:215–231.

Giesler GJ, Yezierski RP, Gerhart KD, Willis WD. Spinothalamic tract neurons that project to medial and/or lateral thalamic nuclei: evidence for a physiologically novel population of spinal cord neurons. *J Neurophysiol* 1981; 46:1285–1308.

Gildenberg PL, Hirshberg RM. Limited myelotomy for the treatment of intractable cancer pain. *Neurol Neurosurg Psychiatry* 1984; 47:94–96.

Graziano A, Jones EG. Widespread thalamic terminations of fibers arising in the superficial medullary dorsal horn of monkeys and their relation to calbindin immunoreactivity. *J Neurosci* 2004; 24:248–256.

Gybels JM, Sweet WH. Neurosurgical treatment of persistent pain. In: Gildenberg PL (Ed). *Neurosurgical Treatment of Persistent Pain,* Pain and Headache, Vol. 11. Basel: Karger, 1989.

Hirshberg RM, Al-Chaer ED, Lawand NB, Westlund KN, Willis WD. Is there a pathway in the posterior funiculus that signals visceral pain? *Pain* 1996; 67:291–305.

Hitchcock E. Stereotaxic cervical myelotomy. *J Neurol Neurosurg Psychiatry* 1970; 33:224–230.

Hitchcock E. Stereotactic myelotomy. *Proc R Soc Med* 1974; 67:771–772.

Hitchcock E. Stereotaxic spinal surgery. *Neurol Surg* 1977; 433:271–280.

Houghton AK, Kadura S, Westlund KN. Dorsal column lesions reverse the reduction in homecage activity in rats with pancreatitis. *Neuroreport* 1997; 8:3795–3800.

Kenshalo DR, Isensee O. Responses of primate SI cortical neurons to noxious stimuli. *J Neurophysiol* 1983; 50:1479–1496.

Kenshalo DR, Leonard RB, Chung JM, Willis WD. Responses of primate spinothalamic neurons to graded and to repeated noxious heat stimuli. *J Neurophysiol* 1979; 42:1370–1389.

Kenshalo DR, Giesler GJ, Leonard RB, Willis WD. Responses of neurons in primate ventral posterior lateral nucleus to noxious stimuli. *J Neurophysiol* 1980; 43:1594–1614.

Kenshalo DR, Chudler EH, Anton F, Dubner R. SI cortical nociceptive neurons participate in the encoding process by which monkeys perceive the intensity of noxious thermal stimulation. *Brain Res* 1988; 454:378–382.

Kim YS, Kwon SJ. High thoracic midline dorsal column myelotomy for severe visceral pain due to advanced stomach cancer. *Neurosurgery* 2000; 46:85–90.

LaMotte RH, Shain CN, Simone DA, Tsai EFP. Neurogenic hyperalgesia: Psychophysical studies of underlying mechanisms. *J Neurophysiol* 1991; 66:190–211.

Mehler WR, Feferman ME, Nauta WJH. Ascending axon degeneration following anterolateral cordotomy. An experimental study in the monkey. *Brain* 1960; 83:718–751.

Mendell LM. Physiological properties of unmyelinated fiber projection to the spinal cord. *Exp Neurol* 1966; 16:316–332.

Milne RJ, Foreman RD, Giesler GJ, Willis WD. Convergence of cutaneous and pelvic visceral nociceptive input onto primate spinothalamic neurons. *Pain* 1981; 11:163–183.

Nathan PW, Smith M, Deacon P. The crossing of the spinothalamic tract. *Brain* 2001; 124:793–803.

Nauta HJW, Hewitt E, Westlund KN, Willis WD. Surgical interruption of a midline dorsal column visceral pain pathway. *J Neurosurg* 1997; 86:538–542.

Nauta HJW, Soukup VM, Fabian RH, et al. Punctate mid-line myelotomy for the relief of visceral cancer pain. *J Neurosurg* 2000; 92:125–130.

Norrsell U. Behavioral thermosensitivity after unilateral, partial lesions of the lateral funiculus in the cervical spinal cord of the cat. *Exp Brain Res* 1989a; 78:369–373.

Norrsell U. Behavioral thermosensitivity after bilateral lesions of the lateral funiculus in the cervical spinal cord of the cat. *Exp Brain Res* 1989b; 78:374–379.

Owens CM, Zhang, D, Willis WD. Changes in the response states of primate spinothalamic tract cells caused by mechanical damage of the skin or activation of descending controls. *J Neurophysiol* 1992; 67:1509–1527.

Palecek J, Dougherty PM, Kim SH, et al. Responses of spinothalamic tract neurons to mechanical and thermal stimuli in an experimental model of peripheral neuropathy in primates. *J Neurophysiol* 1992; 68:1951–1966.

Palecek J, Paleckova V, Willis WD. The roles of pathways in the spinal cord lateral and dorsal funiculi in signaling nociceptive somatic and visceral stimuli in rats. *Pain* 2002; 96:297–307.

Palecek J, Paleckova V, Willis WD. Fos expression in spinothalamic and postsynaptic dorsal column neurons following noxious visceral and cutaneous stimuli. *Pain* 2003a; 104:249–257.

Palecek J, Paleckova V, Willis WD. Postsynaptic dorsal column neurons express NK1 receptors following colon inflammation. *Neuroscience* 2003b; 116:565–572.

Schvarcz JR. Stereotactic high cervical extralemniscal myelotomy for pelvic cancer pain. *Acta Neurochir* 1984; 33(Suppl):431–435.

Simone DA, Baumann TK, LaMotte RH. Dose-dependent pain and mechanical hyperalgesia in humans after intradermal injection of capsaicin. *Pain* 1989; 38:99–107.

Simone DA, Sorkin LS, Oh U, et al. Neurogenic hyperalgesia: central neural correlates in responses of spinothalamic tract neurons. *J Neurophysiol* 1991; 66:228–246.

Surmeier DJ, Honda CN, Willis WD. Responses of primate spinothalamic neurons to noxious thermal stimulation of glabrous and hairy skin. *J Neurophysiol* 1986a; 56:328–350.

Surmeier DJ, Honda CN, Willis WD. Temporal features of the responses of primate spinothalamic neurons to noxious thermal stimulation of hairy and glabrous skin. *J Neurophysiol* 1986b; 56:351–369.

Wang CC, Westlund KN. Responses of rat dorsal column neurons to pancreatic nociceptive stimulation. *Neuroreport* 2001; 12:2527–2530.

Wang CC, Willis WD, Westlund KN. Ascending projections from the central, visceral processing region of the spinal cord: a PHA-L study in rats. *J Comp Neurol* 1999; 415:341–362.

Wertheimer P, Lecuire J. La myélotomie commissurale postérieure. A propos de 107 observations. *Acta Chir Belg* 1953; 6:568–574.

Willis WD. Neural mechanisms of pain discrimination. In: Lund JS (Ed). *Sensory Processing in the Mammalian Brain*. New York: Oxford University Press, 1989, pp 130–143.

Willis WD. Long-term potentiation in spinothalamic neurons. *Brain Res Rev* 2002; 40:202–214.

Willis WD, Coggeshall RE. *Sensory Mechanisms of the Spinal Cord*. New York: Kluwer Academic/Plenum, 2004.

Willis WD, Westlund KN. Pain system. In: Paxinos G, Mai JK (Eds). *The Human Nervous System,* 2nd ed. Amsterdam, Elsevier, 2004, pp 1125–1170.

Willis WD, Trevino DL, Coulter JD, Maunz RA. Responses of primate spinothalamic tract neurons to natural stimulation of hindlimb. *J Neurophysiol* 1974; 37:358–372.

Willis WD, Leonard RB, Kenshalo DR. The cells of origin of the primate spinothalamic tract. *J Comp Neurol* 1979; 188:543–574.

Willis WD, Al-Chaer ED, Quast MJ, Westlund, KN. A visceral pain pathway in the dorsal column of the spinal cord. *Proc Natl Acad Sci USA* 1999; 96:7675–7679.

Zhang X, Wenk HN, Honda CN, Giesler GJ. Locations of spinothalamic tract axons in cervical and thoracic spinal cord white matter in monkeys. *J Neurophysiol* 2000a; 83:2869–2880.

Zhang X, Honda CN, Giesler GJ. Position of spinothalamic tract axons in upper cervical spinal cord of monkeys. *J Neurophysiol* 2000b; 84:1180–1185.

Correspondence to: William D. Willis, MD, PhD, Department of Neuroscience and Cell Biology, University of Texas Medical Branch, 301 University Blvd., Galveston, TX 77555-1069, USA. Fax: 409-772-4687; email: wdwillis@utmb.edu.

Proceedings of the 11th World Congress on Pain,
edited by Herta Flor, Eija Kalso, and Jonathan O.
Dostrovsky, IASP Press, Seattle, © 2006.

25

Visceral Pain and Visceral Hypersensitivity

G.F. Gebhart[a], Klaus Bielefeldt,[b] Khoa Dang,[a] Linjing Xu,[c] R. Carter W. Jones III,[c,d] and Kenneth R. Lamb[c]

*Departments of [a]Anesthesiology, Neurobiology and Pharmacology
and [b]Internal Medicine, the University of Pittsburgh School of Medicine,
Pittsburgh, Pennsylvania, USA; [c]Department of Pharmacology
and [d]Medical Scientist Training Program, Carver College of Medicine,
The University of Iowa, Iowa City, Iowa, USA*

The topic of visceral pain has been addressed in previous congress proceedings (e.g., Cervero 1987; Gebhart and Ness 1991), and revisiting it in the current volume appropriately reflects the growing appreciation by investigators of the importance of understanding the mechanisms of the pain and hypersensitivity that characterize many visceral disorders such as functional dyspepsia, interstitial cystitis/painful bladder syndrome, and irritable bowel syndrome. Fig. 1 documents the exponential increase in publications appearing in the peer-reviewed literature over the past 25 years. The top panel illustrates the results of a search in the Science Citation database using "visceral" AND "pain", and the bottom panel show results of an expanded search using "visceral" AND "pain" OR "nociception." Significantly, more than 50% of the publications in this area of investigation have appeared in the past 5–6 years, a reflection of the commitment by many basic-science investigators to develop models of visceral nociception and methods to study visceral neurons and central processing of visceral input. Notably, clinical investigators have built impressively upon basic findings, confirming many basic findings and extending understanding into central mechanisms of visceral hypersensitivity and supraspinal processing of visceral pain (e.g., Sarkar et al. 2000; Strigo et al. 2003; Hobson et al. 2004, 2006; Dunckley et al. 2005). Despite these impressive basic and clinical science advances, effective clinical management of visceral hypersensitivity remains elusive in most cases, spurring continuing investigation to determine the molecules and mediators that contribute to these visceral pain states.

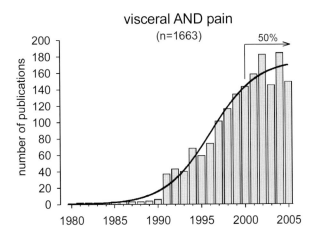

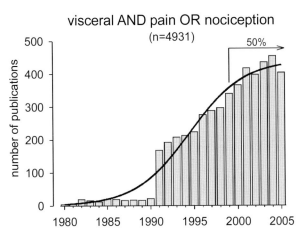

Fig. 1. Illustration of numbers of publications on visceral pain by year from 1980 through 2005 using two search strategies, "visceral" AND "pain" (top) and "visceral" AND "pain" OR "nociception" (bottom), applied in the ISI Web of Knowledge Science Citation database (http://portal.isiknowledge.com).

This chapter will summarize, for the sake of completeness, those features of visceral pain that distinguish it from non-visceral, "somatic" pain, and focus thereafter on peripheral mechanisms of sensitization, implications of innervation of viscera by two nerves, and molecules that contribute to mechanosensation in the viscera. Several comprehensive reviews of visceral pain (Ness and Gebhart 1990; Cervero 1994) and recent updates (e.g., Foreman 1999; Blackshaw and Gebhart 2002; Cervero and Laird 2004; Gebhart et al. 2004; Bielefeldt and Gebhart 2005; Bielefeldt et al. 2005; Ness and Gebhart 2005) have been published to which the reader is directed for more detailed information.

Visceral pain is diffuse in nature, is not felt at the source, is typically difficult to accurately localize, and is commonly referred to non-visceral structures such as the muscles and skin. These characteristics of visceral pain can be explained in large measure by the extent and organization of visceral innervation. Visceral afferents projecting into the spinal cord represent less that 10% of all spinal afferent input. Spinal visceral afferents spread extensively along the rostrocaudal axis of the spinal cord, forming synapses with many second-order neurons over several segments. Each viscus is innervated by two different nerves, typically the vagus nerve and a spinal ("splanchnic") nerve. Second-order spinal neurons upon which visceral afferents terminate also receive convergent non-visceral input as well as input from other viscera.

VISCERAL AFFERENT PLASTICITY

The vast majority of visceral afferent input to the central nervous system (CNS) is not consciously perceived. However, recent studies show that even subliminal stimuli extensively activate cortical structures in humans (Lawal et al. 2005, 2006), providing us with an inner landscape of the body's functional state and potentially contributing to an overall sense of well-being. Conscious perception of distinct visceral stimuli is often associated with negative emotional reactions and interpreted as uncomfortable or even painful (Strigo et al. 2002). Visceral events that can produce discomfort and pain include mechanical stimuli such as hollow organ distension or traction on the mesentery, as well as inflammation and ischemia. Because mechanical stimuli can reliably produce discomfort or pain in humans (and pain-like behaviors in laboratory animals; see Ness and Gebhart 1990 for citations and discussion) and are easily controlled experimentally, mechanosensitive visceral afferents have been studied most with respect to visceral pain and hypersensitivity. Visceral afferent chemosensitivity has been less widely studied. While potentially noxious chemicals, such as protons, can trigger aversive responses or pain (Fass et al. 1998; Lamb et al. 2003), exposure to different nutrients and luminal contents typically does not give rise to conscious sensation (e.g., Mei 1985; Sengupta and Gebhart 1994).

Contributions by many investigators between 1980 and 1995, a time during which the existence of visceral nociceptors was argued (and settled), established that the viscera were innervated by mechanoreceptor endings with low (physiological) response thresholds or with high response thresholds in the noxious range (~30 mmHg) (see Bielefeldt and Gebhart 2005 for citations). These high-threshold mechanosensitive afferents (usually 20–25% of the mechanosensitive population) doubtless convey to the CNS information that may be interpreted as pain. Graded hollow organ distension in many animal species, including humans, produces stimulus-response or psychophysical functions, respectively, that suggest the existence of different populations of mechanosensitive visceral afferents. Consistent with activation of high-threshold afferents, only high-intensity stimuli trigger pain or aversive responses. However, pharmacological interventions that alter biomechanical properties of viscera and thus indirectly affect pain thresholds similarly shift thresholds for low-intensity stimuli (Tack et al. 2004), thus calling into question the unique role of specialized nociceptive afferents in the experience of visceral pain. Further, when tested, mechanosensitive visceral afferents were determined also to be thermosensitive (to heat and/or cold) and/or chemosensitive, and in that sense similar to cutaneous polymodal nociceptors. Notably, visceral mechanosensitive afferents are like nociceptors in another very important way—they sensitize.

A distinguishing characteristic of cutaneous mechano-, thermo-, and polymodal nociceptors is their ability to sensitize (i.e., an increase in response magnitude, typically after tissue insult; see Perl 1996 for discussion), whereas cutaneous mechanoreceptors, which have low thresholds for response, do not sensitize. It is not surprising that high-threshold mechanosensitive visceral afferents sensitize. It was unexpected to find that their low-threshold counterparts, which constitute ~75% of the population of visceral mechanosensitive afferents, also sensitize, suggesting a potentially important role in functional visceral disorders. One interpretation of these findings (see Gebhart et al. 2004 for review and citations) is that most, if not perhaps all, mechanosensitive visceral afferent fibers, regardless of response threshold, have the potential under some circumstances (such as inflammation) to contribute to visceral discomfort and pain. Sensitization of low-threshold mechanosensitive afferent fibers, for example, means that mechanical stimuli in the physiological range could provide significantly increased input to spinal cord second-order neurons.

The viscera are also innervated by mechanically insensitive, "silent" afferents. The percentage of the total visceral afferent input to the spinal cord that is "silent" is unknown, but is estimated to range between 35% and 80%. Regardless, it appears that a significant proportion of the visceral afferent input can be categorized as mechanically insensitive fibers that after organ insult typically acquire spontaneous activity and mechanosensitivity (see Cervero 1996 for citations and discussion). In consideration of experimental evidence suggesting that organ insult contributes to sensitization of both low- and high-threshold mechanosensitive visceral afferents and activation of previously mechanically insensitive visceral afferents, plasticity of visceral organ innervation (and second-order and higher CNS neurons to which such information is conveyed) may be of greater consequence than plasticity of cutaneous afferents.

FUNCTIONAL IMPLICATIONS OF VISCERAL INNERVATION

Each viscus receives dual afferent innervation, and the function of each nerve is distinct, even if not fully understood. Innervation of the viscera is unique among all tissues in the body; each organ is innervated either by the vagus nerve and a spinal nerve, or by the pelvic nerve and a spinal nerve. The vagus nerve innervates all the thoracic viscera, most if not all of the abdominal viscera, and some of the pelvic viscera; spinal and pelvic nerves are distributed from cervical to sacral spinal segments.

VAGUS NERVE

The nociceptive role of the vagus nerve, which is the largest visceral sensory nerve in the body, is neither fully appreciated nor well understood. It has long been considered that the vagus nerve conveys no nociceptive information to the CNS. This view developed principally because vagal neurectomies failed to resolve visceral pain conditions (e.g., angina; Meller and Gebhart 1992), and is supported by reports that nocifensive responses to gastric distension in the rat are unaffected by vagotomy (but blocked by gastric splanchnectomy; Ozaki et al. 2002). Evidence continues to accumulate (e.g., Schuligoi et al. 1998; Michl et al. 2001; Lamb et al. 2003; Kollarik and Undem 2004; Yu et al. 2005), however, to suggest that *chemo*-nociceptive information is mediated by the vagus nerve. Not surprisingly, gastric ulceration produces a long-lasting behavioral hypersensitivity to gastric distension that, as indicated above, is abolished by splanchnectomy (Ozaki et al. 2002). In contrast, nocifensive responses produced by intragastric administration of hydrochloric acid are unaffected by splanchnectomy, but abolished by vagotomy (and also by capsaicin treatment; Lamb et al. 2003). These results, in addition to further supporting a role for vagal afferents in chemonociception, suggest that the gastric vagal afferent innervation, like the much better studied innervation of the viscera by spinal afferents, sensitizes. We studied this phenomenon in two ways: by recording of single vagal afferent fibers and by whole-cell patch clamp of gastric sensory neurons.

To address this issue at the single-fiber level, we examined the effects of acute thermal and chemical stimuli and gastric ulceration on mechanosensitive gastric vagal afferent fibers in the cervical vagus nerve, which were identified by response to gastric distension (Kang et al. 2004). Responses to gastric balloon distension (5–60 mmHg) in the rat were determined before and after intragastric exposure to thermal or chemical stimuli. Intragastric instillation of heated saline (46°C) significantly increased resting activity and sensitized responses to distension, whereas intragastric instillation of hydrochloric acid decreased resting activity (in a concentration-dependent manner), but also sensitized subsequent responses to distension. In contrast, intragastric instillation of the bile acid glycocholic acid desensitized responses to gastric distension (while increasing resting activity). Vagal afferent fibers recorded in rats with gastric ulcers had significantly greater resting activity and responses to gastric distension than sham ulcer rats. These responses were further increased in magnitude after intragastric instillation of a combination of hydrochloric acid and glycocholic acid. These results reveal that acute gastric thermal and chemical stimuli alter the activity and response characteristics of mechanosensitive vagal afferents in the absence of gastric inflammation or structural damage. Accordingly, acute sensitization of gastric afferents through different stimulus modalities may contribute to development of dyspeptic symptoms. In the presence of gastric inflammation, mechanosensitive vagal afferents exhibit a further increase in excitability.

We examined potential mechanisms by which gastric inflammation increases peripheral neuron excitability by studying voltage- and ligand-dependent currents in cells from gastric nodose (vagal innervation) and thoracic (spinal innervation) dorsal root ganglia (DRG).

Sodium currents. Compared to gastric nodose ganglion neurons, a higher fraction of spinal gastric sensory neurons had tetrodotoxin (TTX)-resistant action potentials, pointing to a functional difference between these two afferent pathways (Dang et al. 2005b). Ulceration enhanced neuron excitability, as shown by the presence of spontaneous activity and a decrease in threshold for action potential generation. This finding was associated with an increase in the fraction of neurons with TTX-resistant action potentials in nodose ganglion neurons. Consistent with these findings, the TTX-resistant sodium current contributed more to the peak sodium current. Moreover, gastric inflammation accelerated the recovery from inactivation of voltage-dependent sodium currents (Bielefeldt et al. 2002). In addition, the recovery kinetics of the TTX-sensitive sodium current were significantly faster in cells taken from rats with gastric ulcers. Together with a leftward shift of the voltage dependence of activation of the TTX-resistant current, these changes in voltage-dependent sodium currents are consistent with an enhanced excitability of gastric sensory neurons, and they probably contribute to the process of sensitization.

Potassium currents. Gastric inflammation significantly decreased the A-type potassium current density in gastric DRG and nodose ganglion sensory neurons, whereas the sustained current was not altered (Dang et al. 2004). There was also a significant shift in the steady-state inactivation to more hyperpolarized potentials in nodose ganglion neurons, associated with an acceleration of inactivation kinetics. These results suggest that a reduction in potassium currents in gastric sensory neurons contributes, in part, to increased neuron excitability that—in concurrence with changes in sodium currents described above—can lead to development of sensitization.

Ligand-gated currents. In these experiments, differences between the vagal and spinal innervations of the stomach became more apparent, attesting to functional differences between the two pathways of gastric innervation. Almost all control nodose ganglion neurons (90%), compared with significantly fewer DRG neurons (~38%), responded to the purinergic agonists adenosine triphosphate (ATP) or α,β-methylene ATP (Dang et al. 2005b). Gastric ulceration increased the fraction of DRG cells that responded to purinergic agonists, doubled the current density evoked by the P2X receptor agonist α,β-methylene ATP, and slowed decay of the slowly desensitizing component of the current (without affecting the concentration dependence of the response). These results reveal that gastric ulceration sensitizes both vagal and spinal gastric sensory neurons by affecting both voltage- and ligand-gated channels. In other studies (Sugiura et al. 2005), we characterized acid-elicited currents in DRG and nodose ganglion neurons that innervate the rat stomach and examined their modulation after induction of gastric ulcers. In whole-cell voltage-clamp recordings, all gastric DRG neurons and 55% of gastric nodose ganglion neurons exhibited transient, amiloride-sensitive, acid-sensing ion-channel (ASIC) currents. In the remaining 45% of nodose ganglion neurons, protons activated a slow, sustained current that was attenuated by the transient receptor potential vanilloid subtype 1 (TRPV1) antagonist capsazepine. The kinetics and proton sensitivity of amiloride-sensitive ASIC currents differed between nodose ganglion and DRG neurons. Gastric nodose ganglion neurons had a lower proton sensitivity and faster kinetics, suggesting expression of specific subtypes of ASICs in the vagal and spinal innervations of the stomach. Effects of ASIC modulators on acid-elicited currents suggest contributions of ASIC1a and ASIC2a subunits. Gastric ulcers altered the properties of acid-elicited currents by increasing pH sensitivity and current density and changing current kinetics in gastric DRG neurons.

Collectively, the above summary clearly demonstrates distinct properties of gastric nodose ganglion and DRG neurons and their modulation after gastric inflammation, suggesting differential contributions of vagal and spinal afferent neurons to visceral sensation and nociception. The data confirm a role for vagal afferent neurons in chemonociception, but also show that vagal mechanosensitive sensory neurons are sensitized by non-injurious exposure of the gastric lumen to endogenous chemicals (hydrochloric and glycocholic acid) as well as by gastric ulceration.

SPINAL NERVES

Pelvic organs (the bladder, colon, and uterus) are innervated by the pelvic and splanchnic nerves. This dual innervation of the distal colon and urinary bladder also has been the subject of investigation. In conjunction with collaborators in Australia (Brierley et al. 2004), we directly compared the pelvic nerve and lumbar splanchnic nerve innervations of the mouse distal colon, noting significant differences in type and sensitivity of mechanosensitivity and in the topographical distribution of mechanoreceptive endings in the colon between the two nerves. To obtain a detailed functional characterization of these afferent fibers innervating the mouse colon, experiments were conducted using an in vitro organ-nerve attached preparation. The colon was opened along the antimesenteric border and pinned flat in a perfusion chamber, thus permitting application of a series of defined mechanical stimuli (Fig. 2). Based on their response profiles, five different classes of mechanosensitive afferent fibers were recorded from the lumbar splanchnic and pelvic nerves. Three of these classes of afferent fibers (serosal, muscular, and mucosal) were conserved between both pathways; however, their respective proportions, receptive field distributions, and response properties differed significantly. In general, the mechanosensitivity of pelvic nerve afferent fibers was greater than that of the same classes of fibers recorded in the splanchnic innervation of the colon. Serosal, muscular, and mucosal afferent fibers recorded from the pelvic nerve (Fig. 3) responded

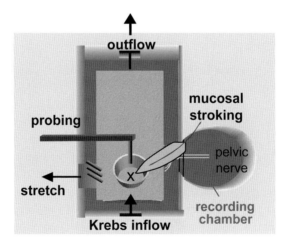

Fig. 2. Representation of the in vitro colon-nerve attached preparation used for study of properties of the afferent innervation of the colon. The terminal 5 cm of the mouse colon with either the pelvic nerve or lumbar splanchnic nerve is removed, opened longitudinally, and pinned flat (mucosal surface up) in a chamber perfused with oxygenated Krebs solution. The nerve is placed in an adjacent, mineral-oil-filled recording chamber from which small filaments are successively teased to isolate single fibers. Mechanical stimuli applied include blunt probing, circumferential stretch, or stroking of the mucosa. The receptive ending (X) can be physically isolated by placing a metal ring over it, withdrawing the Krebs solution, and replacing it with another solution (e.g., one that contains a chemical stimulant or receptor antagonist). This preparation was adopted by us through the courtesy of L. Ashley Blackshaw, Adelaide, Australia (see Brierley et al. 2004).

to lower stimulation intensities, displayed greater response magnitudes to mechanical stimulation, and adapted less completely to mechanical stimulation than did their lumbar splanchnic nerve counterparts. In addition, each nerve contained a specialized class of afferents unique to their respective pathway. Mechanosensitive mesenteric afferents were present in the splanchnic innervation of the colon (but not in the pelvic nerve innervation), and mechanosensitive muscular-mucosal afferents (Fig. 3) were present in the pelvic nerve innervation of the colon (but not in the splanchnic innervation of the colon).

Similarly, the pelvic nerve and lumbar splanchnic nerve innervation of the mouse urinary bladder reveal significant differences in type and sensitivity of mechanosensitivity and in the topographical distribution of mechanoreceptive endings in the bladder between the two nerves (Linjing Xu and G.F. Gebhart, unpublished data). As in the mouse colon, mechanical stimulation of the mouse bladder in vitro reveals four different classes of mechanosensitive afferent fibers, three of which are present in both pathways. Mechanosensitive endings of the lumbar splanchnic innervation of the bladder are located predominantly near the base of the bladder, 67% of which are serosal and 30% muscular (responsive to stretch). No urothelial receptive endings were found in this sample. In contrast, mechanosensitive endings of the pelvic nerve innervation of the bladder

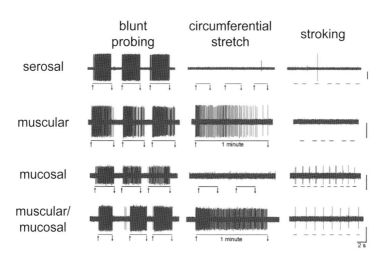

Fig. 3. Responses of mechanosensitive endings innervating the mouse colon. Single colonic pelvic nerve afferent fibers were activated by applying different mechanical stimuli to the colon (see Fig. 2 and Brierley et al. 2004). All mechanosensitive endings respond to blunt probing (>1 g), and endings in the serosa respond only to probing. Muscular receptors respond to circumferential stretch (1–5 g), but not to stroking of the mucosa. Mucosal receptors respond to repetitive stroking of the mucosa (10 mg; lines below the record), but not to stretch. Muscular-mucosal afferents respond to both stroking of the mucosa and circumferential stretch. (Reproduced from Brierley et al. 2004, with permission from the American Gastroenterological Association.)

were distributed throughout the bladder, with endings classed as serosal (14%), muscular (63%), urothelial (14%), and muscular-urothelial (9%). As was found for the mouse colon, a significant majority of stretch-responsive muscular and muscular-urothelial endings are contained in the pelvic nerve innervation of the organ, suggesting a role in sensing organ filling and distension.

In related studies of rat bladder thoracolumbar and lumbosacral DRG neurons (Dang et al. 2005a), representing lumbar splanchnic and pelvic nerve innervations, respectively, we explored functional differences on a cellular level, investigating responses to purinergic agonists, protons, and capsaicin. Most (93%) of the bladder neurons in the pelvic innervation were sensitive to α,β-methylene ATP compared with 50% of bladder neurons in the lumbar splanchnic innervation. Based on inactivation kinetics, a slowly desensitizing current evoked by α,β-methylene ATP predominated in lumbosacral, pelvic nerve neurons (86%) compared with mixed components that characterized lumbar splanchnic neuron responses (58%). The density of this slowly desensitizing current also was greater in pelvic nerve DRG neurons than in lumbar splanchnic nerve DRG neurons. Cystitis enhanced the excitability of bladder afferent neurons and increased the peak current density and fraction of lumbar splanchnic nerve neurons responding to purinergic agonists. Almost all neurons in both pathways responded to protons and to capsaicin, and the density of sustained proton- and capsaicin-activated currents was significantly greater in pelvic nerve neurons than in lumbar splanchnic nerve neurons.

These complementary experiments support the premise that pelvic and lumbar splanchnic pathways are functionally distinct and most likely mediate different sensations from the colon and urinary bladder. Considering the role of purinergic signaling in micturition (Cockayne et al. 2000), our findings may explain the observation that thoracolumbar afferents do not contribute to the regulation of micturition under normal conditions, but play an important role in sensitization during cystitis (Mitsui et al. 2001). As more investigators attend to the differences between nerves innervating the same organ, better understanding of functions will emerge that could lead to improved targeting of treatments for visceral pain disorders.

MODULATION OF MECHANOSENSATION

Because mechanical stimuli in the gastrointestinal tract and urinary bladder can trigger conscious perception of events in these organs, such as fullness, discomfort, or pain, gaining an understanding of the molecules that mediate mechanotransduction is central to developing efficacious treatments for visceral pain. The availability of genetically mutated mice (knockout mice) provides the opportunity to investigate the potential contributions of selected gene products to questions related to visceral sensitivity and hypersensitivity. An increasing number of candidate molecules have been studied that may serve roles as either mechanotransducers or modulators of mechanotransduction in the viscera, including the capsaicin or vanilloid receptor (TRPV1); purinergic receptors (P2X); acid-sensing ion channels (ASICs), which are mammalian homologues of the degenerin/epithelial sodium channel (DEG/ENaC) superfamily; and voltage-gated Na^+ channels (e.g., $Na_V 1.8$) (see above and Cervero and Laird 2003). Protein expression of both TRPV1 and ASIC3, one of six ASIC proteins derived from four genes, is increased in biopsy specimens from patients with inflammatory bowel disease (Yiangou et al. 2001a,b). Modulation of mechanosensory function by TRPV1 and/or ASIC3 in peripheral neurons has recently been shown for the bladder (Dinis et al. 2004) and in a model of muscle pain (Sluka et al. 2003). Thus, several studies have already focused on these molecules in both visceral and non-visceral tissues.

In visceral tissues, Blackshaw and colleagues (Page et al. 2004) recorded different classes of colonic lumbar splanchnic nerve and vagal gastroesophageal afferent fibers, finding that deletion of ASIC1a increased mechanical sensitivity of all classes of afferents studied in both locations. They (Page et al. 2005) also studied ASIC2 knockout mice, but effects of deletion of this gene product on mechanosensitivity of visceral afferent fibers were varied. We (Jones et al. 2005) and they (Page et al. 2005) both examined mechanosensitivity in ASIC3 knockout mice, and independently found that colonic lumbar splanchnic nerve (Page et al. 2005) and pelvic nerve (Jones et al. 2005) afferent fibers exhibited markedly reduced mechanosensitivity relative to control mice. In our study (Jones et al. 2005), we also examined the hypothesis that TRPV1 (in addition to ASIC3) contributes to colon mechanosensation, assessing the effects of gene deletion on both nocifensive responses to colon distension and responses of colonic pelvic nerve afferent fibers to mechanical probing and circumferential stretch. Colon distension (15–60 mmHg) produced graded nocifensive (visceromotor) responses in control (C57BL/6) and both knockout mice strains, but TRPV1 and ASIC3 knockout mice were significantly less sensitive to distension, with an average response magnitude of only 58% and 50% of control, respectively. The behavioral deficits observed in both strains of knockout mice were associated with a significant and selective reduction in afferent fiber sensitivity to circumferential stretch of the colon, an effect that was mimicked in control preparations by pretreatment with capsazepine, a TRPV1-receptor antagonist, but not amiloride, a nonselective ASIC antagonist. In addition, whereas stretch-evoked afferent fiber responses were enhanced by chemical inflammatory mediators in control mice, this effect was differentially impaired in both knockout mouse strains. These results, along with those from

Blackshaw's group, reveal a peripheral mechanosensory role for TRPV1 and ASIC3 in the mouse colon that contributes to nocifensive behavior and possibly neuron sensitization that arises as a consequence of tissue insult. However, considering the biophysical properties of these channels and results obtained by other groups (e.g., Rong et al. 2004; Mogil et al. 2005), TRPV1 and ASIC3 probably modulate mechanosensory function rather than directly transducing the mechanical stimulus energy.

Because ATP is released from urinary bladder epithelial cells (urothelium) in response to stretch or organ distension (e.g., Sun et al. 2001; Rong et al. 2002; Wang et al. 2005), it has been proposed that ATP acting at P2X receptors contributes to bladder mechanosensation and pain, which is supported by several findings. $P2X_2$ and $P2X_3$ receptors are increased in the urothelium of interstitial cystitis patients (Tempest et al. 2004), and $P2X_3$-receptor expression is increased during stretch of urothelial cells taken from cystitis patients (Sun et al. 2001). It has also been reported that $P2X_{2-3}$ knockout mice exhibit bladder hyporeflexia (Cockayne et al. 2000, 2005). In studies with $P2X_3$ knockout mice, although the distribution of receptive endings and their proportions are not different from control C57BL/6 mice, we (Linjing Xu and G.F. Gebhart, unpublished data) found that the absence of $P2X_3$ receptors was associated with significantly reduced mechanosensitivity of bladder pelvic nerve afferent fibers (Fig. 4).

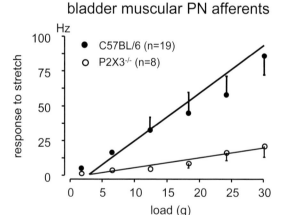

Fig. 4. Stimulus-response functions to stretch (1–30 g) applied to the urinary bladder in control C57BL/6 and $P2X_3$ knockout mice. Responses to stretch (vertical axis) were significantly attenuated in $P2X_3$ knockout mice (L. Xu and G.F. Gebhart, unpublished data). PN = pelvic nerve.

SUMMARY

Interest in and studies addressing visceral pain have increased significantly over the past 5–6 years. In this brief overview, we have focused on only two of many important features of visceral pain: functional roles of the visceral innervation and molecules that may play roles in mechanotransduction in the viscera. Other topics are of equal interest and importance, including emerging evidence that one visceral sensory cell soma in the DRG may generate axons that innervate different organs (Christianson et al. 2004; Malykhina et al. 2004). Moreover, silent visceral nociceptors, which appear to represent a greater proportion of the visceral innervation than has been reported in skin, have not been addressed here.

Although it has long been appreciated that the innervation of the viscera is unique, and that each pathway is associated with different functions, functional differences of visceral innervation have not been widely studied. Determining functional differences between the two pathways innervating an organ is fundamental to understanding visceral disorders and developing strategies to target therapies for them, particularly functional disorders for which insight into pathophysiology and options for treatment remain limited. It is clear for every organ studied that the different innervations have distinct and not always overlapping functions. Considering only mechanosensation, the pelvic nerve innervation of the mouse colon and urinary bladder contain many more stretch-responsive, muscular endings that the lumbar splanchnic nerve innervation, which dominates innervation of the serosal and colonic mesenteric attachment. That information alone suggests strategies for management of some bladder and colon disorders. Presumably, these endings in muscle or serosa are invested with molecules appropriate to the functions they subserve. We know too little about this topic at present, but the available data suggest differences in distribution, for example, of P2X and ASIC channels.

Because mechanical stimuli are among those that most commonly generate conscious appreciation of visceral events, determining which molecules transduce or modulate transduction of mechanical energies into action potentials is fundamental to understanding visceral mechanosensation. The use of knockout mice has led to new knowledge about putative visceral mechanotransducers. For example, as briefly reviewed above, it would appear that ASIC3 is critical to mechanosensitivity in colonic visceral afferent fibers. The presence of other ASICs (e.g., ASIC1a) appears to contribute an inhibitory role, whereas ASIC2 contributes inhibitory and facilitatory functions in different classes of visceral afferents. These findings in studies of visceral afferents diverge from what has been reported for these same channels in skin, suggesting important differences of the same molecule between different tissues. More importantly, these outcomes suggest that targeting molecules such as ASIC3, which appears to have uniform and pronounced effects on visceral mechanosensitivity, could lead to novel and useful therapies more selective for viscera than those presently available. It must be appreciated, however, that this strategy is simplistic in the sense that most molecules of interest (e.g., ASICs, P2X) are composed of multiple subunits and are thus heteromultimeric, which begs the question whether subunit composition changes in the presence of a visceral disorder (or perhaps causes the disorder).

REFERENCES

Bielefeldt K, Gebhart GF. Visceral pain—basic mechanisms. In: Koltzenburg M, McMahon S (Eds). *Textbook of Pain*, 5th ed. Edinburgh: Churchill-Livingstone, 2005, pp 721–736.

Bielefeldt K, Ozaki N, Gebhart GF. Experimental ulcers alter voltage-sensitive sodium currents in rat gastric sensory neurons. *Gastroenterology* 2002; 122:394–405.

Bielefeldt K, Christianson JA, Davis BM. Basic and clinical aspects of visceral sensation: transmission in the CNS. *Neurogastroenterol Motil* 2005; 17:488–499.

Blackshaw LA, Gebhart GF. The pharmacology of gastrointestinal nociceptive pathways. *Curr Opin Pharmacol* 2002; 2:642–649.

Brierley, SM, Jones III, RCW, Gebhart GF, Blackshaw LA. Splanchnic and pelvic mechanosensory afferents signal different qualities of colonic stimuli in mice. *Gastroenterology* 2004; 127:166–178.

Cervero F. Visceral pain. In: Dubner R, Gebhart GF, Bond M (Eds). *Proceedings of the 5th World Congress on Pain*. Amsterdam: Elsevier, 1987, pp 216–226.

Cervero F. Sensory innervation of the viscera: peripheral basis of visceral pain. *Physiol Rev* 1994; 74(1):95–138.

Cervero F. Visceral nociceptors. In: Belmonte C, Cervero F (Eds). *Neurobiology of Nociceptors*. New York: Oxford University Press, 1996, pp 220–240.

Cervero F, Laird JM. Role of ion channels in mechanisms controlling gastrointestinal pain pathways. *Curr Opin Pharmacol* 2003; 3:608–612.

Cervero F, Laird JM. Understanding the signaling and transmission of visceral nociceptive events. *J Neurobiol* 2004; 61:45–54.

Christianson JA, Liang R, Davis BM, Fraser MO, Pezzone MA. Retrograde labeling of urinary bladder and distal colon afferents: a potential role of dichotomizing afferents in the overlap of chronic pelvic pain disorders. *Gastroenterology* 2004; 126:A–115.

Cockayne DA, Hamilton SG, Zhu Q-M, et al. Urinary bladder hyporeflexia and reduced pain-related behaviour in $P2X_3$-deficient mice. *Nature* 2000; 407:1011–1015.

Cockayne DA, Dunn PM, Zhong Y, et al. $P2X_2$ knockout mice and $P2X_2/P2X_3$ double knockout mice reveal a role for the $P2X_2$ receptor subunit in mediating multiple sensory effects of ATP. *J Physiol* 2005; 567:621–639.

Dang K, Bielefeldt K, Gebhart GF. Gastric ulcers reduce A-type potassium currents in rat gastric sensory ganglion neurons. *Am J Physiol* 2004; 286:G573–579.

Dang K, Bielefeldt K, Gebhart GF. Differential responses of bladder lumbosacral and thoracolumbar dorsal root ganglion neurons to purinergic agonists, protons and capsaicin. *J Neurosci* 2005a; 25:3973–3984.

Dang K, Bielefeldt K, Lamb K, Gebhart GF. Gastric ulcers evoke hyperexcitability and enhance P2X receptor function in rat gastric sensory neurons. *J Neurophysiol* 2005b; 93:3112–3119.

Dinis P, Charrua A, Avelino A, et al. Anandamide-evoked activation of vanilloid receptor 1 contributes to the development of bladder hyperreflexia and nociceptive transmission to spinal dorsal horn neurons in cystitis. *J Neurosci* 2004; 24:11253–11263.

Dunckley P, Wise RG, Aziz Q, et al. Cortical processing of visceral and somatic stimulation: differentiating pain intensity from unpleasantness. *Neuroscience* 2005; 133:533–542.

Fass R, Naliboff B, Higa L, et al. Differential effect of long-term esophageal acid exposure on mechanosensitivity and chemosensitivity in humans. *Gastroenterology* 1998; 115:1363–1373.

Foreman RD. Mechanisms of cardiac pain. *Annu Rev Physiol* 1999; 61:143–167.

Gebhart GF, Ness TJ. Mechanisms of visceral pain. In: Bond MR, Charlton JE, Woolf CJ (Eds). *Proceedings of the 7th World Congress on Pain.* Amsterdam: Elsevier, 1991, pp 351–363.

Gebhart GF, Kuner R, Jones III RCW, Bielefeldt K. Visceral hypersensitivity. In: Brune K, Handwerker HO (Eds). *Hyperalgesia: Molecular Mechanisms and Clinical Implications,* Progress in Pain Research and Management, Vol. 30. Seattle: IASP Press, 2004, pp 87–104.

Hobson AR, Khan RW, Sarkar S, Furlong PL, Aziz Q. Development of esophageal hypersensitivity following experimental duodenal acidification. *Am J Gastroenterol* 2004; 99:813–820.

Hobson AR, Furlong PL, Sarkar S, et al. Neurophysiologic assessment of esophageal sensory processing in noncardiac chest pain. *Gastroenterology* 2006; 130:80–88.

Jones III RCW, Xu L, Gebhart GF. Mechanosensitivity of mouse colon afferent fibers and their sensitization by inflammatory mediators require TRPV1 and ASIC3. *J Neurosci* 2005; 25:10981–10989.

Kang Y-M, Bielefeldt K, Gebhart GF. Sensitization of mechanosensitive gastric vagal afferent fibers by thermal and chemical stimuli and gastric ulcers. *J Neurophysiol* 2004; 91:1981–1989.

Kollarik M, Undem BJ. Activation of bronchopulmonary vagal afferent nerves with bradykinin, acid and vanilloid receptor agonists in wild-type and TRPV1-/- mice. *J Physiol* 2004; 555:115–123.

Lamb K, Kang Y-M, Gebhart GF, Bielefeldt K. Gastric inflammation triggers hypersensitivity to acid in awake rats. *Gastroenterology* 2003; 125:1410–1418.

Lawal A, Kern M, Sanjeevi A, Hofmann C, Shaker R. Cingulate cortex: a closer look at its gut-related functional topography. *Am J Physiol* 2005; 289:G722–G730.

Lawal A, Kern M, Sidhu H, Hofmann C, Shaker R. Novel evidence for hypersensitivity of visceral sensory neural circuitry in irritable bowel syndrome patients. *Gastroenterology* 2006; 130:26–33.

Malykhina AP, Chao Q, Foreman RD, Akbarali HI. Colonic inflammation increases Na^+ currents in bladder sensory neurons. *Neuroreport* 2004; 15:2601–2605.

Mei N. Intestinal chemosensitivity. *Physiol Rev* 1985; 65(2):211–237.

Meller ST, Gebhart GF. A critical review of the afferent pathways and the potential chemical mediators involved in cardiac pain. *J Neurosci* 1992; 48:501–524.

Michl T, Jocic M, Heinemann A, Schuligoi R, Holzer P. Vagal afferent signaling of a gastric mucosal acid insult to medullary, pontine, thalamic, hypothalamic and limbic, but not cortical, nuclei of the rat brain. *Pain* 2001; 92:19–27.

Mitsui T, Kakizaki H, Matsuura S, et al. Afferent fibers of the hypogastric nerves are involved in the facilitating effects of chemical bladder irritation in rats. *J Neurophysiol* 2001; 86:2276–2284.

Mogil JS, Breese NM, Witty M-F, et al. Transgenic expression of a dominant-negative ASIC3 subunit leads to increased sensitivity to mechanical and inflammatory stimuli. *J Neurosci* 2005; 25:9893–9901.

Ness TJ, Gebhart GF. Visceral pain: a review of experimental studies. *Pain* 1990; 41:167–234.

Ness TJ, Gebhart GF. Mechanisms of visceral pain. In: Pappagallo M (Ed). *The Neurologic Basis of Pain.* New York: McGraw-Hill, 2005, pp 95–103.

Ozaki N, Bielefeldt K, Sengupta J, Gebhart GF. Models of gastric hyperalgesia in the rat. *Am J Physiol* 2002; 283:G666–G676.

Page A, Brierley S, Martin C, et al. The ion channel ASIC1 contributes to visceral but not cutaneous mechanoreceptor function. *Gastroenterology* 2004; 127:1739–1747.

Page A, Brierley S, Martin C, et al. Different contributions of ASIC channels 1a, 2 and 3 in gastrointestinal mechanosensory function. *Gut* 2005; 54:1408–1415.

Perl ER. Cutaneous polymodal receptors: characteristics and plasticity. In: Kumazawa T, Kruger L, Mizumura K (Eds). *The Polymodal Receptor: A Gateway to Pathological Pain,* Progress in Brain Research, Vol. 113. Amsterdam: Elsevier Science, 1996, pp 21–37.

Rong W, Spyer M, Burnstock G. Activation and sensitisation of low and high threshold afferent fibres mediated by P2X receptors in the mouse urinary bladder. *J Physiol* 2002; 541:591–600.

Rong W, Hillsley K, Davis JB, et al. Jejunal afferent nerve sensitivity in wild-type and TRPV1 knockout mice. *J Physiol (Lond)* 2004; 560:867–881.

Sarkar S, Aziz Q, Woolf CJ, Hobson AR, Thompson DG. Contribution of central sensitisation to the development of non-cardiac chest pain. *Lancet* 2000; 356:1154–1159.

Schuligoi R, Jocic M, Heinemann A, et al. Gastric acid-evoked c-fos messenger RNA expression in rat brainstem is signaled by capsaicin-resistant vagal afferents. *Gastroenterology* 1998; 115:649–660.

Sengupta JN, Gebhart GF. Gastrointestinal afferent fibers and sensation. In: Jacobsen ED, Johnson LR, Christensen J, Alpers DH, Walsh JH (Eds). *Physiology of the Gastrointestinal Tract.* New York: Raven Press, 1994, pp 483–519.

Sluka KA, Price MP, Breese NM, et al. Chronic hyperalgesia induced by repeated acid injections in muscle is abolished by the loss of ASIC3, but not ASIC1. *Pain* 2003; 106:229–239.

Strigo IA, Bushnell MC, Boivin M, Duncan GH. Psychophysical analysis of visceral and cutaneous pain in human subjects. *Pain* 2002; 97:235–246.

Strigo IA, Duncan GH, Boivin M, Bushnell MC. Differentiation of visceral and cutaneous pain in the human brain. *J Neurophysiol* 2003; 89:3294–303.

Sugiura T, Dang K, Lamb K, Bielefeldt K, Gebhart GF. Acid-sensing properties in rat gastric sensory neurons from normal and ulcerated stomach. *J Neurosci* 2005; 25:2617–2627.

Sun Y, Keay S, De Deyne PG, Chai TC. Augmented stretch activated adenosine triphosphate release from bladder uroepithelial cells in patients with interstitial cystitis. *J Urol* 2001; 166:1951–1956.

Tack J, Bisschops R, Sarnelli G. Pathophysiology and treatment of functional dyspepsia. *Gastroenterology* 2004; 127:1239–1255.

Tempest HV, Dixon AK, Turner WH, Elneil S, Ferguson DR. P2X and P2X receptor expression in human bladder urothelium and changes in interstitial cystitis. *BJU Int* 2004; 93(9):1344–1348.

Wang ECY, Lee J-M, Ruiz WG, et al. ATP and purinergic receptor-dependent membrane traffic in bladder umbrella cells. *J Clin Invest* 2005; 115:2412–2422.

Yiangou Y, Facer P, Dyer NHC, et al. Vanilloid receptor 1 immunoreactivity in inflamed human bowel. *Lancet* 2001a; 357:1338–1339.

Yiangou Y, Facer P, Smith JAM, et al. Increased acid-sensing ion channel ASIC-3 in inflamed human intestine. *Eur J Gastroenterol Hepatol* 2001b; 13:891–896.

Yu S, Undem BJ, Kollarik M. Vagal afferent nerves with nociceptive properties in guinea-pig oesophagus. *J Physiol* 2005; 563:831–842.

Correspondence to: G.F. Gebhart, PhD, Department of Neurobiology, University of Pittsburgh School of Medicine, W1444 BSTWR, Pittsburgh, PA 15261, USA. Email: gf-gebhart@uiowa.edu.

Proceedings of the 11th World Congress on Pain,
edited by Herta Flor, Eija Kalso, and Jonathan O.
Dostrovsky, IASP Press, Seattle, © 2006.

26

The Effects of Gonadal Hormones on Pain

Anna Maria Aloisi,[a] Rebecca M. Craft,[b]
and Serge Marchand[c]

*[a]Department of Physiology, Neuroscience and Applied Physiology Section,
University of Siena, Italy; [b]Department of Psychology, Washington State
University, Pullman, Washington, USA; [c]Faculty of Medicine, Neurosurgery,
University of Sherbrooke, Sherbrooke, Quebec, Canada*

Gonadal hormones influence many aspects of neurobiology and behavior in both males and females, during development and in adulthood. Androgens, estrogens, and progesterone appear to play important roles in pain and analgesia. In this chapter we refer to them as "sex hormones" rather than "gonadal hormones" to emphasize that they are also produced by structures other than the gonads. In fact, they are continuously produced in the central nervous system (CNS), where they act through their receptors. The classic genomic action of steroids is now known to be accompanied by nongenomic actions, which include fast-acting and short-lasting effects that are very seldom considered in pain physiology. Understanding the role of sex hormones in endogenous pain modulation will help us to better understand the neurophysiological mechanisms underlying the development and persistence of various chronic pain conditions.

Clinical and epidemiological data have long indicated that women differ from men in the occurrence of chronic painful syndromes. The increased prevalence of several chronic pain conditions in women (Berkley 1997), together with the fact that experimental pain threshold is generally lower in women than in men and varies during the menstrual cycle (Riley et al. 1999), provides evidence of the important role of sex hormones in pain. In adult females, plasma estrogen and progesterone levels change cyclically across the menstrual phases. Thus, a close relationship between ovarian hormones and pain is suggested by the occurrence of pain syndromes that fluctuate across menstrual cycle phases. In fact, the ability of estrogens to decrease the response of muscle cells to norepinephrine

(NE) and to modify the production of many vasoactive substances, such as prostacyclin and nitric oxide, has been hypothesized to contribute to premenstrual migraine attacks (Marcus 1995). There have also been reports that fibromyalgia symptoms fluctuate throughout the menstrual cycle, with increased levels of pain, perceived stress, and depression during the luteal phase, when estrogen and progesterone levels are high (see Korszun et al. 2000).

Experimental pain studies conducted in animals have yielded results similar to those obtained in humans: females have lower nociceptive thresholds than males in the majority of experimental modalities (Mogil 2000). Sex hormones, together with genes, are considered important determinants of these sex differences (Craft et al. 2004a). The presence of estrogen-sensitive neurons in the superficial dorsal horn laminae of the spinal cord as well as estrogen's involvement in the transcriptional control of opioid synthesis and of δ- and κ-opioid receptor expression suggest additional mechanisms by which changing levels of estrogen can regulate pain sensitivity (Amandusson and Blomqvist 2001). The distribution of estrogen-receptor-expressing cells in lamina II corresponds to the localization of preproenkephalin-expressing neurons (Amandusson et al. 1995). Kappa-opioid receptors, which occur at a high density in the lumbosacral spinal cord of both rats and humans (Gouarderes et al. 1985), have been found to mediate sex-steroid-induced antinociception. A recent experiment in which male rats were injected intracerebroventricularly with estradiol found that formalin-induced licking (a supraspinally mediated response) was increased, while paw-jerk (a more spinally mediated reflex) was lower than in controls (Aloisi and Ceccarelli 2000). Similarly, simulation of pregnancy (high plasma levels of estrogens and progesterone in ovariectomized rats) resulted in an increased nociceptive threshold when a spinally mediated response was measured (Dawson-Basoa and Gintzler 1998). Interestingly, this analgesic effect of ovarian hormones also occurs in males (Liu and Gintzler 2000). Both of these studies showed that the complete hormonal profile of gestation is necessary in female (and even in male) rats to obtain the typical opioid-mediated analgesia normally observed during gestation. Indeed, the ratio between estrogen and progesterone, and most probably testosterone as well, probably plays a major role in pain modulation, considering that systemic (intraperitoneal) supplementation of 17β-estradiol or progesterone alone produced opposite effects as compared to supplementation with a physiological level of both hormones in gonadectomized male or female rats (Gaumond et al. 2005).

On the other hand, it was recently shown that the increased responses of nucleus gracilis neurons during proestrus (Bradshaw and Berkley 2000) are partly due to contemporaneous increases in estrogen levels, possibly acting on dorsal root ganglion cells whose estrogen receptors also increase with estrogen replacement (Taleghany et al. 1999). Thus, it appears that while in some structures estrogens can decrease nociceptive sensitivity, in others they can increase nociceptive sensitivity. This is an important aspect of research involving hormones because these substances, like many other neurotransmitters, could act differently depending on the nature of their receptors (i.e., whether they are nuclear or membrane-bound) and on where these receptors are localized.

DEVELOPMENT OF SEX DIFFERENCES IN PAIN AND ANALGESIA

Historically, gonadal steroid hormone effects have been considered to fall into one of two categories: organizational or activational (Cooke et al. 1998). Organizational effects of hormones are those that, during development of the organism, result in permanent structural and functional differences in the CNS. Organizational effects are further divided into masculinizing or defeminizing effects. Masculinizing effects are those that promote male characteristics, and defeminizing effects are those that suppress female characteristics. Typically, male mammals are considered to be masculinized and defeminized due to their higher levels of testosterone during development. In contrast, activational hormone effects are considered temporary and reversible and result from steroids activation (or inhibition) on existing circuits in the adult. That is, hormones continue to promote male or female characteristics in the adult by acting on neural circuits that were organized during development.

As shown in Fig. 1, sexual differentiation of neurobiological substrates mediating pain and opioid analgesia appears to be attributable to the influence of gonadal hormones acting both organizationally and activationally. For example, sex differences in sensitivity to a noxious thermal stimulus can be eliminated by manipulating gonadal hormones during the neonatal period (R.M. Craft, unpublished data) or during adulthood (e.g., Stoffel et al. 2003). Specifically, whereas adult female rats respond more quickly than adult males to a noxious thermal stimulus in the 50°C tail-withdrawal test, this sex difference can be eliminated by castrating male rats on postnatal day (PND) 1 or by treating females with testosterone on PND2, and then testing them as adults (R.M. Craft, unpublished data).

This "male to female" and "female to male" plasticity can be demonstrated in terms of rats' sensitivity to morphine analgesia as well. Depriving males of testosterone from PND1 to adulthood or exposing females to testosterone on PND2 changes their adult sensitivity to morphine analgesia, such that neonatally castrated males are less sensitive to morphine than normal males (i.e., neonatally castrated males are similar to normal adult females) and neonatally androgenized females are more sensitive to morphine than normal females (i.e., neonatally androgenized females are similar to normal adult males) (Cicero et

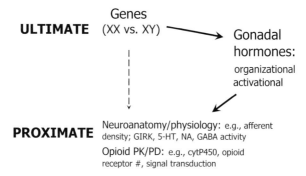

Fig. 1. Schematic representation of the ultimate vs. proximate causes for sex differences in pain and opioid analgesia. According to the classic dogma of mammalian sexual differentiation, the genetic sex of the individual (XX or XY) determines the gonad type. The gonads secrete steroid hormones, which during development (organizational effects) and during adulthood (activational effects) can affect the neural substrates underlying pain and opioid analgesia. Gonadal hormones can modify pain by altering specific neural substrates and neurotransmitters involved in the pain response and can modify opioid analgesia by altering various aspects of drug pharmacokinetics (PK) and pharmacodynamics (PD).

al. 2002; Krzanowska et al. 2002; R.M. Craft, unpublished data). Thus, testosterone exposure early in life appears to be responsible for the development of the male phenotype in terms of sensitivity to pain and opioid analgesia. The normal developmental window for this sexual differentiation is probably *before* the early neonatal period: although males castrated on PND1 responded like females to morphine in adulthood, a brief (2-week) exposure to testosterone in adulthood was sufficient to restore them to the male phenotype (R.M. Craft, unpublished data). The fact that males retained their ability to respond to testosterone indicates that by the time they were castrated on PND1, male pups were already masculinized in terms of their morphine sensitivity. Recent research in fact demonstrates that male mice show greater morphine sensitivity than females, even at 1 week of age (Sternberg et al. 2004).

Gonadal hormones can also modulate pain and opioid analgesia in adult animals. For example, in adult Sprague-Dawley rats, sex differences in sensitivity to a noxious thermal stimulus, the 50°C hotplate test, are estradiol-dependent (e.g., Stoffel et al. 2003), and sex differences in morphine analgesia may be both estradiol- and testosterone-dependent (Craft et al. 2004a). Activational effects of gonadal hormones have also been demonstrated in the formalin test: whereas gonadally intact females had increased nociceptive responses than gonadally intact males, gonadectomized male and female rats had the same nociceptive responses (Gaumond et al. 2002). It was also possible to reproduce a "female response" in males by supplementing castrated males with estrogen and progesterone; conversely, a "male response" could be reproduced by supplementing ovariectomized females with testosterone (Gaumond et al. 2005). However, sex hormones may act differently in different phases of the formalin test. Gonadectomized females had significantly reduced nociceptive responses compared to normal females, but only during the interphase, whereas castrated male rats presented significantly more nociceptive responses than normal males in all phases except the interphase. These results suggest that female sex hormones (progesterone and/or estrogen) are hyperalgesic and that male sex hormones (testosterone) are hypoalgesic. However, this hormonal modulation of pain depends on the type of pain, an observation that may help explain why some, but not all, chronic pain conditions display sex and hormone dependency. The activational effects of gonadal hormones on pain and opioid analgesia are still much debated, and they are very likely to depend in part on the strain of rodent and on the particulars of the hormone manipulation protocol (dose, timing, and duration of gonadectomy or hormone administration).

ENDOGENOUS PAIN MECHANISMS AND SEX HORMONES

As illustrated in Fig. 1, there are a number of ways in which gonadal hormones, either organizationally or activationally (or both), can modulate the biological substrates mediating pain and opioid analgesia. First, gonadal hormones can influence the activity of neurons known to be involved in pain responsiveness: estradiol blunts the increase in firing of on-cells and the decrease in firing of off-cells in the rostral ventromedial medulla of female rats exposed to a noxious thermal stimulus (Craft et al. 2004b). Thus, estradiol may alter pain sensitivity in females by altering the activity of nociceptive neurons. The mechanisms of persistent pain have been mainly hypothesized to be the result of peripheral or central hyperalgesia. However, pain is a dynamic phenomenon resulting from the activity of both inhibitory and excitatory endogenous modulatory systems (Millan 2002). In animals, lesion of the spinal dorsolateral funiculus, a pathway responsible for descending inhibition of serotonin (5-HT) and NE, produces hyperalgesia (Abbott et al. 1996). The reduction of 5-HT and/or NE in certain chronic pain conditions raises the possibility that a deficit of diffuse noxious inhibitory controls (DNIC) is responsible for the experience of diffuse chronic pain syndrome or fibromyalgia (Julien et al. 2005). In a recent study, the percentage of pain reduction by DNIC was evaluated in a group of fibromyalgia patients (S. Marchand et al., unpublished data). The DNIC inhibition was greater during the luteal and ovulatory phases as compared to the follicular phase of the menstrual cycle. These findings are in agreement with previous results showing a menstrual cycle-dependent pain perception in fibromyalgia patients (Korszun et al. 2000). They thus suggest a relationship between sex hormones and endogenous pain inhibition in women suffering from fibromyalgia. One mechanism that may underlie sex differences in (and gonadal hormone effects on) the activity of nociceptive neurons is G-protein-activated, inwardly rectifying potassium channel 2 (GIRK2). A recent study found that GIRK2 knockout mice were more sensitive to noxious thermal stimuli and less sensitive to analgesia than wild-type mice and that sex differences were diminished in knockout mice (Blednov et al. 2003).

There is evidence that sex differences in morphine analgesic sensitivity are due to sex differences in (or gonadal hormone effects on) morphine pharmacokinetics both the extent to which morphine enters the brain (Candido et al. 1992; Craft et al. 1996; but see Cicero et al. 1997) and the extent to which morphine is metabolized to active or inactive metabolites (Ratka 1995; South et al. 2001; Baker and Ratka 2002). Finally, studies have shown that sex differences in morphine analgesic sensitivity are due to sex differences in morphine pharmacodynamics. For example, greater morphine analgesia after central administration may be due to a greater density of μ-opioid receptors in the brains of males compared to females (Mogil et al. 1994; Craft et al. 2001; Duncan and Murphy 2005). Mu-opioid receptor density is known to be modulated by gonadal hormones, especially estrogen, in the adult animal (e.g., Weiland and Wise 1990; Lagrange et al. 1997; Eckersell et al. 1998).

Other neurotransmitters playing a major role in pain modulation also are affected by sex hormones. For example, NE-responsive neurons express both estrogen (Simonian and Herbison 1997) and progesterone receptors (Simonian and Herbison 1997; Haywood et al. 1999), and both estrogen and progesterone alter the expression of 5-HT and NE in neurons of the nucleus raphe magnus and locus ceruleus, respectively (Schutzer and Bethea 1997). Moreover, castration of male rats reduces the expression of 5-HT and NE, suggesting a role for both male and female sex hormones in NE and 5-HT expression in the CNS (Das and Chaudhuri 1995). The activity of gamma-aminobutyric acid (GABA), an inhibitory neurotransmitter involved in modulating pain transmission in the CNS, is also influenced by sex hormones. The $GABA_A$ receptor has a specific site for the binding of neurosteroids such as progesterone, testosterone, deoxycorticosterone, and some steroid metabolites (Zinder and Dar 1999). When neurosteroids bind to $GABA_A$, they modulate the duration and frequency of channel opening. Thus, like benzodiazepines and barbiturates, neurosteroids can potentiate the actions of GABA, resulting in anxiolytic and anaesthetic effects (Pan et al. 1998).

Taken together, these studies indicate that sensitivities to pain and opioid analgesia begin to sexually differentiate very early in development, although gonadal hormones can continue to modulate sensitivities to pain and opioid analgesia well into adulthood. There are multiple neurobiological mechanisms by which gonadal hormones may modulate pain and analgesia, including alteration of nociceptive neuron activity, modification of opioid pharmacokinetics and opioid pharmacodynamics, and changes in other endogenous pain-modulatory mechanisms implicated in the development and persistence of various chronic pain conditions.

REFERENCES

Abbott FV, Hong Y, Franklin KB. The effect of lesions of the dorsolateral funiculus on formalin pain and morphine analgesia: a dose-response analysis. *Pain* 1996; 65:17–23.

Aloisi AM, Ceccarelli I. Role of gonadal hormones in formalin-induced pain responses of male rats: modulation by estradiol and naloxone administration. *Neuroscience* 2000; 95:559–566.

Amandusson A, Blomqvist A. Estrogen receptors can regulate pain sensitivity. Possible explanation of certain chronic pain conditions. *Lakartidningen* 2001; 98:1774–1778.

Amandusson A, Hermanson O, Blomqvist A. Estrogen receptor-like immunoreactivity in the medullary and spinal dorsal horn of the female rat. *Neurosci Lett* 1995; 196:25–28.

Baker L, Ratka A. Sex-specific differences in levels of morphine, morphine-3-glucuronide, and morphine antinociception in rats. *Pain* 2002; 95:65–74.

Berkley KJ. Sex differences in pain. *Behav Brain Sci* 1997; 20:371–380.

Blednov YA, Stoffel M, Alva H, Harris RA. A pervasive mechanism for analgesia: activation of GIRK2 channels. *Proc Natl Acad Sci USA* 2003; 100:277–282.

Bradshaw HB, Berkley KJ. Estrous changes in responses of rat gracile nucleus neurons to stimulation of skin and pelvic viscera. *J Neurosci* 2000; 20:7722–7727.

Candido J, Lufty K, Billings B, et al. Effect of adrenal and sex hormones on opioid analgesia and opioid receptor regulation. *Pharmacol Biochem Behav* 1992; 42:685–692.

Cicero TJ, Nock B, Meyer ER. Sex-related differences in morphine's antinociceptive activity: relationship to serum and brain morphine concentrations. *J Pharmacol Exp Ther* 1997; 282:939–944.

Cicero TJ, Nock B, O'Connor L, Meyer ER. Role of steroids in sex differences in morphine-induced analgesia: activational and organizational effects. *J Pharmacol Exp Ther* 2002; 300:695–701.

Cooke B, Hegstrom CD, Villeneuve LS, Breedlove SM. Sexual differentiation of the vertebrate brain: principles and mechanisms. *Front Neuroendocrinol* 1998; 19:323–362.

Craft RM, Kalivas PW, Stratmann JA. Sex differences in discriminative stimulus effects of morphine in the rat. *Behav Pharmacol* 1996; 7:764–778.

Craft RM, Tseng AH, McNiel DM, Furness MS, Rice KC. Receptor-selective antagonism of opioid antinociception in female versus male rats. *Behav Pharmacol* 2001; 12:591–602.

Craft RM, Mogil JS, Aloisi AM. Sex differences in pain and analgesia: the role of gonadal hormones. *Eur J Pain* 2004a; 8:397–411.

Craft RM, Morgan MM, Lane DA. Oestradiol dampens reflex-related activity of on- and off-cells in the rostral ventromedial medulla of female rats. *Neuroscience* 2004b; 125:1061–1068.

Dawson-Basoa M, Gintzler AR. Gestational and ovarian sex steroid antinociception: synergy between spinal kappa and delta opioid systems. *Brain Res* 1998; 794:61–67.

Das A, Chaudhuri SK. Effects of sex steroids on the concentrations of some brain neurotransmitters in male and female rats: some new observations. *Indian J Physiol Pharmacol* 1995; 39:223–230.

Duncan KA, Murphy AZ. Sex-linked differences in mu opiate receptor distribution in the rat brain. *Soc Neurosci Abstr* 2005.

Eckersell CB, Popper P, Micevych PE. Estrogen-induced alteration of µ-opioid receptor im-
    munoreactivity in the medial preoptic nucleus and medial amygdala. *J Neurosci* 1998;
    18:3967–3976.
Gaumond I, Arsenault P, Marchand S. The role of sex hormones on formalin-induced nociceptive
    responses. *Brain Res* 2002; 958:139–145.
Gaumond I, Arsenault P, Marchand S. Specificity of female and male sex hormones on excita-
    tory and inhibitory phases of formalin-induced nociceptive responses. *Brain Res* 2005;
    1052:105–111.
Gouarderes C, Cros J, Quirion R. Autoradiographic localization of mu, delta and kappa opioid
    receptor binding sites in rat and guinea pig spinal cord. *Neuropeptides* 1985; 6:331–342.
Haywood SA, Simonian SX, van der Beek EM, Bicknell RJ, Herbison AE. Fluctuating estrogen
    and progesterone receptor expression in brainstem norepinephrine neurons through the rat
    estrous cycle. *Endocrinology* 1999; 140:3255–3263.
Julien N, Goffaux P, Arsenault P, Marchand S. Widespread pain in fibromyalgia is related to a
    deficit of endogenous pain inhibition. *Pain* 2005; 114:295–302.
Korszun A, Young EA, Engleberg NC, et al. Follicular phase hypothalamic-pituitary-gonadal
    axis function in women with fibromyalgia and chronic fatigue syndrome. *J Rheumatol* 2000;
    27:1526–1530.
Krzanowska EK, Ogawa S, Pfaff DW, Bodnar RJ. Reversal of sex differences in morphine analgesia
    elicited from the ventrolateral periaqueductal gray in rats by neonatal hormone manipulations.
    Brain Res 2002; 929:1–9.
Lagrange AH, Rønnekleiv OK, Kelly MJ. Modulation of G protein-coupled receptors by an estrogen
    receptor that activates protein kinase A. *J Pharmacol Exp Ther* 1997; 51:605–612.
Liu NJ, Gintzler AR. Prolonged ovarian sex steroid treatment of male rats produces antinociception:
    identification of sex-based divergent analgesic mechanisms. *Pain* 2000; 85:273–281.
Marcus DA. Interrelationships of neurochemicals, estrogen, and recurring headache. *Pain* 1995;
    62:129–139.
Millan MJ. Descending control of pain. *Prog Neurobiol* 2002; 66:355–474.
Mogil JS. Interactions between sex and genotype in the mediation and modulation of nocicep-
    tion in rodents. In: Fillingim RB (Ed). *Sex, Gender and Pain,* Progress in Pain Research and
    Management, Vol. 17. Seattle: IASP Press, 2000, pp 25–40.
Mogil JS, Marek P, O'Toole LA, et al. µ-Opiate receptor binding is up-regulated in mice selectively
    bred for high stress-induced analgesia. *Brain Res* 1994; 653:16–22.
Pan EC, Bohn LM, Belcheva MM, et al. Kappa-opioid receptor binding varies inversely with tumor
    grade in human gliomas. *Cancer* 1998; 83:2561–2566.
Ratka A. Effects of estradiol and testosterone on pharmacodynamics and pharmacokinetics of
    morphine in male rats. *J Idaho Acad Sci* 1995; 31:11–24.
Riley JL III, Robinson ME, Wise EA, Price DD. A meta-analytic review of pain perception across
    the menstrual cycle. *Pain* 1999; 81:225–235.
Schutzer WE, Bethea CL. Lack of ovarian steroid hormone regulation of norepinephrine transporter
    mRNA expression in the non-human primate locus coeruleus. *Psychoneuroendocrinology*
    1997; 22:325–336.
Simonian SX, Herbison AE. Differential expression of estrogen receptors and neuropeptide Y by
    brainstem A1 and A2 noradrenaline neurons. *Neuroscience* 1997; 76:517–529.
South SM, Wright AW, Lau M, Mather LE, Smith MT. Sex-related differences in antinocicep-
    tion and tolerance development following chronic intravenous infusion of morphine in the
    rat: modulatory role of testosterone via morphine clearance. *J Pharmacol Exp Ther* 2001;
    297:446–457.
Sternberg WF, Smith L, Scorr L. Nociception and antinociception during the first week of life in
    mice: sex differences and test dependence. *J Pain* 2004; 5:420–426.
Stoffel EC, Ulibarri CM, Craft RM. Gonadal steroid hormone modulation of nociception, morphine
    antinociception and reproductive indices in male and female rats. *Pain* 2003; 103:285–302.

Taleghany N, Sarajari S, DonCarlos LL, et al. Differential expression of estrogen receptor alpha and beta in rat dorsal root ganglion neurons. *J Neurosci Res* 1999; 57:603–615.

Von Korff M, Dworkin SF, LeResche L, Kruger A. An epidemiologic comparison of pain complaints. *Pain* 1988; 32:173–183.

Zinder O, Dar DE. Neuroactive steroids: their mechanism of action and their function in the stress response. *Acta Physiol Scand* 1999; 167:181–188.

Weiland NG, Wise PM. Estrogen and progesterone regulate opiate receptor densities in multiple brain regions. *Endocrinology* 1990;126:804–808.

Correspondence to: Prof. Anna Maria Aloisi, MD, Dipartimento di Fisiologia, Polo Scientifico Universitario San Miniato, Via Aldo Moro 2, 53100, Siena, Italy. Fax: 39-0577234037; email: aloisi@unisi.it.

Proceedings of the 11th World Congress on Pain,
edited by Herta Flor, Eija Kalso, and Jonathan O.
Dostrovsky, IASP Press, Seattle, © 2006.

27

Rethinking the PAG and RVM: Supraspinal Modulation of Nociception by Opioids and Non-Opioids

Martin W. Wessendorf,[a] Christopher W. Vaughan,[b] and Horacio Vanegas[c]

[a]Department of Neuroscience, University of Minnesota, Minneapolis, Minnesota, USA; [b]Pain Management Research Institute, University of Sydney at Royal North Shore Hospital, St. Leonards, New South Wales, Australia; [c]Venezuelan Institute for Scientific Research, Caracas, Venezuela

Opioid and non-opioid analgesics are thought to exert their actions in part by activating neurons in the periaqueductal gray matter (PAG) that project to the rostral portion of the ventromedial medulla (RVM); such analgesics can also act directly upon the RVM (Fields 2004). In either case, a subpopulation of spinally projecting neurons in the RVM would in turn inhibit nociception (Fig. 1). The same system of PAG and RVM neurons has been proposed to mediate the analgesia induced by electrical or chemical stimulation of the PAG.

Opioids typically inhibit neurons rather than excite them (Duggan and North 1983), thus the administration of opioids to brainstem structures is thought to increase the activity of output neurons by inhibiting their GABAergic inhibitory inputs (Fig. 1, black neurons), i.e., by "disinhibiting" them (Vaughan et al. 1997). In the PAG, activation of the μ-opioid receptor would thus disinhibit excitatory neurons projecting to the RVM. In the RVM, spinally projecting neurons that mediate pain inhibition would be activated from the PAG and/or disinhibited by local μ-opioid action.

In addition to descending antinociceptive circuits, there are spinally projecting RVM neurons that facilitate nociception (Fields 2004; Vanegas and Schaible 2004). This facilitatory pathway was revealed, for example, by selective lesioning of RVM neurons that express μ-opioid receptors, which prevents the development of hyperalgesia and allodynia after spinal nerve ligation. The

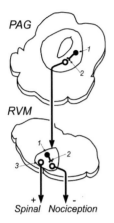

PAG

RVM

Spinal   Nociception

Fig. 1. Brainstem structures involved in descending control of pain. Cross-sections of the midbrain and the medulla highlight the periaqueductal gray matter (PAG) and the rostral ventrome-dial medulla (RVM). Local circuit GABAergic neurons have a black soma, and output neurons have a white soma. Numbers 1–3 indicate proposed sites of μ-opioid action. Plus and minus signs, respectively, indicate facilitation and inhibition of pain transmission within the spinal cord.

spinally projecting RVM neurons that express μ-opioid receptors (Fig. 1, no. 3) may therefore mediate the observed descending facilitation of pain (Fields 2004; Vanegas and Schaible 2004). The mechanisms by which descending facilitatory pathways enhance pain transmission in the spinal cord remain to be determined, but the most efficient model would be that those cells express excitatory neurotransmitters and synapse onto spinal nociceptive neurons.

DOES THE ANATOMY SUPPORT THE MODEL?

Several anatomical hypotheses arise from this model. They include the fol-lowing: (1) μ-opioid receptors should be expressed in the PAG and RVM; (2) GABAergic neurons expressing μ-opioid receptors should exist in the PAG and RVM; (3) μ-opioid receptors should be expressed on GABAergic synaptic ter-minals in those regions; (4) PAG neurons projecting to the RVM, which mediate opioid analgesia, should not express μ-opioid receptors, because inhibition of these cells would decrease descending inhibition of pain; (5) spinally projecting RVM neurons that express μ-opioid receptors (and thus should facilitate pain) should also express excitatory neurotransmitters. Some experimental findings agree with the proposed model, whereas others disagree.

ANATOMICAL DATA THAT AGREE WITH THE MODEL

First, the cloned μ-opioid receptor has been demonstrated in both the PAG and RVM. Both immunocytochemistry (Arvidsson et al. 1995; Kalyuzhny et al. 1996) and in situ hybridization (Mansour et al. 1994a,b; Wang and Wessen-dorf 1999, 2002) suggest that this result is not a technical artifact. Single-cell electrophysiological studies have shown that functional opioid receptors are present in both regions (Pan et al. 1990; Osborne et al. 1996; Marinelli et al. 2002). Second, the cloned μ-opioid receptor is expressed by GABAergic neurons both in the PAG and in the RVM (Kalyuzhny and Wessendorf 1997). These PAG neurons may be local circuit neurons, because very few PAG neurons that project to the RVM (identified by retrograde labeling) are GABAergic. Third, light-microscopic and electron-microscopic studies have shown that the cloned μ-opioid receptor is expressed on synaptic terminals in both the PAG and RVM (Abbadie et al. 2000; Commons et al. 2000). Finally, bulbospinal RVM neurons express the cloned μ-opioid receptor, as shown by both immunocytochemistry and in situ hybridization histochemistry, again suggesting that the finding is not a technical artifact (Kalyuzhny et al. 1996; Wang and Wessendorf 1999). Thus it appears that many of the key anatomical demands of the model have been fulfilled.

ANATOMICAL DATA THAT DO NOT AGREE WITH THE MODEL

PAG neurons that have been retrogradely labeled from the RVM often express μ-opioid receptors. Although this observation was not initially made using light microscopic immunocytochemistry (Kalyuzhny et al. 1996), μ receptors have been found in these cells using in situ hybridization (Wang and Wessendorf 2002) and have been found on their distal dendritic trees using immunocytochemistry at the electron microscopic level (Commons et al. 2000). Moreover, electrophysiological studies have shown that the μ receptors on these PAG neurons are functional (Osborne et al. 1996). These data suggest that some neurons in the PAG that project to the RVM are inhibited, not disinhibited, by opioids.

Although there are bulbospinal RVM neurons that express μ receptors, many contain γ-aminobutyric acid (GABA) or serotonin (Kalyuzhny et al. 1996; Kalyuzhny and Wessendorf 1998). In the case of serotonergic neurons, the finding has been confirmed by in situ hybridization (Wang and Wessendorf 1999), and the μ receptors have been reported to be functional (Marinelli et al. 2002). Although serotonin can be facilitatory, its effects on spinal nociceptive mechanisms, like those of GABA, are thought to be predominantly inhibitory. Thus, it appears that a population of inhibitory, spinally projecting RVM neurons are inhibited by opioids.

RECONCILING THE ANATOMICAL DATA WITH THE MODEL

At present the significance of these discrepancies is unclear, but there are several possibilities. With regard to the PAG, it is possible that the direct inhibitory effect of μ agonists on the PAG neurons that project to the RVM is overwhelmed by the indirect opioid disinhibition of the same cells; indeed, the number of directly inhibited output neurons is rather small (less than 15%). A second possibility is that these directly inhibited PAG neurons selectively innervate RVM cells that facilitate pain, whereas those that do not express μ receptors selectively innervate antinociceptive RVM neurons. If that were the case, administration of opioids to the PAG might both excite antinociceptive RVM neurons and de-facilitate ("inhibit") pronociceptive RVM neurons.

Another discrepancy refers to the RVM neurons that express μ receptors and were thought to facilitate nociception but contain GABA or serotonin (5HT). However, descending serotonergic projections facilitate nociception via the spinal $5HT_3$ receptor (Vanegas and Schaible 2004), and in some circumstances GABA can also be excitatory. Also, some RVM neurons might inhibit spinal inhibitory neurons, thus disinhibiting ("facilitating") nociceptive mechanisms. Whatever the case, reconciliation of the available data to the model will require further investigation.

DOES THE ELECTROPHYSIOLOGY SUPPORT THE MODEL?

In addition to the anatomical data, there are electrophysiological data in favor of, but also in disagreement with, our current model of opioid action upon brainstem pain-modulating circuits.

EFFECTS OF OPIOIDS ON SYNAPTIC TRANSMISSION

The cellular mechanisms of disinhibition have recently been examined using in vitro whole-cell patch-clamp recordings from identified PAG and RVM neurons in isolated brain slices. Experiments on synaptic transmission have demonstrated that activation of both μ-opioid receptors and cannabinoid CB1 receptors inhibits electrically evoked, $GABA_A$-mediated inhibitory postsynaptic currents in neurons throughout the PAG and RVM (Pan et al. 1990; Chieng and Christie 1994; Vaughan et al. 1999, 2003). Experiments using tetrodotoxin, which restricts drug effects to the presynaptic terminal and the postsynaptic membrane, indicate that both opioids and cannabinoids act presynaptically (Fig. 1, no. 2) because they reduce the rate, but have no effect on the amplitude and kinetics, of miniature inhibitory postsynaptic currents. The actions of opioids and cannabinoids are mediated by calcium-independent mechanisms in both brain regions, and opioid inhibition in the PAG is mediated by a lipoxygenase-coupled 4-aminopyridine-sensitive potassium conductance (Vaughan et al. 1997) (Fig. 2).

There are, however, a number of complicating factors. First, μ-opioid and cannabinoid CB1-receptor agonists also inhibit glutamatergic synaptic transmission in both the PAG and the RVM. Second, there are species and brain region

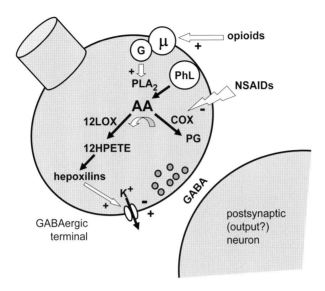

Fig. 2. Synapse of a GABAergic terminal upon an output neuron of the periaqueductal gray matter (see Fig. 1, PAG, no. 2). The action of opioids upon the G-protein-coupled μ-opioid receptor activates phospholipase A$_2$ (PLA$_2$), which cleaves arachidonic acid (AA) from membrane phospholipids (PhL). Under the action of cyclooxygenases (COX) and subsequent enzymes, AA yields prostaglandins (PG). Under the action of 12-lipoxygenases (12LOX) and subsequent enzymes, AA yields 12-hydroperoxyeicosatetraenoic acid (12HPETE) and hepoxilins. These molecules induce an increase in potassium conductance, thus hyperpolarizing the terminal and decreasing GABA release. Nonsteroidal anti-inflammatory drugs (NSAIDs) inhibit COX and thus leave more AA for the 12LOX pathway, which further decreases GABA release.

differences; for example, κ opioids also inhibit GABAergic transmission in the mouse PAG (Vaughan et al. 2003) and inhibit glutamatergic transmission in the rat RVM (Ackley et al. 2001). Finally, the effect of analgesics on synaptic transmission onto descending projection neurons has not yet been examined.

DIRECT SOMATIC EFFECTS OF OPIOIDS

The circuitry underlying the direct postsynaptic actions of opioid analgesics within the PAG and RVM has been studied in more detail. The majority (80–90%) of non-projection neurons within the lateral-ventrolateral PAG and the RVM are directly inhibited (Fig. 1, no. 1) by the activation by μ opioids of an inwardly rectifying potassium conductance, K_{ir} (Pan et al. 1990; Chieng and Christie 1994; Marinelli et al. 2002). In the RVM, 30% of these neurons are also inhibited by δ opioids (Marinelli et al. 2005). The majority of the non-projection neurons within the RVM are non-serotonergic (Marinelli et al. 2002), although it remains to be directly determined whether these opioid-sensitive putative interneurons are GABAergic. Taken together, these experiments show that local circuit neurons within the PAG and RVM are directly inhibited by opioids (Fig. 1, no. 1). This conclusion parallels the above findings of opioidergic reduction of presynaptic GABA release (Fig. 1, no. 2). In contrast to opioids, cannabinoids have no direct somatic effects on neurons in the PAG and RVM, including neurons that do and do not respond to opioids (Vaughan et al. 1999, 2000).

The responses of descending projection neurons in the PAG and RVM have been examined using a combination of in vitro electrophysiology and retrograde tract tracing. Mu opioids directly inhibit less than 15% of the neurons that project from the ventrolateral PAG (a major site of opioid-mediated analgesia) to the RVM (Osborne et al. 1996). In contrast, nearly equal proportions of RVM neurons that project to the dorsal horn of the spinal cord are directly inhibited by μ, δ, and κ opioids (60%, 45%, and 55%, respectively), and these neurons comprise mixed populations of serotonergic and non-serotonergic neurons (Marinelli et al. 2002).

AN EXPANDED UNDERSTANDING OF DISINHIBITION

The in vitro experiments described here support the disinhibition hypothesis, but only partly. The results suggest that μ-opioid disinhibition is produced both *presynaptically,* by inhibition of neurotransmitter release from the terminals of GABAergic neurons that synapse onto descending projection neurons in the PAG and the RVM (Fig. 1, no. 2), and *postsynaptically,* by direct inhibition of local circuit neurons that might be GABAergic (Fig. 1, no. 1). In addition, the overlapping μ- and δ-opioid postsynaptic inhibition of non-spinally projecting RVM neurons provides a potential cellular substrate for antinociceptive synergy between μ and δ opioids. Cannabinoids, however, only have presynaptic actions, and thus they partly differ from μ opioids. Finally, μ-, δ-, and κ-opioid postsynaptic actions on spinally projecting RVM neurons and on synaptic transmission in PAG and RVM are complex and do not easily fit into the disinhibition hypothesis.

DO NON-OPIOID ANALGESICS FIT IN THE MODEL?

Non-opioid analgesics, such as the traditional non-steroidal anti-inflammatory drugs (NSAIDs), may also induce antinociception by acting upon the PAG. This action, like that of opioids, is naloxone-reversible and may lead to tolerance and withdrawal.

Indeed, PAG microinjection and systemic administration of NSAIDs such as dipyrone (metamizol) or lysine-acetylsalicylate (LASA) produces antinociception, as shown by increased tail-flick and paw-withdrawal latencies to noxious heat, increased latencies in the hot-plate test, and decreased spinal dorsal horn neuronal responses to noxious stimulation within their receptive fields (Tortorici and Vanegas 1994, 1995; Tortorici et al. 1996; Vasquez and Vanegas 2000; Hernandez and Vanegas 2001; Pernia-Andrade et al. 2004; Vazquez et al. 2005). This finding suggests that clinically administered NSAIDs induce analgesia by acting not only at the peripheral tissues and the spinal cord (Campbell and Halushka 1996; Vanegas and Schaible 2001), but also directly at the PAG.

Interestingly, antinociception induced by dipyrone or LASA, whether microinjected into the PAG or administered systemically, is reversed when naloxone is administered either systemically or specifically to the PAG, the RVM, or the spinal cord. These findings suggest that the analgesic action of NSAIDs upon the PAG depends upon local endogenous opioids, and that activation of the PAG then triggers opioidergic circuits downstream along the descending pain control system, i.e., at the RVM and the spinal dorsal horn (Fig. 1).

Repeated administration of opioids carries the risk of inducing tolerance and of a potential withdrawal syndrome. Repeated administration of dipyrone or LASA, whether systemically or by PAG microinjection, induces both tolerance to the NSAID and cross-tolerance to morphine (Tortorici and Vanegas 2000; Pernia-Andrade et al. 2004). Furthermore, systemic administration of naloxone to NSAID-tolerant rats precipitates a withdrawal syndrome. Repeated administration of NSAIDs therefore causes some of the problems of repeated administration of opioids. These NSAID/opioid interactions may explain several clinical and experimental reports of tolerance to NSAIDs, warranting a warning against the possibility of a withdrawal syndrome in patients under chronic NSAID treatment.

The neuropeptide cholecystokinin is known to be involved in tolerance to opioids, and its antagonists can prevent or reverse opioid tolerance (Wiesenfeld-Hallin et al. 1999; Tortorici et al. 2003). Interestingly, cholecystokinin antagonists also prevent or reverse tolerance to dipyrone and its cross-tolerance to morphine (Tortorici et al. 2004), thus again showing a striking similarity between the actions of opioid and non-opioid analgesics at the PAG.

These findings reveal that the central antinociceptive action of NSAIDs is intimately associated with endogenous opioids, raising questions about the nature of the NSAID/opioid relationship within the PAG. Perhaps NSAIDs, whether administered systemically to patients or experimentally microinjected into the PAG of rats, activate the release of endogenous opioids at the PAG; these opioids would then induce analgesia, as described above. However, induction of opioid release by NSAIDs has never been investigated. An additional possibility for the NSAID/opioid interaction involves arachidonic acid processing along molecular pathways proposed some years ago for GABAergic neurons in the PAG (Vaughan et al. 1997; Vaughan 1998) and depicted in Fig. 2. According to this view, opioids promote the release of arachidonic acid from membrane phospholipids. Arachidonic acid can yield prostaglandins when acted upon by the cyclooxygenases and subsequent enzymes, and it can yield hepoxilins when acted upon by 12-lipoxygenases and subsequent enzymes. Hepoxilins are eicosanoids that increase potassium conductance, thereby hyperpolarizing the terminal and decreasing GABA release (Fig. 1, no. 2). As we have described in this chapter, a decrease in GABAergic inhibition in the PAG induces antinociception. When NSAIDs act upon the PAG, the cyclooxygenases are inhibited, thus leaving more arachidonic acid available for the hepoxilin pathway and thereby further decreasing GABAergic inhibition and inducing antinociception.

CONCLUSIONS

Not surprisingly, the neuronal and molecular interactions that support the descending inhibition of nociception have become more complex than was originally thought. This complexity poses new questions and offers new interpretations for the effects of both opioid and non-opioid analgesics. The considerable variety of potential interactions both in the PAG and the RVM has slowly become apparent. Finding out which pathways and synapses are boosted and which are damped by opioid and non-opioid analgesics should inspire much research in the years to come. Further, finding out how such pathways and synapses affect, and are affected by, chronic pain states and how this situation can be handled with analgesics for the patient's benefit promises to provide new strategies for pain management in these difficult conditions.

REFERENCES

Abbadie C, Pan YX, Pasternak GW. Differential distribution in rat brain of mu opioid receptor carboxy terminal splice variants MOR-1C-like and MOR-1-like immunoreactivity: evidence for region-specific processing. *J Comp Neurol* 2000; 419:244–256.

Ackley MA, Hurley RW, Virnich DE, Hammond DL. A cellular mechanism for the antinociceptive effect of a kappa opioid receptor agonist. *Pain* 2001; 91:377–388.

Arvidsson U, Riedl M, Chakrabarti S, et al. Distribution and targeting of a mu-opioid receptor (MOR1) in brain and spinal cord. *J Neurosci* 1995; 15:3328–3341.

Campbell WB, Halushka PV. Lipid-derived autacoids. Eicosanoids and platelet-activating factor. In: Hardman JG, Limbird LE, Molinoff PB, et al. (Eds). *Goodman & Gilman's The Pharmacological Basis of Therapeutics.* New York: McGraw-Hill, 1996, pp 601–616.

Chieng B, Christie MJ. Hyperpolarization by opioids acting on mu-receptors of a sub-population of rat periaqueductal grey neurones in vitro. *Br J Pharmacol* 1994; 113:121–128.

Commons KG, Aicher SA, Kow LM, Pfaff DW. Presynaptic and postsynaptic relations of mu-opioid receptors to gamma-aminobutyric acid-immunoreactive and medullary-projecting periaqueductal gray neurons. *J Comp Neurol* 2000; 419:532–542.

Duggan AW, North RA. Electrophysiology of opioids. *Pharmacol Rev* 1983; 35:219–281.

Fields H. State-dependent opioid control of pain. *Nat Rev Neurosci* 2004; 5:565–575.

Hernandez N, Vanegas H. Antinociception induced by PAG-microinjected dipyrone (metamizol) in rats: involvement of spinal endogenous opioids. *Brain Res* 2001; 896:175–178.

Kalyuzhny AE, Wessendorf MW. CNS GABA neurons express the mu-opioid receptor: immuno-cytochemical studies. *Neuroreport* 1997; 8:3367–3372.

Kalyuzhny AE, Wessendorf MW. Relationship of μ- and δ-opioid receptors to GABAergic neurons in the central nervous system, including antinociceptive brainstem circuits. *J Comp Neurol* 1998; 392:528–547.

Kalyuzhny AE, Arvidsson U, Wu W, Wessendorf MW. Mu-opioid and delta-opioid receptors are expressed in brainstem antinociceptive circuits: studies using immunocytochemistry and retrograde tract-tracing. *J Neurosci* 1996; 16:6490–6503.

Mansour A, Fox CA, Burke S, et al. Mu, delta, and kappa opioid receptor mRNA expression in the rat CNS: an in situ hybridization study. *J Comp Neurol* 1994a; 350:412–438.

Mansour A, Thompson RC, Akil H, Watson SJ. Mu-opioid receptor mRNA expression in the rat CNS: comparison to mu-receptor binding. *Brain Res* 1994b; 643:245–265.

Marinelli S, Vaughan CW, Schnell SA, Wessendorf MW, Christie MJ. Rostral ventromedial medulla neurons that project to the spinal cord express multiple opioid receptor phenotypes. *J Neurosci* 2002; 22:10847–10855.

Marinelli S, Connor M, Schnell SA, et al. δ-Opioid receptor-mediated actions on rostral ventro-medial medulla neurons. *Neuroscience* 2005; 132:239–244.

Osborne PB, Vaughan CW, Wilson HI, Christie MJ. Opioid inhibition of rat periaqueductal grey neurones with identified projections to rostral ventromedial medulla in vitro. *J Physiol (Lond)* 1996; 490:383–389.

Pan ZZ, Williams JT, Osborne PB. Opioid actions on single nucleus raphe magnus neurons from rat and guinea-pig *in vitro*. *J Physiol (Lond)* 1990; 427:519–532.

Pernia-Andrade AJ, Tortorici V, Vanegas H. Induction of opioid tolerance by lysine-acetylsalicylate in rats. *Pain* 2004; 111:191–200.

Tortorici V, Vanegas H. Putative role of medullary off- and on-cells in the antinociception produced by dipyrone (metamizol) administered systemically or microinjected into PAG. *Pain* 1994; 57:197–205.

Tortorici V, Vanegas H. Antinociception induced by systemic or PAG-microinjected lysine-ace-tylsalicylate in rats. Effects on tail-flick related activity of medullary off- and on-cells. *Eur J Neurosci* 1995; 7:1857–1865.

Tortorici V, Vanegas H. Opioid tolerance induced by metamizol (dipyrone) microinjections into the periaqueductal gray of rats. *Eur J Neurosci* 2000; 12:4074–4080.

Tortorici V, Vasquez E, Vanegas H. Naloxone partial reversal of the antinociception produced by dipyrone microinjected in the periaqueductal gray of rats. Possible involvement of medullary off- and on-cells. *Brain Res* 1996; 725:106–110.

Tortorici V, Nogueira L, Salas R, Vanegas H. Involvement of local cholecystokinin in the toler-ance induced by morphine microinjections into the periaqueductal gray of rats. *Pain* 2003; 102:9–16.

Tortorici V, Nogueira L, Aponte Y, Vanegas H. Involvement of cholecystokinin in the opioid toler-ance induced by dipyrone (metamizol) microinjections into the periaqueductal gray matter of rats. *Pain* 2004; 112:113–120.

Vanegas H, Schaible H-G. Prostaglandins and cyclooxygenases in the spinal cord. *Prog Neurobiol* 2001; 64:327–363.

Vanegas H, Schaible H-G. Descending control of persistent pain: inhibitory or facilitatory? *Brain Res Rev* 2004; 46:295–309.

Vaughan CW. Enhancement of opioid inhibition of GABAergic synaptic transmission by cyclo-oxygenase inhibitors in rat periaqueductal grey neurones. *Br J Pharmacol* 1998; 123:1479–1481.

Vaughan CW, Ingram SL, Connor MA, Christie MJ. How opioids inhibit GABA-mediated neuro-transmission. *Nature (Lond)* 1997; 390:611–614.

Vaughan CW, McGregor IS, Christie MJ. Cannabinoid receptor activation inhibits GABAergic neurotransmission in rostral ventromedial medulla neurons in vitro. *Br J Pharmacol* 1999; 127:935–940.

Vaughan CW, Connor M, Bagley EE, Christie MJ. Actions of cannabinoids on membrane proper-ties and synaptic transmission in rat periaqueductal gray neurons in vitro. *Mol Pharmacol* 2000; 57:288–295.

Vaughan CW, Bagley EE, Drew GM, et al. Cellular actions of opioids on periaqueductal grey neurons from C57B16/J mice and mutant mice lacking MOR-1. *Br J Pharmacol* 2003; 139:362–367.

Vasquez E, Vanegas H. The antinociceptive effect of PAG-microinjected dipyrone in rats is mediated by endogenous opioids of the rostral ventromedial medulla. *Brain Res* 2000; 854:249–252.

Vazquez E, Hernandez N, Escobar W, Vanegas H. Antinociception induced by intravenous di-pyrone (metamizol) upon dorsal horn neurons: involvement of endogenous opioids at the periaqueductal gray matter, the nucleus raphe magnus, and the spinal cord in rats. *Brain Res* 2005; 1048:211–217.

Wang H, Wessendorf MW. μ- and δ-Opioid receptor mRNAs are expressed in spinally projecting serotonergic and nonserotonergic neurons of the rostral ventromedial medulla. *J Comp Neurol* 1999; 404:183–196.

Wang H, Wessendorf MW. μ- and δ-opioid receptor mRNAs are expressed in periaqueductal gray neurons projecting to the rostral ventromedial medulla. *Neuroscience* 2002; 109:619–634.

Wiesenfeld-Hallin Z, Alster P, Grass S, et al. Opioid sensitivity in antinociception: role of anti-opioid systems with emphasis on cholecystokinin and NMDA receptors. In: Kalso E, McQuay HJ, Wiesenfeld-Hallin Z (Eds). *Opioid Sensitivity of Chronic Noncancer Pain,* Progress in Pain Research and Management, Vol. 14. Seattle: IASP Press, 1999, pp 237–252.

Correspondence to: Prof. Dr. Horacio Vanegas, Institut für Physiologie I, Friedrich-Schiller-Universität, Teichgraben 8, 07740 Jena, Germany. Email: hvanegas@ivic.ve.

Proceedings of the 11th World Congress on Pain,
edited by Herta Flor, Eija Kalso, and Jonathan O.
Dostrovsky, IASP Press, Seattle, © 2006.

28

Corticothalamic Feedback from the Primary Somatosensory Cortex: A Link for Bottom-Up and Top-Down Processing of Innocuous and Noxious Inputs

Lénaïc Monconduit, Alberto Lopez-Avila, Jean-Louis Molat, Maryse Chalus, and Luis Villanueva

INSERM E-216, University of Clermont, Clermont-Ferrand, France

Anatomical, physiological, and clinical data implicate several cortical regions in pain perception, but their precise roles in pain processing remain poorly understood. This is especially the case for the primary somatosensory cortex (S1). The proposal that S1 plays a major role in the localization and discrimination of pain is still controversial (Bushnell et al. 1999). A powerful endogenous control of nociception probably originates from S1. Cortical activity must be highly dependent on reciprocal interactions with thalamic relays because there are nearly 10 times as many fibers projecting back from S1 to the ventrobasal thalamus as there are in the forward direction from thalamus to cortex (Deschênes et al. 1998). The function of this massive feedback network in pain has not been fully studied. Although numerous findings indicate a substantial influence of S1 on the processing of tactile information at a thalamic level, there has been no definitive demonstration of a major influence of S1 on the response properties to noxious inputs to the ventroposterolateral (VPL) thalamic nucleus, which is a major nociceptive relay in the spinothalamic system of the rat (Albe-Fessard et al. 1985).

This chapter summarizes a study in which we examined the fine anatomical and functional organization of the VPL/S1 network by combining electrophysiological, high-resolution anatomical tracing and simultaneous extracellular recordings in the S1 cortex and the VPL nucleus.

METHODS

A total of 67 male Sprague-Dawley rats weighing 220–250 g were used in this study. All the animal experiments were approved by our local animal care committee and were in accordance with the guidelines of the IASP.

IN VIVO SINGLE-CELL TRACING AND ELECTROPHYSIOLOGICAL CHARACTERIZATION IN THE VPL

Surgery, stimulation, recordings of neuronal activity, and individual labeling of VPL neurons were performed as described previously (Monconduit and Villanueva 2005). A systematic search was performed for units responding to cutaneous tactile and/or noxious thermal stimulation of the contralateral hindpaw. Once a VPL neuron was characterized, it was individually labeled by juxtacellular iontophoresis of biotin-dextran. This technique combines the functional characterization of extracellularly recorded VPL neurons and the staining, in a Golgi-like manner, of their perikarya, dendritic, and axonal fields. Following postoperative survival of 2–3 days, the animals were re-anesthetized with an overdose of chloral hydrate and perfused with phosphate buffered solution containing paraformaldehyde, glutaraldehyde, and picric acid. Their brains were then removed and processed for biotin-dextran histochemistry. Digitized gray-scale images were built using a computer-assisted reconstruction of the biotin-dextran labeling technique. In other experimental series, to clarify the extent and organization of the S1/VPL loop, we made iontophoretic injections of the high-resolution anterograde/retrograde tracer tetramethylrhodamine-labeled dextran, under electrophysiological control, with the aim of labeling the VPL area containing the neurons activated by innocuous and noxious cutaneous inputs from the hindpaw.

EXTRACELLULAR RECORDINGS

In rats anesthetized with halothane, local field potential and multi-unit recordings were obtained in layers V–VI of the hindpaw representation area of the S1 cortex and in the VPL thalamic nucleus. A systematic search was made for VPL units responding to innocuous stimulation (rubbing, gentle stroking) of the extremity of the hindpaw. Calibrated brushing of the extremity of the hindpaw was performed with a computer-driven, motorized, 360°-turning paintbrush. Thermal stimuli were produced with a 13-mm^2 circular thermode whose temperature was controlled by thermoelectric Peltier elements that were driven by a computer. Tonic noxious thermal stimuli consisted of 30-second 44°–55°–44°C ramps that were applied to the extremity of the hindpaw in an area adjacent to the brushing. We tested the effects of microinjections within layer VI of S1 (see Fig. 3A), on background and evoked cortical and thalamic neuronal responses. The drugs employed were DL-homocysteic acid (10 mM, 200 nL dissolved in saline), muscimol (8.7 mM, 500 nL dissolved in saline), and a subconvulsive dose of bicuculline (50 μM, 500 nL dissolved in saline).

RESULTS

STRUCTURE-FUNCTION PROPERTIES OF VPL NEURONS

All the VPL neurons had receptive fields that could be activated by natural cutaneous stimulation of the paws. As in previous studies, the cells were classified as nociceptive-specific (NS) cells if they were responsive only to noxious heat (48°C), as non-nociceptive (NN) cells if they were responsive only to innocuous brushing, and as wide-dynamic range (WDR) cells if they were responsive to both noxious heat and brushing. As shown in the individual examples in Fig. 1, none of the functional categories was associated with cells of a particular morphology, size, or dendritic tree. Cumulative data in Fig. 1 show that most of the neurons were multipolar with dense dendritic arbors of variable length and orientations. All the axons of NS, NN, and WDR cells turned rostrally through the internal capsule, often after giving off collaterals in the thalamic reticular nucleus. These axons then entered the globus pallidus and striatum, the corpus callosum, crossed the forceps minor, and terminated mainly within layer IV of the primary somatosensory cortex. Terminal labeling was in the form of thin collateral fibers that innervated a common area of S1.

Injections of tetramethylrhodamine-labeled dextran into the physiologically defined area of the VPL (Fig. 2A) produced dense labeling of efferents, which terminated mainly as patches in layer IV of the rostral S1 cortex and extended superficially to layer III (Fig. 2B). Fig. 2C shows, at high magnification, a reconstruction of labeling in S1, in the form of a dense network of thin afferent fibers with small varicosities in the centralmost aspect of layer IV. Moreover, numerous retrogradely labeled neurons with apical dendrites were observed in layer VI. These corticothalamic cells occupied the same area as that covered by the band of afferent labeling in layer IV. Interestingly, the densest labeling was located in the same S1 zone that contained the afferents of physiologically identified neurons as shown in Fig. 1.

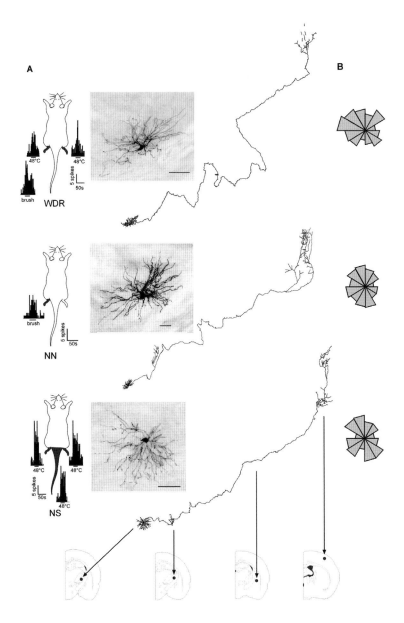

Fig. 1. (A) Digital photomicrographs of the perikaryon and proximal processes of three different functional classes of juxtacellularly stained nociceptive-specific (NS), non-nociceptive (NN), and wide-dynamic range (WDR) neurons of the ventroposterolateral thalamic nucleus (VPL). For each cell, the response characteristics to peripheral cutaneous stimuli and the receptive fields are presented. Camera-lucida drawings represent cells with their axonal processes and terminal innervation in a common area within S1. Scale bars represent 50 μm. (B) Cumulative data showing the topographic distribution of dendritic arbors of juxtacellularly labeled VPL cells. Areas representing the percentage of the total length of the dendrites within 30° sections show the widespread, multipolar orientation of the dendritic trees.

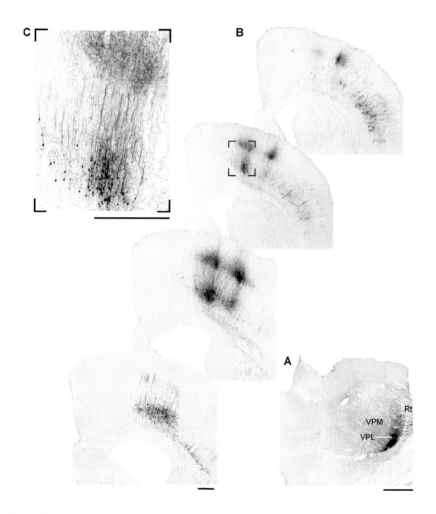

Fig. 2. Digital photomicrographs of labeling in coronal sections of the primary somatosensory (S1) cortex (B) following the tetramethylrhodamine-labeled dextran injection into the ventro-posterolateral (VPL) thalamic nucleus shown in panel A. Panel C shows higher magnification of the layer IV afferent labeling from the VPL and layer VI efferent labeling in the region delineated in panel B. Note the numerous retrogradely labeled cells in layer VI, which occupy the same area covered by the patches of anterograde labeling in layer IV. Scale bars = 500 μm. Rt = reticular thalamic nucleus; VPM = ventroposteromedial thalamic nucleus.

CORTICOTHALAMIC MODULATION OF VPL RESPONSES TO SOMATOSENSORY STIMULI IS MODALITY-SPECIFIC

The strong convergence of spinal and lemniscal afferents to the VPL (Ma et al. 1987), together with the close correspondence between afferents and efferents within the ventrobasal thalamus-S1 network, suggests the existence of functionally related thalamocortical circuits that are involved in the modulation of innocuous and noxious inputs. To investigate this possibility, we examined corticothalamic effects on calibrated, innocuous mechanical (brushing) and noxious heat-evoked responses of VPL cells. We made simultaneous multi-unit recordings of the responses of VPL and local field potential recordings of layers V–VI of S1 following innocuous and noxious cutaneous stimulation of neighboring areas on the hindpaw (Fig. 3A). Corticothalamic activity was depressed or enhanced following microinjections in the layer V–VI zone that innervates VPL neurons driven from receptive fields on the hindpaw (Fig. 3B–D).

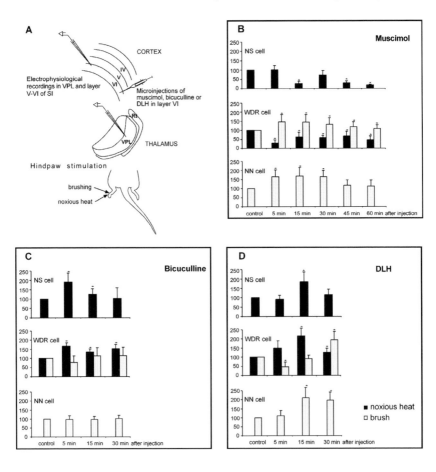

Fig. 3. (A) Experimental setup for the multi-unit, multisite recordings and cortical microinjections. Summary of the experiments investigating the effects on the responses of nociceptive-specific (NS), non-nociceptive (NN) and wide-dynamic range neurons (WDR) of the ventroposterolateral (VPL) thalamus of microinjections of (B) muscimol, (C) bicuculline, or (D) DL-homocysteic acid (DLH) in layers V–VI of the primary somatosensory cortex (S1). Results are expressed as percentages of control responses recorded before the microinjection ($P < 0.05$).

Microinjections of the GABA$_A$ agonist muscimol strongly reduced cortical activity in deep layers of S1 15 minutes after the injection, and concomitantly, brushing-evoked responses were enhanced and noxious heat-evoked responses of VPL neurons were depressed (Fig. 3B). Bicuculline enhanced noxious heat-evoked responses of NS and WDR cells without affecting innocuous-stimulation-evoked responses of NN and WDR neurons 5 minutes after the injection (Fig. 3C). The background activity and thresholds for peripheral activation of VPL neurons were not significantly affected by either muscimol or bicuculline.

Glutamatergic activation of corticothalamic output following microinjections of the excitatory amino acid DL-homocysteic acid (DLH) into layers V–VI enhanced noxious-stimulation-evoked responses of both WDR and NS neurons and responses of NN cells (Fig. 3D). Innocuous-evoked responses of WDR were affected in a biphasic way, with a depression followed by a facilitation. As shown in Fig. 3D, the effects of DLH were significant between 5–30 minutes following microinjection.

DISCUSSION

The findings described in this chapter demonstrate that top-down influences from the S1 cortex can differentially affect the responses of VPL neurons to innocuous and noxious cutaneous inputs. Importantly, our data provide evidence that corticothalamic feedback from S1 to VPL is in part stimulus-driven. Thus, VPL responses to somatosensory inputs are defined at least in part by GABAergic and glutamatergic-mediated, excitatory and inhibitory corticofugal mechanisms.

We found that glutamatergic enhancement of corticofugal feedback elicits a selective facilitation of WDR and NS noxious-stimulation-evoked responses, a facilitation of the NN evoked responses, and biphasic effects on innocuous-stimulation-evoked responses of WDR cells. It is possible that the effects observed not only are due to corticothalamic feedback, but are mediated by corticobulbar/corticospinal influences.

Former studies in the somatosensory system have demonstrated that S1 can selectively modulate thalamic spatial responses through specific excitatory or inhibitory mechanisms that either sharpen or enlarge thalamic receptive fields (Rauscheker 1998). Our findings show that the sensory-discriminative properties of S1 are more widespread because S1 is also able to selectively modulate different somatosensory submodalities. Indeed, under some experimental conditions, the effects of somatosensory-driven corticothalamic feedback are highly specific, consisting of either an enhancement of cutaneous responses evoked by innocuous stimulation or a reduction of those evoked by noxious stimulation.

CONCLUSIONS

Earlier human brain-imaging studies revealed that noxious heat applied to regions of the forearm elicited either an increase, a decrease, or a lack of modification of activity in the S1 cortex (Bushnell et al. 1999). Recent studies showed that these discrepancies were due mostly to the fact that S1 activation by either tactile or painful stimuli is strongly modulated by cognitive factors that modify somatosensory perception (Meyer et al. 1991; Hofbauer et al. 2001). Modulation of S1 activity in humans seems to occur only with the concurrent presence of somatosensory activation. Although it is still unknown how the cortex "knows" that inputs are nociceptive or innocuous, part of the modulation observed in human studies may be subserved by corticofugal mechanisms driven by peripheral stimuli that are modality specific, such as those described here. Taken together, human and animal studies indicate that stimulus-evoked responses of S1 corticofugal neurons can contribute to somatosensory discrimination by selecting thalamic responses to preferred versus non-preferred inputs, in a modality-specific fashion. In conjunction with mechanisms underlying topographic response sharpening, heightened activity in corticofugal S1 neurons may create a circumscribed zone of enhanced activity within the thalamocortical loop that mediates discrimination between tactile and painful sensations.

ACKNOWLEDGMENTS

This work was supported by the Fondation pour la Recherche Médicale, Institut UPSA de la Douleur, and Société Française d'Etude et de Traitement de la Douleur. We are grateful to Dr. S.W. Cadden for advice in the preparation of the manuscript.

REFERENCES

Albe-Fessard D, Berkley KJ, Kruger L, Ralston HJ, Willis WD. Diencephalic mechanisms of pain sensation. *Brain Res Rev* 1985; 9:217–296.

Bushnell MC, Duncan GH, Hofbauer RK, et al. Pain perception: is there a role for primary somatosensory cortex? *Proc Natl Acad Sci USA* 1999; 96:7705–7709.

Deschênes M, Veinante P, Zhang ZW. The organization of corticothalamic projections: reciprocity versus parity. *Brain Res Rev* 1998; 28:286–308.

Hofbauer RK, Rainville P, Duncan GH, Bushnell MC. Cortical representation of the sensory dimension of pain. *J Neurophysiol* 2001; 86:402–411.

Ma W, Peschanski M, Ralston HJ. The differential synaptic organization of the spinal and lemniscal projections to the ventrobasal complex of the rat thalamus. Evidence for convergence of the two systems upon single thalamic neurons. *Neuroscience* 1987; 3:925–934.

Meyer E, Ferguson SS, Zatorre RJ, et al. Attention modulates somatosensory cerebral blood flow response to vibrotactile stimulation as measured by positron emission tomography. *Ann Neurol* 1991; 29:440–443.

Monconduit L, Villanueva L. The lateral ventromedial thalamic nucleus spreads nociceptive signals from the whole body surface to layer I of the frontal cortex. *Eur J Neurosci* 2005; 12:3395–3402.

Rauscheker JP. Cortical control of the thalamus: top-down processing and plasticity. *Nat Neurosci* 1998; 1:179–180.

Correspondence to: Luis Villanueva, DDS, PhD, INSERM E-216, Université de Clermont-1, 11 Boulevard Charles de Gaulle, 63000 Clermont-Ferrand. Email: luis. villanueva@u-clermont1.fr.

Proceedings of the 11th World Congress on Pain,
edited by Herta Flor, Eija Kalso, and Jonathan O.
Dostrovsky, IASP Press, Seattle, © 2006.

29

Pain and Body Protection: Sensory, Autonomic, Neuroendocrine, and Behavioral Mechanisms in the Control of Inflammation and Hyperalgesia

Wilfrid Jänig,[a] C. Richard Chapman,[b] and Paul G. Green[c]

[a]Department of Physiology, University of Kiel, Kiel, Germany; [b]Pain Research Center, Department of Anesthesiology, University of Utah School of Medicine, Salt Lake City, Utah, USA; [c]Department of Oral and Maxillofacial Surgery, University of California San Francisco, National Institutes of Health Pain Center, San Francisco, California, USA

Mechanisms of inflammation, pain, and hyperalgesia cannot be reduced to peripheral local processes involving cells of the immune system, the vasculature, peripheral nociceptive afferent fibers, and sympathetic fibers. How are these cellular and subcellular processes, which form the basis of inflammation, pain, and hyperalgesia, orchestrated by the brain as part of the continuous protection of the body against agents from outside as well as from within the body?

This chapter presents data obtained in various experimental approaches that show that the brain plays an important role in controlling protective body reactions via the neuroendocrine system (the hypothalamo-pituitary axis and the sympatho-adrenal system) and the autonomic (sympathetic) nervous system. Feedback to the brain occurs via various signaling molecules (e.g., interleukins), hard-wired nociceptive afferents, and other afferent neurons (Fig. 1). The three bodily domains (cutaneous, deep somatic, and visceral) participate in this process in an integrated fashion. Ideas presented in this chapter will show how experimental studies on humans and in animal models relate to clinical pain conditions. These ideas might contribute to the understanding of various clinical pain syndromes, such as fibromyalgia, chronic fatigue syndrome, sickness behavior, irritable bowel syndrome, and functional dyspepsia. This chapter summarizes human studies involving the interaction of the nervous, endocrine,

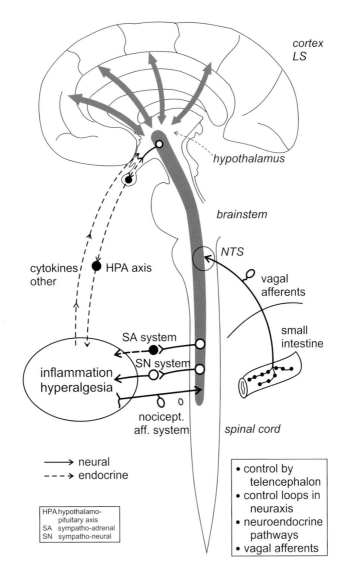

Fig. 1. The neuraxis contains neuronal circuits (shaded area) that control nociceptor sensitivity and inflammation in the periphery of the body via the sympatho-adrenal (SA) system and the hypothalamo-pituitary-adrenal (HPA) system. Feedback information from the peripheral inflammatory process occurs via nociceptive primary afferent neurons and cytokines. Abdominal vagal afferents signal events from the inner defense line of the body (gut-associated lymphoid tissue) to the lower brainstem (NTS = nucleus tractus solitarii). The telencephalon controls inflammation and sensitivity of nociceptors via the circuits in the neuraxis (see shaded double arrows). LS = limbic system.

and immune systems, and then describes rat studies of integrated neural and neuroendocrine control of experimental joint inflammation and of bradykinin-induced mechanical hyperalgesic behavior.

THE DEFENSE RESPONSE: BRAIN-BODY MECHANISMS

The defense response is a complex systemic response to threat that enhances the probability of survival. Because pain as a phenomenal experience is the awareness of tissue trauma, the defense response tends to accompany events that cause pain. At the physiological level, the nociception occasioned by an injury triggers a complex protective reaction that involves nervous, endocrine, and immune responses.

Response to nociception involves multiple levels of the nervous system (Byers and Bonica 2001). Peripherally, injury activates nociceptors, and the chemical processes that comprise inflammation sensitize nociceptive endings. Centrally, complex modulatory processes come into play at the level of the dorsal horn (Vanegas and Schaible 2004). Higher-level noradrenergic circuits originating at the locus ceruleus generate processes that ultimately produce a sense of threat (Charney and Deutch 1996). The periaqueductal gray system rapidly readies the organism for immediate fight or flight and may activate descending pathways that inhibit nociceptive traffic (Bandler et al. 2000). The frontal-amygdala system also contributes heavily to defense, integrating interpretation of potentially threatening events and other higher-order cognitive processes (Hariri et al. 2003).

The endocrine system, in addition to controlling growth, development, and reproduction, contributes to defense, working in concert with the sympathetic nervous system to provide the protective stress response. The main mediators of the stress response are (1) the hypothalamo-pituitary-adrenocortical (HPA) axis, including the corticotrophin-releasing hormone (CRH) system, and (2) the noradrenergic locus ceruleus system and the sympatho-adrenal system (Tsigos and Chrousos 2002). Activation of central noradrenergic neurons, e.g., in the locus ceruleus or in the lower brainstem (Rassnick et al. 1994; Dayas et al. 2001), stimulates several peripheral sympathetic pathways. In humans, this response manifests as increased heart rate and stroke volume, sweaty palms, and rapid respiration together with a sense of threat, hypervigilance, and a readiness to fight or flee.

The immune system perceives threats that the nervous system cannot detect, namely the invasion of microorganisms, and reacts by mounting local inflammatory responses, such as around a wound (Blalock 2005). Many elements of the immune system provide immediate host defense, including pro-inflammatory cytokines acting peripherally and centrally (O'Connor et al. 2003). Evidence suggests that cytokines may directly activate or sensitize nociceptive fibers (Sommer and Kress 2004) and that they act upon the hypothalamus. During stress, microglia can sensitize central pathways and create allodynia (Watkins and Maier 2002). If the nervous, endocrine, and immune systems work in concert to mount a defense response, how do they communicate with one another? Below, we briefly review communication between the nervous and immune systems, the nervous and endocrine systems, and the immune and endocrine systems. The reciprocal communication of these three systems involves many messenger molecules, and the role of most of them is poorly understood (Fig. 2).

Communication between the nervous system and the immune system can occur, in part, via the sympathetic innervation of all lymphoid organs (Vizi and Elenkov 2002; Mignini et al. 2003). The axon terminals of the sympathetic nervous system release norepinephrine and neuropeptide Y, and the adrenal

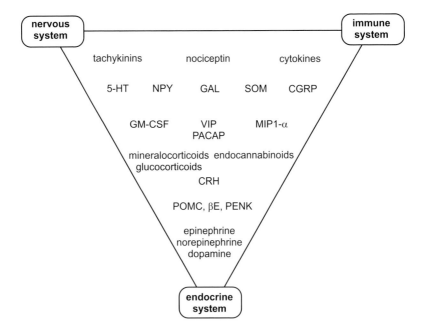

Fig. 2. The nervous, immune, and endocrine systems continuously interact through a common chemical language. All three systems produce and bind hormones, peptides, cytokines, and neurotransmitters that, in addition to their other functions, serve as inter-system messenger substances. This figure illustrates some of these messenger substances: 5-HT (serotonin), NPY (neuropeptide Y), GAL (galanin), SOM (somatostatin), CGRP (calcitonin-gene-related peptide), GM-CSF (granulocyte macrophage colony stimulation factor), VIP (vasoactive intestinal peptide), PACAP (pituitary adenylate cyclase-activating peptide), MIP1-α (macrophage inflammatory protein 1 alpha), CRH (corticotrophin-releasing hormone), POMC (pro-opiomelanocortin), β-E (beta-endorphin), and PENK (preproenkephalin).

medulla releases epinephrine into the systemic circulation. These substances presumably exert a strong influence on many immune cells, principally through adrenoreceptors and possibly the via the neuropeptide Y1 and Y2 receptors that such cells bear (Torres et al. 2005).

Neuropeptides and their receptors are involved in both nervous and immune systems (ten Bokum et al. 2000; Mignini et al. 2003). T lymphocytes express receptors for substance P, calcitonin-gene-related peptide, somatostatin, and vasoactive intestinal peptide, and macrophages express receptors for pituitary adenylate cyclase-activating polypeptide (PACAP). Afferent C fibers within lymphoid organs release these same peptides (ten Bokum et al. 2000; Delgado et al. 2003). Vasoactive intestinal peptide and PACAP exert an anti-inflammatory influence on the immune system by inhibiting the production of pro-inflammatory cytokines (Delgado et al. 2004).

Perhaps the best studied link between the nervous and immune systems is the cytokine connection. Cytokines act at the hypothalamus (Dunn et al. 1999), and electrical stimulation of the vagus nerve induces interleukin 1-β in the hypothalamus and hippocampus (Hosoi et al. 2000). The lipid signaling molecules of the endocannabinoid system act at receptors CB1 and CB2. Immune cells express these cannabinoid receptors (Klein et al. 2003). Endocannabinoids decrease neurotoxicity and inhibit the release of pro-inflammatory cytokines from microglia (Walter and Stella 2004).

The hypothalamus plays a central role in endocrine responses (Tsigos and Chrousos 2002; Raffin-Sanson et al. 2003). The hypothalamic periventricular nucleus produces CRH and arginine vasopressin, which act as both neurotransmitters and neurohormones (De Kloet 2004). During stress, CRH activates serotonergic neurons in the caudal dorsal raphe nucleus, which may facilitate modulation of nociceptive signals (Hammack et al. 2002). Activation of these serotonergic neurons also stimulates the HPA axis, invoking the synthesis and secretion of CRH (Jorgensen et al. 2002; Itoi et al. 2004). Yet another aspect of neuroendocrine communication is the pro-opiomelanocortin system (Raffin-Sanson et al. 2003). The endocrine stress response acts powerfully at multiple levels of the nervous system and yet is under the control of the nervous system.

Coordination of the endocrine and immune systems involves cannabinoids that activate the HPA axis (Wenger et al. 2003). In addition, cytokines regulate the HPA axis, which in turn regulates the immune system through cortisol (Turnbull and Rivier 1999).

NEUROENDOCRINE PATHWAYS MODULATE
THE INFLAMMATORY RESPONSE

Inflammation is a protective, beneficial response to injury, irritation, or infection. It is a multicomponent response consisting of increased blood flow, vascular permeability, attraction of leukocytes, and sensitization of primary afferent neurons. Together, these inflammatory components help in clearing invading microorganisms, releasing potent bactericidal cytotoxic agents (e.g., reactive oxygen species), and promoting tissue repair. The inflammatory response constitutes a positive feedback inflammatory cascade that, if allowed to continue unchecked, results in tissue damage due to an excess of cytotoxic mediators. While removal or cessation of the stimulus that initiated an inflammatory response may be sufficient to terminate inflammation, the noxious component of inflammation may play a role as a generator of negative feedback control mechanisms of the inflammatory response.

NOXIOUS SOMATIC STIMULATION: ROLE OF THE
HYPOTHALAMIC-PITUITARY-ADRENAL AND
SYMPATHOADRENAL AXES

The effect of noxious somatic stimulation on the magnitude of plasma extravasation was tested in a rat model of synovial inflammation, produced by application of the potent endogenous inflammatory mediator, bradykinin (BK). Continuous perfusion of BK through the rat knee joint (Fig. 3A) produced a large, sustained increase in plasma extravasation (Fig. 3B, filled circles). The BK-induced plasma extravasation response is largely dependent on the

---

Fig. 3. Experimental inflammation is controlled by the hypothalamo-pituitary-adrenal axis. (A) Bradykinin (BK)-induced plasma extravasation was determined in the knee joint of anesthetized rats. Skin overlying the knee was excised to expose the joint capsule, and rats were then given an intravenous injection of Evans blue dye (50 mg/kg); 30-gauge inflow and 25-gauge outflow needles were then inserted into the knee joint cavity for administration of perfusion fluid (0.9% saline at 250 µL/min). Perfusion fluid was collected every 5 minutes for up to 120 minutes, and dye concentration was determined spectrophotometrically at 620 nm. The absorbance at this wave length is linearly related to the dye concentration and therefore to the degree of plasma extravasation of the synovia (see ordinate scale in panel B). Following collection of the first three samples to establish baseline plasma extravasation levels, BK and other substances are added to the perfusing fluid. (B) Addition of BK (160 nM) to the perfusion fluid produced a rapid and sustained increase in the magnitude of plasma extravasation (filled circles, $n = 8$). Noxious transcutaneous electrical stimulation (25 mA, 3 Hz, 0.25-ms pulses) applied to one hindpaw after sample 8 produced a rapid decrease in the magnitude of plasma extravasation (open triangles, $n = 7$). This inhibition produced by noxious electrical stimulation was prevented in animals that had been adrenalectomized 1 week prior to the perfusion study (inverted open triangles, $n = 7$). Data are mean ± SEM. Panel B is adapted from Green et al. (1995). →

postganglionic sympathetic neuron terminal; surgical sympathectomy reduced the magnitude of response by 60–70%, but acute sympathetic decentralization (section of the preganglionic axons) had no significant effect (Miao et al. 1996a,b; Green et al. 1997).

Noxious, but not non-noxious, somatic electrical stimulation to the hindpaw markedly inhibited the magnitude of plasma extravasation (Fig. 3B, open triangles). Destruction of the peripheral terminals of primary afferent neurons by neonatal treatment with neurotoxic doses of capsaicin markedly reduced the effect of electrical stimulation (Green et al. 1995). This phenomenon was not

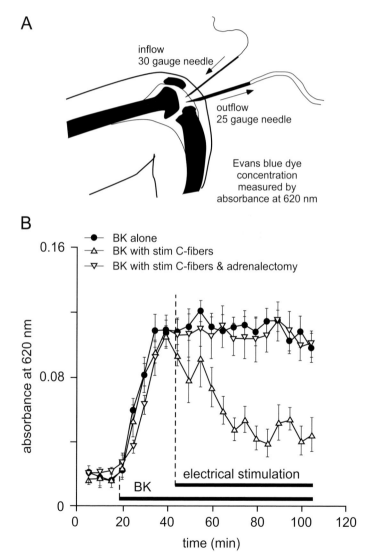

due to reflex activation of sympathetic efferents supplying the synovia, since acute decentralization of the lumbar sympathetic chain (denervation of the sympathetic postganglionic neurons by interruption of the preganglionic axons), while leaving the sympathetic terminals intact, did not prevent the inhibition of plasma extravasation.

Acute transection of the spinal cord at the T2 level prevented inhibition of plasma extravasation, suggesting the participation of ascending spinal pathways. The effect of noxious electrical stimulation applied to the forepaw was not blocked by T2 level spinal transection, suggesting that supraspinal mechanisms are involved in the inhibition. The inhibition of plasma extravasation by noxious stimulation was also markedly attenuated by hypophysectomy and by adrenal-ectomy (inverted open triangles in Fig. 3B). This finding suggests a role for the HPA axis. In support of this suggestion, intravenous corticosterone also sup-pressed bradykinin-induced plasma extravasation (Green et al. 1997). Adrenal enucleation, as well as adrenal denervation, partially attenuated the inhibition, suggesting a contribution from the adrenal medulla (Green et al. 1995).

Interestingly, when intraplantar capsaicin was used as a noxious stimulus in the hindpaw, the dose-dependent inhibition of BK-induced plasma extravasation was only partially inhibited by hypophysectomy, but it was virtually abolished after ablation of adrenal medulla function (Miao and Levine 1999; Miao et al. 2000). This model contrasts with electrical stimulation, in which hypophy-sectomy completely blocked the inhibition of plasma extravasation, whereas ablation of adrenal medulla function produced only a partial attenuation. There are qualitative differences in the somatic noxious stimulation by capsaicin and electrical stimulation. Electrical stimulation indiscriminately and synchronously activates all afferents including $A\beta$ and all $A\delta$ fibers, while capsaicin activates predominantly C fibers and a subpopulation of $A\delta$ fibers, asynchronously and at a lower intensity. This differential pattern of activation of nociceptive afferents could be responsible for specific encoding of nociceptive signals to selectively activate specific neuroendocrine circuits. In other words, both HPA and sym-pathoadrenal neuroendocrine pathways are activated by noxious stimulation, and the relative activation of one pathway may be dependent on qualitative or quantitative differences of nociceptive input.

VAGAL AFFERENT ACTIVITY MODULATES THE NOXIOUS STIMULATION FEEDBACK OF INFLAMMATION

Following complete subdiaphragmatic vagotomy, the dose-response curves for inhibition of plasma extravasation due to somatic stimulation are markedly shifted to the left, with a maximal effect occurring 7–14 days after vagotomy (Miao et al. 1997b) (Fig. 4). This finding suggests that activity in vagal afferents

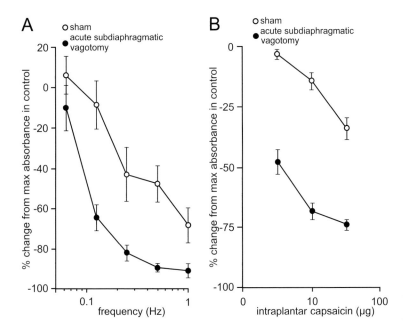

Fig. 4. Vagotomy enhances noxious-stimulation-induced inhibition of plasma extravasation. Noxious stimulation of the hindpaw by either (A) electrical stimulation (25 mA) or (B) capsaicin depresses bradykinin-induced plasma extravasation. Compared to control rats (A, n = 7; B, n = 9) that received sham surgery (open circles), acute subdiaphragmatic vagotomy (filled circles) markedly potentiated the effect of noxious electrical (n = 6) or capsaicin (n = 9) stimulation, shifting the dose-response curve significantly to the left. Data are mean ± SEM. Adapted from Miao et al. (1997, 2004).

tonically inhibits ascending impulse transmission in the neuraxis projecting to both the hypothalamus and the adrenal medulla, and that vagotomy removes central inhibition acting on these neuroendocrine pathways, thus leading to the release of hormonal signals from the adrenal medulla and cortex.

Recent studies found that celiac branch vagotomy or surgical removal of the duodenum mimicked the effect of total subdiaphragmatic vagotomy in potentiating the effect of noxious stimulation-induced inhibition of BK-induced plasma extravasation (Miao et al. 1997a, 2004). Fasting, to unload mechanically sensitive polymodal afferents in the proximal gastrointestinal tract, produced a similar leftward shift in the dose-response curve for the inhibitory effect of capsaicin, an effect that was reversed by balloon distension in the duodenum in fasting rats, while balloon distension had no effect after vagotomy.

THE GASTROINTESTINAL TRACT AS AN EARLY DEFENSE SYSTEM

Mechanosensitive duodenal vagal afferents may play an integral role in the body's defense against toxic insults. The gastrointestinal tract is an early line of defense against ingested infectious agents and toxic substances. Although the stomach is the first segment of the gastrointestinal tract with which orally ingested substances stay in contact for any period of time, toxic insults may be dealt with by being exposed to a high concentration of hydrogen ions (i.e., acidic pH). Toxic substances that pass through the stomach reach the duodenum, which is the first segment of the gastrointestinal tract that has an absorptive function and is, therefore, also a potential portal for the entry of toxic agents into the body. The polymodal duodenal vagal afferents are, therefore, ideally situated to rapidly communicate the presence of noxious or toxic insults and to coordinate specific neural and endocrine signals that can differentially regulate vascular and immune function in different parts of the body. Vagal afferent activity also contributes to modulation of pain, fever, and other signs and symptoms, collectively referred to as "illness symptoms" (Goehler et al. 2000; Jänig 2005). It will be important to examine the role of polymodal duodenal vagal afferents in illness symptoms.

BIOLOGICAL ROLE FOR A VAGALLY MODULATED NOCICEPTIVE FEEDBACK CIRCUIT

What are the functions of the complex neuronal network that regulates the final sympathetic pathway to the release of epinephrine by the adrenal medullary cells and the final pathway to the release of glucocorticoids by the adrenal cortical cells, in the inhibitory control of experimental joint inflammation? Teleologically, it makes sense to attenuate and terminate protective inflammatory reactions, since ongoing inflammation may lead to pathological tissue changes and finally tissue destruction. Inflammation may be abolished by activation of the sympathoadrenal system or the HPA axis. Most inflammatory processes are accompanied by stimulation of nociceptors, which activates the central nociceptive positive-feedback reflex circuit and in turn the neuroendocrine final pathways.

Many questions have yet to be answered. For example, the joint inflammation model has specifically determined that noxious input activates circuits that inhibit a sympathetic dependent inflammatory response, but we do not know whether this feedback system can be generalized to nonsympathetic dependent inflammatory responses. While there may be something unique about the sympathetic nervous system, this possibility does not diminish the significance of this circuit. While we only evaluated the plasma extravasation component of inflammation, there is increasing appreciation that the sympathetic nervous system is involved in other aspects of the inflammatory response; for example, it has recently been shown that the sympathetic nervous system powerfully modulates bacterial dissemination (Straub et al. 2005).

We are still in the early days of understanding the peripheral and central mechanisms that underlie the regulation of inflammation by the coordinated sensory, autonomic, and neuroendocrine control system. This control system can regulate not only the inflammatory response, but also hyperalgesia. Regulation of both inflammation and pain by this control system indicates interdependent protective processes. Future research will show how this control system, and in particular vagal afferent activity, may underlie the pathology of chronic painful inflammatory diseases.

MECHANICAL HYPERALGESIC BEHAVIOR IS CONTROLLED BY THE SYMPATHO-ADRENAL SYSTEM

EFFECT OF VAGOTOMY AND ACTIVATION OF THE ADRENAL MEDULLA ON BRADYKININ-INDUCED MECHANICAL HYPERALGESIC BEHAVIOR

The paw-withdrawal threshold to mechanical stimulation of the dorsal skin of the rat hindpaw with a linearly increasing mechanical stimulus decreases dose-dependently after intradermal injection of bradykinin (BK; open and closed circles in Fig. 5A). This response is called BK-induced mechanical hyperalgesic behavior. The decrease in paw-withdrawal threshold is generated by sensitization of cutaneous nociceptors by BK. It is dependent on the presence of sympathetic terminals in the dermis but not on activity in the sympathetic neurons, and is prevented by indomethacin (injected locally or systemically) and mediated by the B2-receptor. The BK-induced mechanical hyperalgesic behavior is significantly enhanced in rats with subdiaphragmatic vagotomy, performed at least 7 days before the measurements (open triangles in Fig. 5A). Furthermore, the baseline threshold is decreased. A small part of this enhancement is due to removal of inhibition in the dorsal horn, maintained by activity in vagal afferents and mediated by an inhibitory bulbospinal descending system (Fig. 5C) as predicted from the literature (see Foreman 1989; Randich and Gebhart 1992). However, the largest part of this enhancement is related to the activation of the adrenal medulla after vagotomy. After denervation of the adrenal medulla, subdiaphragmatic vagotomy has only a small effect on BK-induced decrease of paw-withdrawal threshold (compare open squares with open triangles in Fig. 5A). This experiment argues that vagotomy leads to release of epinephrine (probably by activation of sympathetic premotor neurons), which in turn sensitizes nociceptors and enhances the sensitization of nociceptors for mechanical stimulation by BK. Two groups of experiments support this conclusion.

First, in vagotomized rats the decreased paw-withdrawal threshold to intra-cutaneously injected BK and the decreased baseline paw-withdrawal threshold are reversed after denervation of the adrenal medulla (section of the pregan-glionic axons innervating the adrenal medulla; Fig. 5C). The development of enhanced mechanical hyperalgesic behavior and its reversal have a slow time course of 1–2 weeks (Khasar et al. 1998b).

Second, chronic administration of epinephrine (10.8 µg/h, using a subcuta-neously implanted micro-osmotic pump) generates the same effect as vagotomy, i.e., the BK-induced paw-withdrawal threshold to mechanical stimulation significantly decreases. This decrease is delayed and reaches its peak effect 14 days after the start of epinephrine infusion. After chronic infusion of the β_2-ad-renoceptor blocker ICI 118,551, the BK-induced decrease of paw-withdrawal threshold following vagotomy is significantly attenuated. Plasma levels of epinephrine following vagotomy significantly increase 3, 7, and 14 days after subdiaphragmatic vagotomy compared to sham-vagotomized animals (Khasar et al. 2003).

Fig. 5. Long-term enhancement of bradykinin (BK)-induced mechanical hyperalgesia after vagotomy and its disappearance after denervation of the adrenal medulla. (A) Decrease of paw-withdrawal threshold to mechanical stimulation of the dorsum of the rat hindpaw induced by BK (BK-induced behavioral mechanical hyperalgesia) in naive control rats (open circles, $n = 26$), vagotomized rats (open triangles, $n = 16$; 7 days after subdiaphragmatic vagotomy), sham-vagotomized rats (closed circles, $n = 18$), and vagotomized rats with denervated adrenal medullas (open squares, $n = 6$). Cutaneous nociceptors on the dorsum of the paw are stimulated by a linearly increasing mechanical force. Paw-withdrawal threshold is defined as the mean ($\pm$ SEM) minimum force (in grams, ordinate scale) at which the rat withdraws its paw. Abscissa scale: log dose of BK (in nanograms) injected in a volume of 2.5 µL of saline into the dermis of the skin. (B) Total change of paw-withdrawal threshold in response to intradermal injection of 1 ng BK in rats before and 3 to 35 days after vagotomy (open triangles, $n = 6$), before and 7–35 days after sham vagotomy (closed circles, $n = 8$) and in rats whose adrenal medullas were denervated 14 days after vagotomy and measurements taken up to 35 days after initial surgery (closed normal triangles, rats tested after vagotomy and denervation of the adrenal medulla [$n = 6$]; inverted closed triangles, rats tested only after additional denervation of the adrenal medulla [$n = 4$]). * $P < 0.01$, ▲/△ vs. sham-vagotomized rats on day 7; + $P > 0.05$, ▲/▼ vs. sham-vagotomized rats on days 28 and 35; # $P < 0.01$, ▲/▼ vs. vagotomized rats (△) on days 28 and 35. (C) Schematic diagram showing the proposed neural circuits in the spinal cord and brainstem that modulate nociceptor sensitivity via the sympatho-adrenal system. Sensitivity of cutaneous nociceptors for mechanical stimulation is modulated by epinephrine from the adrenal medulla. Activation of the adrenal medulla increases the sensitivity of the nociceptors. Activity in preganglionic neurons innervating the adrenal medulla depends on activity in vagal afferents from the small intestine which has an inhibitory influence on the central pathways to these preganglionic (preggl) neurons. Thus, interruption of the vagal afferents leads to activation of the adrenal medulla. It is hypothesized that these neuronal (reflex) circuits in the brainstem are under the control of upper brainstem, hypothalamus, and telencephalon. Dotted thin lines: Axons of sympathetic premotor neurons in the brainstem that project through the dorsolateral funiculi of the spinal cord to the preganglionic neurons of the adrenal medulla. –, inhibition; NTS = nucleus tractus solitarii; SDV = subdiaphragmatic vagotomy. Modified from Khasar et al. (1998b). ⟶

INTERPRETATION OF THE RESULTS

These results suggest that vagotomy not only removes ongoing inhibition of nociceptive impulses transmission in the dorsal horn but also triggers the activation of sympathetic preganglionic neurons innervating the adrenal medulla, probably by removing central inhibition acting at this sympathetic pathway. This situation leads to an increased release of epinephrine from the adrenal medulla and consequently to higher levels of epinephrine in the plasma. Interruption of the sympathetic preganglionic axons innervating the adrenal medulla stops the release of epinephrine. It therefore prevents the decrease of baseline mechanical paw-withdrawal threshold and the enhancement of BK-induced decrease of paw-withdrawal threshold to mechanical stimulation; it reverses both in rats that were vagotomized 2 weeks previously. This new finding implies that the sensitivity of nociceptors to mechanical stimulation is potentially under control of the

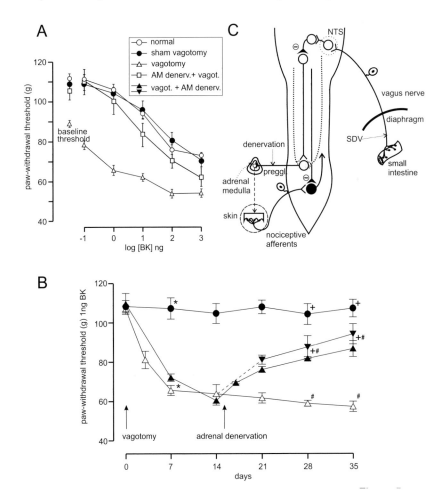

sympatho-adrenal system and that nociceptor sensitivity can be regulated from remote body domains by way of the brain and this neuroendocrine pathway. This novel mechanism has several implications and raises several interesting questions and problems (Jänig et al. 2000):

1) The vagal afferents that are involved in modulation of hyperalgesic behavior project through the celiac branches of the abdominal vagus nerves (Khasar et al. 1998a) and supply the small and large intestines, but probably not the liver and stomach. These vagal afferents may monitor toxic and other events at the inner defense line of the body, namely the gut-associated lymphoid tissue. The physiological stimuli activating these vagal afferents are unknown (Jänig 2005).

2) The changes following vagotomy (decreased mechanical baseline threshold and enhanced BK-induced mechanical hyperalgesic behavior) are generated by the *interruption* of vagal afferents. Thus, the vagal afferents involved must be tonically active.

3) The mechanism of the slow time course of the changes in paw-withdrawal threshold is unknown. Epinephrine obviously must act over a long period of time to induce changes in the micromilieu of the nociceptor population, leading in turn to their sensitization (see Khasar et al. 2003). We hypothesize that it does not act *directly* on the nociceptors but that it acts on other cells (e.g., macrophages, mast cells, keratinocytes), which then release substances that sensitize nociceptors, particularly since prostaglandin E_2-induced mechanical hyperalgesic behavior is *not* changed after vagotomy (Khasar et al. 1998a).

4) A change in sensitivity of a population of cutaneous nociceptors that is generated by epinephrine and regulated by the brain would be a novel mechanism of sensitization. This novel mechanism of nociceptor sensitization would be different from mechanisms that lead to activation or sensitization of nociceptors by sympathetic-afferent coupling under pathophysiological conditions (see Jänig 2002).

Which central pathways are involved in the activation of preganglionic sympathetic neurons that innervate the adrenal medulla after subdiaphragmatic vagotomy? Are only sympathetic neurons that innervate the adrenal medulla activated, or are other functional types of sympathetic neuron activated as well? (Jänig and McLachlan 2002; Jänig 2006). Experimental investigations performed on rats show that sympathetic preganglionic neurons innervating cells of the adrenal medulla that release epinephrine are connected to distinct neuronal circuits in the neuraxis that are different from those connected to preganglionic neurons that are involved in regulating other autonomic functions (Morrison and Cao 2000; Morrison 2001).

CONCLUSIONS

The body is continuously exposed to potentially injurious events from both the external environment and the internal environment of the gastrointestinal tract. This exposure leads to activation of local and coordinated protective mechanisms in the body involving the brain, immune system, and neuroendocrine systems and results in inflammation, pain, and hyperalgesia. Regulation of these protective mechanisms occurs in the short term (seconds to minutes) and long term (hours to days). Defense may involve rapid mechanisms (fight or flight) involving fast nociceptive signaling and the hypothalamo-mesencephalic system, as well as slow recuperation and healing, involving the immune system in particular (Maier and Watkins 1998; Jänig and Levine 2005). This chapter has discussed some of the principles of integration of central and peripheral neural, immune, and endocrine mechanisms that mediate fast defense and slow recuperation.

ACKNOWLEDGMENTS

Supported by the German Research Foundation, the Federal Ministry of Education and Research (Germany; Jänig), and the National Institutes of Health (Chapman, Green).

REFERENCES

Bandler R, Keay KA, Floyd N, Price J. Central circuits mediating patterned autonomic activity during active vs. passive emotional coping. *Brain Res Bull* 2000; 53:95–104.

Blalock JE. The immune system as the sixth sense. *J Intern Med* 2005; 257:126–138.

Byers MR, Bonica JJ. Peripheral pain mechanisms and nociceptor plasticity. In: Loeser JD, Butler SH, Chapman CR, Turk DC (Eds). *Bonica's Management of Pain.* 3rd ed. Philadelphia: Lippincott Williams and Wilkins, 2001, pp 26–72.

Charney DS, Deutch A. A functional neuroanatomy of anxiety and fear: implications for the pathophysiology and treatment of anxiety disorders. *Crit Rev Neurobiol* 1996; 10:419–446.

Dayas CV, Buller KM, Day TA. Medullary neurones regulate hypothalamic corticotropin-releasing factor cell responses to an emotional stressor. *Neuroscience* 2001; 105:707–719.

De Kloet ER. Hormones and the stressed brain. *Ann NY Acad Sci* 2004; 1018:1–15.

Delgado M, Abad C, Martinez C, et al. PACAP in immunity and inflammation. *Ann NY Acad Sci* 2003; 992:141–157.

Delgado M, Pozo D, Ganea D. The significance of vasoactive intestinal peptide in immunomodulation. *Pharmacol Rev* 2004; 56:249–290.

Dunn AJ, Wang J, Ando T. Effects of cytokines on cerebral neurotransmission. Comparison with the effects of stress. *Adv Exp Med Biol* 1999; 461:117–127.

Foreman RD. Organization of the spinothalamic tract as a relay for cardiopulmonary sympathetic afferent fiber activity. *Prog Sensory Physiol* 1989; 9:1–51.

Goehler LE, Gaykema RP, Hansen MK, et al. Vagal immune-to-brain communication: a visceral chemosensory pathway. *Auton Neurosci* 2000; 85:49–59.

Green PG, Miao FJP, Jänig W, Levine JD. Negative feedback neuroendocrine control of the inflammatory response in rats. *J Neurosci* 1995; 15:4678–4686.

Green PG, Jänig W, Levine JD. Negative feedback neuroendocrine control of inflammatory response in the rat is dependent on the sympathetic postganglionic neuron. *J Neurosci* 1997; 17:3234–3238.

Hammack SE, Richey KJ, Schmid MJ, et al. The role of corticotropin-releasing hormone in the dorsal raphe nucleus in mediating the behavioral consequences of uncontrollable stress. *J Neurosci* 2002; 22:1020–1026.

Hariri AR, Mattay VS, Tessitore A, Fera F, Weinberger DR. Neocortical modulation of the amygdala response to fearful stimuli. *Biol Psychiatry* 2003; 53:494–501.

Hosoi T, Okuma Y, Nomura Y. Electrical stimulation of afferent vagus nerve induces IL-1 beta expression in the brain and activates HPA axis. *Am J Physiol Regul Integr Comp Physiol* 2000; 279:R141–R147.

Itoi K, Jiang YQ, Iwasaki Y, Watson SJ. Regulatory mechanisms of corticotropin-releasing hormone and vasopressin gene expression in the hypothalamus. *J Neuroendocrinol* 2004; 16:348–355.

Jänig W. Pain in the sympathetic nervous system: pathophysiological mechanisms. In: Mathias CJ, Bannister R (Eds). *Autonomic Failure,* 4th ed. New York: Oxford University Press, 2002, pp 99–108.

Jänig W. Vagal afferents and visceral pain. In: Undem B, Weinreich D (Eds). *Advances in Vagal Afferent Neurobiology.* Boca Raton: CRC Press, 2005, pp 461–489.

Jänig W. *The Integrative Action of the Autonomic Nervous System. Neurobiology of Homeostasis.* Cambridge: Cambridge University Press, 2006.

Jänig W, Levine JD. Autonomic-neuroendocrine-immune responses in acute and chronic pain. In: McMahon SB, Koltzenburg M (Eds). *Textbook of Pain.* Edinburgh: Elsevier Churchill Livingstone, 2005, pp 205–218.

Jänig W, McLachlan EM. Neurobiology of the autonomic nervous system. In: Mathias CJ, Bannister R (Eds). *Autonomic Failure,* 4th ed. New York: Oxford University Press, 2002, pp 3–15.

Jänig W, Khasar SG, Levine JD, Miao FJP. The role of vagal visceral afferents in the control of nociception. *Prog Brain Res* 2000; 122:273–287.

Jorgensen H, Knigge U, Kjaer A, Moller M, Warberg J. Serotonergic stimulation of corticotropin-releasing hormone and pro-opiomelanocortin gene expression. *J Neuroendocrinol* 2002; 14:788–795.

Khasar SG, Miao FJP, Jänig W, Levine JD. Modulation of bradykinin-induced mechanical hyperalgesia in the rat by activity in abdominal vagal afferents. *Eur J Neurosci* 1998a; 10:435–444.

Khasar SG, Miao FJP, Jänig W, Levine JD. Modulation of bradykinin-induced mechanical hyperalgesia in the rat skin by activity in the abdominal vagal afferents. *Eur J Neurosci* 1998b; 10:435–444.

Khasar SG, Green PG, Miao FJ, Levine JD. Vagal modulation of nociception is mediated by adrenomedullary epinephrine in the rat. *Eur J Neurosci* 2003; 17:909–915.

Klein TW, Newton C, Larsen K, et al. The cannabinoid system and immune modulation. *J Leukoc Biol* 2003; 74:486–496.

Maier SF, Watkins LR. Cytokines for psychologists: implications of bidirectional immune-to-brain communication for understanding behavior, mood, and cognition. *Psychol Rev* 1998; 105:83–107.

Miao FJ, Levine JD. Neural and endocrine mechanisms mediating noxious stimulus-induced inhibition of bradykinin plasma extravasation in the rat. *J Pharmacol Exp Ther* 1999; 291:1028–1037.

Miao FJP, Jänig W, Levine JD. Role of sympathetic postganglionic neurons in synovial plasma extravasation induced by bradykinin. *J Neurophysiol* 1996a; 75:715–724.

Miao FJ, Green PG, Coderre TJ, Jänig W, Levine JD. Sympathetic-dependence in bradykinin-induced synovial plasma extravasation is dose-related. *Neurosci Lett* 1996b; 205:165–168.

Miao FJP, Jänig W, Levine JD. Vagal branches involved in inhibition of bradykinin-induced synovial plasma extravasation by intrathecal nicotine and noxious stimulation in the rat. *J Physiol (Lond)* 1997a; 498:473–481.

Miao FJP, Jänig W, Green PG, Levine JD. Inhibition of bradykinin-induced synovial plasma extravasation produced by noxious cutaneous and visceral stimuli and its modulation by activity in the vagal nerve. *J Neurophysiol* 1997b; 78:1285–1292.

Miao FJ, Jänig W, Levine JD. Nociceptive neuroendocrine negative feedback control of neurogenic inflammation activated by capsaicin in the rat paw: role of the adrenal medulla. *J Physiol (Lond)* 2000; 527:601–610.

Miao FJ, Green PG, Levine JD. Mechano-sensitive duodenal afferents contribute to vagal modulation of Inflammation in the Rat. *J Physiol (Lond)* 2004; 554:227–235.

Mignini F, Streccioni V, Amenta F. Autonomic innervation of immune organs and neuroimmune modulation. *Auton Autacoid Pharmacol* 2003; 23:1–25.

Morrison SF. Differential control of sympathetic outflow. *Am J Physiol Regul Integr Comp Physiol* 2001; 281:R683–R698.

Morrison SF, Cao WH. Different adrenal sympathetic preganglionic neurons regulate epinephrine and norepinephrine secretion. *Am J Physiol Regul Integr Comp Physiol* 2000; 279: R1763–R1775.

O'Connor KA, Johnson JD, Hansen MK, et al. Peripheral and central proinflammatory cytokine response to a severe acute stressor. *Brain Res* 2003; 991:123–132.

Raffin-Sanson ML, de Keyzer Y, Bertagna X. Proopiomelanocortin, a polypeptide precursor with multiple functions: from physiology to pathological conditions. *Eur J Endocrinol* 2003; 149:79–90.

Randich A, Gebhart GF. Vagal afferent modulation of nociception. *Brain Res Rev* 1992; 17:77–99.

Rassnick S, Sved AF, Rabin BS. Locus coeruleus stimulation by corticotropin-releasing hormone suppresses in vitro cellular immune responses. *J Neurosci* 1994; 14:6033–6040.

Sommer C, Kress M. Recent findings on how proinflammatory cytokines cause pain: peripheral mechanisms in inflammatory and neuropathic hyperalgesia. *Neurosci Lett* 2004; 361:184–187.

Straub RH, Pongratz G, Weidler C, et al. Ablation of the sympathetic nervous system decreases gram-negative and increases gram-positive bacterial dissemination: key roles for tumor necrosis factor/phagocytes and interleukin-4/lymphocytes. *J Infect Dis* 2005; 192:560–572.

ten Bokum AM, Hofland LJ, van Hagen PM. Somatostatin and somatostatin receptors in the immune system: a review. *Eur Cytokine Netw* 2000; 11:161–176.

Torres KC, Antonelli LR, Souza AL, et al. Norepinephrine, dopamine and dexamethasone modulate discrete leukocyte subpopulations and cytokine profiles from human PBMC. *J Neuroimmunol* 2005; 166:144–157.

Tsigos C, Chrousos GP. Hypothalamic-pituitary-adrenal axis, neuroendocrine factors and stress. *J Psychosom Res* 2002; 53:865–871.

Turnbull AV, Rivier CL. Regulation of the hypothalamic-pituitary-adrenal axis by cytokines: actions and mechanisms of action. *Physiol Rev* 1999; 79:1–71.

Vanegas H, Schaible HG. Descending control of persistent pain: inhibitory or facilitatory? *Brain Res Brain Res Rev* 2004; 46:295–309.

Vizi ES, Elenkov IJ. Nonsynaptic noradrenaline release in neuro-immune responses. *Acta Biol Hung* 2002; 53:229–244.

Walter L, Stella N. Cannabinoids and neuroinflammation. *Br J Pharmacol* 2004; 141:775–785.

Watkins LR, Maier SF. Beyond neurons: evidence that immune and glial cells contribute to pathological pain states. *Physiol Rev* 2002; 82:981–1011.

Wenger T, Ledent C, Tramu G. The endogenous cannabinoid, anandamide, activates the hypothalamo-pituitary-adrenal axis in CB1 cannabinoid receptor knockout mice. *Neuroendocrinology* 2003; 78:294–300.

Correspondence to: Prof. Dr. Wilfrid Jänig, Dr. med, Physiologisches Institut, Christian-Albrechts-Universität zu Kiel, Olshausenstr. 40, 24098 Kiel, Germany. Tel: 431-8802036; Fax: 431-8805256; email: w.janig@physiologie.uni-kiel.de.

Proceedings of the 11th World Congress on Pain,
edited by Herta Flor, Eija Kalso, and Jonathan O.
Dostrovsky, IASP Press, Seattle, © 2006.

30

Chronic Pain and Descending Facilitation

Stephen P. Hunt,[a] Rie Suzuki,[b] Wahida Rahman,[b] and Anthony H. Dickenson[b]

*Departments of [a]Anatomy and Developmental Biology and [b]Pharmacology,
University College London, London, United Kingdom*

Chronic pain, particularly neuropathic pain, has remained difficult to treat effectively, with only around one in three patients experiencing adequate pain relief (Sindrup and Jensen 1999). In part, the success rate remains poor because we have yet to understand the underlying pathology that gives rise to pain, particularly when the original injury is thought to have resolved. Research has concentrated on both peripheral and central areas of the nervous system, with particular focus on the peripheral nervous system as a source of chronic pain. Despite the recent explosion of knowledge of peripheral pharmacology and the cloning of large numbers of receptor genes specifically expressed by nociceptors, new treatments have not been forthcoming (Basbaum and Fields 1984). Targeted knockout or disruption of identified genes has suggested that particular nociceptor-specific transcripts may well be involved in maintaining abnormally high levels of nociceptive sensitivity following either inflammation or nerve injury, but specific drugs that mimic these molecular interventions have yet to be successfully developed (Wood et al. 2004). However, two widely used treatment approaches for neuropathic pain, the drugs gabapentin and pregabalin and the tricyclic antidepressants, have a significant central action, and recent studies have emphasized the central control of pain processing, in particular the influence of descending pathways on nociceptive signals passing through the dorsal horn (Urban and Gebhart 1999; Porreca et al. 2002). These descending influences can be inhibitory or facilitatory and originate from the brainstem (Millan 2002; Vanegas and Schaible 2004). The presence of descending excitatory influences that facilitate nociception is now attracting attention as a possible target for chronic pain control. Following peripheral nerve injury, damaged axons and neurons frequently become highly excitable and give rise to spontaneous or ectopic discharges that may account for some of the earliest reports of pain. However, ectopic firing of neurons is rarely seen more than 7 days after the initial nerve damage and cannot therefore explain long-term chronic pain (Chaplan et al. 1994; Han et al. 2000; Liu et al. 2000a,b). It may be that damage to the peripheral nervous system resulting in a high-intensity barrage into the superficial dorsal horn gives rise to long-term changes in the dorsal horn that outlives the period of stimulation (Klein et al. 2004). This memory of the initial insult, if retained over long periods of time, would result in all subsequent activation of the dorsal horn through peripheral nerve activation being misinterpreted by the central nervous system, leading to symptoms typical of neuropathic pain. For many years this plasticity of the dorsal horn was thought to be an intrinsic function of the dorsal horn and unrelated to brain processing, but this seems not to be the case, at least in experimental models of neuropathic and inflammatory pain. Ablation or inactivation of descending pathways from the brainstem alleviates pain states (Pertovaara 2000; Millan 2002; Porreca et al. 2002), a repeated finding that suggests that the maintenance of chronic pain states requires the cooperation of descending pathways, and also that the inappropriate activation of brain systems that modulate nociception is in some way contributing to the pathology.

DESCENDING FACILITATION

The hypothesis that descending control is inappropriately activated in chronic pain states raises a number of questions about how the brain processes nociceptive information. What is the function of descending facilitation in the normal life of the animal before pathology develops, and how are descending pathways triggered by incoming nociceptive signals?

Pain is essential for survival. Under normal circumstances, the ability to tolerate pain and to predict harmful consequences of our actions is essential; the brain has to compute a "cost/benefit" analysis. Are the rewards of taking a particular line of action greater than the possible threat to survival? There is now a growing body of evidence to suggest that one of the main ways by which the brain modulates levels of perceived pain is through activation of descending pathways that run from the brainstem to the dorsal horn of the spinal cord. These pathways can reduce or enhance the flow of nociceptive signals through the dorsal horn. Many of the numerous descending pathways from the brainstem to the spinal cord have been implicated in regulating pain sensitivity (Millan 2002). There are significant noradrenergic projections from the pontine A7 group of neurons that are largely inhibitory to dorsal horn neurons, and a group of neurons in the dorsal medullary reticular formation provides excitatory input to the dorsal horn (Lima and Almeida 2002; Monconduit et al. 2002). Descending facilitation has been emphasized as a function of the cell groups within the rostroventral medulla (RVM) (Porreca et al. 2002). Stimulation of the RVM can inhibit or facilitate both nociceptive and non-nociceptive input and mediates many of the well-documented effects of periaqueductal gray (PAG) stimulation. Neurons in the RVM have been designated as "on" or "off" cells depending on their response to noxious stimulation; they show an anticipatory pain-related activity, probably under forebrain control (Fields 2004). Many of these neurons are serotonergic. Analgesia or enhanced nociception can be generated by activation of these pathways under the direction of forebrain motivational, cognitive, or affective systems. For example, recovery from a significant injury requires the absence of further damage and a period of recuperation. Fight or flight behaviors are thought to be accompanied by a temporary period of stress-induced analgesia as, for example, was recorded in Beecher's (1956) accounts of the Normandy landings when severely injured soldiers rarely took significant amounts of analgesics. Generally, the survival value of intrinsically generated analgesia consists of allowing an animal to escape or attack without significant distraction from the pain of an injury inflicted by a predator. In contrast, the period of convalescence following injury is accompanied by a heightened sensitivity at the site of damage that is essential to prevent further injury. Convalescence is also accompanied by a period of reduced motor activity and loss of appetite, implying an interaction of the pain matrix with motivational centers in the brain. Increased motivational drive has also been implicated in producing analgesia, as has suckling or ingestion of sucrose solution. Increased production of dopamine, a neurotransmitter central to the generation of motivational states, can also enhance analgesia (Blass et al. 1987; Bucher et al. 1995; Segato et al. 1997; Burkey et al. 1999; Ohara et al. 2003; Fields 2004). Recent brain-imaging studies have shown that the learned prediction of either painful or pleasurable, pain-relieving events, when variably associated with a visual stimulus, can be processed at a largely unconscious level and that the perception of intensity is modulated by the learned expectancies acquired through such conditioning. The prediction of aversive events seems to be coded for by the lateral orbitofrontal cortex and the anterior cingulate cortex, whereas pleasurable events (in this case the reduction of pain) are coded for in the amygdala and midbrain (Seymour et al. 2005). The anterior cingulate cortex has also been implicated in placebo-generated analgesia (Petrovic et al. 2002) and in the learning of an association between noxious stimulation and a particular environmental context (Johansen and Fields 2004). In almost all of these studies, an association was made between forebrain areas that perceive the level of pain and the context of the animal's environment at a particular moment in time. In most cases the level of pain perceived was thought to be coordinated by the activation of descending pathways from the midbrain PAG and subsequently the RVM, which projects upon the dorsal horn. For example, recent human imaging studies during noxious stimulation of somatic or visceral sites has implicated the PAG, the nucleus cuneiformis (which lies ventral to the PAG), and the parabrachial area in nociceptive processing, with a strong correlation between activation of the right PAG and anxiety during visceral but not somatic stimulation (Dunckley et al. 2005). In summary, it seems likely that descending facilitation modulates nociception, protecting the coherence of ongoing behavior and preparing the animal for future encounters informed by past experience.

WHAT TRIGGERS DESCENDING FACILITATION?

It seems clear that forebrain systems concerned with many aspects of an animal's behavior can activate descending facilitatory controls and modulate nociception at the level of the spinal cord. However, activation of descending pathways is closely coupled to incoming nociceptive information (Fig. 1). Evidence indicates that subsets of dorsal horn projection neurons have privileged access to descending controls and that their activity is closely coupled (Hunt 2000). The pathways that carry nociceptive information from the dorsal horn have been intensively studied, at least in the rat. Essentially, there are two

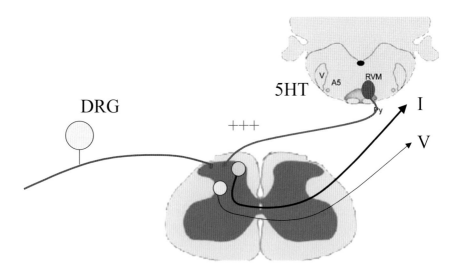

Fig. 1. Overview of the ascending nociceptive pathways arising from laminae I and V and the descending facilitatory serotonergic pathway originating from the rostroventral medulla (RVM) and modulating nociception at the 5-HT$_3$ receptor on primary afferents and dorsal horn interneurons. DRG = dorsal root ganglion.

populations of projection neurons, the first situated in laminae I and III and the second in lamina V. Lamina I neurons are nocispecific, receive peptidergic primary afferent input (particularly substance P and calcitonin gene-related peptide), express the substance P-preferring neurokinin-1 (NK1) receptor, and project to a number of brainstem sites, including the thalamus, that relay nociceptive information to regions of the forebrain concerned with affect, cognition, and motivation (Hunt 2000; Hunt and Mantyh 2001; Ikeda et al. 2003; Gauriau and Bernard 2004). In contrast, lamina V neurons respond over a wide dynamic range to noxious and non-noxious stimulation and project to those parts of the brainstem and forebrain largely concerned with motor activity and arousal. Lamina V neurons and lamina I NK1-positive projection neurons have been shown to support long-term potentiation, a long-term change in synaptic efficacy generated by low- or high-frequency, high-threshold stimulation (Rygh et al. 2002; Ikeda et al. 2003; Suzuki et al. 2004a).

Recently a technique was developed to ablate lamina I NK1-positive neurons selectively using a substance P-saporin (SP-SAP) conjugate that only targets NK1-expressing neurons (Mantyh et al. 1997; Nichols et al. 1999). Given that the majority of lamina I NK1-positive neurons express the NK1 receptor, this technique allows us for the first time to determine whether lamina I NK1-positive and lamina V projections have separate functions in pain control. Nichols et al. (1999) studied rats in which lamina I-NK1-positive projection neurons had been ablated and found that normal pain behavior appeared to be intact; behavioral responses to noxious mechanical, chemical, and heat stimuli were normal. However, once a pain state had been established by inflaming the hindpaw or by causing peripheral nerve damage, the usual development of an increased sensitivity to pain was reduced. Also, an established neuropathic pain state was attenuated by a subsequent ablation of lamina I NK1-positive projection neurons. These results imply that lamina I NK1-positive projection neurons inform the brain of the ongoing pain and are required for the maintenance of a pain state. Furthermore, the absence of a pain state after ablation of lamina I NK1-positive projection neurons implies that descending facilitatory pathways had not been engaged in the usual way. These speculations have received substantial experimental support.

In the lamina I-NK1-positive neuron-lesioned rats it was possible to record from lamina V neurons and to detect how their responses changed (Suzuki et al. 2002). There are two possible routes of communication between lamina I-NK1-positive cells and lamina V projection neurons: segmentally through direct axon collaterals or interneurons, or through long ascending and descending pathways. In fact, subsequent research has demonstrated that the response of lamina V neurons is an index of the contribution made by descending facilitation in both normal animals and animals in which a pain state has been induced.

Following lamina I NK1-positive neuron lesions (Fig. 2), the response of deep dorsal horn neurons showed changes in the fidelity with which these neurons encoded thermal and mechanical stimuli, as well as reduced receptive field size, lost wind-up response to high-threshold stimulation, and an attenuated second phase of response to formalin injection of the hindpaw (Suzuki et al. 2002). The second phase of the formalin response is usually taken as an index of "central sensitization," which is the degree to which the response properties of dorsal horn neurons have increased, and it accompanies the development of behavioral allodynia and hyperalgesia. In a separate set of experiments we asked how neuropathic pain states alter the activity of lamina V neurons and whether such changes depend on an intact lamina I NK1-positive neuronal projection to the brainstem (Suzuki et al. 2005). In control rats subjected to ligation of spinal nerves L5 and L6 to produce a neuropathic pain state, lamina V neurons were consistently more spontaneously active, had enlarged receptive fields to

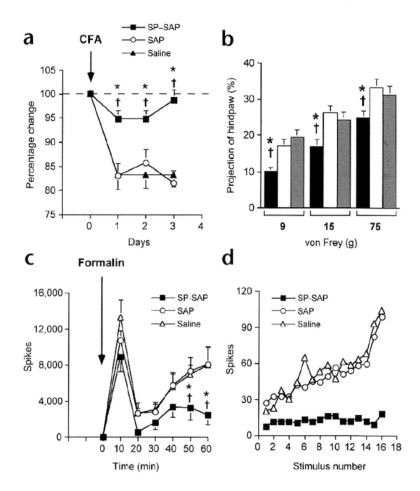

high-intensity stimulation, and showed an enhanced response to cooling stimuli applied to the hindpaw. In contrast, in rats in which the lamina I NK1-positive neuron projection pathway had been ablated, most of the changes in lamina V neurons associated with neuropathy were attenuated or lost.

The importance of the lamina I NK1-positive pathway in supporting the electrophysiological enhancement of the activity of lamina V neurons suggested that activation of brainstem descending pathways to the spinal cord was impaired after disruption of the lamina I projection system. Extensive activation of RVM neurons following hindpaw injection of formalin was detected using c-fos immunohistochemistry (Fig. 3). Many of these neurons co-stained for serotonin (5-HT). Ablation of the lamina I NK1-positive pathway resulted in reduced activation of the RVM, including neurons that contained 5-HT (Suzuki et al. 2002). This finding suggested that serotonergic pathways had been activated by noxious stimulation of the periphery and that serotonin may have been providing the excitatory drive to the dorsal horn, facilitating nociception. A similar conclusion has been reached following direct ablation of a subpopulation of RVM neurons using saporin conjugated to the μ-opioid-receptor agonist dermorphin or following injection of a local anesthetic (Porreca et al. 2001; Burgess et al. 2002). A proportion of the neurons ablated were thought to be "on" cells that should give rise to a descending facilitatory drive. This ablation resulted in an

---

← **Fig. 2.** Substance P and saporin (SP-SAP) attenuates complete Freund's adjuvant (CFA)-induced mechanical hyperalgesia, receptive field size, formalin-evoked activity, and wind-up of deep dorsal horn neurons. (a) Treatment with SP-SAP ($n = 10$) significantly attenuates mechanical hyperalgesia induced by CFA, compared to SAP or saline-injected animals; * and † indicate a significant difference ($P < 0.05$) from SAP- and saline-treated animals, respectively. (b) A comparison of the mean receptive field size of spinal neurons in SP-SAP (black bars), SAP (white bars) and saline-injected animals (gray bars), mapped using von Frey filaments of three different intensities. Neurons of SP-SAP-treated rats displayed significantly smaller receptive field sizes compared to those of SAP- or saline-injected rats. Data are expressed as a mean percentage of projected area ± SEM; * and † indicate a significant difference ($P < 0.05$) from SAP- and saline-treated groups, respectively. (c) The responses of spinal neurons to intraplantar formalin injection, in SP-SAP-treated (black squares), SAP-treated (open circles), and saline-treated animals (open triangles). The first phase was defined as the neuronal activity in the first 10 minutes following formalin injection, whilst the second phase was quantified as the subsequent neuronal activity lasting up to 60 minutes. The second phase of the formalin-evoked activity was significantly attenuated in rats treated with SP-SAP; * and † indicate a significant difference ($P < 0.05$) from SAP- and saline-treated animals, respectively. (d) The responses of spinal neurons to repetitive electrical stimulation in SP-SAP-treated (black squares), SAP-treated (open circles), and saline-treated rats (open triangles). Trains of 16 electrical stimuli (0.5 Hz) were given at three times the threshold current for C fibers. The number of action potentials evoked per stimulus in the train of 16 stimuli was plotted against the stimulus number. The marked increase in neuronal response ("wind-up") observed after repetitive electrical stimulation in SAP- and saline-treated rats was absent in SP-SAP rats. (From Suzuki et al. 2002.)

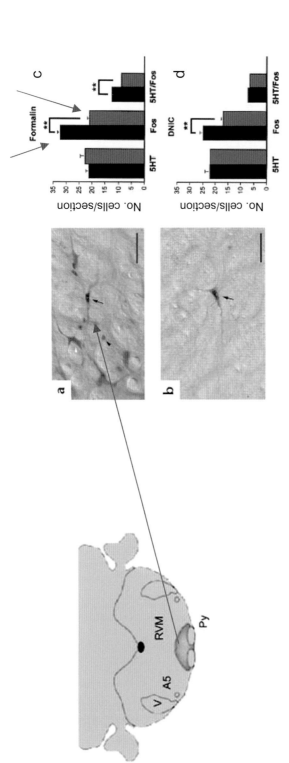

Fig. 3. (a) Immuno-histochemical visualization of Fos, 5-HT, and 5-HT/Fos immunoreactive neurons in the nucleus raphe magnus (RMg) following peripheral formalin injection in a saporin (SAP)-treated rat. Black arrows represent double-labeled cells, the black arrowhead represents Fos, and the white arrow represents 5-HT alone. (b) High-power photomicrograph of a double-labeled neuron in the RMg of a rat treated with substance P and saporin (SP-SAP) following peripheral formalin injection. (c) Histogram of the mean number of Fos-immunoreactive (Fos-IR) neurons in the RMg following peripheral formalin injection, comparing SP-SAP (gray bars) and SAP rats (black bars). There was a marked reduction in the number of Fos and 5-HT/Fos neurons in rats treated with SP-SAP. Data are expressed as mean number ± SEM per section (**$P < 0.005$). (d) Histogram of the mean number of Fos-IR neurons evoked in the ipsilateral lumbar spinal cord following peripheral noxious thermal stimulation, comparing SP-SAP-treated (gray bars) and SAP-treated rats (black bars). Cells immunoreactive for Fos were significantly reduced in SP-SAP rats; however, unlike the case with formalin injection, the proportion of double-labeled neurons (5-HT/Fos) remained comparable in SP-SAP- and SAP-treated rats. Data are expressed as mean number ± SEM per section (**$P < 0.005$). From Suzuki et al. (2002).

attenuation of neuropathic pain behaviors, although normal nociceptive responses were intact. Finally, if descending serotonergic function were crucial for the development of chronic pain states, it should be possible to replicate the effects of lamina I NK1-positive lesions with 5-HT-receptor antagonists, both behaviorally and electrophysiologically, and to ameliorate pain states by selectively depleting 5-HT locally within the lumbar spinal cord. Although multiple 5-HT receptors are expressed both by dorsal horn neurons and by primary afferent fibres, the $5-HT_3$ receptor was found to be a major candidate for the mediation of descending facilitation (Suzuki et al. 2002, 2004b, 2005). 5-HT is excitatory at the $5-HT_3$ receptor, a ligand-gated ion channel localized to both subsets of dorsal horn neurons and small-diameter primary afferent fibres (Miquel et al. 2002; Zeitz et al. 2002; Maxwell et al. 2003). Previous work has suggested that neurons that express the $5-HT_3$ receptor may include a population of Aδ primary afferent nociceptors (Zeitz et al. 2002; Maxwell et al. 2003). Application of the $5-HT_3$-receptor antagonist ondansetron directly to the spinal cord replicated many of the effects of lamina I-NK1 neuron ablation. Ondansetron treatment attenuated the second-phase formalin response and disrupted coding of mechanical and thermal stimuli. Similarly, in rats in which a neuropathic pain state had been established by spinal nerve ligation, a low dose of ondansetron was particularly effective in reducing neuronal activity in neuropathic rats but had no effect in sham animals, suggesting that descending facilitatory drive is enhanced in the deep dorsal horn (Suzuki et al. 2002, 2005).

The effects of local spinal 5-HT depletion have been studied in a model of at-level pain produced by partial or complete section of the spinal cord (Fig. 4). In this model, lesion of the spinal cord or disruption of the incoming sensory input (Zhang et al. 1993) results in a local "sprouting" of 5-HT-positive axons. Depletion of 5-HT-positive axons with the toxin 5,7-dihydroxytryptamine or local treatment with ondansetron successfully attenuated the allodynic pain state (Oatway et al. 2004). Finally, some treatment efficacy of ondansetron was seen in human neuropathic pain patients following a single intravenous injection of the drug (McCleane et al. 2003).

All these results suggest that descending facilitation of nociceptive processing is mediated, in part, by 5-HT pathways from the RVM acting at spinal $5-HT_3$ receptors and triggered by activity in the lamina I NK1-positive projection pathway. The site of interaction between the ascending and descending pathway presumably involves multiple forebrain areas, but direct innervation of the PAG by ascending nociceptive pathways could rapidly trigger descending facilitation through the RVM. Furthermore, activity in both ascending and descending pathways appears to be essential for the maintenance of chronic pain states (Nichols et al. 1999; Porreca et al. 2002).

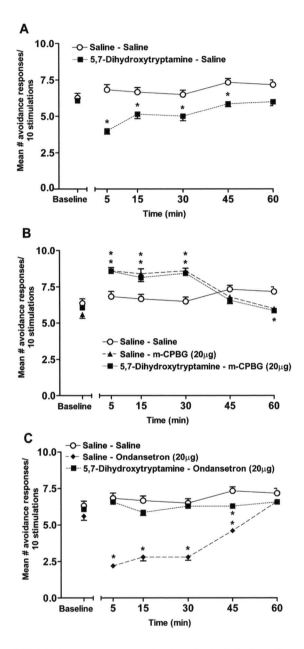

Fig. 4. Effect of 5,7-DHT pretreatment on at-level mechanical allodynia 5 weeks post-spinal cord injury. 5,7-DHT or saline was intrathecally administered 28 days after spinal cord injury, and mechanical allodynia was assessed 3–7 days later following acute injection of (A) saline, (B) m-CPBG (a 5-HT$_3$ agonist), or (C) ondansetron (a 5-HT$_3$ antagonist). The values shown represent the mean number of avoidance responses to 10 stimulations $\pm$ SEM. *, $P < 0.05$ compared to saline-treated controls. From Oatway et al. (2004).

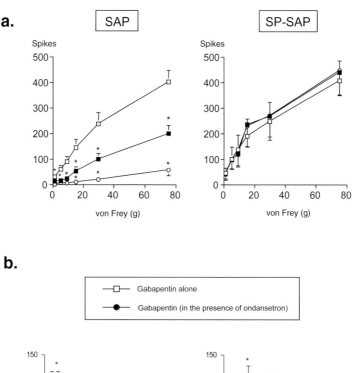

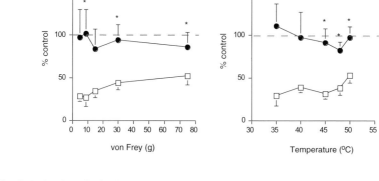

Fig. 5. Activation of spinal 5-HT$_3$ receptors is necessary for full gabapentin (GBP) efficacy. (a) Comparison of the effect of systemic GBP administration on spinal neuronal responses to mechanical punctate stimulation in rats treated with saporin and spinal nerve ligation (SAP-SNL, left panel) and in rats treated with substance P-saporin and SNL (SP-SAP SNL, right panel). Open squares represent pre-drug baseline values, while closed squares and open circles indicate neuronal responses after GBP administration (10 mg/kg and 100 mg/kg, respectively). (b) Systemic administration of GBP (100 mg/kg) produced pronounced inhibition of the mechanical and heat-evoked responses of deep dorsal horn neurons in SNL rats (open squares). The inhibitory effects of the drug were completely abolished in the presence of ondansetron (i.t.), a 5-HT$_3$-receptor antagonist (closed circles). Significance level is taken as * $P < 0.05$. From Suzuki et al. (2005).

GABAPENTIN AND DESCENDING FACILITATION

Our analysis of the role of the brainstem in maintaining pain states suggests novel strategies for the treatment of chronic pain states. But how do currently available drugs such as gabapentin and pregabalin interact with the spinal-brainstem-spinal loops that maintain chronic pain states? Gabapentin, licensed for the treatment of chronic pain, binds to a unique site on the $\alpha_2\delta$ subunit common to all voltage-dependent calcium channels (Gee et al. 1996; Luo et al. 2001). In animals, the actions of gabapentin are state dependent, and the drug only modulates abnormal pain function without influencing acute nociceptive activity. After ablation of lamina I NK1-positive projection neurons or local treatment with ondansetron, dorsal horn activity and neuropathic pain behaviors were blunted, as described above. Even though ondansetron itself reduced neuronal activity, the addition of gabapentin failed to produce a further inhibitory response (Fig. 5). In this series of experiments, Suzuki at al. (2005) found that activation of the 5-HT$_3$ receptor with the specific agonist 2-methyl-5-HT produced modest increases in the activity of deep dorsal horn neurons in naive rats. However, subsequent treatment with gabapentin dramatically inhibited the mechanical and thermal evoked responses of spinal neurons. In other words, the pharmacological activation of the 5-HT$_3$ receptor enables the antinociceptive activity of gabapentin in naive rats, which would suggest that the actions of this drug rely on an interaction between 5-HT$_3$ receptors and gabapentin-binding sites. A similar approach was used to test whether the lack of gabapentin efficacy in SP-SAP-treated rats was due to a loss of descending facilitation. In rats with ablation of lamina I-NK1-positive projection neurons and spinal nerve injury, gabapentin efficacy was minimal, as expected. However, the effects of gabapentin were fully restored when the drug was administered in combination with local application of the 5-HT$_3$-receptor agonist 2-methyl 5-HT to the spinal cord. Gabapentin now produced a strong inhibition of spinal neuronal responses. These results suggest that gabapentin requires an excitatory serotonergic influence from the brainstem for its efficacy.

FINAL COMMENTS

Descending facilitation is undoubtedly of considerable importance in the maintenance of chronic pain states. Descending serotonergic action at the 5-HT$_3$ receptor is a major component of descending facilitation, and activity in this pathway seems essential for the full efficacy of drugs such as gabapentin. However, we do not yet understand the dynamics of 5-HT release during the development or maintenance of a chronic pain state. As originally reported by Nichols et al. (1999), neuropathic pain can be alleviated by a subsequent ablation of lamina I NK1-positive projection neurons, implying that sustained activity by these neurons is necessary to maintain the pain state. Lamina I projection neurons are innervated by 5-HT-positive fibers from the brainstem (Polgar et al. 2002), and some primary afferent nociceptors express 5-HT$_3$ receptors. Abnormally high levels of activity maintained in lamina I NK1-positive neurons and primary afferents by increased descending facilitation may well result in prolonged excitation in the nociceptive pathway. This finding would suggest the hypothesis that the drive to maintain the chronic pain state originates in the brainstem or higher centers, similar to recent hypotheses concerning the etiology of migraine (Goadsby 2005).

REFERENCES

Basbaum AI, Fields HL. Endogenous pain control systems: brainstem spinal pathways and endorphin circuitry. *Annu Rev Neurosci* 1984; 7:309–338.

Beecher HK. Relationship of significance of wound to pain experienced. *JAMA* 1956; 161:1609–1613.

Blass E, Fitzgerald E, Kehoe P. Interactions between sucrose, pain and isolation distress. *Pharmacol Biochem Behav* 1987; 26:483–489.

Bucher HU, Moser T, von Siebenthal K, et al. Sucrose reduces pain reaction to heel lancing in preterm infants: a placebo-controlled, randomized and masked study. *Pediatr Res* 1995; 38:332–335.

Burgess SE, Gardell LR, Ossipov MH, et al. Time-dependent descending facilitation from the rostral ventromedial medulla maintains, but does not initiate, neuropathic pain. *J Neurosci* 2002; 22: 5129–5136.

Burkey AR, Carstens E, Jasmin L. Dopamine reuptake inhibition in the rostral agranular insular cortex produces antinociception. *J Neurosci* 1999; 19:4169–4179.

Chaplan SR, Bach FW, Pogrel JW, Chung JM, Yaksh TL. Quantitative assessment of tactile allodynia in the rat paw. *J Neurosci Methods* 1994; 53:55–63.

Dunckley P, Wise RG, Fairhurst M, et al. A comparison of visceral and somatic pain processing in the human brainstem using functional magnetic resonance imaging. *J Neurosci* 2005; 25:7333–7341.

Fields H. State-dependent opioid control of pain. *Nat Rev Neurosci* 2004; 5:565–575.

Gauriau C, Bernard JF. A comparative reappraisal of projections from the superficial laminae of the dorsal horn in the rat: the forebrain. *J Comp Neurol* 2004; 468:24–56.

Gee NS, Brown JP, Dissanayake VU, et al. The novel anticonvulsant drug, gabapentin (Neurontin), binds to the alpha-2-delta subunit of a calcium channel. *J Biol Chem* 1996; 271: 5768–5776.

Goadsby PJ. Migraine pathophysiology. *Headache* 2005; 45(Suppl 1):S14–24.

Han HC, Lee DH, Chung JM. Characteristics of ectopic discharges in a rat neuropathic pain model. *Pain* 2000; 84:253–261.

Hunt SP. Pain control: breaking the circuit. *Trends Pharmacol Sci* 2000; 21:284–287.

Hunt SP, Mantyh PW. The molecular dynamics of pain control. *Nat Rev Neurosci* 2001; 2:83–91.

Ikeda H, Heinke B, Ruscheweyh R, Sandkuhler J. Synaptic plasticity in spinal lamina I projection neurons that mediate hyperalgesia. *Science* 2003; 299:1237–1240.

Johansen JP, Fields HL. Glutamatergic activation of anterior cingulate cortex produces an aversive teaching signal. *Nat Neurosci* 2004; 7:398–403.

Klein T, Magerl W, Hopf HC, Sandkuhler J, Treede RD. Perceptual correlates of nociceptive long-term potentiation and long-term depression in humans. *J Neurosci* 2004; 24:964–971.

Lima D, Almeida A. The medullary dorsal reticular nucleus as a pronociceptive centre of the pain control system. *Prog Neurobiol* 2002; 66:81–108.

Liu CN, Wall PD, Ben-Dor E, et al. Tactile allodynia in the absence of C-fiber activation: altered firing properties of DRG neurons following spinal nerve injury. *Pain* 2000a; 85:503–521.

Liu X, Eschenfelder S, Blenk KH, Jänig W, Habler H. Spontaneous activity of axotomized afferent neurons after L5 spinal nerve injury in rats. *Pain* 2000b; 84:309–318.

Luo ZD, Chaplan SR, Higuera ES, et al. Upregulation of dorsal root ganglion (alpha)2(delta) calcium channel subunit and its correlation with allodynia in spinal nerve-injured rats. *J Neurosci* 2001; 21:1868–1875.

Mantyh PW, Rogers SD, Honore P, et al. Inhibition of hyperalgesia by ablation of lamina I spinal neurons expressing the substance P receptor. *Science* 1997; 278:275–279.

Maxwell DJ, Kerr R, Rashid S, Anderson E. Characterisation of axon terminals in the rat dorsal horn that are immunoreactive for serotonin 5-HT$_{3A}$ receptor subunits. *Exp Brain Res* 2003; 149:114–124.

McCleane GJ, Suzuki R, Dickenson AH. Does a single intravenous injection of the 5HT$_3$ receptor antagonist ondansetron have an analgesic effect in neuropathic pain? A double-blinded, placebo-controlled cross-over study. *Anesth Analg* 2003; 97:1474–1478.

Millan MJ. Descending control of pain. *Prog Neurobiol* 2002; 66:355–474.

Miquel MC, Emerit MB, Nosjean A, et al. Differential subcellular localization of the 5-HT$_3$-As receptor subunit in the rat central nervous system. *Eur J Neurosci* 2002; 15:449–457.

Monconduit L, Desbois C, Villanueva L. The integrative role of the rat medullary subnucleus reticularis dorsalis in nociception. *Eur J Neurosci* 2002; 16:937–944.

Nichols ML, Allen BJ, Rogers SD, et al. Transmission of chronic nociception by spinal neurons expressing the substance P receptor. *Science* 1999; 286:1558–1561.

Oatway MA, Chen Y, Weaver LC. The 5-HT$_3$ receptor facilitates at-level mechanical allodynia following spinal cord injury. *Pain* 2004; 110:259–268.

Ohara PT, Granato A, Moallem TM, et al. Dopaminergic input to GABAergic neurons in the rostral agranular insular cortex of the rat. *J Neurocytol* 2003; 32:131–141.

Pertovaara A. Plasticity in descending pain modulatory systems. *Prog Brain Res* 2000; 129:231–242.

Petrovic P, Kalso E, Petersson KM, Ingvar M. Placebo and opioid analgesia—imaging a shared neuronal network. *Science* 2002; 295:1737–1740.

Polgar E, Puskar Z, Watt C, Matesz C, Todd AJ. Selective innervation of lamina I projection neurones that possess the neurokinin 1 receptor by serotonin-containing axons in the rat spinal cord. *Neuroscience* 2002; 109:799–809.

Porreca F, Burgess SE, Gardell LR, et al. Inhibition of neuropathic pain by selective ablation of brainstem medullary cells expressing the mu-opioid receptor. *J Neurosci* 2001; 21:5281–5288.

Porreca F, Ossipov MH, Gebhart GF. Chronic pain and medullary descending facilitation. *Trends Neurosci* 2002; 25:319–325.

Rygh LJ, Tjolsen A, Hole K, Svendsen F. Cellular memory in spinal nociceptive circuitry. *Scand J Psychol* 2002; 43:153–159.

Segato FN, Castro-Souza C, Segato EN, Morato S, Coimbra NC. Sucrose ingestion causes opioid analgesia. *Braz J Med Biol Res* 1997; 30:981–984.

Seymour B, O'Doherty JP, Koltzenburg M, et al. Opponent appetitive-aversive neural processes underlie predictive learning of pain relief. *Nat Neurosci* 2005; 8:1234–1240.

Sindrup SH, Jensen TS. Efficacy of pharmacological treatments of neuropathic pain: an update and effect related to mechanism of drug action. *Pain* 1999; 83:389–400.

Suzuki R, Morcuende S, Webber M, Hunt SP, Dickenson AH. Superficial NK1-expressing neurons control spinal excitability through activation of descending pathways. *Nat Neurosci* 2002; 5:1319–1326.

Suzuki R, Rygh LJ, Dickenson AH. Bad news from the brain: descending 5-HT pathways that control spinal pain processing. *Trends Pharmacol Sci* 2004a; 25:613–617.

Suzuki R, Rahman W, Hunt SP, Dickenson AH. Descending facilitatory control of mechanically evoked responses is enhanced in deep dorsal horn neurones following peripheral nerve injury. *Brain Res* 2004b; 1019:68–76.

Suzuki R, Rahman W, Rygh LJ, et al. Spinal-supraspinal serotonergic circuits regulating neuropathic pain and its treatment with gabapentin. *Pain* 2005; 117:292–303.

Urban MO, Gebhart GF. Supraspinal contributions to hyperalgesia. *Proc Natl Acad Sci USA* 1999; 96:7687–7692.

Vanegas H, Schaible HG. Descending control of persistent pain: inhibitory or facilitatory? *Brain Res Brain Res Rev* 2004; 46:295–309.

Wood JN, Abrahamsen B, Baker MD, et al. Ion channel activities implicated in pathological pain. *Novartis Found Symp* 2004; 261:32–40; discussion 40–54.

Zeitz KP, Guy N, Malmberg AB, et al. The $5-HT_3$ subtype of serotonin receptor contributes to nociceptive processing via a novel subset of myelinated and unmyelinated nociceptors. *J Neurosci* 2002; 22:1010–1019.

Zhang B, Goldberger ME, Murray M. Proliferation of SP- and 5HT-containing terminals in lamina II of rat spinal cord following dorsal rhizotomy: quantitative EM-immunocytochemical studies. *Exp Neurol* 1993; 123:51–63.

Correspondence to: Professor Stephen P. Hunt, PhD, Department of Anatomy and Developmental Biology, University College London, London WC1E 6JP, United Kingdom. Tel: 44-207-6791332; email: hunt@ucl.ac.uk.

Proceedings of the 11th World Congress on Pain,
edited by Herta Flor, Eija Kalso, and Jonathan O.
Dostrovsky, IASP Press, Seattle, © 2006.

31

Genetic Tracing of Ascending Nociceptive Circuits

João Manuel Braz and Allan I. Basbaum

*Departments of Anatomy and Physiology and W.M. Keck Foundation Center
for Integrative Neuroscience, University of California, San Francisco,
California, USA*

To date, two major classes of unmyelinated primary afferent nociceptors have been identified (Snider and McMahon 1998). The peptidergic population expresses substance P and calcitonin gene-related peptide, projects primarily to lamina I and the outer part of lamina II of the substantia gelatinosa, and contacts projection neurons that transmit nociceptive messages to brainstem and thalamus. By contrast, the nonpeptidergic population that binds the isolectin IB4 terminates mainly in the inner part of lamina II, a region characterized by a distinct subset of interneurons that express the gamma isoform of protein kinase C (PKCγ). These fundamental differences in the pattern of primary afferent termination suggest that different information is conveyed by peptidergic and nonpeptidergic sensory neurons and that these two classes of primary afferent nociceptors engage separate ascending "pain" pathways in the central nervous system (CNS). To begin to address this question, we used a novel genetic tracing method that permits labeling of multisynaptic CNS circuits after transneuronal transfer of an endogenously expressed tracer in specific subsets of neurons (Horowitz et al. 1999; Yoshihara et al. 1999).

This chapter summarizes an analysis that was performed in a transgenic mouse line (Braz et al. 2002), in which expression of the transneuronal tracer wheat germ agglutinin (WGA) is both temporally and spatially inducible. A full description of our analysis has been published elsewhere (Braz et al. 2005). Fig. 1 illustrates the construct that we used to generate the ZW transgenic mice, so named because the expression vector includes a lox-P-flanked LacZ gene (the Z of the ZW) inserted upstream of a cDNA that codes for WGA (the W of the ZW). Both the Z and W genes are activated by a cytomegalovirus-enhanced β-actin promoter. In this arrangement, the cells constitutively produce β-galactosidase,

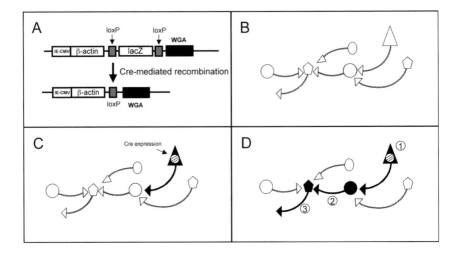

Fig. 1. A genetic approach to transneuronal tracing of complex circuits in the central nervous system (CNS). (A) Construct used to generate the ZW mice. Under normal conditions, ZW mice should express β-galactosidase in every CNS neuron. At the appropriate time and in the desired region of the CNS, the floxed lacZ sequence is excised by Cre-mediated recombination. This procedure initiates expression of the wheat germ agglutinin (WGA) gene in Cre-expressing cells. (B) This diagram represents cell labeling in the ZW mice, prior to Cre-mediated recombination. All neurons express the lacZ gene (white cell bodies) (C) When Cre is induced, it is translocated to the nucleus (hatched); this translocation, in turn, leads to the recombination event, resulting in the expression of the WGA protein tracer (black). (D) Subsequent transneuronal transport and transfer of the WGA tracer reveals the relevant circuit (black neurons) from within the large population of neurons that are not part of the circuit. Second-order (2) and third-order (3) neurons contain WGA after its transneuronal transfer from the first-order WGA-expressing neuron (1).

which is the protein product of the LacZ gene. To induce expression of the WGA, one must first excise the LacZ gene. This is accomplished by taking advantage of a bacterial enzyme, called Cre-recombinase, which recognizes specific sequences that surround the LacZ (called loxP sites), and cuts out anything in between. To achieve Cre-recombination, we cross the ZW mice with others in which Cre expression is directed by a promoter that is uniquely present in a subset of neurons. Excision of the LacZ gene results in synthesis of the WGA protein and its subsequent transneuronal transport into circuits engaged by the neuronal population in which Cre was induced. Importantly, the WGA synthesis is sustained for the life of the animal.

In our first studies of nociceptive circuits, we crossed the ZW mice with other mice that synthesize the Cre protein in dorsal root ganglion neurons that express the voltage-gated, tetrodotoxin-resistant Na$^+$ channel, Na$_v$1.8 (Stirling et al. 2005). The resultant ZW/Na$_v$1.8 Cre double transgenic mice synthesize

WGA exclusively in a subpopulation of primary afferent nociceptors. Unexpectedly, however, we found that there was a mosaic, rather than ubiquitous, expression of the ZW transgene, resulting in a preferential induction of WGA in the IB4-positive, nonpeptide class of primary afferent nociceptors (Braz et al. 2005).

WGA EXPRESSION, TRANSPORT, AND TRANSNEURONAL TRANSFER TO THE SPINAL CORD DORSAL HORN

As illustrated in Fig. 2, WGA expression in doubly transgenic mice was induced preferentially in small-diameter $Na_V1.8$-positive neurons of the IB4 class; 75% of these neurons expressed the $P2X_3$ purinoceptor. When we followed the transneuronal transport and transfer of WGA to the spinal cord, we observed labeling in a wide range of second- and third-order neurons, extending from lamina I to lamina V. Fig. 2A illustrates the typical pattern of transneuronal label in the spinal cord of a 3-week-old $Na_V1.8$-ZW animal. We observed a dense band of WGA-immunoreactive terminals and small cell bodies in a region corresponding to lamina II within the superficial dorsal horn. This finding was not surprising, given the extensive overlap of WGA and IB4 staining in the dorsal root ganglia. In addition, we observed WGA-immunoreactive neuronal cell bodies in deeper regions of the dorsal horn, laminae III, IV, and V and around the central canal. Only rarely did we find labeled neurons in lamina I. Interestingly, in postnatal day 0 (P0) mice, the WGA labeling was restricted to terminals and cell bodies in the superficial dorsal horn. In fact, we detected WGA immunolabeling of deeper laminae only in animals older than 3 weeks, suggesting that the pattern of labeling observed in deeper laminae resulted from transneuronal transport of the WGA from second-order interneurons in the superficial dorsal horn.

Double-labeling experiments provided some surprising insights into the nature of the neurons targeted by IB4-positive nociceptors. We did not find neurons expressing neurokinin-1 receptors, which mark a major population of projection neurons in the superficial dorsal horn. More surprisingly perhaps, we did not find double labeling of interneurons that express PKCγ. In fact, the $Na_V1.8$ subset of nonpeptidergic afferents clearly terminates dorsal to the band of PKCγ interneurons (Fig. 2B). These results illustrate that the IB4-positive nociceptors do not terminate in the part of inner lamina II where the PKCγ neurons reside (an observation recently reported by Zylka et al. 2005), and they also show that the PKCγ interneurons do not even receive a polysynaptic input from this nonpeptide subset of nociceptors.

WGA TRANSPORT AND TRANSNEURONAL
TRANSFER TO SUPRASPINAL SITES

We first observed WGA transneuronal transport to the brain in 3-week-old mice. In fact, despite the presence of significant labeling in primary afferents and in the superficial dorsal horn, we never observed WGA-positive neurons in the brain of younger animals. This observation provides further evidence that the brain labeling in adults resulted from transneuronal transfer from deeper spinal laminae. In general, we observed a consistent pattern of staining within regions previously recognized as major targets of spinal cord nociresponsive neurons (Cliffer et al. 1991; Newman et al. 1996; Gauriau and Bernard 2004). These regions included the hypothalamus, the amygdala, the bed nucleus of the stria terminalis (Fig. 2C), and, most unexpectedly, the lateral aspect of the globus pallidus (Fig. 2D), where we found extensive transneuronal labeling of neurons. As previous studies reported very limited labeling from the spinal cord, the magnitude of the labeling in the globus pallidus was unexpected. Furthermore, although the spinothalamic and spinoparabrachial pathways are considered to be the main ascending spinal routes for the transmission of nociceptive messages from the spinal cord, it was surprising that we did not find transneuronal labeling in the thalamus or the parabrachial nuclei.

Taken together, our results suggest that interneurons of lamina II receive a direct input from IB4-positive nociceptors. These interneurons target projection neurons in lamina V (to a greater extent than in lamina I), and the lamina V neurons in turn project to various limbic and striatal areas of the brain.

We considered it essential to show that synthesis of the WGA only occurs in the primary afferent nociceptors and that labeling in forebrain regions was not the result of brain expression after local Cre recombination. To address this question, we crossed the $Na_V1.8$-Cre mice with the ROSA26 Cre reporter mouse (Soriano 1999) and generated doubly transgenic animals that express the lacZ gene in neurons where Cre recombination occurs. In these mice, we only found β-galactosidase activity in sensory neurons. The lack of brain labeling ruled out transient expression of $Na_V1.8$ during development and confirmed that the WGA immunoreactivity detected in supraspinal neurons of the $Na_V1.8$-ZW mice resulted from transneuronal transfer of the lectin tracer from the spinal cord. This transneuronal tracing analysis provides the first description of the CNS circuits engaged by the "nonpeptide" population of sensory neurons. Our findings suggest that the two classes of primary afferent nociceptors are at the origin of parallel pathways for the transmission of "pain" messages. Although the information conveyed by the two populations of nociceptors may converge at higher levels of the CNS, it appears that the circuits engaged at the level of the spinal cord are remarkably segregated. The results are summarized in Fig.

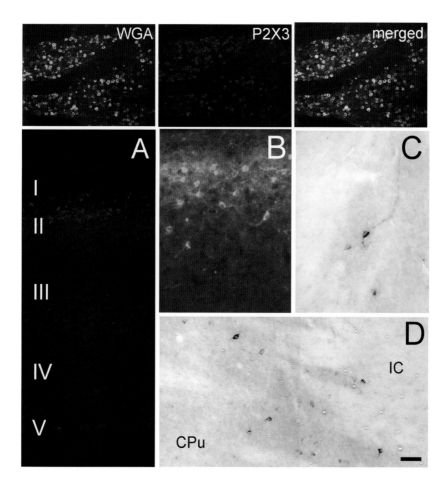

Fig. 2. Expression, transneuronal transport, and transfer of wheat germ agglutinin (WGA) in Na$_V$1.8-ZW mice. WGA expression was preferentially induced in small-diameter, non-peptidergic nociceptors, as revealed by double labeling of WGA (green) and P2X$_3$ (red) in Na$_V$1.8-ZW dorsal root ganglion neurons. (A) Typical transneuronal labeling pattern in the spinal cord of Na$_V$1.8-ZW mice. We found that a wide range of spinal interneurons and likely projection neurons receive inputs from the Na$_V$1.8 subpopulation of nonpeptidergic sensory neurons, but (B) these do not include PKCγ interneurons (green). (C–D) We found transneuronal transfer of WGA primarily in limbic areas (C, bed nucleus of the stria terminalis) and striatal areas (D, globus pallidus). IC: internal capsule; CPu: caudate putamen. Adapted from Braz et al. (2005), with permission.

3. The peptide-containing nociceptors communicate with lamina I projection neurons, which target the thalamus and parabrachial nuclei. By contrast, the Na$_V$1.8-expressing subset of the IB4 population of nociceptors primarily engages limbic regions of the brain, via a trisynaptic circuit that includes lamina II interneurons and lamina V projection neurons. For several reasons, we do not

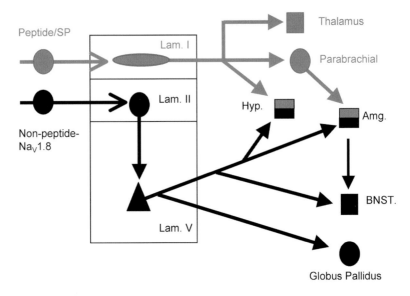

Fig. 3. Parallel, and largely independent, circuits are engaged by the two major primary afferent nociceptor populations. The major output from the $Na_V 1.8$ population of nonpeptidergic nociceptors is via connections with second-order interneurons in lamina II. Transneuronally labeled (third-order) lamina V neurons project, in part directly, to several limbic and striatal regions (fourth-order neurons), including the globus pallidus. In contrast, lamina I neurons, which receive a peptidergic input, project heavily to the brainstem (parabrachial nuclei) and thalamus, but these latter regions were not labeled in the $Na_V 1.8$-ZW mice. Inputs from the two nociceptor populations may converge at supraspinal levels (e.g., the hypothalamus and amygdala), but the routes to these sites differ, in effect constituting parallel pathways for the transmission of "pain" messages. Abbreviations: Amg = amygdala, BNST = bed nucleus of the stria terminalis; Hyp = hypothalamus; Lam = lamina. Adapted from Braz et al. (2005), with permission.

believe that the lamina I neurons are part of this circuit. First, very few lamina I neurons contained the WGA tracer. Second, we did not record any WGA transneuronal transport in the parabrachial nucleus, a major relay to the amygdala from lamina I projection neurons. Third, we made injections of the retrograde tracer Fluorogold into parabrachial nuclei, and only rarely did we find Fluorogold-labeled lamina I WGA-positive cells. We presume that these cells arose from the small number (8%) of peptide-containing nociceptors that carried the ZW transgene. Taken together, our results suggest that the projection of the IB4 population of nociceptors to lamina I neurons is very limited. We propose that lamina I neurons and the supraspinal regions that they target receive inputs predominantly from the Trk-A-expressing, peptidergic population of primary afferent nociceptors. The spino-parabrachial-amygdala pathway (Bernard and Besson 1990; Jasmin et al. 1997), involving primarily neurokinin-1-expressing spinal neurons that receive input from the peptidergic population of nociceptors, is thus paralleled by a direct spino-amygdalar pathway involving deep dorsal horn projection neurons that receive inputs from the nonpeptidergic population of nociceptors. Whether there is a functional distinction between these two circuits remains to be determined.

One of the inherent limitations of this genetic tracing method is the dilution of the tracer after it crosses multiple synapses, making it more difficult to detect the tracer in higher order cells. We assume that extensive convergence of spinal afferents arising from all levels of the spinal cord effectively concentrated the tracer in the different limbic and striatal areas where transneuronal label was readily observed. Conversely, some areas of the brain may be topographically organized to such an extent that conventional immunocytochemical methods are not sensitive enough to detect very low amounts of tracer transferred to these areas. This possibility may explain the lack of labeling of the traditional targets of spinal cord neurons, including the ventroposterolateral nuclei of the thalamus and the parabrachial nuclei.

Our studies suggest that the information transmitted by this subset of nociceptors contributes mainly to the affective component of the pain experience, while the peptidergic population contributes more to its sensory discriminative component. The labeling of striatal (motor) regions of the brain also underscores the fact that the experience of pain rarely occurs independently from a behavior (i.e., from a motor output). In this regard, it is of interest that many patients with persistent clinical pain conditions, such as complex regional pain syndromes, have concurrent severe motor disturbances (Oaklander 2004). Conceivably, the spino-pallidal circuits that are engaged by the nonpeptidergic afferents are critical to activating those complex behaviors.

ACKNOWLEDGMENTS

This work was supported by NIH grants NS-14627 NS-048499 and DE-08973 and by an unrestricted gift from Bristol Myers Squibb.

REFERENCES

Bernard JF, Besson JM. The spino(trigemino)pontoamygdaloid pathway: electrophysiological evidence for an involvement in pain processes. *J Neurophysiol* 1990; 63:473–490.

Braz JM, Rico B, Basbaum AI. Transneuronal tracing of diverse CNS circuits by Cre-mediated induction of wheat germ agglutinin in transgenic mice. *Proc Natl Acad Sci USA* 2002; 99:15148–15153.

Braz JM, Nassar MA, Wood JN, Basbaum AI. Parallel "pain" pathways arise from subpopulations of primary afferents nociceptors. *Neuron* 2005; 47:787–793.

Cliffer KD, Burstein R, Giesler GJ Jr. Distributions of spinothalamic, spinohypothalamic, and spinotelencephalic fibers revealed by anterograde transport of PHA-L in rats. *J Neurosci* 1991; 11:852–868.

Gauriau C, Bernard JF. A comparative reappraisal of projections from the superficial laminae of the dorsal horn in the rat: the forebrain. *J Comp Neurol* 2004; 468:24–56.

Horowitz LF, Montmayeur JP, Echelard Y, Buck LB. A genetic approach to trace neural circuits. *Proc Natl Acad Sci USA* 1999; 96:3194–3199.

Jasmin L, Burkey AR, Card JP, Basbaum AI. Transneuronal labeling of a nociceptive pathway, the spino-(trigemino)-parabrachio-amygdaloid, in the rat. *J Neurosci* 1997; 17:3751–3765.

Newman HM, Stevens RT, Apkarian AV. Direct spinal projections to limbic and striatal areas: anterograde transport studies from the upper cervical spinal cord and the cervical enlargement in squirrel monkey and rat. *J Comp Neurol* 1996; 365:640–658.

Oaklander AL. Progression of dystonia in complex regional pain syndrome. *Neurology* 2004; 63:751.

Snider WD, McMahon SB. Tackling pain at the source: new ideas about nociceptors. *Neuron* 1998; 20:629–632.

Soriano P. Generalized lacZ expression with the ROSA26 Cre reporter strain. *Nat Genet* 1999; 21:70–71.

Stirling LC, Forlani G, Baker MD, et al. Nociceptor-specific gene deletion using heterozygous $Na_V1.8$-Cre recombinase mice. *Pain* 2005; 113:27–36.

Yoshihara Y, Mizuno T, Nakahira M, et al. A genetic approach to visualization of multisynaptic neural pathways using plant lectin transgene. *Neuron* 1999; 22:33–41.

Zylka MJ, Rice FL, Anderson DJ. Topographically distinct epidermal nociceptive circuits revealed by axonal tracers targeted to Mrgprd. *Neuron* 2005; 45:17–25.

Correspondence to: João Manuel Braz, Department of Anatomy, University of California San Francisco, 1550 Fourth Street, San Francisco, CA 94143-2722, USA. Email: bjoao@phy.ucsf.edu.

Proceedings of the 11th World Congress on Pain,
edited by Herta Flor, Eija Kalso, and Jonathan O.
Dostrovsky, IASP Press, Seattle, © 2006.

32

Neuropathic Pain:
A Neurodegenerative Disease

Joachim Scholz and Clifford J. Woolf

*Neural Plasticity Research Group, Department of Anesthesia and Critical Care,
Massachusetts General Hospital and Harvard Medical School, Charlestown,
Massachusetts, USA*

MULTIPLE DISORDERS OF THE PERIPHERAL NERVOUS SYSTEM PRODUCE PERSISTENT PAIN

Chronic pain is a feature of many diseases involving injury of a peripheral nerve or spinal nerve root (peripheral neuropathic pain). Compression of a spinal nerve caused by a slipped intervertebral disk, entrapment of the median nerve at the wrist in carpal tunnel syndrome, inadvertent cutting of a nerve during surgery, and strain caused by a blunt trauma are examples of mechanical nerve damage associated with ongoing pain. Persistent pain also occurs in metabolic disorders of the peripheral nervous system, predominantly diabetic neuropathies; after toxic nerve damage as induced by chemotherapy; and in infectious diseases of the peripheral nervous system, such as herpes zoster or acquired immunodeficiency syndrome (AIDS).

NEUROPATHIC PAIN COMES IN MANY GUISES

Pain caused by diseases of the nervous system manifests with a complex variety of signs and symptoms. Spontaneous pain may be constantly present or manifest in episodes interspersed with pain-free intervals. Peripheral nerve lesions inevitably lead to a loss of sensation that reflects the degree of sensory fiber damage. However, in addition to sensory loss, patients with neuropathic pain have hypersensitivity to mechanical and thermal stimuli. Normally innocuous touch or dynamic mechanical stimulation, such as the movement of a shirt on the surface of the skin, may evoke pain (tactile allodynia). Likewise, pain may be elicited by a normally nonpainful cold sensation, as from a cool breeze (cold allodynia). In addition, stimuli that are already painful under normal circumstances such as a pinprick or a very hot shower may produce pain of a disproportional intensity (hyperalgesia). Sensory loss and evoked pain may occur in neighboring or overlapping body areas (Fields et al. 1998; Gottrup et al. 1998).

One difficulty in understanding neuropathic pain, which also causes problems for its treatment, is the persistence of the pain. Even when the cause is a discrete trauma or a transient condition like the reactivation of herpes zoster virus, chronic pain that lasts for years may develop. Currently, no pharmacological treatment prevents the transition from acute pain after nerve injury to chronic neuropathic pain, with one exception: patients vaccinated against varicella-zoster virus have a reduced risk of postherpetic neuralgia if they do develop herpes zoster; the vaccine reduced the incidence of herpes zoster by 51.3% and decreased the incidence of postherpetic neuralgia by 66.5% (Oxman et al. 2005). All other drugs for neuropathic pain do not target the actual nerve-damaging disease process; they only provide symptomatic relief. Recommendations for a first-line therapy include gabapentin or pregabalin, tricyclic antidepressants (nortriptyline, amitriptyline, and desipramine), dual reuptake inhibitors of serotonin and norepinephrine, opioid analgesics, tramadol, and topical lidocaine (Dworkin et al. 2003; Goldstein, et al. 2005). The efficacy of these drugs is modest. Between 2.5 and 5.5 patients must be treated before pain relief of at least 50% is achieved in one patient (Backonja 2002; Eisenberg et al. 2005; Finnerup et al. 2005). Moreover, most of these drugs have undesirable side effects. A disease-modifying treatment that preempts or aborts chronic pain after nerve injury is needed. However, developing such a preemptive treatment first requires an explanation for the persistence of neuropathic pain.

MECHANISMS OF NEUROPATHIC PAIN

The lack of a direct relationship between pain mechanisms and disease etiology prevents inference of operating mechanisms from the clinical diagnosis. A particular mechanism may operate in many diseases, and a single disease may prompt activation of multiple mechanisms. Moreover, neuropathic pain is a dynamic disorder, with more than one mechanism operating at any time, and with mechanisms that change over the course of a disease.

Immediately following a nerve lesion, injured primary sensory neurons produce a short-lived surge of spontaneous activity, termed injury discharge. This transient rise in frequency of action potentials is followed by a second increase in spontaneous (ectopic) activity that also involves uninjured neighboring neurons; this second wave of activity is sustained for several weeks after the injury (Devor 2006). Changes in the expression, phosphorylation, and membrane distribution of receptors of the transient receptor potential (TRP) family that transduce chemical and thermal stimuli may produce increased responses of sensory neurons to these stimuli (peripheral sensitization). Sympathetic nerve fibers sprout into the neuroma that forms at the proximal stump of an injured nerve and into the dorsal root ganglia (DRG), where they surround the cell bodies of primary afferents. Norepinephrine released from these sympathetic fibers can modify the activity of sensory neurons. Cytokines produced by immune cells infiltrating the lesion site and invading the DRG have a similar effect, producing an increase in spontaneous and stimulus-evoked discharges. Finally, sensory neurons change their chemical phenotype and begin to express new ion channels, receptors, and transmitter peptides (Fig. 1).

Peripheral nerve injury provokes a marked change in the responsiveness of the central nervous system to primary afferent input that has profound consequences for the processing of sensory information, including pain (Hökfelt et al. 2006). Activity-dependent opening of the ionotropic N-methyl-D-aspartate (NMDA)-type glutamate receptor, as well as its phosphorylation and increased expression, lead to potentiated synaptic transmission in the dorsal horn of the spinal cord (central sensitization). Enhanced recruitment of α-amino-3-hydroxy-5-methyl-4-isoxazole propionate (AMPA) receptors at postsynaptic synapses further augments glutamatergic activation of dorsal horn neurons. New synapses may form between sprouting low-threshold sensory fibers and transmission neurons in lamina II of the superficial dorsal horn; as a consequence, input from nonpainful stimulation would become more effective. This and other possible mechanisms can lead to innocuous mechanical stimulation mistakenly eliciting a painful response, corresponding to the tactile allodynia observed in many patients with neuropathic pain. Peripheral nerve lesions also provoke a marked neuroimmune reaction in the dorsal horn, including microglial activation and cytokine release (Fig. 1). This neuroimmune response plays a major role in the development of neuropathic pain (Tsuda et al. 2005), but the precise pathways of communication between primary sensory afferents, microglia, and dorsal horn neurons still need to be resolved.

Normally, local interneurons and descending fiber tracts originating in brainstem nuclei maintain a balanced processing of sensory input that reflects the nature and intensity of environmental stimuli. However, after nerve injury, descending control shifts toward facilitation. We find that peripheral nerve injury triggers a slow process of neurodegeneration in the dorsal horn that continues for several weeks, causes a substantial loss of inhibitory interneurons, and consequently leads to spinal disinhibition (Scholz et al. 2005). This irreversible disinhibition is an important contributor to the persistence of neuropathic pain.

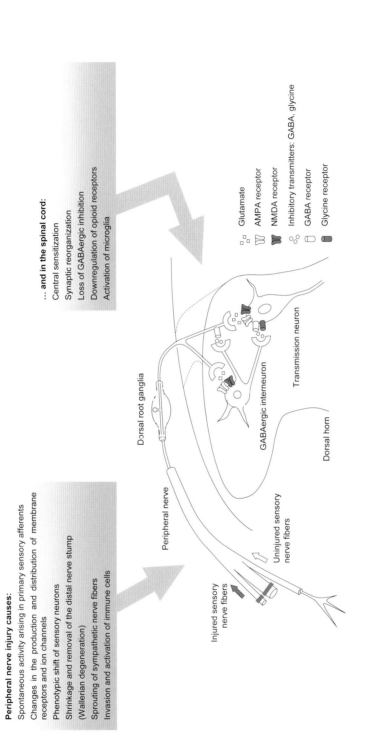

Peripheral nerve injury causes:

Spontaneous activity arising in primary sensory afferents

Changes in the production and distribution of membrane receptors and ion channels

Phenotypic shift of sensory neurons

Shrinkage and removal of the distal nerve stump (Wallerian degeneration)

Sprouting of sympathetic nerve fibers

Invasion and activation of immune cells

... and in the spinal cord:

Central sensitization

Synaptic reorganization

Loss of GABAergic inhibition

Downregulation of opioid receptors

Activation of microglia

Injured sensory nerve fibers

Uninjured sensory nerve fibers

Peripheral nerve

Dorsal root ganglia

GABAergic interneuron

Transmission neuron

Dorsal horn

Glutamate

AMPA receptor

NMDA receptor

Inhibitory transmitters: GABA, glycine

GABA receptor

Glycine receptor

Fig. 1. Multiple mechanisms are responsible for the manifestation and persistence of pain after nerve injury. Some of these mechanisms involve injured primary afferents, while others operate in uninjured neighboring fibers or in the spinal cord.

SPINAL CONTROL OF SENSORY TRANSMISSION

Sensory input from the periphery leads to a parallel activation of transmission neurons and inhibitory interneurons in the superficial laminae of the spinal cord. Activation of these interneurons creates a negative feedback, downregulating the transmitter release from sensory nerve fibers (presynaptic inhibition) and reducing the excitability of transmission neurons (postsynaptic inhibition). Dorsal horn interneurons synthesize two main inhibitory transmitters: γ-aminobutyric acid (GABA) and glycine. Presynaptic inhibition is mediated by GABA acting on $GABA_A$ and $GABA_B$ receptors, while postsynaptic inhibition of transmission neurons involves GABA and glycine. The two components of inhibitory action can be separated pharmacologically, using the drugs bicuculline and strychnine, which block the activation of $GABA_A$ or glycine receptors, respectively.

In whole-cell patch-clamp recordings from isolated slices of the spinal cord (Fig. 2A), pharmacological blockade of GABAergic inhibition leads to a sharp increase in polysynaptic excitatory postsynaptic currents (EPSCs) (Fig. 2B–D). The increase includes recruitment of Aβ-fiber afferents (Fig. 2B, E). In comparison, blocking glycinergic inhibition has only a slight effect (Baba et al. 2003). In vivo, injections of bicuculline or strychnine produce an exaggeration of withdrawal reflexes and pain-related behavior (Sugimoto et al. 1990; Sivilotti and Woolf 1994; Malan et al. 2002), demonstrating the significance of spinal inhibition for controlling the transmission of nociceptive input. Although GABA, after nerve injury, anomalously produces excitation in a subgroup of lamina I neurons (Coull et al. 2003), the predominant GABAergic effect in lamina II of the spinal cord is still to produce inhibition (Scholz et al. 2005). Intrathecal administration of GABA agonists decreases behavioral indications of pain in animal models of peripheral nerve injury (Malan et al. 2002; Scholz et al. 2005).

NERVE-INJURY-INDUCED LOSS OF SPINAL INHIBITION

Normally, inhibitory postsynaptic currents (IPSCs) are present in more than 95% of lamina II neurons, indicating that virtually all these neurons are held under tight control to prevent runaway excitation. However, following nerve injury the number of superficial dorsal horn neurons with inhibitory currents is significantly diminished such that only 70% of the neurons receive inhibitory input. Moreover, the currents are much smaller and shorter because of a marked decrease in the GABAergic component, whereas the glycinergic component of the currents remains largely intact (Fig. 3A). Consequently, inhibitory control of spinal cord neurons after nerve injury is severely weakened, mainly due to

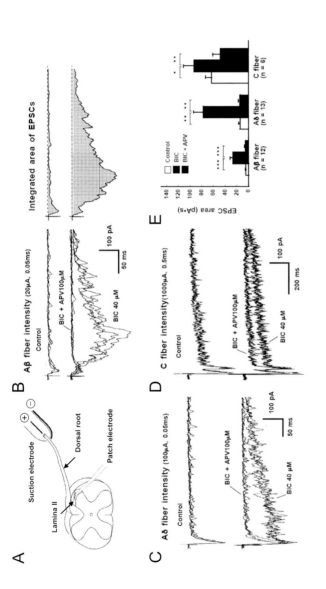

Fig. 2. Blocking GABAergic inhibition with bicuculline (BIC) enhances polysynaptic excitatory transmission. (A) Scheme illustrating the technique of whole-cell patch clamp recording in slices of the rat lumbar spinal cord that have the L4 dorsal root attached for afferent stimulation. (B, C) Stimulation at A-fiber intensity evoked mono- and polysynaptic excitatory postsynaptic currents (EPSCs) of short duration. Bath-applied bicuculline (40 μM) resulted in repetitive, long-lasting (300–1000 ms) polysynaptic EPSCs, which were eliminated by the NMDA-receptor antagonist DL-2-amino-5-phosphonovalerate (APV; 100 μM). (D) Bicuculline enhanced long-lasting polysynaptic components of EPSCs evoked by C-fiber stimulation. (E) The effects of bicuculline and APV on the integrated area of EPSCs. * P < 0.05, ** P < 0.01, *** P < 0.001. Reprinted from Baba et al. (2003), copyright 2003, with permission from Elsevier.

a specific loss of GABAergic input. GABA receptors are still present (Moore et al. 2002) and functional (Scholz et al. 2005). The loss of inhibition has to be caused by a reduction in either the synthesis or release of GABA by inhibitory interneurons.

APOPTOSIS OF DORSAL HORN NEURONS

In the early 1990s, Peter Watson at the University of Toronto examined the spinal cords of patients who had suffered from postherpetic neuralgia during their lifetimes, in one case for 18 years (Watson et al. 1991). He found a substantial reduction in the size of the dorsal horn in spinal segments that were supplied by sensory fibers innervating the affected dermatomes, a first hint that diseases associated with peripheral neuropathic pain may provoke neurodegeneration in the dorsal horn. At the same time, Gary Bennett's group at the National Institutes of Health observed the occurrence of abnormal "dark" neurons in the dorsal horn of animals after a partial nerve injury (Sugimoto et al. 1990). Bennett's group interpreted the appearance of these neurons as a sign of degeneration in response to the injury; however, they did not show whether these neurons actually died. Based on his observation, Bennett postulated that injury-induced discharge elicits an immediate massive inflow of sensory stimuli to the spinal cord, producing a level of excitation high enough to cause a rapid loss of dorsal horn neurons.

Glutamate, the most prominent transmitter released by sensory nerve fibers, is a prime candidate for causing excitotoxic insult. High levels of glutamate are responsible for the death of neurons following spinal cord trauma or stroke. These massive direct lesions result primarily in necrosis (passive cell death), followed by a second wave of apoptotic cell death. Activation of glutamate receptors leads to depolarization of neurons and calcium influx. The involvement of calcium in many vital cell functions demands careful buffering of its intracellular concentrations. Mitochondria are the cell organelles watching over intracellular calcium levels by taking up excess calcium ions. However, in the presence of abnormally increased glutamate release and sustained activation of glutamate receptors, the calcium-buffering capacity of mitochondria quickly becomes exhausted. When overloaded with calcium, the membrane of mitochondria begins to leak, triggering the release of cytochrome c, which initiates the self-destruction (apoptosis) of critically damaged cells by activating caspases, a family of protein-cleaving enzymes.

Following partial injury of the rat sciatic nerve, we saw no evidence of necrosis in the dorsal horn. However, 7 days after injury, apoptotic cell profiles occurred in the superficial dorsal horn (laminae I–III), where sensory fibers

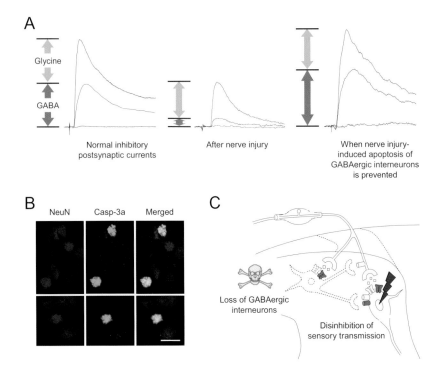

Fig. 3. Loss of inhibitory interneurons causes spinal disinhibition after peripheral nerve injury. (A) Representative traces of afferent stimulation-evoked inhibitory postsynaptic currents (IPSCs) recorded in lamina II neurons of the rat dorsal horn. These IPSCs have two elements: a glycinergic component (blocked by strychnine) and a GABAergic component (blocked by the GABA$_A$-receptor antagonist bicuculline). Two weeks after spared nerve injury, the IPSC amplitude and the decay time were substantially reduced. Recordings in the presence of strychnine (0.5 µmol/L) and bicuculline (5–10 µmol/L) revealed a particularly marked reduction in the GABAergic IPSC component. Continuous intrathecal delivery of zVAD, a caspase activity blocker, starting at the time of nerve injury, prevented the decrease in afferent-evoked IPSCs. (B) Active caspase-3 (Casp-3a) in dorsal horn neurons (immunolabeled for neuronal nuclear protein, NeuN) after spared nerve injury. (C) Nerve-injury-induced loss of GABAergic inhibitory interneurons leads to disinhibition of sensory transmission in the dorsal horn. Modified from Scholz et al. (2005), with permission from the Society of Neuroscience.

conveying nociceptive information terminate. While the number of apoptotic cells was small at any time, we observed apoptosis over an extended period of 3 weeks. When we compared different types of peripheral nerve injury associated with pain-like behavior—spared nerve injury (Decosterd and Woolf 2000), chronic constriction injury of the sciatic nerve (Bennett and Xie 1988) and spinal nerve ligation (Kim and Chung 1992)—we found the same protracted temporal pattern of apoptosis induction. At the peak of apoptosis induction, we detected active caspase-3 in neurons (Fig. 3B). The cumulative effect of this protracted degeneration was substantial: 4 weeks after the injury, thousands of dorsal horn neurons (more than 20%) were lost (Scholz et al. 2005).

Nerve-injury-induced apoptosis was reduced by the NMDA-receptor antagonist dizocilpine (MK-801), supporting the hypothesis that glutamate is the major culprit responsible for the death of dorsal horn neurons. The delayed peak and protracted time course of apoptosis induction suggested a sustained form of excitotoxic insult. To elucidate the role of sensory input, we applied microspheres loaded with the local anesthetic bupivacaine proximal to the injured nerve. The bupivacaine microspheres released the anesthetic slowly so that sensory nerve fiber activity originating at the lesion site was prevented from reaching the spinal cord for 7 days. This sustained blockade of sensory input reduced the number of apoptotic profiles very efficiently, supporting the concept that excitotoxic levels of glutamate result from abnormal afferent activity. However, as soon as the nerve block was released, apoptosis induction set in again, although the nerve injury was now 7 days old (Scholz et al. 2005). Obviously, the degeneration of dorsal horn neurons results from a persistently increased activity of sensory nerve fibers and is not caused by the short-lived injury discharge that immediately follows a nerve lesion.

GABAERGIC INHIBITORY INTERNEURONS ARE AMONG THE DORSAL HORN NEURONS THAT DEGENERATE

To determine whether GABAergic inhibitory interneurons degenerate after nerve injury, we employed in situ hybridization of glutamic acid decarboxylase (GAD67) messenger RNA, an enzyme required for GABA synthesis (Mackie et al. 2003). Four weeks after injury, the number of GAD67 mRNA-positive neurons was decreased by 25%, indicating that the nerve-injury-induced loss of GABAergic inhibition is caused by death of inhibitory interneurons. The loss of these interneurons was dependent on caspase activation, because continuous treatment with benzyloxycarbonyl-Val-Ala-Asp(OMe)-fluoromethylketone (zVAD), a drug that blocks caspase activity, reduced the number of apoptotic cells and prevented the death of GABAergic interneurons. Importantly, the interneurons maintained their inhibitory function if they were protected against apoptosis. When caspase activity was blocked with zVAD, inhibitory currents were preserved after nerve injury (Fig. 3A). Averting neuronal death and the loss of spinal inhibition with zVAD reduced pain hypersensitivity after nerve injury. This neuroprotective treatment did not resolve neuropathic pain-like behavior completely, probably because other pain mechanisms operated independently of interneuron degeneration. However, apoptosis of GABAergic interneurons is likely to be a prominent factor contributing to the persistence of pain, because neurons in the adult nervous system lack the ability to regenerate. Loss of spinal interneurons creates a chronic state of disinhibition; it destroys the delicate balance between excitation and inhibition (Fig. 3C). The result is ongoing pathological hyperexcitability in the dorsal horn, comparable to an epileptic focus, but one that produces pain rather than seizures. Neuroprotection with zVAD had a sustained effect on pain-like behavior that outlasted termination of the treatment, indicating that blocking neuronal apoptosis prevents pain persistence.

CONCLUSION

Neuroprotection is a novel, disease-modifying concept for the treatment of chronic neuropathic pain: it targets an underlying pain mechanism rather than suppressing painful symptoms. Correct timing of the therapeutic intervention will be crucial for successful translation of our findings into clinical practice. Two approaches are conceivable, and a combination of both is likely to provide the best results. First, abnormally increased sensory input needs to be effectively reduced in order to curtail the sensory inflow that leads to the induction of apoptosis. Such analgesia has to be maintained not just for a few days after nerve injury, but for several weeks or longer. Second, viable strategies for neuroprotection are required to improve the resistance of dorsal horn neurons to excitotoxicity. In patients, it will not be possible to block apoptosis by caspase inhibition, because apoptosis is involved in the constant physiological turnover of tissues and plays an important role in tumor defense. Other strategies for intervention are needed. Regrettably, treatment with glutamate receptor antagonists is hampered by severe side effects, as glutamate is an almost ubiquitous neurotransmitter in the central nervous system. Overcoming these obstacles and finding efficient strategies to prevent the nerve-injury-induced loss of dorsal horn neurons will be worth the effort, since for the first time, we have an opportunity to modify the course of neuropathic pain.

ACKNOWLEDGMENTS

This work was supported by a Feodor-Lynen fellowship from the Alexander von Humboldt-Foundation (J. Scholz), research grants from the National Institute of Neurological Disorders and Stroke (NINDS), and the Swiss National Science Foundation. We thank Charles B. Berde for providing the bupivacaine-loaded microspheres.

REFERENCES

Baba H, Ji RR, Kohno T, Moore KA, et al. Removal of GABAergic inhibition facilitates polysynaptic A fiber-mediated excitatory transmission to the superficial spinal dorsal horn. *Mol Cell Neurosci* 2003; 24:818–830.

Backonja MM. Use of anticonvulsants for treatment of neuropathic pain. *Neurology* 2002; 59: S14–S17.

Bennett GJ, Xie YK. A peripheral mononeuropathy in rat that produces disorders of pain sensation like those seen in man. *Pain* 1988; 33:87–107.

Coull JA, Boudreau D, Bachand K, et al. Trans-synaptic shift in anion gradient in spinal lamina I neurons as a mechanism of neuropathic pain. *Nature* 2003; 424:938–942.

Decosterd I, Woolf CJ. Spared nerve injury: an animal model of persistent peripheral neuropathic pain. *Pain* 2000; 87:149–158.

Devor M. Response of nerves to injury in relation to neuropathic pain. In: McMahon SB, Koltzenburg M (Eds). *Wall and Melzack's Textbook of Pain*. Elsevier Churchill Livingstone, 2006, pp 905–927.

Dworkin RH, Backonja M, Rowbotham MC, et al. Advances in neuropathic pain: diagnosis, mechanisms, and treatment recommendations. *Arch Neurol* 2003; 60:1524–1534.

Eisenberg E, McNicol ED, Carr DB. Efficacy and safety of opioid agonists in the treatment of neuropathic pain of nonmalignant origin: systematic review and meta-analysis of randomized controlled trials. *JAMA* 2005; 293:3043–3052.

Fields HL, Rowbotham M, Baron R. Postherpetic neuralgia: irritable nociceptors and deafferentation. *Neurobiol Dis* 1998; 5:209–227.

Finnerup NB, Otto M, McQuay HJ, Jensen TS, Sindrup SH. Algorithm for neuropathic pain treatment: an evidence based proposal. *Pain* 2005; 118:289–305.

Goldstein DJ, Lu Y, Detke MJ, Lee TC, Iyengar S. Duloxetine vs. placebo in patients with painful diabetic neuropathy. *Pain* 2005; 116:109–118.

Gottrup H, Nielsen J, Arendt-Nielsen L, Jensen TS. The relationship between sensory thresholds and mechanical hyperalgesia in nerve injury. *Pain* 1998; 75:321–329.

Hökfelt T, Zhang X, Xiaojun X, Wiesenfeld-Hallin Z. Central consequences of peripheral nerve damage. In: McMahon SB, Koltzenburg M (Eds). *Wall and Melzack's Textbook of Pain*. Elsevier Churchill Livingstone, 2006, pp 947–959.

Kim SH, Chung JM. An experimental model for peripheral neuropathy produced by segmental spinal nerve ligation in the rat. *Pain* 1992; 50:355–363.

Mackie M, Hughes DI, Maxwell DJ, Tillakaratne NJ, Todd AJ. Distribution and colocalisation of glutamate decarboxylase isoforms in the rat spinal cord. *Neuroscience* 2003; 119:461–472.

Malan TP, Mata HP, Porreca F. Spinal GABA(A) and GABA(B) receptor pharmacology in a rat model of neuropathic pain. *Anesthesiology* 2002; 96:1161–1167.

Moore KA, Kohno T, Karchewski LA, et al. Partial peripheral nerve injury promotes a selective loss of GABAergic inhibition in the superficial dorsal horn of the spinal cord. *J Neurosci* 2002; 22:6724–6731.

Oxman MN, Levin MJ, Johnson GR, et al. A vaccine to prevent herpes zoster and postherpetic neuralgia in older adults. *N Engl J Med* 2005; 352:2271–2284.

Scholz J, Broom DC, Youn DH, et al. Blocking caspase activity prevents transsynaptic neuronal apoptosis and the loss of inhibition in lamina II of the dorsal horn after peripheral nerve injury. *J Neurosci* 2005; 25:7317–7323.

Sivilotti L, Woolf CJ. The contribution of GABAA and glycine receptors to central sensitization: disinhibition and touch-evoked allodynia in the spinal cord. *J Neurophysiol* 1994; 72:169–179.

Sugimoto T, Bennett GJ, Kajander KC. Transsynaptic degeneration in the superficial dorsal horn after sciatic nerve injury: effects of a chronic constriction injury, transection, and strychnine. *Pain* 1990; 42:205–213.

Tsuda M, Inoue K, Salter MW. Neuropathic pain and spinal microglia: a big problem from molecules in "small" glia, *Trends Neurosci* 2005; 28:101–107.

Watson CP, Deck JH, Morshead C, Van der Kooy D, Evans RJ. Post-herpetic neuralgia: further post-mortem studies of cases with and without pain. *Pain* 1991; 44:105–117.

Correspondence to: Clifford J. Woolf, MD, PhD, Neural Plasticity Research Group, Department of Anesthesia and Critical Care, Massachusetts General Hospital and Harvard Medical School, 149 13th Street, Room 4309, Charlestown, MA 02129, USA. Fax: 617-724-3632; email: woolf.clifford@mgh.harvard.edu.

Part IV

Imaging Pain

Proceedings of the 11th World Congress on Pain,
edited by Herta Flor, Eija Kalso, and Jonathan O.
Dostrovsky, IASP Press, Seattle, © 2006.

33

Recent Advances in Imaging Pain

Karen D. Davis

*Toronto Western Research Institute, Toronto Western Hospital,
University Health Network, and Department of Surgery,
University of Toronto, Toronto, Ontario, Canada*

Over the last 15 years there has been a dramatic increase in public awareness of the importance of pain research. In fact, the U.S. government declared
the 1990s as the "Decade of the Brain" and the 2000s as the "Decade of Pain
Control and Research." In 2004, the Canadian government declared the first
week in November of each year as "National Pain Awareness Week." Concurrent with this public attention toward pain research has been greater recognition
and support for the utility of brain imaging technologies to study basic and
clinical neuroscience, psychology, and psychiatry. Therefore, it is an opportune
time to study the mechanisms of acute and chronic pain with brain imaging
technologies.

Numerous imaging studies have identified sites of activation during application of noxious stimuli within a distributed network including the primary and
secondary somatosensory cortices (S1, S2), the anterior cingulate cortex (ACC),
the insula, and the prefrontal cortex (for review see Apkarian et al. 2005). This
network provides a general framework from which to begin to study the cortical
mechanisms of pain. As described below, pain is a complex multidimensional
experience, and the cortical mechanisms underlying specific aspects of this
experience and the impact of individual factors and behavioral context are just
beginning to be unraveled. Before considering the pain experience itself, this
chapter will introduce some basic concepts concerning brain imaging itself.
Then, some more sophisticated approaches to imaging pain will be described
that consider the myriad of perceptual, behavioral, attentional, and personality
factors that influence brain responses (Fig. 1).

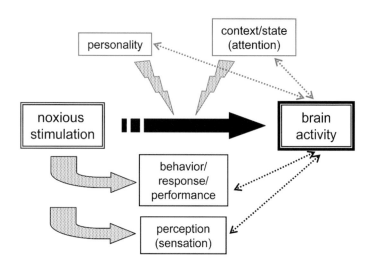

Fig. 1. Brain imaging analysis approaches for pain studies. A simple approach in fMRI pain studies is to find the loci of brain activity that show increased responses during application of a noxious stimulus. However, more sophisticated approaches can be used to interrogate the evoked brain activity for responses that correlate with specific aspects of the subject's evoked response such as a particular sensation or behavior. Each subject's personality or attentional state or other contextual components of the experimental session can also be used as regressors to identify trait-specific activations.

IMAGING BASICS AND CORRELATION APPROACHES

Modern neuroimaging has contributed to our understanding of the forebrain mechanisms of pain. The most common neuroimaging technologies that have been used to study pain are positron emission tomography (PET), functional magnetic resonance imaging (fMRI), magnetoencephalography (MEG), and electroencephalography (EEG). The latter techniques (EEG and MEG) are electrical-magnetic-based imaging methods that can identify brain activity with excellent temporal accuracy (milliseconds) and spatial accuracy (millimeters); the capabilities of each method vary depending on the number of detectors or channels. The resolution of these methods is beneficial to study response latencies of particular brain regions to painful stimuli. On the other hand, PET and fMRI are vascular-based, indirect methods of acquiring information pertaining to brain activity evoked by a stimulus or task. This chapter will focus on the most popular imaging method used in pain research, fMRI.

The basic premise of fMRI is that neuronal activity increases metabolic demand. This increased metabolic demand results in hemodynamic changes that alter MRI magnetic fields. The resultant MRI signal changes are known as BOLD (blood-oxygen-level-dependent) signals, and they form the basis of fMRI (Arthurs and Boniface 2002). Because fMRI studies rely on identifying BOLD signal differences within voxels (brain volumes) between conditions (e.g., rest versus stimulation), they are known as "activation studies." Voxels that show statistically significant signal differences across conditions are typically color-coded and are overlaid on high-resolution MRI images.

In a simple block experimental design, a stimulus is held on for blocks of time, say 15–30 seconds, interleaved with blocks of a control or rest period. For this type of experiment, it is common to use a simple "boxcar" predictor model to locate brain areas that respond to the stimulus. Essentially, the MRI signals in all voxels in the brain are assessed to locate those responses that increase and decrease (i.e., in a sawtooth pattern) as the stimulus is repeatedly applied and removed.

A more sophisticated approach to fMRI analysis is to specifically correlate the activity within a defined cortical region (i.e., region of interest) to a quantifiable factor associated with the subject's evoked sensation (e.g., pain intensity), response (e.g., autonomic, emotion), experimental context or state (e.g., attention), or personality (e.g., neuroticism, catastrophizing) (see Fig. 1). In these types of studies, the stimulus intensity can be held constant for all trials in the experiment, or it can be varied, in which case the stimulus intensity can also be included as a regression factor.

Another type of correlation analysis is based on the temporal dynamics of the evoked sensation. The hemodynamic response function to a brief stimulus characteristically takes the form of a 10–12-second gamma variate function with a 2–4-second lag and a peak at approximately 6 seconds (Heeger and Ress 2002). Therefore, the time course of the task or stimuli can be convolved with the gamma variate function to create a predictor function that can then be used in the analysis of brain-imaging data to locate brain regions whose activity correlates with the predictor. This approach extracts brain responses that more closely correlate with the hemodynamic response to the stimulus, or alternatively with the time course of the evoked sensation. This "percept-related fMRI" approach, described in more detail below, can be used to identify brain activity related to specific types of sensation (Davis et al. 2002, 2004).

PAIN AS A MULTIDIMENSIONAL EXPERIENCE

Nearly 40 years ago, Melzack and Casey (1968) described pain as a multidimensional experience. This conceptual framework described pain as an experience that includes different qualities and quantities of sensation, as well as evaluative, perceptual, motivational, and affective reactions to painful stimuli.

The McGill Pain Questionnaire (MPQ) expanded this concept and listed specific words that described sensory and affective qualities and evaluative aspects of the multidimensional pain experience (Melzack 1975). The MPQ has been particularly useful in the study of chronic pain because certain descriptors or constellations of qualities tend to characterize particular types of pains. For example, central pain is most commonly described as burning, aching, lancinating, pricking, lacerating, and/or pressing (Boivie 2002). Therefore it is important to understand how specific qualities of pain arise.

THE DISCONNECT BETWEEN A NOXIOUS STIMULUS, NOCICEPTION, AND PAIN

Typically a noxious stimulus excites nociceptors, produces nociception (a neurophysiological event), and leads to the subjective experience of pain. However, it is well known that a noxious stimulus can evoke different sensory and emotional experiences in different individuals. Furthermore, there are instances when the intensity and temporal properties of a noxious stimulus and pain do not coincide. For example, some pains become attenuated (i.e., they show habituation) (e.g., Milne et al. 1991), while others increase with repeated or maintained noxious stimulation (i.e., they show temporal summation) (e.g., Arendt-Nielsen et al. 1994; Lautenbacher et al. 1995; Vierck et al. 1997; Sarlani and Greenspan 2002). Additionally, a maintained noxious stimulus may also evoke multiple sensory qualities, each with a different time course (e.g., Davis and Pope 2002). There are also many clinical conditions characterized by discordance between the stimulus and the pain, as is exemplified in situations of allodynia, hyperalgesia, or hyperpathia. Conversely, there are conditions in which patients experience chronic pain but are insensitive to externally applied stimuli. For example, we have reported that chronic pain patients with hysterical anesthesia can exhibit abnormal brush-evoked and noxious stimulus-evoked responses in the S1 and S2 cortices, the posterior parietal cortex, the ACC, and the prefrontal cortex contralateral to the body region in which they do not perceive stimuli (Mailis-Gagnon et al. 2003). Therefore, the standard approach used in most fMRI studies, which relies on a hemodynamic response function derived from a stimulus predictor, may not be adequate to extract the cortical responses that underlie different aspects of the pain experience and the relationship between that experience and the evoking stimulus. One solution to this problem is to incorporate the temporal properties of an individual's specific pain experience into the predictors used in the statistical analysis of fMRI data. Examples of the utility of this percept-related fMRI approach (Davis et al. 2002) are described below.

IDENTIFYING CORTICAL ACTIVITY RELATED TO PAIN EXPERIENCES: THE PERCEPT-RELATED fMRI APPROACH

Recent advances in fMRI studies of pain include greater sophistication in study design and more advanced analysis and approaches to data interpretation. One strategy is based on the consideration of temporal response attributes and perceptual responses to a noxious stimulus. There are two important elements of a percept-related fMRI study: sensory ratings and unique sensory experiences. Concerning the former, the most effective way to conduct a percept-related fMRI study is to obtain each subject's ratings (continuous, if possible) of the sensation of interest. An offline psychophysical session can be used to collect ratings of sensations that are evoked in a predictable fashion. However, the results should be viewed only as an approximation of the sensation-related responses during acquisition of fMRI data because the investigators cannot know with certainty whether the subjects' responses outside the fMRI session mirror those experienced during the fMRI session. The second important aspect of a percept-related fMRI study is that the sensation of interest occurs in relative temporal isolation compared to other sensations evoked by the stimulus.

Percept-related fMRI and other correlative approaches have been used to delineate forebrain activations associated with the salience, intensity, and various other qualities of acute and chronic pains. Examples of these qualities are given below.

Cold-evoked prickle sensation and paradoxical heat. Cooling the skin down to near 0°C evokes a myriad of sensations including cold, pain, ache, prickling, and, especially upon rewarming, paradoxical heat (Davis and Pope 2002). However, the prickle sensations and paradoxical heat sensations do not usually occur in synchrony with the other sensations and the time course tends to be quite variable within and across subjects. Therefore, brain responses could be found that coincide with individual reports of either prickle or paradoxical heat. These experiments revealed prickle-related responses in areas associated with pain and touch (ACC, S2, and insula), with motor planning (supplementary motor area, premotor cortex, and caudate nucleus), and with attention/awareness and evaluative functions (prefrontal cortex, posterior parietal cortex, and ACC) (Davis et al. 2002). The paradoxical heat reports were uniquely correlated with activity in the right anterior insula (Davis et al. 2004). This finding is in accord with recent studies implicating the insula in thermosensory and interoceptive functions (Craig et al. 2000; Craig 2002; Bechara and Naqvi 2004).

Stimulus salience. In a series of experiments, Downar et al. (2000, 2001, 2002, 2003) searched for brain responses to attention-grabbing stimuli across multiple sensory modalities, including prolonged pain. The findings across the experiments converged on a frontal-parietal-cingulate salience network.

Interestingly, several nodes in this network, such as the temporoparietal junction, inferior frontal gyrus, and ACC have also been implicated as important in pain mechanisms. However, our studies suggest that such areas may act to detect the salience of pain, rather than its quality or intensity. Conversely, it was shown that responses in the S1, S2, and anterior insula were more likely to contribute to stimulus intensity. The concept of the ACC as a salience detector across multiple modalities is further supported by our electrophysiological findings of human ACC neurons responsive to pain and various attention tasks (mental arithmetic or the Stroop test) with salient features (Hutchison et al. 1999; Davis et al. 2000, 2005).

Rectal pain in irritable bowel syndrome. Normally, repeated rectal distension evokes painful sensations that begin at the onset of each distension and subside immediately after the cessation of distension (Kwan et al. 2002). However, patients with irritable bowel syndrome have rectal hypersensitivity exhibited by a lower pain threshold and prolonged pain to rectal distension. These patients can continue to experience pain long after each distension (Kwan et al. 2005a). Therefore, we used percept-related fMRI to distinguish brain responses evoked by the rectal distension itself from the responses associated with the reported perception of pain (Fig. 2). We found that compared to healthy controls, patients with irritable bowel syndrome had heightened responses in some brain areas that most likely were related to rectal hypersensitivity (S1) and affect (the medial thalamus and hippocampus) and attenuated responses in the insula and rostral ACC that were possibly related to interoceptive or homeostatic functions (Kwan et al. 2005b).

PAIN-ATTENTION INTERACTIONS: IMPACT OF INDIVIDUAL ATTRIBUTES

Another consideration in brain-imaging studies of pain is the context in which the pain is experienced. It is well known from behavioral, clinical, and neurophysiological studies that the pain and attention systems overlap and affect each other (Eccleston 1995; Peyron et al. 2000; Pincus and Morley 2001; Petrovic and Ingvar 2002; Villemure and Bushnell 2002). Several laboratories have begun to integrate cognitive tasks into pain studies to examine the interaction and interference effects between pain-related and cognitive, attention-related activations. Our laboratory has demonstrated an attenuation of pain-evoked activity in areas encoding pain intensity and affect (including S1, S2, and the anterior insula) when there is a competing cognitive load. Interestingly, this attenuation was confined to a subset of subjects whose behavioral performance improved during concomitant pain (Seminowicz et al. 2004). These findings

A: rectal pressure-related S2 response

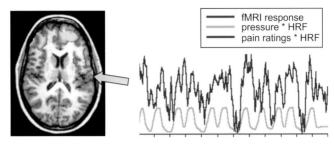

B: rectal pain-related ACC response

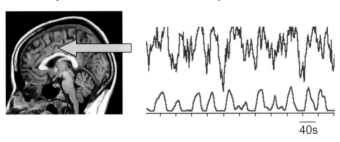

40s

Fig. 2. Example of percept-related fMRI in a rectal distension study. Panel A shows an example of an activation in the secondary somatosensory cortex (S2) correlated to noxious rectal distension pressure stimuli. Panel B shows an example of an activation in the anterior cingulate cortex (ACC) id entified by interrogating the fMRI data with a predictor function constructed from the subject's pain ratings, convolved with a hemodynamic response function (HRF).

suggest that attenuation of pain-evoked responses during cognitive performance may relate to different coping strategies or to shifts of attentional resources. This possibility raises the issue of personality attributes and their impact on the pain experience. Several recent studies have correlated behavioral measures with brain-imaging findings on responses to pain within particular cortical regions in individual subjects. For example, a recent study by Gracely et al. (2004) highlights the effect of pain catastrophizing on pain-evoked cortical responses in patients with fibromyalgia. We recently demonstrated that personality factors such as neuroticism and pain catastrophizing can also affect pain-evoked behavioral and cortical responses (particularly in the rostral ACC, dorsolateral prefrontal cortex, and insula) in normal healthy subjects (Seminowicz and Davis, in press). Correlation of brain-imaging responses with some measure of behavior, performance, or personality is commonly performed in studies of psychological functions such as memory and cognition (for an overview see Wilkinson and Halligan 2004). Similarly, we might gain further insight into an individual's pain response by incorporating psychological and behavioral factors into fMRI studies of pain.

CONCLUSIONS

Recent advances in the neuroimaging of pain are now considering how specific aspects of the pain experience, such as pain qualities, are represented in the brain. Furthermore, investigators are now considering the impact of individual traits and of the context of the pain experience (e.g., attention or distraction) on forebrain activity evoked by noxious stimuli. These and other new correlation analysis approaches are being incorporated into pain-imaging studies to better identify abnormalities in chronic pain conditions.

ACKNOWLEDGMENTS

These studies were funded by the Canadian Institutes of Health Research, the Ontario Mental Health Foundation, and the Canada Research Chair Program. K.D. Davis is a Canada Research Chair in Brain and Behavior. I am grateful for scientific contributions made by my trainees Dr. Jonathan Downar, Chun L. Kwan, and David Seminowicz, and for the technical contributions of Mr. Geoff Pope.

REFERENCES

Apkarian AV, Bushnell MC, Treede RD, Zubieta JK. Human brain mechanisms of pain perception and regulation in health and disease. *Eur J Pain* 2005; 9:463–484.

Arendt-Nielsen L, Brennum J, Sindrup S, Bak P. Electrophysiological and psychophysical quantification of temporal summation in the human nociceptive system. *Eur J Appl Physiol* 1994; 68:266–273.

Arthurs OJ, Boniface S. How well do we understand the neural origins of the fMRI BOLD signal? *Trends Neurosci* 2002; 25:27–31.

Bechara A, Naqvi N. Listening to your heart: interoceptive awareness as a gateway to feeling. *Nat Neurosci* 2004; 7:102–103.

Boivie J. Central pain. In: Melzack R, Wall PD (Eds) *The Textbook of Pain.* Edinburgh: Churchill Livingstone, 2002, pp 879–914.

Craig AD. How do you feel? Interoception: the sense of the physiological condition of the body. *Nat Rev Neurosci* 2002; 3:655–666.

Craig AD, Chen K, Bandy D, Reiman EM. Thermosensory activation of insular cortex. *Nat Neurosci* 2000; 3:184–190.

Davis KD, Pope GE. Noxious cold evokes multiple sensations with distinct time courses. *Pain* 2002; 98:179–185.

Davis KD, Hutchison WD, Lozano AM, Tasker RR, Dostrovsky JO. Human anterior cingulate cortex neurons modulated by attention-demanding tasks. *J Neurophysiol* 2000; 83:3575–3577.

Davis KD, Pope GE, Crawley AP, Mikulis DJ. Neural correlates of prickle sensation: a percept-related fMRI study. *Nat Neurosci* 2002; 5:1121–1122.

Davis KD, Pope GE, Crawley AP, Mikulis DJ. Perceptual illusion of "paradoxical heat" engages the insular cortex. *J Neurophysiol* 2004; 92:1248–1251.

Davis KD, Taylor KS, Hutchison WD, et al. Human anterior cingulate cortex neurons encode cognitive and emotional demands. *J Neurosci* 2005; 25:8402–8406.

Downar J, Crawley AP, Mikulis DJ, Davis KD. A multimodal cortical network for the detection of changes in the sensory environment. *Nat Neurosci* 2000; 3:277–283.

Downar J, Crawley AP, Mikulis DJ, Davis KD. The effect of task-relevance on the cortical response to changes in visual and auditory stimuli: an event-related fMRI study. *Neuroimage* 2001; 14:1256–1267.

Downar J, Crawley AP, Mikulis DJ, Davis KD. A cortical network sensitive to stimulus salience in a neutral behavioral context across multiple sensory modalities. *J Neurophysiol* 2002; 87:615–620.

Downar J, Mikulis DJ, Davis KD. Neural correlates of the prolonged salience of painful stimulation. *Neuroimage* 2003; 20:1540–1551.

Eccleston C. The attentional control of pain: methodological and theoretical concerns. *Pain* 1995; 63:3–10.

Gracely RH, Geisser ME, Giesecke T, et al. Pain catastrophizing and neural responses to pain among persons with fibromyalgia. *Brain* 2004; 127:835–843.

Heeger DJ, Ress D. What does fMRI tell us about neuronal activity? *Nat Rev Neurosci* 2002; 3:142–151.

Hutchison WD, Davis KD, Lozano AM, Tasker RR, Dostrovsky JO. Pain-related neurons in the human cingulate cortex. *Nat Neurosci* 1999; 2:403–405.

Kwan CL, Mikula K, Diamant NE, Davis KD. The relationship between rectal pain, unpleasantness, and urge to defecate in normal subjects. *Pain* 2002; 97:53–63.

Kwan CL, Diamant NE, Mikula K, Davis KD. Characteristics of rectal perception are altered in irritable bowel syndrome. *Pain* 2005a; 113:160–171.

Kwan CL, Diamant NE, Pope G, et al. Abnormal forebrain activity in functional bowel disorder patients with chronic pain. *Neurology* 2005b; 65:1268–1277.

Lautenbacher S, Roscher S, Strian F. Tonic pain evoked by pulsating heat: temporal summation mechanisms and perceptual qualities. *Somatosens Mot Res* 1995; 12:59–70.

Mailis-Gagnon A, Giannoylis I, Downar J, et al. Altered central somatosensory processing in chronic pain patients with "hysterical" anesthesia. *Neurology* 2003; 60:1501–1507.

Melzack R. The McGill Pain Questionnaire: major properties and scoring methods. *Pain* 1975; 1:277–299.

Melzack R, Casey KL. Sensory, motivational, and central control determinants of pain: a new conceptual model. In: Kenshalo D (Ed). *The Skin Senses*. Springfield: C.C. Thomas, 1968, pp 423–439.

Milne RJ, Kay NE, Irwin RJ. Habituation to repeated painful and non-painful cutaneous stimuli: a quantitative psychophysical study. *Exp Brain Res* 1991; 87:438–444.

Petrovic P, Ingvar M. Imaging cognitive modulation of pain processing. *Pain* 2002; 95:1–5.

Peyron R, Laurent B, Garcia-Larrea L. Functional imaging of brain responses to pain. A review and meta- analysis. *Neurophysiol Clin* 2000; 30:263–288.

Pincus T, Morley S. Cognitive-processing bias in chronic pain: a review and integration. *Psychol Bull* 2001; 127:599–617.

Sarlani E, Greenspan JD. Gender differences in temporal summation of mechanically evoked pain. *Pain* 2002; 97:163–169.

Seminowicz DA, Davis KD. Cortical responses to pain in healthy individuals depends on pain catastrophizing. *Pain* 2006; 120:297–306.

Seminowicz DA, Mikulis DJ, Davis KD. Cognitive modulation of pain-related brain responses depends on behavioral strategy. *Pain* 2004; 112:48–58.

Vierck CJ Jr, Cannon RL, Fry G, Maixner W, Whitsel BL. Characteristics of temporal summation of second pain sensations elicited by brief contact of glabrous skin by a preheated thermode. *J Neurophysiol* 1997; 78:992–1002.

Villemure C, Bushnell MC. Cognitive modulation of pain: how do attention and emotion influence pain processing? *Pain* 2002; 95:195–199.

Wilkinson D, Halligan P. The relevance of behavioural measures for functional-imaging studies of cognition. *Nat Rev Neurosci* 2004; 5:67–73.

Correspondence to: Karen D. Davis, PhD, Toronto Western Hospital, University Health Network, 399 Bathurst Street, Room MP14-306, Toronto, Ontario, Canada M5T 2S8. Tel: 416-603-5662; Fax: 416-603-5745; email: kdavis@uhnres.utoronto.ca.

Proceedings of the 11th World Congress on Pain,
edited by Herta Flor, Eija Kalso, and Jonathan O.
Dostrovsky, IASP Press, Seattle, © 2006.

34

The Time-Course of Sensory and Affective Pain Processing: Evidence from Laser-Evoked Potentials

Deborah E. Bentley,[a] Ulf Baumgärtner,[b] Alison Watson,[a] Geoff Barrett,[c] Bhavna Kulkarni,[a] Paula D. Youell,[a,d] Tanja Schlereth,[b] Anthony K.P. Jones,[a] and Rolf-Detlef Treede[b]

[a]University of Manchester Human Pain Research Group, Hope Hospital, Salford, United Kingdom; [b] Institute of Physiology and Pathophysiology, Johannes Gutenberg University, Mainz, Germany; [c]Human Sciences Team, Defence Science and Technology Laboratory, Fareham, United Kingdom; [d]Laser Photonics, Department of Physics and Astronomy, University of Manchester, Manchester, United Kingdom

It is now clear that there is a network of structures in the brain that mediates the perception of pain (Apkarian et al. 2005). Pain has sensory-discriminative, affective-motivational, and cognitive-evaluative dimensions (Melzack and Casey 1968). Increasing evidence suggests that these different aspects of pain are processed by distinct, but integrated, brain systems. It seems that the medial pain system, including the anterior cingulate cortex, orbitofrontal cortex, and parts of the insular cortex, is responsible for the affective (emotional) aspects of pain, whereas the lateral pain system, comprising the primary (S1) and secondary (S2) somatosensory and inferior parietal cortices, subserves the sensory-discriminative aspects of pain. Recent anatomical and functional data suggest that the dorsal and anterior part of the insula also belong to the lateral pain system (Craig 2003). We recently used positron emission tomography (PET) to image brain function during the experience of pain, while healthy participants paid attention to different aspects of the pain sensation (Kulkarni et al. 2005a). We found that when participants attended to the spatial location (sensory aspect) of a painful stimulus, the contralateral S1 and inferior parietal cortices increased in activation. In contrast, when they attended to the unpleasantness (affective aspect) of the same stimulus, activations increased in areas including the perigenual cingulate, orbitofrontal, and posterior insular cortices. These findings are supported by the work of other groups (Rainville et al. 1997; Tölle et al. 1999).

Functional brain-imaging techniques such as PET and functional magnetic resonance imaging provide information regarding the brain areas activated under certain conditions, but they do not have sufficient temporal resolution to assess the sequence of activation of these areas, and so very early, transient events may not be detected at all. Cortical evoked potentials, on the other hand, provide information about brain activation on a millisecond time-scale. Laser-evoked potentials (LEPs) reflect electrical brain activity in response to radiant heat stimuli delivered by a laser, which selectively activate Aδ- and C-fiber nociceptors that mediate the sensation of pain (Bromm et al. 1984; see Treede 1994 for an overview of LEPs). The main LEP components are named after the electroencephalogram surface potentials: the first response (N1) is a negativity recorded bilaterally at temporal leads (T3, T4), and the main potential (N2–P2) is a biphasic waveform that can be recorded from the vertex (Cz). The brain generators of scalp-recorded LEPs, and their time-courses of activation, can be estimated using electrical source modeling techniques (Garcia-Larrea et al. 2003).

In this chapter we describe the results of studies that used LEPs to investigate the sequence of brain activation whilst manipulating different aspects of the pain experience, in order to gain further insight into the neurophysiological mechanisms of human pain perception. All studies were approved by the appropriate research ethics committees and were carried out in accordance with the Declaration of Helsinki. All participants gave their written informed consent prior to taking part.

METHODS

In the first study, we recorded LEPs from 10 healthy participants while they either performed spatial and intensity discrimination tasks involving painful stimuli delivered to both hands or were actively distracted from the stimuli by a mental arithmetic task (Schlereth et al. 2003). Brain electrical source analysis revealed that the LEP data were well explained by four sources that were activated in the following sequence: the contralateral operculo-insular cortex, the ipsilateral operculo-insular cortex, the mid-cingulate gyrus (early response), and the contralateral postcentral gyrus (S1) and mid-cingulate gyrus (late response) (Fig. 1). The mid-cingulate gyrus is the cytoarchitectonically and functionally distinct (posterior) part of what is traditionally called the anterior cingulate

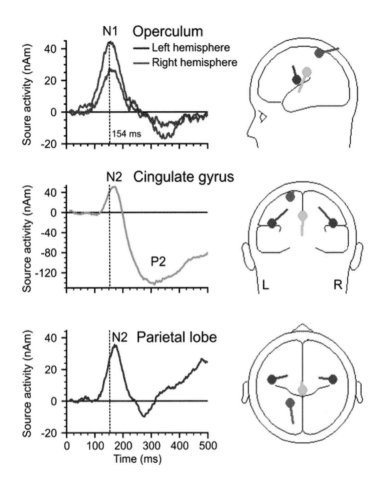

Fig. 1. Source analysis of laser-evoked potentials after stimulation of the right hand. Blue, left operculo-insular cortex; red, right operculo-insular cortex; green, cingulate gyrus; pink, contralateral postcentral gyrus (S1). Reprinted from Schlereth et al. (2003), with permission from Elsevier.

cortex (Vogt et al. 1995). The activity of all sources was enhanced during the sensory discrimination tasks compared with the distraction task, although this effect was most pronounced for the operculo-insular sources (an increase of, on average, about 40%). In addition, source strength in the left operculo-insular cortex was significantly greater than that in the right hemisphere (on average by 23%), regardless of the side of stimulation. These data suggest a dominant role of the left frontal operculum and adjacent dorsal insula in the early sensory-discriminative aspects of pain processing.

LEP amplitude at ~300 ms at T7

N300-T7 group (n=11)

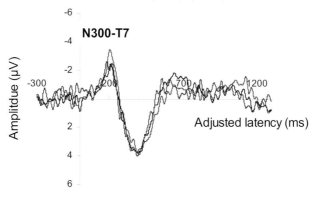

N300-T7 group (n=11)

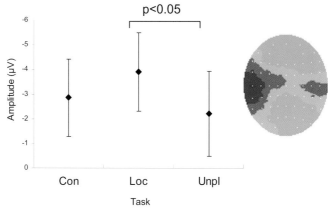

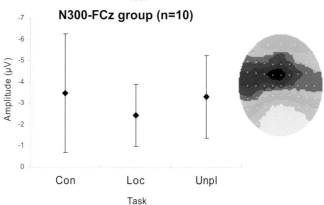

In the second study, we compared brain processing of the sensory and affective dimensions of pain (Bentley et al. 2004). LEPs were recorded from 21 healthy participants while they performed a pain localization task (sensory), a pain unpleasantness rating task (affective), and a pain detection task (to control for generalized attention to the pain). The participants were divided into two subgroups on the basis of different topographic scalp distributions of the early negative LEP peak (Fig. 2). For 11 participants (the N300-T7 subgroup), the N300 peak was maximal over the contralateral temporal scalp region (electrode T7). For the remaining 10 participants (the N300-FCz subgroup), this peak was maximal at electrode FCz, overlying the midline centrofrontal scalp region. Evidence suggests that the N300 (N2) LEP peak is generated by sources in bilateral operculo-insular cortices (e.g., Schlereth et al. 2003). The lateralization of this peak in the N300-T7 subgroup may be caused by the superimposition on N2 of the earlier lateralized N1 LEP peak, thought to be generated by a source in the contralateral operculo-insular cortex, with a possible contribution from contralateral S1. This finding suggests a greater early involvement of contralateral LEP generators for the N300-T7 subgroup compared with the N300-FCz subgroup.

RESULTS

N300 peak amplitude was significantly greater when volunteers performed pain localization compared with rating pain unpleasantness, but only for the N300-T7 subgroup (Fig. 2), despite almost identical performance on the pain localization task for the two subgroups (around 88% in both cases). The task effect on N300 peak amplitude was statistically more likely to be due to an increase in the localization task compared to the control, rather than to decreased peak amplitude in the unpleasantness rating task; see Bentley et al. (2004) for details. Participants in the N300-T7 subgroup retrospectively rated a lower percentage of stimuli as painful during the localization task than did those in the N300-FCz subgroup (although not significantly so). Thus, we concluded that perhaps the N300-T7 subgroup had to pay more attention to the localization

---

◄─── **Fig. 2.** N300 laser-evoked potential (LEP) peak amplitude (mean ± standard deviation) was significantly greater during pain localization (Loc) than unpleasantness rating (Unpl) tasks (Con, control task), but only for the subgroup of participants who had a lateralized N300 (N300-T7, corresponding to N1), and not for the subgroup who had a midline N300 (N300-FCz, corresponding to N2) as shown by the topographic maps on the right of each plot. The upper figure shows average LEPs for this subgroup (red, Loc; blue, Unpl; black, Con). Reprinted from Bentley et al. (2004), with permission from the International Federation of Clinical Neurophysiology.

task than the other subgroup, in order to achieve the same performance. This difference in the allocation of spatial attention between the two subgroups may have caused increased activation of the contralateral generator(s) of the N300 peak (left operculo-insular cortex and maybe S1), giving rise to an increase in N300 peak amplitude. These findings are consistent with an early role of the contralateral operculo-insular cortex and possibly S1 in the localization of pain. Since in this study we only stimulated the right hand, we cannot determine to what extent the left-hemisphere dominance for processing the sensory dimension of pain contributed to this finding.

We recently performed a source analysis of the data report in Bentley et al. (2004), using the four-source model of Schlereth et al. (2003). This model explained the data well, as shown by the mean goodness-of-fit of 84%, and revealed the same activation sequence of sources as that reported by Schlereth et al. (Bentley et al. 2005). Table I illustrates that absolute latencies were different, because CO_2 lasers yield slower intracutaneous temperature ramps than thulium lasers (Spiegel et al. 2000). When the task effects were investigated, we found that the ipsilateral (right) operculo-insular source was significantly more active during the unpleasantness rating task than during the control task across the whole group (40.0 ± 5.0 versus 28.1 ± 5.4 nAm). This effect was most marked for the N300-T7 subgroup, although not significantly so. Although not statistically significant, the contralateral (left) operculo-insular source was

Table I
Latencies of laser-evoked potentials and dipole source
activities using different infrared lasers (mean ± SEM)

	Thulium	CO_2 Laser
Wavelength (μm)	2.01	10.60
Pulse duration (ms)	3	150
Global field power peaks (ms)		
Latency 1	147 ± 6	299 ± 6
Latency 2	248 ± 10	448 ± 6
Dipole activity peaks (ms)		
OIC contralateral	158 ± 6	280 ± 5
OIC ipsilateral	164 ± 6	289 ± 5
MCC early	172 ± 8	291 ± 5
S1 contralateral	181 ± 1	297 ± 4
MCC late	306 ± 13	450 ± 6

Notes: Global field power is an overall measure of electroencephalogram activity. OIC = operculo-insular cortex; MCC = mid-cingulate cortex (the posterior part of what is traditionally called the anterior cingulate cortex); S1 = primary somatosensory (parietal) cortex.

more active in the localization task than during the other tasks for the N300-T7 subgroup, consistent with the greater N300-T7 peak amplitude in these participants reported in Bentley et al. (2004). The N300-T7 subgroup had much less active cingulate and postcentral gyrus sources than the N300-FCz subgroup for all tasks (significant for the postcentral gyrus source and the early cingulate response).

These results suggest a role of the ipsilateral (right) operculo-insular cortex in processing the unpleasant nature of pain. This finding is consistent with our PET study (Kulkarni et al. 2005a) and with other functional imaging studies of negative affect (e.g., Canli et al. 1998; Brooks et al. 2002; Phillips et al. 2003), but the temporal resolution of LEPs has, in addition, shown that processing of the unpleasant aspect occurs at the earliest stages of pain processing. Our findings also support those of Schlereth et al. (2003) in suggesting an involvement of the left operculo-insular cortex in the sensory-discriminative component of pain, in this case localization. Our findings therefore provide evidence that the affective aspects of pain may be processed in the brain as early as the sensory aspects. This finding goes against the widely held assumption that the processing of affect occurs relatively late compared with the processing of the sensory aspects of a painful stimulus.

SUMMARY

The results of our studies using LEPs suggest that both the sensory and affective dimensions of pain are processed at the earliest stages of pain processing, at least in part by the operculo-insular cortices. Further work is needed to assess the possible hemispheric lateralization of the responses related to pain unpleasantness, although evidence to date is consistent with a role of the left operculo-insular cortex in sensory-discriminative aspects (Schlereth et al. 2003) and a role of the right operculo-insular cortex in processing negative emotions (Canli et al. 1998).

These findings suggest that the emotional aspects of pain are evaluated as quickly as the sensory qualities, and are therefore just as important, even in healthy participants responding to an acute painful stimulus. This situation might be expected to be even more relevant in patients suffering from chronic pain, which has a greater emotional salience. This supposition is consistent with findings from our group that patients with fibromyalgia syndrome, who suffer from chronic widespread pain in the absence of any apparent nociceptive input, seem to be less able than healthy subjects to switch their attention away from the emotional aspects of pain when instructed to perform a pain localization task (Kulkarni et al. 2005b). However, these findings were obtained in a

PET study, so further work is required to determine the timing of sensory and affective pain processing in these patients. Studies of LEP sources may prove useful in investigating the pathophysiological mechanisms of pain perception in patients with different chronic pain disorders.

ACKNOWLEDGMENTS

The work described in this chapter was supported by the Arthritis Research Campaign (United Kingdom), the Dr Hadwen Trust for Humane Research (United Kingdom), the Human Sciences Domain of the U.K. Ministry of Defence Scientific Research Programme, the Deutsche Forschungsgemeinschaft (DFG Tr 236/13-3), and the NIH (NS038493). We thank Gertud Schatt for technical assistance.

REFERENCES

Apkarian AV, Bushnell MC, Treede RD, Zubieta JK. Human brain mechanisms of pain perception and regulation in health and disease. *Eur J Pain* 2005; 9:463–484.

Bentley DE, Watson A, Treede R-D, et al. Differential effects on the laser evoked potential of selectively attending to pain localisation versus pain unpleasantness. *Clin Neurophysiol* 2004; 115:1846–1856.

Bentley DE, Baumgärtner U, Watson A, et al. Early involvement of right operculo-insular cortex in processing pain unpleasantness: evidence from laser evoked potentials. *Brain Topogr* 2005; 17:180–181.

Bromm B, Jahnke MT, Treede R-D. Responses of human cutaneous afferents to CO_2 laser stimuli causing pain. *Exp Brain Res* 1984; 55:158–166.

Brooks JCW, Nurmikko TJ, Bimson WE, Singh KD, Roberts N. fMRI of thermal pain: effects of stimulus laterality and attention. *Neuroimage* 2002; 15:293–301.

Canli T, Desmond JE, Zhao Z, Glover G, Gabrieli JD. Hemispheric asymmetry for emotional stimuli detected with fMRI. *Neuroreport* 1998; 9:3233–3239.

Craig AD. Pain mechanisms: labeled lines versus convergence in central processing. *Annu Rev Neurosci* 2003; 26:1–30.

Garcia-Larrea L, Frot M, Valeriani M. Brain generators of laser-evoked potentials: from dipoles to functional significance. *Neurophysiol Clin* 2003; 33:279–292.

Kulkarni B, Bentley DE, Elliott R, et al. Attention to pain localisation and unpleasantness discriminates the functions of the medial and lateral pain systems. *Eur J Neurosci* 2005a; 21:3133–3142.

Kulkarni B, Boger E, Watson A, et al. Attentional dysfunction in fibromyalgia. *Rheumatology (Oxford)* 2005b; 44(Suppl 1):i94.

Melzack R, Casey KL. Sensory, motivational and central control determinants of pain: a new conceptual model. In: Kenshalo DR (Ed). *The Skin Senses*. Springfield, IL: Charles C. Thomas, 1968, pp 423–443.

Phillips ML, Gregory LJ, Cullen S, et al. The effect of negative emotional context on neural and behavioural responses to oesophageal stimulation. *Brain* 2003; 126:669–684.

Rainville P, Duncan GH, Price DD, Carrier B, Bushnell MC. Pain affect encoded in human anterior cingulate but not somatosensory cortex. *Science* 1997; 277:968–971.

Schlereth T, Baumgärtner U, Magerl W, Stoeter P, Treede RD. Left-hemisphere dominance in early nociceptive processing in the human parasylvian cortex. *Neuroimage* 2003; 20:441–454.

Spiegel J, Hansen C, Treede RD. Clinical evaluation criteria for the assessment of impaired pain sensitivity by thulium-laser evoked potentials. *Clin Neurophysiol* 2000; 111:725–735.

Tölle TR, Kaufmann T, Siessmeier T, et al. Region-specific encoding of sensory and affective components of pain in the human brain: a positron emission tomography correlation analysis. *Ann Neurol* 1999; 45:40–47.

Treede R-D. Evoked potentials related to pain. In: Hansson P, Lindblom U (Eds). *Touch, Temperature, and Pain in Health and Disease: Mechanisms and Assessments,* Progress in Pain Research and Management, Vol. 3. Seattle: IASP Press, 1994, pp 473–489.

Vogt BA, Nimchinsky EA, Vogt LJ, Hof PR. Human cingulate cortex: surface features, flat maps, and cytoarchitecture. *J Comp Neurol* 1995; 359:490–506.

Correspondence to: Ulf Baumgärtner, Dr. med, Institute of Physiology and Pathophysiology, Johannes Gutenberg University, Duesbergweg 6, D-55099 Mainz, Germany. Tel: 49-6131-3925219; Fax: 49-6131-3925902; email: baumgaer@uni-mainz.de.

Proceedings of the 11th World Congress on Pain,
edited by Herta Flor, Eija Kalso, and Jonathan O.
Dostrovsky, IASP Press, Seattle, © 2006.

35

Brain Opioid Receptor Availability Differs in Central and Peripheral Neuropathic Pain

Joseph Maarrawi,[a,b] Roland Peyron,[a,c] and Luis Garcia-Larrea[a]

[a]INSERM EMI-342 (Central Integration of Pain), Lyon and St-Etienne, France;
[b]Functional Neurosurgery Department, Neurological Hospital, Lyon, France;
[c]Neurology Department, Bellevue Hospital, St-Etienne, France

The endogenous opioid system, which includes opioid peptides and receptor-bearing neurons, is one of the most potent neurochemical systems for the modulation of pain processing. Its activation by exogenous opioids (i.e., morphine or its derivatives) has analgesic effects on nociceptive pain and, under some conditions, on neuropathic pain (Bowsher 1992; Attal et al. 2002). Despite extensive clinical use of exogenous opioids, the pathophysiology of the endogenous opioid system in chronic pain conditions is far from being fully understood. Studies in animals (Iadarola et al. 1988; Zangen et al. 1998), in healthy humans (Stacher et al. 1988; Zubieta et al. 2002), and in patients with inflammatory pain (Jones et al. 1994) suggest that painful conditions are associated with endogenous opioid release, which is seen as a compensatory mechanism that would tend to lessen the sensory and affective aspects of the pain experience.

In contrast to nociceptive pain, possible changes in the endogenous opioid system in chronic neuropathic pain have received little attention to date. Using positron emission tomography (PET) scans and opioid ligands, Willoch et al. (2004) and Jones et al. (2004) recently described reduced opioid receptor binding in five and four patients, respectively, with central neuropathic pain. The decrease in opioid receptor binding clearly predominated in the hemisphere contralateral to pain, when the pain was unilateral. The decrease in opioid binding was interpreted differently in these two studies, either as reflecting a genuine loss of opioid receptors (Jones et al. 2004) or resulting from an increased (reactive) secretion of endogenous opioids (Willoch et al. 2004).

To sort out these interpretive ambiguities, we investigated the changes in central opioid binding in two groups of patients, one with a peripheral and the other with a central form of neuropathic pain. We hypothesized that, if opioid receptor decrease was due to a genuine decrease of opioid receptors in the brain, it should be present in central pain but not in peripheral neuropathic pain. Further, we predicted that the decrease in opioid binding should predominate in the damaged or functionally altered hemisphere, i.e., contralateral to the pain.

METHODS

Opioid receptor binding was studied in 15 patients suffering from chronic neuropathic pain, which was of central supraspinal origin in eight patients with central post-stroke pain (CPSP), and of peripheral origin in seven patients (four with proximal nerve injuries, two with plexus avulsions, and one with spinal root injury). In all patients, pain was refractory to medical therapy, with subjective pain intensity ratings >5/10 on a visual analogue scale despite appropriate pharmacological polytherapy. Pain was matched for intensity (Mann-Whitney $Z = -0.302$ for continuous pain and -1.455 for paroxysmal pain ratings; n.s.) and duration ($Z = -0.2$; n.s.) in the central and peripheral groups. All patients had been off opioid medication for at least 2 months before entering the study, and remained so during the entire study. All patients gave their written informed consent to the study, which was conducted according to the Declaration of Helsinki (Rickham 1964), and approved by the local medical ethics committee at University Hospital, St Etienne, France.

Opioid receptors were studied using the nonselective opioid antagonist [^{11}C]diprenorphine. After intravenous injection of high-specific-activity [^{11}C]diprenorphine, data acquisition using PET scans progressed for 70 minutes, comprising 37 contiguous time-frames. Scan duration increased progressively from 20 seconds in the first time-frame to 5 minutes in the last, yielding a total scan time of 70 minutes. Early frames (1–20) essentially reflecting blood flow were discarded, and the remaining ones, reflecting diprenorphine fixation to opioid receptors, were submitted to parametric computation of ligand binding to opioid receptors using the standardized reference tissue model (Frost et al. 1989; Willoch et al. 2004). Parametric images from each patient were then normalized into the standardized space of the International Consortium for Brain Mapping (www.loni.ucla.edu/ICBM/, McGill University, Montreal, Quebec). These transformations yielded a standardized set of images mutually comparable on a voxel-to-voxel basis by applying statistical tests after smoothing.

Two approaches were used for comparison: in the first (intergroup comparison), opioid binding in the whole brain was compared between the groups of patients with central pain and peripheral pain. In the second (interhemispheric comparison), opioid binding was contrasted between the hemispheres contralateral and ipsilateral to pain, so as to quantify and localize possible lateralized changes in opioid binding, separately in each group of patients.

OPIOID RECEPTOR BINDING IN CENTRAL VERSUS PERIPHERAL NEUROPATHIC PAIN

GROUP COMPARISON: CENTRAL VERSUS PERIPHERAL PAIN

Direct comparison between the CPSP and peripheral neuropathic pain groups revealed several regions with a significant decrease of opioid binding in CPSP patients, relative to patients with peripheral neuropathic pain. Opioid binding decrease in CPSP patients exclusively involved the hemisphere contralateral to pain. Specific regions with a significant decrease were the insular cortex (mean 18% decrease), the posterior temporal region (16% decrease), and the lateral prefrontal cortex (30% decrease) (Fig. 1). Conversely, patients with peripheral neuropathic pain did not exhibit any region with a significant decrease of opioid binding relative to CPSP patients.

INTER-HEMISPHERIC COMPARISON OF OPIOID RECEPTOR BINDING

CPSP patients.   Side-to-side comparisons in the 8 patients with CPSP revealed significant ($P < 0.001$) relative decrease in opioid binding in several regions of the hemisphere contralateral to pain. Binding decrease was maximal in the lateral prefrontal cortex (32% decrease), the posterior temporal cortex (13% decrease), the insular cortex (16% decrease), the posteromedial thalamus (20% decrease), and the posterior midbrain (20% decrease). No significant increase in binding was observed in any regions of the hemisphere contralateral to pain.

Peripheral neuropathic pain patients.   In the group with peripheral forms of pain, side-to-side comparisons revealed no significant inter-hemispheric changes (either decrease or increase) in opioid binding.

A NEUROCHEMICAL DIFFERENCE BETWEEN CENTRAL AND PERIPHERAL NEUROPATHIC PAIN?

Differences in opioid binding between central and peripheral neuropathic pain could not be explained by tissue loss from anatomical brain lesions (see Fig. 2), as binding decrease was not restricted to the lesion sites, but rather distributed within cortical and subcortical structures. Differences did not appear

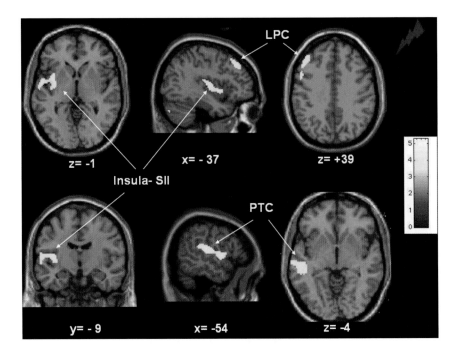

Fig. 1. Clusters of significantly reduced diprenorphine binding potential contralateral to pain in the group of patients with central post-stroke pain relative to patients with peripheral neuropathic pain, superimposed onto a T1-weighted magnetic resonance image. Note that all significant differences between groups were restricted to the hemisphere contralateral to pain. Stereotactic coordinates (in millimeters) are relative to the AC-PC (anterior commissure-posterior commissure) line, with AC as the origin of the coordinates. The color scale (right) corresponds to the T-score values of displayed clusters. LPC = lateral prefrontal cortex; PTC = posterior temporal cortex; SII = secondary somatic area.

to result from changes in the intensity or duration of pain or from drug intake in the two groups of patients; both the mean pain intensity ratings and disease duration were comparable in the two groups, as were the number of patients on each medication and the corresponding dosages. Pain had been classified as refractory to pharmacological therapy in all patients, and all had entered a program of motor cortex or spinal cord stimulation, so the intrusive and distressing character of pain was comparable between the two groups. Hence, the differences in opioid binding between the central and peripheral groups were likely to reflect a genuine neurochemical difference between patients with central or peripheral forms of neuropathic pain.

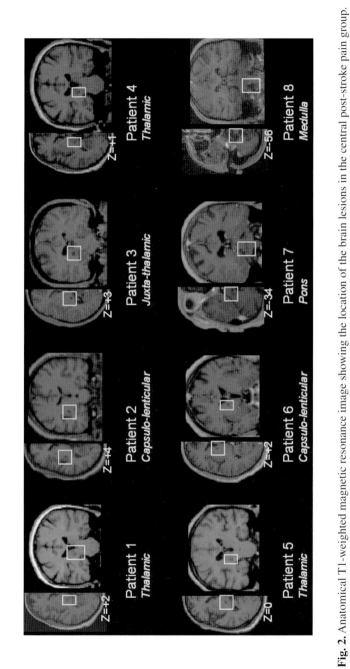

Fig. 2. Anatomical T1-weighted magnetic resonance image showing the location of the brain lesions in the central post-stroke pain group.

THE SIGNIFICANCE OF DECREASED OPIOID BINDING IN CENTRAL NEUROPATHIC PAIN

Opioid binding decrease in CPSP is most likely attributable to a reduction in the number of available receptors. Such a decrease in opioid receptor availability in CPSP might be attributable to at least two different mechanisms: it could be secondary to actual receptor loss (Jones et al. 2004), or it might reflect increased endogenous peptides occupying binding sites, rendering them unavailable to the exogenous ligand (Willoch et al. 2004). The present findings, showing that opioid receptor changes occurred *exclusively* in the central forms of neuropathic pain, make a case for a genuine loss of opioid receptors in CPSP. Endogenous opioid secretion is considered part of a defensive (antinociceptive) reaction to painful input (Fields 2004) that occurs largely independent of the etiology of pain or the lesion site. Therefore, had opioid receptor changes been due to a reactive endogenous secretion, it would have been highly unexpected to find them solely in central pain, and not in peripheral forms of pain with equal intensity and duration.

Decrease of opioid binding in our CPSP patients was most probably related to loss, or metabolic inactivation, of receptor-bearing neurons. While direct neuronal damage cannot explain receptor loss, as cerebral structures with decreased opioid binding largely exceeded the lesion sites (compare Figs. 1 and 2), metabolic diaschisis and transneuronal degeneration in regions interconnected with lesion sites might explain such a pattern. Focal lesions can entail metabolic depression at distant but interconnected sites in the same hemispheric network (Feeney and Baron 1986; Baron et al. 1992), as well as anterograde and retrograde degeneration (Chung et al. 1990). Diaschisis or transneuronal changes may have resulted in local loss or metabolic inactivation of opioidergic synapses at regions connected with the damaged areas. Consistent with this hypothesis is the predominance of opioid-binding decrease within the same hemisphere as the lesions causing pain, as well as the localization of the opioid-binding decrease in regions of the nociceptive system (such as the thalamus, the insula or the periaqueductal gray) interconnected with the lesion sites.

POSSIBLE CLINICAL IMPLICATIONS

Differences in brain opioid receptor availability in central and peripheral neuropathic pain suggest differences in the clinical response of these two types of pain to exogenous opioids. In particular, loss or inactivation of central binding sites in CPSP would predict this condition to be less responsive to opioid analgesia than peripheral neuropathic pain, where binding sites are more numerous. Previous literature on opioid analgesia in neuropathic pain has shown beneficial effects essentially in peripheral forms, such as nerve injury or postherpetic neuralgia (Rowbotham et al. 1991; Kalso et al. 2004). In the largest series reported so far, Rowbotham et al. (2003) tested the efficacy of oral opioids in 81 neuropathic pain patients, and reported 16% responders among patients with CPSP and 30–39% of responders among patients with peripheral and spinal-related neuropathic pain. Similarly, in our series, 5/7 (71.4%) patients with peripheral neuropathic pain, but only 3/8 (37.5%) patients with central neuropathic pain, had responded partially to oral opioids. Our PET results lend support to the notion that relative loss of opioid sensitivity in CPSP may be due to a decrease in brain receptors available for exogenous opioid.

ACKNOWLEDGMENTS

This work was supported by a Projet Hospitalier de Recherche Clinique (PHRC), and by grants from the Fondation CNP and from the Fonds Benoît, a branch of the Roi Baudouin Foundation.

REFERENCES

Attal N, Guirimand F, Brasseur L, et al. Effects of IV morphine in central pain: a randomized placebo-controlled study. *Neurology* 2002; 58:517–518.

Baron JC, Levasseur M, Mazoyer B, et al. Thalamocortical diaschisis: positron emission tomography in humans. *J Neurol Neurosurg Psychiatry* 1992; 55:935–942.

Bowsher D. Responsiveness of chronic pain to morphine. *Lancet* 1992; 339:1367–1371.

Chung SK, Cohen RS, Pfaff DW. Transneuronal degeneration in the midbrain central gray following chemical lesions in the ventromedial nucleus: a qualitative and quantitative analysis. *Neuroscience* 1990; 38:409–426.

Feeney DM, Baron JC. Diaschisis. *Stroke* 1986; 17:817–830.

Fields H. State-dependent opioid control of pain. *Nat Rev Neurosci* 2004; 5:565–575.

Frost JJ, Douglass KH, Mayberg HS, et al. Multicompartmental analysis of [^{11}C]carfentanil binding to opiate receptors in humans measured by positron emission tomography. *J Cereb Blood Flow Metab* 1989; 9:398–409.

Iadarola MJ, Brady LS, Draisci G, et al. Enhancement of dynorphin gene expression in spinal cord following experimental inflammation: stimulus specificity, behavioral parameters and opioid receptor binding. *Pain* 1988; 35:313–326.

Jones AKP, Cunningham VJ, Ha-Kawa S, et al. Changes in central opioid receptor binding in relation to inflammation and pain in patients with rheumatoid arthritis. *Br J Rheumatol* 1994; 33:909–916.

Jones AKP, Watabe H, Cunningham VJ, et al. Cerebral decreases in opioid receptor binding in patients with central neuropathic pain measured by [^{11}C]diprenorphine binding and PET. *Eur J Pain* 2004; 8:479–485.

Kalso E, Edwards JE, Moore RA, et al. Opioids in chronic non-cancer pain: systematic review of efficacy and safety. *Pain* 2004; 112:372–380.

Rickham PP. Human experimentation. Code of ethics of the World medical association. Delaration of Helsinki. *BMJ* 1964; 5402:177.

Rowbotham MC, Reisner-Keller LA, Fields HL. Both intravenous lidocaine and morphine reduce the pain of postherpetic neuralgia. *Neurology* 1991; 41:1024–1028.

Rowbotham MC, Twilling L, Davies PS, et al. Oral opioid therapy for chronic peripheral and central neuropathic pain. *N Engl J Med* 2003; 348:1223–1232.

Stacher G, Abatzi TA, Schulte F, et al. Naloxone does not alter the perception of pain induced by electrical and thermal stimulation of the skin in healthy humans. *Pain* 1988; 34:271–276.

Willoch F, Schindler F, Wester HJ, et al. Central poststroke pain and reduced opioid receptor binding within pain processing circuitries: a [^{11}C]diprenorphine PET study. *Pain* 2004; 108:213–220.

Zangen A, Herzberg U, Vogel Z, et al. Nociceptive stimulus induces release of endogenous beta-endorphin in the rat brain. *Neuroscience* 1998; 85:659–662.

Zubieta JK, SmithYR, Bueller JA, et al. Mu-opioid receptor-mediated antinociceptive responses differ in men and women. *J Neurosci* 2002; 22:5100–5107.

Correspondence to: Joseph Maarrawi, MD, MSc, INSERM EMI-342 (Central Integration of Pain), 59 Boulevard Pinel, 69394 Lyon, France. Email: joseph.maarrawi@chu-lyon.fr; jomaarrawi@hotmail.com.

Proceedings of the 11th World Congress on Pain,
edited by Herta Flor, Eija Kalso, and Jonathan O.
Dostrovsky, IASP Press, Seattle, © 2006.

36

Pain Processing and Modulation in the Cingulate Gyrus

Brent A. Vogt,[a] Carlo A. Porro,[b]
and Marie-Elisabeth Faymonville[c]

*[a]Cingulum NeuroSciences Institute and Department of Neuroscience and
Physiology, SUNY Upstate Medical University, Syracuse, New York, USA;
[2]Department of Biomedical Science, University of Modena, Modena, Italy;
[3]Department of Anesthesiology and Reanimation,
University of Liège, Liège, Belgium*

The cingulate cortex occupies a large part of the medial surface of the brain and has become an important region of interest in acute and chronic pain studies. Although it is among the most frequently activated regions in human functional imaging research, no part of the cingulate gyrus can be referred to as a "pain center" because none has been shown to have mainly pain-processing functions. For example, the midcingulate cortex (MCC), which is usually activated during acute noxious stimulation, has important skeletomotor functions through the two cingulate motor areas and becomes activated in numerous tasks that do not involve noxious stimuli, including the Stroop and Flanker interference tests, complex movements, and word generation tasks. Logical study of pain processing in this context requires a clear statement of the functions of each cingulate region in general brain function, followed by an assessment of how these functions are redirected to resolve problems of anticipated or actual pain experiences. This chapter describes the structural connections and functional organization of the cingulate gyrus, outlines its top-down role in anticipation of pain, and discusses the application of hypnosis to engage cingulate-mediated processing for hypnotic sedation.

STRUCTURAL ORGANIZATION OF THE CINGULATE CORTEX IN THE CONTEXT OF PAIN PROCESSING

REGIONS, SUBREGIONS, AND AREAS

Reports of the location of human nociceptive cingulate cortex have become progressively more confusing because different studies provide many different names for each activation site. For example, one part of the cingulate gyrus dorsal to the genu of the corpus callosum has been termed the dorsal anterior cingulate cortex (with or without the gyral surface included), the rostral anterior cingulate cortex, the anterior anterior cingulate cortex, and the mid-cingulate anterior cingulate cortex. None of these designations refers to any histological observation in the tradition of Brodmann, Rose, and C. and O. Vogt (Vogt et al. 2004), but rather to places/coordinates on the cingulate gyrus. Confusion arises because no specific limits, connections, or functions are associated with these sites, and ambiguities will grow with each new terminology based on neuron-free, structural imaging coordinates.

Using histological methods, we have identified four regions in the cingulate gyrus: the anterior cingulate cortex (ACC), the MCC, the posterior cingulate cortex (PCC), and the retrosplenial cortex (RSC). We have divided the first three regions into six subregions: the subgenual and pregenual ACC (sACC, pACC), the anterior and posterior MCC (aMCC, pMCC), and the dorsal and ventral PCC (dPCC, vPCC). Each of the subregions is comprised of a few cytoarchitectural areas, and each area has specific neuron markers/types and unique projections. The critical difference between histologically defined areas, regions, and subregions and the proliferating nomenclatures in the imaging literature is that the former can evaluate border locations, circuits, and brain functions in the broader context of a neurobiological model rather than just stating that activity is in the "rostral anterior cingulate cortex." Most importantly for pain research, neuron cytology affects our view of the role of the cingulate cortex in pain processing.

Let us take an example of a functional system that has clear histological correlates: the rostral cingulate motor area (rCMA, anatomical review by Vogt et al. 2004). Fig. 1 shows a circle over the cingulate sulcus in the aMCC and a pair of arrows showing a coronal section through the cingulate gyrus. On the coronal section, four areas are identified with area 33´ in the callosal sulcus, areas a24a´ and a24b´ on the gyral surface, and area a24c´ on the ventral bank of the cingulate sulcus. In humans, the dorsal bank also has a large part of area a24c´. This latter area is further magnified in the figure to show its laminar architecture including layer Vb with the large neurons that are known to have corticospinal projections. These neurons were stained with an antibody that is specific for neuronal nuclei to avoid confusing them with glia and vascular

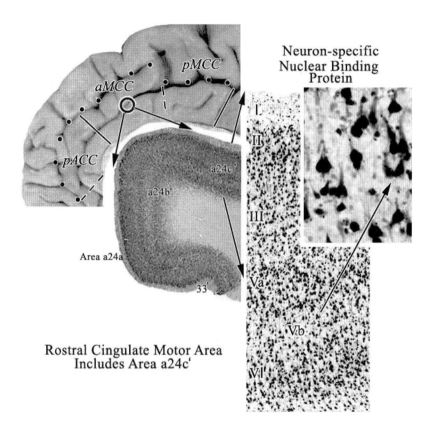

Fig. 1. Histological analysis of the anterior midcingulate cortex (aMCC) with four levels of magnification: (1) medial surface; (2) coronal section reacted for neuron-specific nuclear binding protein; (3) "strip" through area a24c′ in the cingulate sulcus showing layers from I below the pia (top) to VI next to the white matter (bottom); (4) layer Vb contains large, cingulospinal projection neurons in the rostral cingulate motor area (Vogt et al. 2004). aMCC = anterior midcingulate cortex; pMCC = posterior midcingulate cortex.

elements. Finally, the aMCC region is completed with area 32′ that lies dorsal to the rCMA.

Fig. 2A presents an overview of the entire cingulate gyrus with its regions and subregions marked. Onto this have been plotted peak voxels of activation in studies of acute noxious cutaneous stimulation (white dots) and noxious visceral stimulation (black dots) according to recent studies of the literature (Vogt et al. 2003; see Vogt 2005 for citations). Most cutaneous activations are in the MCC, while those associated with visceral activity are most often located in the pACC. In view of the functional dichotomy between ACC with its visceral integrative functions and MCC with its skeletomotor and response selection functions, it appears that pain processing in different parts of the body may be regulated by two different parts of the cingulate gyrus.

A. Regions & Acute Pain Responses

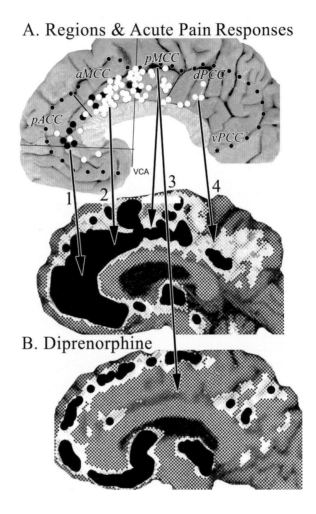

Fig. 2. (A) Distribution of regions, subregions, and areas on the cingulate gyrus with an analysis of peak voxel activations during acute noxious cutaneous stimulation (white dots) and visceral stimulation (black dots) (Vogt et al. 2003; Vogt 2005). (B) Distribution of diprenorphine binding at high (black), moderate (white), and low or non-existent (shaded) levels of binding capacity. The arrows link particular areas and pain activation sites with different levels of opioid receptor binding (Vogt et al. 1995). aMCC = anterior midcingulate cortex; dPCC = dorsal posterior cingulate cortex; pACC = pregenual anterior cingulate cortex; pMCC = posterior midcingulate cortex; vPCC = ventral posterior cingulate cortex.

OPIOID RECEPTOR BINDING

It has been known for four decades that opioid receptor binding is not uniform in the cingulate gyrus. This binding has been evaluated in terms of the four-region model of the cingulate gyrus with trace labeling of

[^{11}C]diprenorphine binding with positron emission tomography (PET; Vogt et al. 1995). Fig. 2B shows this binding in two midsagittal levels with arrows from the cytoarchitectural map above. The binding capacities are coded as high with black, moderate with white, and low to none with background grey. The highest binding is in ACC (arrow #1), although it does extend dorsally into the MCC. The gyral surface in aMCC has a high level of binding (arrow #2), while this is not true for the cortex in the cingulate sulcus. As noted with the pair of arrows at #3, the first also points to high binding on the gyral surface of the pMCC, while the second points to the depths of the cingulate sulcus, where little or no binding was detected. The cingulate motor areas in the MCC do not appear to express opioid receptors, and they are not under opioid ligand control. Although the dPCC has almost no activations during noxious stimulation (Fig. 2A), there is one patch of high diprenorphine binding that does coregister with these few sites on the gyral surface; otherwise, the PCC is relatively free of binding, and the ventral PCC appears to have little or none.

SOURCE OF NOCICEPTIVE DRIVE

Neurons in the cingulate cortex have broad, usually whole-body, sometimes multimodal, nociceptive fields (Sikes and Vogt 1992), and these characteristics apply to neurons in the midline and intralaminar thalamic nuclei (Casey 1966; Dong et al. 1978). It is not surprising, therefore, that the main source of nociceptive information to the cingulate gyrus is the midline and intralaminar thalamic nuclei (Vogt et al. 1979) and that lidocaine block of these neurons abolishes cingulate nociceptive responses (Sikes and Vogt 1992). As shown in Fig. 3, the parafascicular nucleus (Pf) and other midline and intralaminar thalamic nuclei receive inputs from the dorsal horn of the spinal cord, the subnucleus reticularis dorsalis (SRD), and the parabrachial nuclei (Villanueva et al. 1990, 1998; Bester et al. 1999; Saper 2000). These three sources of input to the midline and intralaminar thalamic nuclei generate the receptive field properties observed in the cingulate gyrus. Finally, the Pf nucleus projects more intensely to the rCMA than to the caudal CMA (Hatanka et al. 2003), suggesting that the former is more sensitive to nociceptive input.

Thus, the rCMA is heavily activated by excitatory inputs from the nociceptive midline and intralaminar thalamic nuclei but is not regulated by opioid receptors, whereas the ACC is heavily regulated by opioid compounds, drives autonomic motor activity, and stores emotional memories, but has weaker nociceptive excitatory driving. Descending projections from the cingulate gyrus determine its role in anticipation and in the mechanisms of hypnotic intervention in pain processing.

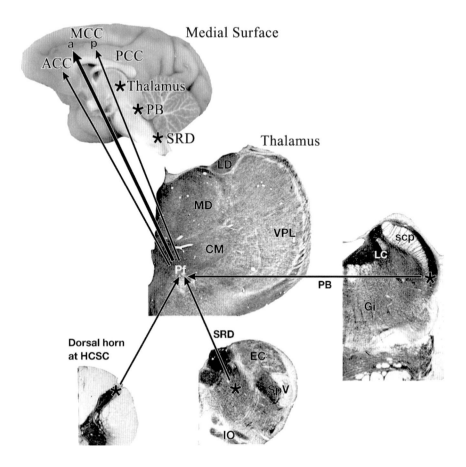

Fig. 3. Summary of projections in the medial pain system from central nervous system nociceptive sites (HCSC, SRD, and PB) to the parafascicular (Pf) nucleus and other midline and
intralaminar thalamic nuclei, and from these nuclei to the ACC and MCC (Vogt 2005). ACC
= anterior cingulate cortex; CM = centrum medianum; EC = external cuneate nucleus; Gi =
gigantocellular nucleus of the reticular formation; HCSC = high cervical level of the dorsal
horn in the spinal cord; IO = inferior olive; LC = locus coeruleus; MCC = midcingulate cortex;
MD = mediodorsal thalamic nucleus; PB = parabrachial nucleus; scp = superior cerebellar
peduncle; SpV = spinal nucleus of the fifth nerve; SRD = subnucleus reticularis dorsalis;
VPL = ventral posterior lateral thalamic nucleus.

ANTICIPATION-RELATED MODULATION OF PAIN
PROCESSING IN THE CINGULATE GYRUS

Anticipation of pain and anticipation of analgesia (placebo) are interesting
models to investigate how complex mental activities can affect pain perception
in humans (Petrovic and Ingvar 2002; Porro 2003; Colloca and Benedetti 2005).
The involvement of the cingulate cortex in anticipatory functions has been

extensively investigated over the last decade (Murtha et al. 1996; Hsieh et al. 1999; Critchley et al. 2001). There is preliminary electrophysiological evidence for neurons related to anticipation of noxious input in the human cingulate cortex (Hutchison et al. 1999), and anticipation effects on cortical activity have been described by several groups using functional magnetic resonance imaging (fMRI; Ploghaus et al. 1999; Sawamoto et al. 2000; Porro et al. 2002, 2003; Jensen et al. 2003; Singer et al. 2004; Koyama et al. 2005).

Using event-related fMRI, Ploghaus et al. (1999) found discrete areas in the medial prefrontal cortex that were selectively activated during anticipation of brief noxious thermal stimuli, but not during pain itself or anticipation of warmth. In individual subjects, anticipation of pain-related foci was located in the aMCC or in dorsal pACC, whereas foci responding to noxious input were in the pMCC. The authors hypothesized that the regions activated during anticipation could be involved in learning to predict pain or in the modulation of autonomic, affective, or motor reactions. Another event-related fMRI study showed that anticipation-related activation in the aMCC occurred regardless of whether the subject could actively avoid the aversive stimulus (Jensen et al. 2003).

A more complex involvement of cingulate areas during anticipation was demonstrated by Porro and colleagues (2002, 2003) using a different experimental paradigm characterized by more prolonged waiting (up to 60 seconds) and stimulation periods. The crucial difference with the above-mentioned studies was that the subjects were not aware of the quality of the impending stimulus (either painful or not painful), and they had not previously experienced the same kind of noxious stimulus (subcutaneous injection of an ascorbic acid solution). These experimental conditions resulted in what has been called "uncertain" anticipation, which has been associated with the emotional state of anxiety and with an increased attentional state. Several lines of evidence suggest that previous knowledge of the stimulus and available information prior to its onset (quality, intensity, and site) are indeed critical for determination of the response during the anticipation period and may influence the subsequent perception of the stimulus itself (Hsieh et al. 1999; Price 1999; Ploghaus et al. 2003). Both the PCC and MCC showed increased mean fMRI signals during the anticipatory phase, but only the MCC showed increased fMRI signals during the period immediately following the tactile or painful stimulation (Porro et al. 2003).

These findings suggest that large populations of neurons in the cingulate cortex are involved during uncertain expectation of pain. No significant *net* fMRI signal changes were found in the pACC, which often displays a composite array of areas showing fMRI increases or decreases during anticipation (Porro et al. 2002, 2003). In a recent event-related fMRI study using another paradigm of "uncertain" anticipation of pain, foci in the right pACC were found that were uniquely active during the anticipatory period, but not following actual noxious stimuli (Lui et al., unpublished manuscript). Thus, activated foci in this area do not appear to be specific for fear-related processes, which are thought to occur during certain expectation (Hsieh et al. 1999). Anticipation is a complex state, and the cognitive factors involved in activity increases in the cingulate cortex are not yet fully understood; selective attention (Mesulam et al. 2001; Bantick et al. 2002; Small et al. 2003), arousal (Critchley et al. 2001; Porro et al. 2003), and mental representation of impending stimuli (Koyama et al. 2005) may play a role. Foci of decreased pACC activity during anticipation may be related to emotional changes (Simpson et al. 2001, Porro et al. 2003).

A key issue with regard to pain mechanisms is whether the cortical pain system can be directly modulated by anticipation. There is now evidence that anticipation modulates both basal and noxious-evoked activity within the cingulate cortex (Sawamoto et al. 2000; Porro et al. 2002, 2003; Singer et al. 2004; Koyama et al. 2005). Clusters encoding pain intensity in the aMCC (as well as in parietal and insular regions) show significant changes of activity during uncertain anticipation, similar to those displayed during pain but approximately one-third as large (Porro et al. 2002, 2003; Fig. 4). Another recent study has shown that as the magnitude of expected pain increases, fMRI signals increase in the aMCC, thalamus, insula, and prefrontal and parietal cortical regions; by contrast, expectations of lower pain intensities powerfully reduced both the subjective experience of pain and the activation of an array of brain regions

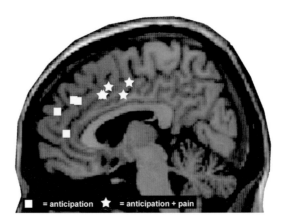

Fig. 4. Peak clusters according to Montreal Neurological Institute (MNI) clusters on the mesial hemispheric wall showing fMRI signal changes during anticipation of pain (squares) or during both anticipation and processing noxious input (stars). Only clusters with peak coordinates within 10 mm from midline were included (data from both hemispheres), projected on the same parasagittal plane ($x = 6$ mm) for the sake of simplicity. Note the segregation of the two response patterns in the pACC (anticipation) and MCC (anticipation + pain), respectively.

partially overlapping with the ones that were involved during pain, including the MCC (Koyama et al. 2005). These findings may explain why anticipation of pain influences the perception of subsequent noxious stimuli, a well-known effect in experimental studies and in the clinical setting. Increased fMRI activity occurring after anticipatory cues in nociceptive clusters of the MCC and anterior insula has also been noted during certain expectation of either one's own pain or others' pain; these foci have therefore been suggested to participate in the neural substrates of empathy for pain (Singer et al. 2004).

Recently, functional imaging studies have also investigated neural circuits involved in anticipation of analgesia (namely, in the placebo analgesic process) and the placebo effects on the pain neuromatrix (Petrovic et al. 2002; Lieberman et al. 2004; Wager et al. 2004). Lieberman et al. (2004) and Wager et al. (2004) provided evidence for distinct foci in the MCC, showing decreased activation during the pain period that correlated with the magnitude of placebo-induced analgesia (likely "sites" of modulation in the pain system). Other clusters in the Wager et al. (2004) study showed positive correlations between fMRI activity during the anticipation phase and the reported placebo effects in behavioral ratings; these foci may be part of an "executive" circuit mediating cognitive control functions. The two populations appear largely intermingled in the aMCC, which thus appears to be at the interface of modulatory and nociceptive systems. On the other hand, converging information from different studies (Ploghaus et al. 1999; Petrovic et al. 2002) suggests that pACC sites probably constitute a higher-order link in the circuits underlying modulation of the pain system due to anticipatory mechanisms.

CINGULATE-MEDIATED MECHANISMS OF HYPNOSIS: APPLICATION TO SURGICAL ANESTHESIA

Just prior to the development of chemical anesthesia in 1846, the Scottish physician Esdaile (1847) documented the use of hypnosis to control surgical pain. He successfully used hypnosis widely in India, and most of his patients survived—a rare event in those days. Opposition to surgery under hypnosis was intense, and the practice died out after chemical anesthesia became available. Throughout the history of hypnosis, speculation about the basic nature and underlying causes of these phenomena has been full of controversies, conflicts, and passion. There are many different theories about hypnosis in the literature, which overlap in many respects yet also have major differences. Some researchers state that hypnotic phenomena cannot be explained without positing a special psychological state (an altered state of consciousness), while others regard all phenomena seen in association with hypnosis as being explainable by using ordinary psychological concepts (role-playing, expectation).

Hypnosis is a naturally occurring state of mind different from sleep (Gorton 1949). A variety of phenomena accompany the hypnotic state, which may be induced by the instruction of a therapist or self-induced. During hypnosis the focus of attention is narrowed and shifted toward an internal cognitive focus, which leads to a reduction in awareness of other sensory inputs. Reduction in critical thinking, reality testing and tolerance of reality distortion, heightened vividness of imagery or reality, alterations in perceptions, voluntary muscle activity, distortion of memory and time perception, and heightening of expectations and motivations are features often reported by subjects under hypnosis.

Hypnosis can facilitate cognitive strategies that are helpful in alleviating pain. Hypnosis combined with conscious intravenous sedation and local anesthesia (also called hypnosedation) has been used at the Department of Anesthesiology-Reanimation at the University of Liège in more than 5,000 surgical patients (Faymonville et al. 1995, 1997, 1999; Meurisse et al. 1999; Defechereux et al. 2000). This form of anesthesia was used instead of general anesthesia for a broad range of procedures including head and neck lift, breast augmentation, correction of mammary ptosis, nasal septorhinoplasty, skin grafting, tubal ligation, hysterectomy, maxillofacial reconstruction, thyroidectomy, and cervicotomy for hyperparathyroidism.

Hypnosis replaces pharmacological unconsciousness during surgery, allowing patient participation, and is associated with faster recovery and a shorter hospital stay. It requires some changes in the working habits of surgeons and anesthesiologists, such as closer teamwork. The credibility of hypnosis and its acceptance by the scientific community will depend on independently confirmed and reproducible criteria for assessing this state. Functional activation of brain regions is thought to be reflected by increases in regional cerebral blood flow in PET studies. This functional brain imaging technique has contributed unique information on the neurophysiological correlates of hypnosis, directly implicating parts of the cingulate cortex. These imaging approaches have also provided strong support for the notion that hypnotic suggestions can modulate auditory perception (Szechtman et al. 1998), pain (Rainville et al. 1997; Lang et al. 2000), and visual perception (Kosslyn et al. 2000).

To better understand what happens in patients in the hypnotic state during surgery, Faymonville et al. (2000) explored brain function in healthy volunteers by determining the distribution of regional cerebral blood flow as an index of local neuronal activity. The group analysis showed that the hypnotic state is related to the activation of a widespread, mainly left-sided, set of cortical areas involving occipital, parietal, precentral, premotor, and ventrolateral prefrontal cortices as well as right-sided regions of the occipital and anterior cingulate area 32. This pattern of activation differs from those induced by simple evocation of autobiographical memories. The deactivation of the precuneus cortex is an important metabolic feature distinguishing the hypnotic state from alert, visual mental imagery (Maquet et al. 1999). The hypnotic state should be distinguished from other types of internally generated, polymodal perception, motor experiences, the functional anatomy of which has been evaluated with PET; from dreams during rapid eye movement sleep in volunteers (Maquet et al. 1996); and from hallucinations in schizophrenic patients (Silbersweig et al. 1995).

These results suggest that hypnosis is a particular cerebral waking state in which the subject, seemingly somnolent, experiences a vivid multimodal, coherent, memory-based mental imagery that invades consciousness. The neural mechanism underlying pain modulation by hypnosis was first reported by Rainville et al. (1997) in a PET study aimed at differentiating cortical areas involved in pain affect. The authors proposed that hypnotic suggestion selectively alters the unpleasantness of noxious stimulation without changing its perceived intensity. This powerful expectation of increased or decreased unpleasantness of the experimental painful stimulation increases or decreases the activity of a rostral part of the aMCC in parallel with increased or decreased subjective pain intensity and unpleasantness.

The hypnotic protocol of Faymonville et al. (2000) was based on the recall of pleasant life experiences without any reference to pain perception, and subjects were not asked to actively induce analgesia. The study had a factorial design with two factors: state (hypnosis, normal alertness with recall of pleasant life experience, rest) and stimulation (thermode applied to the thenar eminence of the right hand and target temperatures that were reproducibly experienced as warm and non-noxious at 39°–40°C or as hot and noxious at 47°–48°C). Two PET scans were obtained with the ^{15}O H_2O technique during each stimulation condition. Volunteers also rated pain intensity and unpleasantness after each scan. Statistical parametric mapping was used to determine the main effects of noxious stimulation and hypnotic state and to highlight brain areas that would be more or less activated in hypnosis than in the control condition, under noxious stimulation. During hypnosis, decreased pain sensation and unpleasantness ratings were observed.

This "hypnoanalgesia" is produced by complex interactions among areas in the pain neuromatrix. The interaction analysis showed that the activity in the aMCC was related to pain intensity and unpleasantness differently in the hypnotic state than in the control state. During hypnosis, blood flow in the aMCC decreased when pain sensation and unpleasantness decreased, as shown in Fig. 5A. The controls had no such correlation in the aMCC (Faymonville et al. 2000).

Hypnosis-induced changes in functional connectivity between the aMCC and a large neural network involved in the different aspects of noxious processing were also assessed. The assessment of functional integration using

A. Hypnotically Sensitive aMCC

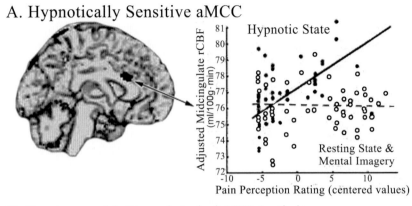

B. Regions with Correlated aMCC Activity

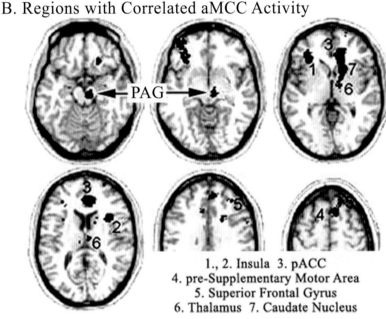

1., 2. Insula 3. pACC
4. pre-Supplementary Motor Area
5. Superior Frontal Gyrus
6. Thalamus 7. Caudate Nucleus

Fig. 5. (A) Location of hypnotically sensitive areas of the aMCC with reports of pain intensity in the hypnotic state and during resting and mental imagery. (B) A correlation study was seeded with voxels in the aMCC activation site during hypnosis, and sites with significant correlation coefficients were identified. In addition to a correlation with the pACC, which most likely was associated with the pleasant imagery used to induce the hypnotic state, an important site can be seen in the midbrain that was probably associated with the periaqueductal gray (PAG) and with activation of the descending noxious inhibitory system that mediates hypnotic sedation during surgical procedures. rCBF = regional cerebral blood flow.

psychophysiological interaction analyses is limited by the known structural connections between the reference region (aMCC) and the rest of the brain. A psychophysiological interaction means that the contribution of one area to another changes significantly with the experimental context (Friston et al. 1997). Compared to normal alertness states (rest and mental imagery), the hypnotic state enhanced the functional modulation between the aMCC and bilateral anterior insular cortices, pACC area 32, the pre-supplementary motor area (area 6), right prefrontal cortex (area 8), right thalamus, right striatum, and brainstem. The latter region appears to include the periaqueductal gray (PAG), as shown in Fig. 5B. At a lower threshold for significance, left prefrontal area 10, right prefrontal areas 9 and 11, and mesiofrontal area 9 were also identified (Faymonville et al. 2003).

In view of the role of the PAG in descending inhibitory mechanisms, we hypothesize that the reduced nociception during hypnosis compared to normal alertness is mediated by an increased functional connectivity between pACC area 32, which is active during pleasant imagery, and the PAG. In addition, cortical regions implicated in the affective, cognitive, and behavioral aspects of nociception are also activated to reduce the general level of pain processing. These observations reinforce the idea that the cingulate cortex plays a pivotal role in cognitive modulation of pain and provide important new avenues for targeting pain control systems.

CONCLUSIONS

The structural and functional heterogeneity of the cingulate gyrus suggests that this region plays a diverse role in pain processing. For example, visceral processing of nociceptive information occurs preferentially in the ACC, a region that directly regulates autonomic outputs, while the MCC region is more closely linked to cutaneous nociceptive processing and directly regulates skeletomotor systems via the cingulate motor areas. The challenge of this system for clinical pain control is to regulate descending projections from different cingulate regions to alleviate acute and chronic pain. Two approaches to this problem are currently available. In one, opiate drugs can be used with greatest influence in ACC and result in modulation of affective and autonomic systems, while much less control is exerted in the MCC and almost none in the PCC and RSC. A second strategy is to modulate pain anticipation to cognitively control unique functional entities. This "top-down" strategy is used in hypnosedation, which appears to operate mainly through projections of parts of the ACC that are activated with pleasant imagery to trigger the diffuse noxious inhibitory system via the PAG. Over the long term, selective functional activation may be used to influence parts of the cingulate gyrus with great precision to control psychiatrically intransigent aspects of chronic pain syndromes.

ACKNOWLEDGMENTS

Supported by NIH, NINDS (RO1 NS44222 to B.A. Vogt), and MIUR (Ministero Istruzione Università e Ricerca, Italy; grants COFIN and FIRB RBNE018ET9 to C.A. Porro).

REFERENCES

Bantick SJ, Wise R, Ploghaus A, et al. Imaging how attention modulates pain in humans using functional MRI. *Brain* 2002; 125:310–319.

Bester H, Bourgeais L, Villanueva L, et al. Differential projections to the intralaminar and gustatory thalamus from the parabrachial area: a PHA-L study in the rat. *J Comp Neurol* 1999; 405:421–449.

Casey KL. Unit analysis of nociceptive mechanisms in the thalamus of awake squirrel monkey. *J Neurophysiol* 1966; 29:727–750.

Colloca L, Benedetti F. Placebos and painkillers: Is mind as real as matter? *Nat Rev Neurosci* 2005; 6:47–54.

Critchley HD, Mathias CJ, Dolan RJ. Neural activity in the human brain relating to uncertainty and arousal during anticipation. *Neuron* 2001; 29:537–545.

Defechereux T, Degauque C, Fumal I, et al. L'hypnosédation, un nouveau mode d'anesthésie pour la chirurgie endocrinienne cervicale. Etude prospective randomisée. *Ann Chir* 2000; 125:539–546.

Dong WK, Ryu H, Wagman IH. Nociceptive responses of neurons in medial thalamus and their relationship to spinothalamic pathways. *J Neurophsyiol* 1978; 41:1592–1613.

Esdaile J. *Mesmerism in India and its Practical Application in Surgery and Medicine*. Hartford, 1847.

Faymonville ME, Fissette J, Mambourg PH, et al. Hypnosis as adjunct therapy in conscious sedation for plastic surgery. *Reg Anesth* 1995; 20:145–151.

Faymonville ME, Mambourg PH, Joris J, et al. Psychological approaches during conscious sedation. Hypnosis versus stress reducing strategies: a prospective randomized study. *Pain* 1997; 73:361–367.

Faymonville ME, Meurisse M, Fissette J. Hypnosedation: a valuable alternative to traditional anaesthetic techniques. *Acta Chir Belg* 1999; 99:141–146.

Faymonville ME, Laureys S, Degueldre C, et al. Neural mechanisms of antinociceptive effects of hypnosis. *Anesthesiology* 2000; 92:1257–1267.

Faymonville ME, Roediger L, Del Fiore G, et al. Increased cerebral functional connectivity underlying the antinociceptive affects of hypnosis. *Cogn Brain Res* 2003; 17:255–262.

Friston KJ, Buechel C, Fink GR. Psychophysiological and modulatory interactions in neuroimaging. *Neuroimage* 1997; 6:218–229.

Gorton BE. "The physiology of hypnosis." *Psychiatr Q* 1949; 23:317–343, 457–385.

Hatanka N, Tokuno H, Hamada I, et al. Thalamocortical and intracortical connections of monkey cingulate motor areas. *J Comp Neurol* 2003; 462:121–138.

Hsieh J, Stone-Elander S, Ingvar M. Anticipatory coping of pain expressed in the human anterior cingulate cortex: a positron emission tomography study. *Neurosci Lett* 1999; 262:61–64.

Hutchison W, Davis K, Lozano A, et al. Pain-related neurons in the human cingulate cortex. *Nat Neurosci* 1999; 2:403–405.

Jensen J, McIntosh AR, Crawley AP, et al. Direct activation of the ventral striatum in anticipation of aversive stimuli. *Neuron* 2003; 40:1251–1257.

Kosslyn SM, Thompson WL, Costantini-Ferrando MF, et al. Hypnotic visual illusion alters color processing in the brain. *Am J Psychiatry* 2000; 157:1279–1284.

Koyama T, McHaffie JG, Laurienti PJ, Coghill RC. The subjective experience of pain: where expectations become reality. *Proc Natl Acad Sci USA* 2005; 102:12951–12955.

Lang EV, Benotsch EG, Fick LJ, et al. Adjunctive non-pharmacological analgesia for invasive medical procedures: a randomised trial. *Lancet* 2000; 355:1486–1490.

Lieberman MD, Jarcho JM, Berman S, et al. The neural correlates of placebo effects: a disruption account. *Neuroimage* 2004; 22:447–455.

Maquet P, Peters J, Aerts J, et al. Functional neuroanatomy of human rapid-eye-movement sleep and dreaming *Nature* 1996; 383:163–166.

Maquet P, Faymonville ME, Degueldre C, et al. Functional neuroanatomy of hypnotic state. *Biol Psychiatry* 1999; 45:327–333.

Mesulam MM, Nobre AC, Kim YH, Parrish TB, Gitelman DR. Heterogeneity of cingulate contributions to spatial attention. *Neuroimage* 2001; 13:1065–1072.

Meurisse M, Hamoir E, Defechereux TH, et al. Bilateral neck exploration under hypnosedation. *Ann Surg* 1999; 229:401–408.

Murtha S, Chertkow H, Beauregard M, Dixon R, Evans A. Anticipation causes increased blood flow to the anterior cingulate cortex. *Hum Brain Mapp* 1996; 4:103–112.

Petrovic P, Ingvar M. Imaging cognitive modulation of pain processing. *Pain* 2002; 95:1–5.

Petrovic P, Kalso E, Petersson KM, Ingvar M. Placebo and opioid analgesia—imaging a shared neuronal network. *Science* 2002; 295:1737–1740.

Ploghaus A, Tracey I, Gati J, et al. Dissociating pain from its anticipation in the human brain. *Science* 1999; 284:1979–1981.

Ploghaus A, Becerra L, Borras C, Borsook D. Neural circuitry underlying pain modulation: expectation, hypnosis, placebo. *Trends Cogn Sci* 2003; 7:197–200.

Porro CA. Functional imaging and pain: behavior, perception, and modulation. *Neuroscientist* 2003; 9:354–369.

Porro CA, Baraldi P, Pagnoni G, et al. Does anticipation of pain affect cortical nociceptive circuits? *J Neurosci* 2002; 22:3206–3214.

Porro CA, Cettolo V, Francescato MP, Baraldi P. Functional activity mapping of the mesial hemispheric wall during anticipation of pain. *Neuroimage* 2003; 19:1738–1747.

Price D. *Psychological Mechanisms of Pain and Analgesia,* Progress in Brain Research and Management, Vol. 15. Seattle: IASP Press, 1999.

Rainville P, Duncan GH, Price DD, et al. Pain affect encoded in human anterior cingulate but not somatosensory cortex. *Science* 1997; 277:968–971.

Saper CB. Pain as a visceral sensation. *Prog Brain Res* 2000; 122:237–243.

Sawamoto N, Honda M, Okada T, et al. Expectation of pain enhances responses to nonpainful somatosensory stimulation in the anterior cingulate cortex and parietal operculum/posterior insula: an event-related functional magnetic resonance imaging study. *J Neurosci* 2000; 20:7438–7445.

Sikes RW, Vogt BA. Nociceptive neurons in area 24 of rabbit cingulate cortex. *J Neurophysiol* 1992; 68:1720–1732.

Silbersweig DA, Stern E, Frith C, et al. A functional neuroanatomy of hallucinations in schizophrenia. *Nature* 1995; 378:176–179.

Simpson JR, Drevets WC, Snyder AZ, Gusnard DA, Raichle ME. Emotion-induced changes in human medial prefrontal cortex: II. During anticipatory anxiety. *Proc Natl Acad Sci USA* 2001; 98: 688–693.

Singer T, Seymour B, O'Doherty J, et al. Empathy for pain involves the affective but not sensory components of pain. *Science* 2004; 303:1157–1162.

Small DM, Gitelman DR, Gregory MD, et al. The posterior cingulate and medial prefrontal cortex mediate the anticipatory allocation of spatial attention. *Neuroimage* 2003; 18:633–641.

Szechtman H, Woody E, Bowers KS, Nahmias C. Where the imaginal appears real: a positron emission tomography study of auditory hallucinations *Proc Natl Acad Sci USA* 1998; 95:1956–1960.

Villanueva L, Cliffer KD, Sorkin LS, et al. Convergence of heterotopic nociceptive information onto neurons of caudal medullary reticular formation in monkey (*Macaca fascicularis*). *J Neurophysiol* 1990; 63:1118–1127.

Villanueva L, Debois C, Le Bars D, Bernard JF. Organization of diencephalic projections from the medullary subnucleus reticularis dorsalis: a retrograde and anterograde tracer study in rat. *J Comp Neurol* 1998; 390:133–160.

Vogt BA. Pain and emotion interactions in subregions of the cingulate gyrus. *Nat Rev Neurosci* 2005; 6:533–545.

Vogt BA, Rosene D L, Pandya DN. Thalamic and cortical afferents differentiate anterior from posterior cingulate cortex in the monkey. *Science* 1979; 204:205–207.

Vogt B, Watanabe H, Grootoonk S, Jones AKP. Topography of diprenorphine binding in human cingulate gyrus and adjacent cortex derived from PET and MR images. *Hum Brain Mapp* 1995; 3:1–12

Vogt BA, Berger GR, Derbyshire SWJ. Structural and Functional dichotomy of human midcingulate cortex. *Eur J Neurosci* 2003; 18:3134–3144.

Vogt BA, Hof PR, Vogt, LJ. Cingulate gyrus. In: Paxinos G, Mai JK (Eds). *The Human Nervous System,* 2nd ed. Academic Press, 2004, pp 915–949.

Wager TD, Rilling JK, Smith EE, et al. Placebo-induced changes in fMRI in the anticipation and experience of pain. *Science* 2004; 303:1162–1167.

Correspondence to: Brent A. Vogt, PhD, Department of Neuroscience and Physiology, SUNY Upstate Medical University, 750 E. Adams Street, Syracuse, NY 13210, USA. Email: vogtb@upstate.edu.

Proceedings of the 11th World Congress on Pain,
edited by Herta Flor, Eija Kalso, and Jonathan O.
Dostrovsky, IASP Press, Seattle, © 2006.

37

Repetitive Pain Exposure: Neuronal Correlates in the Human Brain

Michael Valet,[a] Till Sprenger,[a] Henning Boecker,[b]
Ernst Rummeny,[c] and Thomas R. Tölle[a]

*[a]Neurology Clinic and Polyclinic, [b]Nuclear Medicine Clinic and Polyclinic,
[c]Institute for Radiographic Diagnosis, Technical University of Munich,
Munich, Germany*

The experience of acute pain is an elementary sensation necessary for maintaining individual integrity and well-being in interaction with the environment (Woolf 2004). However, persistent noxious input can induce chronic pain states without any biological advantage. Long-term changes in the excitability of neurons have been shown at the peripheral and spinal cord levels (Woolf 1993), but it is a major challenge to investigate cerebral mechanisms and structures that contribute to pain sensitization. Maladaptive supraspinal reorganization is thought to play an important role in central sensitization, reconfiguring the central pain-processing matrix through learning, extinction, and memory processes. Although neuroimaging studies have been conducted in patients with chronic pain (Flor et al. 1995; Peyron et al. 1998; Maihofner et al. 2003), we are not aware of human experimental imaging results on the dynamic evolution of cerebral sensitization. This chapter describes a study focusing on neuronal activity changes in the brain of healthy volunteers in the course of repetitive noxious heat stimulation over 2 weeks.

METHODS

Fourteen right-handed healthy volunteers participated in this study. Subjects (10 men and 4 women) were between 27 and 62 years old, with a mean age of 43.3 years. All participants received detailed information about the experimental procedures, were free to withdraw from the study at any time, and gave written informed consent. The study protocol was approved by our university's ethics committee.

Volunteers received noxious heat stimulation on 11 consecutive working days; no procedures were conducted on weekends. Each session consisted of a series of eight noxious and eight innocuous heat stimuli in pseudo-randomized order, $1°C$ above and $3°C$ below the individual pain threshold; each stimulus was applied for 40 seconds. Between the stimuli a 20-second neutral stimulus of $35°C$ was used to determine basal neuronal activity. The overall length of the stimulation was about 16 minutes. Stimuli were applied to the inner side of the right forearm with a 30×30 mm thermode using a thermal stimulator. To avoid any skin damage during the 40-second noxious heat stimuli the temperature oscillated at a frequency of 0.5 Hz and amplitude of $1°C$ starting from the individual pain threshold (Lautenbacher et al. 1995) (see also Valet et al. 2004 for a more detailed description and illustration of the noxious heat stimulation protocol). The position of the thermode was changed in pseudo-randomized order every day to one of five possible positions on the forearm to prevent skin sensitization. Although the individual pain threshold was assessed every day to check for changes in pain sensation, the temperature of the noxious heat stimulus the subjects received was that determined on the first day. Subjects were blinded to this fact, believing that they were receiving the newly determined pain threshold temperature each day. Acute perception of pain intensity and unpleasantness were measured separately using an 11-point numerical rating scale and analyzed with a repeated-measures analysis of variance (ANOVA). Additionally, Beck Depression Inventory scores (Beck et al. 1988) and anxiety scores on a 5-point Likert scale (0 = "no anxiety," 4 = "extreme anxiety about painful stimulation") were evaluated on the first and 11th day of pain stimulation with a single-sided Student's t-test.

Functional magnetic resonance imaging (fMRI) was performed on a 1.5-Tesla magnetic resonance scanner using an echo planar imaging technique. We used statistical parametric mapping software for functional imaging analysis (Friston et al. 1995). The fMRI data were realigned to correct for motion artifacts, normalized to standard reference space according to the echo planar imaging template of our statistical parametric mapping software, based on the mean brain of 305 healthy subjects determined at the Montreal Neurological Institute (MNI) (Collins et al. 1994). Finally, data were smoothed to account for anatomical individual variances and to improve the signal-to-noise ratio.

For the statistical analysis, subject-specific statistical parametric maps for noxious and innocuous heat effects of the first and 11th day were calculated using the general linear model approach (using a block design with conditions convolved with the hemodynamic response function) and applied for second-level analysis (random effects analysis, one sample t-test). To check for pain-induced activation changes between the first and 11th day of stimulation, statistical comparisons (paired t-test) were performed. Statistical comparison was also performed for innocuous heat effects to differentiate pain-specific responses from general sensitization phenomena. Statistical parametric maps were thresholded at $P < 0.001$ uncorrected with a minimum cluster size of 135 mm^3, because we expected activation in the previously established pain-processing network (the brainstem, thalamus, primary and secondary somatosensory cortices, and insular, parietal, and prefrontal cortices) (Peyron et al. 2000a; Apkarian et al. 2005). Furthermore, we were interested in brain structures of the limbic lobe and defined the amygdala, hippocampus, and cingulate cortex as regions of interest (Maldjian et al. 2003), because it is known that these structures are involved in memory processes (Phelps 2004). Results of these analyses were corrected for multiple comparisons according to the random field theory with $P < 0.05$ (Worsley et al. 1996).

RESULTS

All volunteers reported the noxious temperature stimulation (mean ± standard deviation = 45.2°C ± 1.0°C) as moderately to severely painful on each day of stimulation. No significant change was detected in individual pain threshold, which we determined daily (mean of 45.2°C the first day to 45.4°C the last day; $F_{10,130} = 0.8627$, n.s.).

The rating of pain unpleasantness increased significantly from 4.2 ± 2.0 to 5.8 ± 1.2 over the 2 weeks (repeated measures one-way ANOVA, $F_{10,130} = 3.585$, $P < 0.0001$) when subjects were stimulated with the same noxious temperature every day. Subjective ratings of pain intensity also increased significantly, but to a lesser extent than for pain unpleasantness, from an average of 5.7 ± 1.8 to 6.1 ± 1.7 ($F_{10,130} = 1.913$, $P = 0.0487$).

No depressive complaints and no significant changes on the self-report scale for the measurement of depression (Beck Depression Inventory) were reported (mean ± SD = 2.5 ± 2.3 on the first day versus 1.5 ± 1.6 on the 11th day; Student's t-test: n.s.). No change in anxiety ratings was detected on a 5-point Likert scale (0.3 ± 0.47 on the first day versus 0.1 ± 0.36 on the 11th day; Student's t-test: n.s.).

The noxious heat stimulation on the first and last day of stimulation induced significant activation in the midbrain, thalamus, secondary somatosensory cortex, anterior cingulate cortex (ACC), insular cortex, frontal cortex, and parietal cortex ($P < 0.001$). The comparison of fMRI data of the first versus the 11th day during noxious stimulation ($P < 0.05$) indicated increased activation of the right amygdala extending to the entorhinal cortex (peak MNI coordinates: 18, –9, –30; $Z = 4.55$), the right and left hippocampal complex (coordinates: 21, –12, –30; $Z = 4.35$ and –27, 0, –24; $Z = 3.93$), and the rostral ACC (coordinates:

9, 36, –3; Z = 3.65) (Fig. 1). No increased brain activation was observed during innocuous heat stimulation when we compared the first versus the 11th day, suggesting that these changes are pain specific.

DISCUSSION

The study described in this chapter demonstrates that repetitive painful stimulation not only increases subjective pain perception over time but also alters the cerebral pain processing. Increased activation was found in multiple parts of the limbic system, namely the amygdala, the hippocampal complex, and the rostral ACC.

The amygdala and the hippocampal complex are two structures of the medial temporal lobe that are engaged in memory processes. As part of the limbic system, the amygdala is known to be specialized in emotional processing, including the evaluation of sensory stimuli as pleasant or aversive (Hamann et al. 1999), but also in the consolidation of memories of emotionally arousing experiences such as fear or disgust (Murphy et al. 2003; McGaugh 2004; Phelps 2004). However, the amygdala's role in pain processing in general and especially in the processing of aversive responses to pain and pain memory is currently under investigation. Because of its neuroanatomical and functional connections with the insular and anterior cingulate cortices (Pitkanen et al. 1997; LeDoux 2000; Price 2000), the amygdala is very likely to participate in the processing of affective components of pain (LeDoux 2000; Bingel et al.

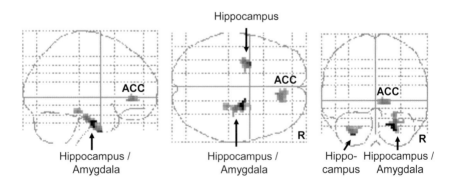

Fig. 1. Pain-induced blood-oxygen-level-dependent signal increases shown by functional magnetic resonance imaging after 2 weeks of pain stimulation compared to the pain activation of the first day. Increased activation is found in the amygdalar and hippocampal region and the rostral anterior cingulate cortex (ACC), as shown on the statistical parametric mapping software's maximum intensity projection at a threshold of P < 0.001 uncorrected for multiple comparisons. According to neurological convention, the right side of the image corresponds to the right side of the brain.

2002). Moreover, the amygdala has widespread connections to the forebrain and brainstem including the periaqueductal grey (PAG) and rostral ventromedial medulla (RVM). As the PAG and RVM are key structures of the descending pain inhibitory system (Fields and Basbaum 1999; LeDoux 2000; Price 2003), one important function of the amygdala is its interaction with the "brain defense system" (Ingvar 1999), thereby leading to pain inhibition (Rhudy and Meagher 2003). This pathway induces direct and indirect changes in affect, such as fear, and also subserves somatic and autonomic reflexive responses to life-threatening stimuli (Cousins 1994; Rosen et al. 1994; Hsieh et al. 1996).

The hippocampal complex plays a central role in the formation of declarative/episodic long-term memory, associated with the possibility of recollecting events at will (Phelps 2004). Aversive events tend to be preferentially memorized, and their recall to be more persistent and vivid than that of memories without emotional content. The enhanced memory capability of emotional events is probably due to the amygdala's influence on encoding and storage of hippocampal-dependent memories (Cahill 1999; Pikkarainen et al. 1999; Richter-Levin 2004). In the context of pain processing, we suggest that the coactivation of the hippocampus and amygdala indicates that these structures act jointly. The function of the amygdala may be to enhance the encoding and retrieval of pain-related memory processes located in the hippocampal complex.

The increased rostral ACC activation on the last day of our study may have different explanations. The first possibility is that the ACC activation reflects the augmented processing of the affective components of pain. Certain parts of the ACC play an important role in processing the affective dimension of pain, as has been demonstrated in previous pain neuroimaging studies (Tölle et al. 1999; Peyron et al. 2000b). This hypothesis is supported by the increased ratings of pain unpleasantness in our study. Second, given the neuroanatomical connections between the hippocampal-amygdalar formation and the rostral ACC (Insausti et al. 1987), the rostral ACC might be involved in hippocampal-amygdalar processing and expression of emotional aspects of pain memory. Third, an alternative explanation of the increased ACC activity arises from the known participation of this brain region in cognitive modulation of pain (Petrovic et al. 2000; Bantick et al. 2002; Petrovic and Ingvar 2002; Valet et al. 2004). In order to execute top-down modulation, the rostral ACC cooperatively inhibits or facilitates pain perception together with the PAG-RVM system (Valet et al. 2004). Given that the volunteers in our study reported increased subjective pain perception, either this system must be insufficient or the theoretical mechanisms described above might compete with the hippocampal-amygdalar amplification, thereby outweighing the "brain defense system."

SUMMARY AND CONCLUSIONS

The study described in this chapter demonstrates cerebral sensitization in an experimental model of repetitive pain exposure in healthy humans. Increasing subjective pain ratings were reflected by increases in the activation of the amygdala, hippocampus, and ACC. We suggest that neuroplasticity in the amygdala and hippocampus contributes to the encoding, consolidation, and retrieval of a pain memory trace. Activation of the rostral ACC might reflect the amplification of emotional pain components. These results have implications for the acute treatment of pain. Therapy should be initiated as early as possible to prevent the development of pain sensitization, which is the first step on the way to chronic pain.

ACKNOWLEDGMENTS

This work was supported by the "German Research Network on Neuropathic Pain," granted by the German Ministry of Education and Research (BMBF) and by the SFB 391 C9 grant from the Deutsche Forschungsgemeinschaft.

REFERENCES

Apkarian AV, Bushnell MC, Treede RD, Zubieta JK. Human brain mechanisms of pain perception and regulation in health and disease. *Eur J Pain* 2005; 9:463–484.

Bantick SJ, Wise RG, Ploghaus A, et al. Imaging how attention modulates pain in humans using functional MRI. *Brain* 2002; 125(Pt 2):310–319.

Beck AT, Steer RA, Garbin MG. Psychometric properties of the Beck Depression Inventory: twenty-five years of evaluation. *Clin Psychol Rev* 1998; 8:77–100.

Bingel U, Quante M, Knab R, et al. Subcortical structures involved in pain processing: evidence from single-trial fMRI. *Pain* 2002; 99:313–321.

Cahill L. A neurobiological perspective on emotionally influenced, long-term memory. *Semin Clin Neuropsychiatry* 1999; 4:266–273.

Collins DL, Neelin P, Peters TM, Evans AC. Automatic 3D intersubject registration of MR volumetric data in standardized Talairach space. *J Comput Assist Tomogr* 1994; 18:192–205.

Cousins M. Acute and postoperative pain. In: Wall PD, Melzack R (Eds). *Textbook of Pain*. Edinburgh: Churchill Livingstone, 1994, pp 357–385.

Fields HL, Basbaum A. Central nervous system mechanisms of pain modulation. In: Wall PD, Melzack R (Eds). *Textbook of Pain*. Edinburgh: Churchill Livingstone, 1999, pp 309–329.

Flor H, Elbert T, Knecht S, et al. Phantom-limb pain as a perceptual correlate of cortical reorganization following arm amputation. *Nature* 1995; 375:482–484.

Friston KJ, Holmes AP, Worsley KJ, et al. Statistical parametric maps in functional imaging: a general linear approach. *Hum Brain Mapp* 1995; 2:189–210.

Hamann SB, Ely TD, Grafton ST, Kilts CD. Amygdala activity related to enhanced memory for pleasant and aversive stimuli. *Nat Neurosci* 1999; 2:289–293.

Hsieh JC, Stahle-Backdahl M, Hagermark O, et al. Traumatic nociceptive pain activates the hypothalamus and the periaqueductal gray: a positron emission tomography study. *Pain* 1996; 64:303–314.

Ingvar M. Pain and functional imaging. *Philos Trans R Soc Lond B Biol Sci* 1999; 354:1347–1358.

Insausti R, Amaral DG, Cowan WM. The entorhinal cortex of the monkey: II. Cortical afferents. *J Comp Neurol* 1987; 264:356–395.

Lautenbacher S, Roscher S, Strian F. Tonic pain evoked by pulsating heat: temporal summation mechanisms and perceptual qualities. *Somatosens Mot Res* 1995; 12:59–70.

LeDoux JE. Emotion circuits in the brain. *Annu Rev Neurosci* 2000; 23:155–184.

Maihofner C, Handwerker HO, Neundorfer B, Birklein F. Patterns of cortical reorganization in complex regional pain syndrome. *Neurology* 2003; 61:1707–1715.

Maldjian JA, Laurienti PJ, Kraft RA, Burdette JH. An automated method for neuroanatomic and cytoarchitectonic atlas-based interrogation of fMRI data sets. *Neuroimage* 2003; 19:1233–1239.

McGaugh JL. The amygdala modulates the consolidation of memories of emotionally arousing experiences. *Annu Rev Neurosci* 2004; 27:1–28.

Murphy FC, Nimmo-Smith I, Lawrence AD. Functional neuroanatomy of emotions: a meta-analysis. *Cogn Affect Behav Neurosci* 2003; 3:207–233.

Petrovic P, Ingvar M. Imaging cognitive modulation of pain processing. *Pain* 2002; 95:1–5.

Petrovic P, Petersson KM, Ghatan PH, Stone-Elander S, Ingvar M. Pain-related cerebral activation is altered by a distracting cognitive task. *Pain* 2000; 85:19–30.

Peyron R, Garcia-Larrea L, Gregoire MC, et al. Allodynia after lateral-medullary (Wallenberg) infarct. A PET study. *Brain* 1998; 121(Pt 2):345–356.

Peyron R, Garcia-Larrea L, Gregoire MC, et al. Parietal and cingulate processes in central pain. A combined positron emission tomography (PET) and functional magnetic resonance imaging (fMRI) study of an unusual case. *Pain* 2000a; 84:77–87.

Peyron R, Laurent B, Garcia-Larrea L. Functional imaging of brain responses to pain. A review and meta-analysis. *Neurophysiol Clin* 2000b; 30:263–288.

Phelps EA. Human emotion and memory: interactions of the amygdala and hippocampal complex. *Curr Opin Neurobiol* 2004; 14:198–202.

Pikkarainen M, Ronkko S, Savander V, Insausti R, Pitkanen A. Projections from the lateral, basal, and accessory basal nuclei of the amygdala to the hippocampal formation in rat. *J Comp Neurol* 1999; 403:229–260.

Pitkanen A, Savander V, LeDoux JE. Organization of intra-amygdaloid circuitries in the rat: an emerging framework for understanding functions of the amygdala. *Trends Neurosci* 1997; 20:517–523.

Price DD. Psychological and neural mechanisms of the affective dimension of pain. *Science* 2000; 288:1769–1772.

Price JL. Comparative aspects of amygdala connectivity. *Ann NY Acad Sci* 2003; 985:50–58.

Rhudy JL, Meagher MW. Negative affect: effects on an evaluative measure of human pain. *Pain* 2003; 104:617–626.

Richter-Levin G. The amygdala, the hippocampus, and emotional modulation of memory. *Neuroscientist* 2004; 10:31–39.

Rosen SD, Paulesu E, Frith CD, et al. Central nervous pathways mediating angina pectoris. *Lancet* 1994; 344:147–150.

Tölle TR, Kaufmann T, Siessmeier T, et al. Region-specific encoding of sensory and affective components of pain in the human brain: a positron emission tomography correlation analysis. *Ann Neurol* 1999; 45:40–47.

Valet M, Sprenger T, Boecker H, et al. Distraction modulates connectivity of the cingulo-frontal cortex and the midbrain during pain—an fMRI analysis. *Pain* 2004; 109:399–408.

Woolf CJ. The pathophysiology of peripheral neuropathic pain—abnormal peripheral input and abnormal central processing. *Acta Neurochir Suppl (Wien)* 1993; 58:125–130.

Woolf CJ. Pain: moving from symptom control toward mechanism-specific pharmacologic management. *Ann Intern Med* 2004; 140:441–451.

Worsley KJ, Marrett S, Neelin P, et al. A unified statistical approach for determining significant signals in images of cerebral activation. *Hum Brain Mapp* 1996; 4:58–73.

Correspondence to: Dr. med. Michael Valet, Neurologische Klinik, Klinikum rechts der Isar, Möhlstr. 28, 81675 München, Germany. Fax: 49-89-4140-4659; email: valet@lrz.tum.de.

Proceedings of the 11th World Congress on Pain,
edited by Herta Flor, Eija Kalso, and Jonathan O.
Dostrovsky, IASP Press, Seattle, © 2006.

38

Cortical Responses to Noxious Stimulation in Preterm Infants

Rebeccah Slater,[a] Anne Cantarella,[b] Alan Worley,[c]
Stewart Boyd,[c] Judith Meek,[b] and Maria Fitzgerald[a]

*[a]The London Pain Consortium, Department of Anatomy and Developmental
Biology, University College London, London, United Kingdom; [b]Neonatal
Intensive Care Unit, Elizabeth Garrett Anderson and Obstetric Hospital,
London, United Kingdom; [c]Department of Clinical Neurophysiology,
Great Ormond Street Hospital, London, United Kingdom*

The poor state of pain management in preterm infants has been increasingly highlighted in recent years. We lack even the most basic information about effective methods of pain control in the youngest patients. To treat infant pain successfully and improve developmental outcomes, we must understand the neurobiological mechanisms of pain processing during development (Fitzgerald 2005). It has been demonstrated that the youngest infants can respond to noxious stimuli and tissue damage (Craig et al. 1993), and more recent research has highlighted some of the long-term consequences of early exposure to pain (Grunau et al. 2001; Peters et al. 2005). Infants undergoing intensive care are subjected to repeated painful procedures. However, because infants are unable to report pain directly, our understanding of pain processing in this vulnerable group has relied heavily upon surrogate measures, such as nociception. The distinction between nociception and pain is a fundamental problem in the study of infants. While nociception reflects the activity of central pathways at the level of primary sensory neurons and spinal and brainstem circuits, true pain perception has an emotional and affective component that requires higher-level cortical processing (Treede et al. 1999).

To date, studies in neonates have used indirect methods to demonstrate that noxious stimulation can activate sensory pathways, resulting in a wide range of physiological, biochemical, and behavioral responses (Franck et al. 2000; McNair et al. 2004). Other more direct neurophysiological approaches use nociceptive spinal flexion reflex responses to study the postnatal development of infant pain processing to single and repetitive noxious stimulation (Andrews and Fitzgerald 1994, 1999, 2002). While these methods have been used to demonstrate the ability of the youngest infants to mount a strong and organized response to noxious stimulation, the question remains as to how much pain human infants actually experience. The strong responses observed in preterm infants may be entirely mediated at the spinal or brainstem level with little or no cortical involvement. A recent study showed that below 32 weeks postconceptional age there was no difference in behavioral and physiological pain scores between infants with parenchymal brain injury (often associated with white matter damage) and normal controls, suggesting that below 32 weeks these responses may largely be mediated subcortically (Oberlander et al. 2002). It is therefore possible that nociceptive afferent input either does not reach the cortex in preterm human infants before 32 weeks, or that the cortical circuits cannot be activated before this time.

Our understanding of pain processing in the adult brain has greatly increased due to the use of advanced imaging techniques developed over the last 15 years (Apkarian et al. 2005). Studies of the hemodynamic correlates of pain have led to a better understanding of pain processing in adults at supraspinal levels, and the analysis of pain-evoked potentials has provided an electrophysiological representation of pain processing (Kakigi et al. 2005). However, the imaging techniques and experimental paradigms adopted for the study of adult pain processing are inappropriate for the study of infants in intensive care. It is particularly challenging to study pain processing in premature infants because ethically studies can only be undertaken when there is a clinical requirement for a painful procedure to be carried out. Furthermore, for research purposes the noxious stimulus must be a clearly defined clinical procedure that is not affected by other aspects of the infant's care. It is therefore not possible to use repetitive painful stimuli at predetermined intervals to assess the development of pain processing throughout early development. Measuring a clearly defined response to noxious stimulation will pave the way for the development of a systematic approach to reduce pain and improve analgesic strategies in this vulnerable population.

This chapter describes a study where we addressed the question of cortical pain processing in very young infants by directly measuring cortical responses to noxious stimulation using near-infrared spectroscopy (NIRS) (Slater et al. 2006) and electroencephalography (EEG). NIRS measures regional changes in oxygenated and deoxygenated hemoglobin concentration, whereas EEG assesses cortical electrical activity. We hypothesized that we could use these techniques to determine whether the immature cortex is functionally activated in response to noxious stimulation. However, it is necessary that the evoked responses are clearly defined, are detectable without the use of extensive averaging techniques, and are specific to a noxious stimulus. Contamination by movement artifacts needs to be addressed, and it is essential to control for the influence of generalized sensory or attention-related responses. Because the exact relationship between the hemodynamic response and underlying electrical activity is both unclear and conceivably different from that in adults, it is advantageous to measure responses simultaneously using both recording modalities.

NIRS is ideal for the study of neonates because it is portable and non-invasive; the benefit of this technique over other optical imaging methods is that studies can be done at the cotside, while the infant remains in intensive care. This technique is widely used in neonatal research and has successfully been applied to detect cortical responses in the newborn brain, such as those evoked by visual, auditory, and olfactory stimuli (Meek et al. 1998; Sakatani et al. 1999; Bartocci et al. 2000). Somatosensory evoked potentials (SEPs) have also been measured in infants, mostly in investigations of the integrity of somatosensory pathways and of prognostic indicators of neurological impairment (Pihko and Lauronen 2004). Most often the stimulus used to activate the median or tibial nerve has been electrical (Taylor et al. 1996; Pike et al. 1997), but other methods, such as tactile stimulation of the fingers, have also been used (Pihko et al. 2004). It has been shown that cortical SEPs can be reliably measured from at least 27 weeks postmenstrual age (PMA) (Taylor et al. 1996) where PMA is defined as the age of the infant measured from the first day of the mothers last menstrual period. However, until now neither NIRS nor SEPs have been used to investigate the onset or development of the cortical response to noxious stimuli. By combining these techniques we were able to assess whether the nociceptive pathways transmit information to the cortex and whether the youngest premature infants are able to display a cortical response to noxious stimulation. Measuring cortical activity produced by noxious stimulation in the preterm infant's brain provides a direct measure of pain processing in the immature cortex.

METHODS

Studies were undertaken on inpatients in the neonatal intensive care unit and the special care baby unit at University College London Hospital, United Kingdom. Approval was obtained to perform the studies from the institutional ethics committee. Parents provided informed written consent for each infant who took part in the study. Infants aged between 25 and 45 weeks PMA were studied during routine heel lancing when blood samples were clinically required.

NEONATAL ASSESSMENT

Medical charts were reviewed for pertinent medical history, and infants included in the study had normal appearances on cranial ultrasound scans. At the time of the study, all infants were assessed as clinically stable. Infant handling was kept to a minimum, so the infants were studied in a variety of positions and sleep states.

HEEL LANCE PROTOCOL

The heel lance was performed when heart rate, oxygen saturation, and hemodynamic cerebral activity were stable. The foot was not squeezed for a period of 30 seconds following the heel lance to ensure that the evoked response occurred only as a result of the initial stimulus.

ASSESSMENT OF SLEEP STATE

Sleep state was assessed according to the Premature Infant Pain Profile using the behavioral state indicator, which categorizes an infant into one of four states: active/awake, quiet/awake, active/asleep, or quiet/asleep (Stevens et al. 1996). Infants in the first two categories were classified as awake and those in the second two categories were classified as asleep.

SOMATOSENSORY EVOKED POTENTIALS

Skin impedances were reduced using EEG prepping gel, and surface electrodes were positioned on the scalp according to the international 10–20 EEG placement system and held in place with conductive EEG paste. Adhesive tape was placed over the electrodes to prevent displacement. EEG activity was recorded on a computer using a high bandwidth data acquisition unit and an isolated pre-amplifier. Activity was continuously recorded for 10 minutes prior to the heel lance, to ensure the stability of the traces.

NEAR-INFRARED SPECTROSCOPY

A double-channel near-infrared spectrophotometer was used to measure regional changes in hemoglobin concentration. The light emitters and detectors (optodes) were positioned symmetrically on either side of the head over the somatosensory cortex, using the international 10–20 EEG placement system to identify key landmarks. Optodes were placed on the head at least 15 minutes prior to recording, and changes in cerebral hemodynamic activity were recorded. The baseline was determined 20 seconds before the stimulus, and the cortical response was measured for 20 seconds post-stimulus. Changes in oxyhemoglobin (HbO_2) and deoxyhemoglobin (HHb) were measured. Total hemoglobin (HbT) concentration change was calculated as $\Delta HbT = \Delta HbO_2 + \Delta HHb$. The maximum change in HbT was defined as the maximum difference from the mean prestimulus recording in the 20-second period post-heel lance. To assess whether the stimulus response was significantly different from the prestimulus baseline within an individual subject, the maximum post-stimulus value was compared with the prestimulus sample mean (two-sample t-test).

Infants were monitored for heart rate and oxygen saturation using a transcutaneous monitor. The infant's behavior and facial expressions were recorded on video throughout the study. Precise triggering was used to ensure that the evoked response in each recording modality was time-locked to the noxious stimulus.

RESULTS

In this study we have shown that there is an increase in total hemoglobin concentration in the contralateral somatosensory cortex following a heel lance in infants aged 25–45 weeks PMA. Fig. 1 presents a sample trace showing an increase in HbT in the contralateral somatosensory cortex of 13.2 µmol/L and a decrease in HbT of 5.12 µmol/L on the side ipsilateral to the stimulus.

The importance of this finding lies in the fact that changes in hemoglobin concentration can be used to identify functionally activated regions of the brain.

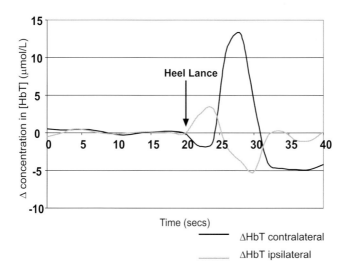

Fig. 1. Sample trace in a single infant (29 + 4 weeks postmenstrual age [PMA]) demonstrating the evoked change in total hemoglobin (HbT) in the contralateral and ipsilateral somatosensory cortex following a painful stimulus given at $t = 20$ seconds.

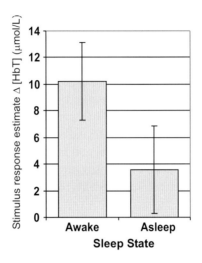

Fig. 2. Comparison between the stimulus response estimate (change in total hemoglobin in the contralateral somatosensory cortex) following heel lance in the awake and asleep state at mean PMA, 35.2 weeks. Error bars represent the 95% confidence interval limits; the mean difference between the two estimates achieves statistical significance. See Slater et al. (2006) for details.

This premise is based on our understanding that increased tissue oxygenation represents an increase in blood flow, which is in turn associated with an increase in underlying neural activity (Logothetis et al. 2001).

Although the stimulus responses in the youngest infants were of low amplitude, even the very youngest infant in the study (25 + 5 weeks PMA) demonstrated a clear and significant response above the prestimulus baseline ($P < 0.005$, two-sample t-test). The data shows that the magnitude of the hemodynamic response is lower in younger infants (Slater et al. 2006) and is dependent upon sleep state (Fig. 2).

Using EEG to measure the electrically evoked activity allows us to establish if reproducible waveforms can be observed, if they correlate with the hemodynamic activity, and if there is an observable change in the amplitude, latency, or onset of the potentials with increasing age. Our preliminary results suggest that it is technically feasible to record time-locked EEG activity following heel lance, indicating that it is possible to identify SEPs that occur as a specific consequence of activation of nociceptive receptors.

DISCUSSION

The results presented in this chapter show that noxious stimulation can evoke specific hemodynamic changes that reflect increased neural activity in the somatosensory cortex of both preterm and term infants. Cortical responses to noxious stimulation tend to be lower in younger infants, perhaps reflecting lower energy requirements due to reduced neuronal activity arising from the immaturity of the thalamocortical input (Rosanova and Timofeev 2005). The results also suggest that the hemodynamic response is attenuated during sleep.

The experimental set-up used in this study enables a number of different recording modalities to be used to investigate the response to noxious stimulation in preterm infants. Simultaneously measuring the time-locked hemodynamic, electrical, physiological, and behavioral activity that occurs during acutely painful procedures provides an excellent experimental paradigm to further our understanding of evoked responses during early development. This integrative approach provides an excellent opportunity to assess the effect of noxious stimuli on the immature nervous system.

ACKNOWLEDGMENTS

This study was funded by the Wellcome Trust and the UCLH Special Trustees. R. Slater is on the Wellcome Trust-funded London Pain Consortium 4-year PhD program.

REFERENCES

Andrews K, Fitzgerald M. The cutaneous withdrawal reflex in human neonates: sensitization, receptive fields, and the effects of contralateral stimulation. *Pain* 1994; 56:95–101.

Andrews K, Fitzgerald M. Cutaneous flexion reflex in human neonates: a quantitative study of threshold and stimulus-response characteristics after single and repeated stimuli. *Dev Med Child Neurol* 1999; 41:696–703.

Andrews K, Fitzgerald M. Wound sensitivity as a measure of analgesic effects following surgery in human neonates and infants. *Pain* 2002; 99:185–195.

Apkarian AV, Bushnell MC, Treede RD, Zubieta JK. Human brain mechanisms of pain perception and regulation in health and disease. *Eur J Pain* 2005; 9:463–484.

Bartocci M, Winberg J, Ruggiero C, et al. Activation of olfactory cortex in newborn infants after odor stimulation: a functional near-infrared spectroscopy study. *Pediatr Res* 2000; 48:18–23.

Craig KD, Whitfield MF, Grunau RV, Linton J, Hadjistavropoulos HD. Pain in the preterm neonate: behavioural and physiological indices. *Pain* 1993; 52:287–299.

Fitzgerald M. The development of nociceptive circuits. *Nat Rev Neurosci* 2005; 6:507–520.

Franck LS, Greenberg CS, Stevens B. Pain assessment in infants and children. *Pediatr Clin North Am* 2000; 47:487–512.

Grunau RE, Oberlander T, Whitfield MF, et al. Pain reactivity in former extremely low birth weight infants at corrected age 8 months compared with term born controls. *Infant Behavior Dev* 2001; 24:41–55.

Kakigi R, Inui K, Tamura Y. Electrophysiological studies on human pain perception. *Clin Neurophysiol* 2005; 116:743–763.

Logothetis NK, Pauls J, Augath M, Trinath T, Oeltermann A. Neurophysiological investigation of the basis of the fMRI signal. *Nature* 2001; 412:150–157.

McNair C, Ballantyne M, Dionne K, Stephens D, Stevens B. Postoperative pain assessment in the neonatal intensive care unit. *Arch Dis Child Fetal Neonatal Ed* 2004; 89:F537–F541.

Meek JH, Firbank M, Elwell CE, et al. Regional hemodynamic responses to visual stimulation in awake infants. *Pediatr Res* 1998; 43:840–843.

Oberlander TF, Grunau RE, Fitzgerald C, Whitfield MF. Does parenchymal brain injury affect biobehavioral pain responses in very low birth weight infants at 32 weeks' postconceptional age? *Pediatrics* 2002; 110:570–576.

Peters JW, Schouw R, Anand KJ, et al. Does neonatal surgery lead to increased pain sensitivity in later childhood? *Pain* 2005; 114:444–454.

Pihko E, Lauronen L. Somatosensory processing in healthy newborns. *Exp Neurol* 2004; 190(Suppl 1):S2–S7.

Pihko E, Lauronen L, Wikstrom H, et al. Somatosensory evoked potentials and magnetic fields elicited by tactile stimulation of the hand during active and quiet sleep in newborns. *Clin Neurophysiol* 2004; 115:448–455.

Pike AA, Marlow N, Dawson C. Posterior tibial somatosensory evoked potentials in very preterm infants. *Early Hum Dev* 1997; 47:71–84.

Rosanova M, Timofeev I. Neuronal mechanisms mediating the variability of somatosensory evoked potentials during sleep oscillations in cats. *J Physiol* 2005; 562:569–582.

Sakatani K, Chen S, Lichty W, Zuo H, Wang YP. Cerebral blood oxygenation changes induced by auditory stimulation in newborn infants measured by near infrared spectroscopy. *Early Hum Dev* 1999; 55:229–236.

Slater R, Cantarella A, Gallella S, et al. Cortical pain responses in human infants. *J Neurosci* 2006; 26:3662–3666.

Stevens B, Johnston C, Petryshen P, Taddio A. Premature Infant Pain Profile: development and initial validation. *Clin J Pain* 1996; 12:13–22.

Taylor MJ, Boor R, Ekert PG. Preterm maturation of the somatosensory evoked potential. *Electroencephalogr Clin Neurophysiol* 1996; 100:448–452.

Treede RD, Kenshalo DR, Gracely RH, Jones AK. The cortical representation of pain. *Pain* 1999; 79:105–111.

Correspondence to: Rebeccah Slater, MSc, The London Pain Consortium, Department of Anatomy and Developmental Biology, University College London, Gower Street, London, WC1E 6BT, United Kingdom. Fax: 020-7383-0929; email: r.slater@ucl.ac.uk.

Part V

Opioids: Mechanisms and Therapy

Proceedings of the 11th World Congress on Pain, edited by Herta Flor, Eija Kalso, and Jonathan O. Dostrovsky, IASP Press, Seattle, © 2006.

39

A Motivation-Decision Model of Pain: The Role of Opioids

Howard L. Fields

Departments of Neurology and Physiology, University of California San Francisco, San Francisco, California, USA

THE PSYCHOPHYSICAL APPROACH TO PAIN

Pain is a sensation, like touch, vision, and olfaction, and it is defined by its subjective properties. Although activation of primary afferent nociceptors initiates a variety of responses (orientation, arousal, autonomic changes, and withdrawal), it is the relation of the noxious stimulus to the psychophysical properties of the subjective experience that has attracted the attention of most researchers. In fact, the official IASP definition of pain is based on psychophysics: it states that pain is "an unpleasant sensory and emotional experience associated with actual or potential tissue damage, or described in terms of such damage" (International Association for the Study of Pain 2005).

Over the past century, the major goal of basic pain research has been to explain how the nervous system generates this psychophysical phenomenon. This approach has been enormously successful. Psychophysical correlates have been used to identify primary afferent nociceptors and some of the transducing molecules that are tuned to specific aspects of tissue-damaging processes (Julius and Basbaum 2001). Psychophysics has also been an important guide and catalyst for research into the central afferent pathways and cortical mechanisms underlying pain perception. Thus, studies that correlate single neuron firing or magnetic resonance imaging of cortical blood oxygen utilization with psychophysical measures such as pain intensity and unpleasantness have revolutionized our thinking about how the central nervous system processes nociceptive inputs (e.g., Craig 2003; Lorenz and Casey 2005). The psychophysics of pain and pain modulation continues to guide our thinking about pain mechanisms and our ability to treat pain patients.

Despite this progress and the promise of future discoveries, the psycho-physical approach does have significant limitations. First, most of the neural activity elicited by noxious stimulation is not accessible to conscious experience. Second, many of the physiological responses (e.g., withdrawal reflexes and autonomic changes) can be dissociated from perceived pain intensity. Finally, it is not yet possible to precisely define a neural substrate that is both necessary and sufficient for the subjective experience of pain. We are ethically limited in what we can directly measure in humans, and animals cannot tell us what they feel. Despite these limitations, a deeper mechanistic understanding of how nociceptive inputs influence behavior can be achieved using behavioral approaches that do not require psychophysical methods or constructs.

PAIN AS MOTIVATION: A BEHAVIORAL APPROACH

Purely behavioral methods provide an alternative that is complementary to the psychophysical approach. Independent of psychophysics, afferent nociceptive pathways can be understood by the behavioral responses they mediate. In most cases, noxious stimuli elicit autonomic, hormonal, and tissue-protective responses (withdrawal, escape, and recuperative behaviors). When the behavioral responses to a noxious stimulus are flexible and goal directed, we can think of the stimulus as inducing a motivational state, i.e., a drive to escape, terminate, and avoid the causative tissue-damaging process (e.g., Fanselow 1986; Craig 2003). While the response to noxious stimulation has a certain unique immediacy, aversive motivational states can be elicited by many different types of stimuli. Avoidance behaviors assist the animal to maintain safety and homeostasis against a variety of perturbations. For example, rats instinctively avoid light and open environments (danger from predators), just as they would avoid environments that have extremes of heat or cold. Aversive motivational states are of value not only because they drive immediate behaviors, but also because they serve as teaching signals so that individuals learn to avoid situations and actions associated with harm to the organism (Johansen and Fields 2004).

MULTIPLE MOTIVATIONS, CONFLICT AND DECISION

One of the great strengths of the motivational approach is that it can encompass a broad understanding of the factors that lead to variability in pain responses. Attention, expectancy, and strong emotional states such as fear and anger can have powerful effects on pain perception; however, one must look for explanations beyond the psychophysical data (i.e., the relation of the subjective experience to the properties of the stimulus). Here is where the behavioral approach shows its value and can inform our biological understanding of psychophysics. For example, the variability in the relation between the strength of a noxious stimulus and the intensity of the resulting pain experience can be understood as the manifestation of a decision process. In an individual, nociceptor activation characteristically occurs in the setting of other motivations (e.g., threat, hunger, and sexual attraction). Since individuals have a limited range of behaviors that can be simultaneously engaged, they are often faced with the choice between responding to the motivation elicited by the noxious stimulus (by withdrawal, escape, or recuperation) or to the motivation that drives a conflicting behavior such as feeding, attack, or mating.

THE ALTERNATIVE TO PAIN: ENDOGENOUS OPIOIDS AND PAIN-MODULATING CIRCUITS

Responding to one of those conflicting motivations typically requires inhibiting the responses to noxious stimulation. Under some circumstances (e.g., fear or anticipated reward), the inhibition of nociceptor-elicited responses is mediated by the well-described descending modulatory control circuit (e.g., Fields 2004). This descending circuit involves neurons in the frontal neocortex, hypothalamus, amygdala, and brainstem that control the nociceptive afferent pathway in the spinal and trigeminal dorsal horn. Under conditions of threat, where overt responses to noxious stimulation could mean death, inhibition of withdrawal reflexes has been shown to involve the release of endogenous opioids acting at μ-opioid receptors on neurons in the descending modulatory circuit, which comprises the amygdala, periaqueductal gray (PAG), and rostral ventromedial medulla (RVM) (Bellgowan and Helmstetter 1998; Foo and Helmstetter 1999).

Examining the role of opioid-mediated pain-modulating circuits in resolving motivational conflict illuminates the variability of pain in a unique and informative way and can lead to a simpler and more general understanding of the various factors (other than stimulus intensity) that alter responses to noxious stimuli (only one of which is the subjective experience of pain). This point was first articulated by Fanselow (1986) in regard to the opioid-mediated analgesic effect of stimuli that elicit innate (e.g., predator-driven) fear and conditioned (learned) fear. He showed that in these situations, threat-related sensory cues block pain responses via opioid release. In other words, pain responses (reflecting a nociceptor-activated motivational state to avoid tissue damage) have been blocked in order to protect against a greater threat (immediate death). I propose that this concept of motivational conflict can be extended in two critical ways:

first, descending control can facilitate as well as inhibit nociceptive transmission systems, and second, opioid inhibition of withdrawal reflexes can be activated by anticipation of reward as well as threat of harm.

BIDIRECTIONAL MODULATORY CONTROL AND THE DECISION PROCESS

A critical assumption for this proposal is that if a noxious stimulus occurs in the presence of a competing motivational state such as hunger, a decision must be made. The decision is whether or not to respond to the noxious stimulus. Either alternative leads to engagement of descending modulatory systems that control afferent nociceptive pathways at the level of the dorsal horn (Fields 2004; Fields et al. 2006). A critical property of this modulatory circuit is that it exerts bidirectional control. If the decision is to respond to the noxious stimulus, descending facilitation is activated, which speeds escape and withdrawal responses. Conversely, inhibition of escape and withdrawal ensues when the decision is to respond to a competing drive (e.g., hunger or threat) rather than to the noxious stimulus. Under a variety of circumstances, this inhibition of acute nociceptor-elicited responses is mediated by endogenous opioids acting on the same circuitry that is activated by opioid analgesics such as morphine.

Studies have indicated that brainstem neurons in the modulatory circuit contribute to a bidirectional decision process. When a noxious stimulus is applied to the tail or paw of a lightly anesthetized rat, two robust patterns of neural activity are observed in midbrain and medullary pain-modulatory nuclei (i.e., the PAG and RVM). In one class of neuron, the OFF cell, spontaneous neuronal activity is abruptly silenced about 0.2–0.4 seconds prior to the withdrawal reflex. Local application of μ-opioid agonists activates OFF cells, prevents their pause, and is sufficient to inhibit the tail-flick or paw-withdrawal reflex. Clearly, OFF cells exert a generalized inhibitory effect on withdrawal reflexes. A second class of neuron, the ON cell, is activated by acute or tonic noxious stimulation and *inhibited* by μ-opioid agonists. With acute noxious stimuli, ON cells also show a burst of activity beginning about 0.2 seconds prior to the onset of the withdrawal reflex. ON-cell activity is sufficient to facilitate withdrawal reflexes (Neubert et al. 2004). Thus, OFF-cell silence *permits* withdrawal reflexes and ON-cell activity facilitates them. Conversely, OFF-cell activity blocks responses to noxious stimuli. As would be expected of an all-or-none (go/no go) decision circuit, the ON and OFF cell populations have reciprocal activity patterns; under a variety of circumstances, when ON cells are active (a pain-facilitating state), OFF cells are silent, and vice versa.

These patterns of ON- and OFF-cell activity, beginning significantly before the onset of escape behavior, are also consistent with a role for these neurons in the "decision" to respond or not to a noxious input. Pharmacological studies of conditioned fear in rats also provide indirect evidence implicating these neurons in a decision task. In the conditioned fear paradigm, rats are placed in a context in which they previously received inescapable shock. This manipulation leads to a transient suppression of withdrawal reflexes that is reversed by μ-opioid antagonists microinjected into the PAG or RVM (Bellgowan and Helmstetter 1998; Foo and Helmstetter 1999). Since OFF cells are the only neurons in these nuclei that are activated by μ-opioid agonists, it is likely that they mediate the observed inhibition of withdrawal reflexes.

Under circumstances of acute tissue injury, for example in an automobile accident, a fight, or a sports injury, the decision process is initiated at short latency after the stimulus and is typically completed prior to any conscious experience of pain. This immediacy is possible despite the fact that short-latency sensory information about the nature of the stimulus must reach the decision center so that an accurate cost/benefit comparison can be made among possible competing motivations and actions (e.g., Should I try to move or remain immobile? Should I run or continue to fight?). The early sensory and contextual information and the decision process that it initiates do not produce a conscious experience of pain (or of deciding). If the competing motivation wins out, responses to noxious stimulation, including the conscious experience of pain, are blocked. One way this occurs is via release of endogenous opioids, with consequent activation of OFF cells leading to inhibition of nociceptive transmission neurons at the level of the dorsal horn. If the competing motivations are less powerful, the noxious input "wins." In this case inhibition is shut down (OFF cells are silent), while facilitating modulation is activated via activation of ON cells. This facilitation speeds and strengthens responses (including withdrawal) to noxious stimulation. It is only after the process of deciding and the activation of modulatory output that the psychophysical consequences of the decision process are manifest. If the decision is to respond, the experience of pain ensues.

It is worth pointing out that because the modulatory system acts at the first central synapse of the pain transmission system, ON- and OFF-cell activity will influence decision making (Fig. 1). With OFF cell activity, the nociceptor-driven motivational state will be weakened, thus biasing the individual to engage in competing behaviors. Conversely, ON-cell activity will enhance the aversive motivational state produced by any level of noxious stimulation and will therefore weaken the influence of conflicting motivations on the decision process. Thus, activation of the brainstem-to-dorsal horn component of the descending modulatory system does more than enact the outcome of the decision

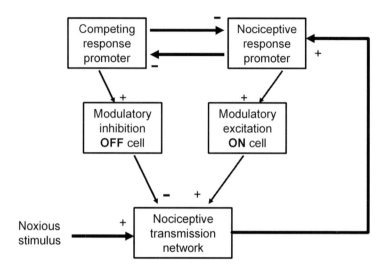

Fig. 1. A motivation-decision model for pain. Pain-modulatory systems exert bidirectional control over the nociceptive transmission network. OFF cells inhibit and ON cells facilitate nociceptive transmission. Nociceptive inputs produce a motivational state that enhances responses to noxious stimulation through activation of a "nociceptive response promoter" circuit. This circuit activates ON cells, which facilitate nociceptive transmission and secondarily enhance the nociceptive response promoter. Activity in this circuit has an inhibitory effect on motivation for responses that conflict with the response to noxious stimulation. The competing motivations activate the "competing response promoter" circuit, which inhibits the nociceptive response promoter and activates OFF cells. OFF cells suppress pain transmission, which leads to reduced activation of the nociceptive response promoter circuit.

process; its activity (involving ON or OFF cells) has a positive feedback effect that enhances and serves to maintain whichever decision is made.

REWARD AND ANALGESIA: THE MESOLIMBIC PATHWAYS AND DECISION

If this proposal is correct, the decision process is critical for the survival of the individual, and elucidating its neurobiology becomes essential. One issue of great clinical importance is that the most effective analgesic drugs, the opioids, have significant addiction potential. A body of evidence indicates that opioids, as well as other addicting substances, play an important role in biasing the decision between escape from pain and approach to reward. In fact, animal and human studies document that, in addition to morphine, most rewarding (addictive) drugs produce analgesia (see Franklin 1998 for review).

For example, inhibition of nociceptor-elicited behaviors can be produced by psychostimulants such as cocaine (Franklin 1998), alcohol (James et al. 1978), and nicotine (Iwamoto 1991; Decker et al. 2004; Girdler et al. 2005). In addition to addictive drugs, natural rewards, notably highly palatable foods such as chocolate, milk, or sucrose, can produce a naloxone-reversible analgesic effect (Dum and Herz 1984; Blass and Fitzgerald 1988). Clearly, a general theme is emerging; the consumption or anticipation of a reward can inhibit responses to pain. The motivation-decision approach makes it clear why this happens: if reward consumption and escape from pain are two incompatible behaviors, anything that facilitates one will inhibit the other.

For the neurobiologist interested in pain, the challenge of this hypothesis is to determine where in the brain the possible alternative behaviors are compared and to then elucidate the neural mechanism of the decision process. The decision process requires information about the homeostatic state of the individual (e.g., hunger, thirst, and inflammation), noxious input, and contextual cues about threats and the availability of rewards. One brain system that has such access is the dopaminergic mesolimbic pathway, which has been implicated in reward and appetitive motivation. Midbrain dopamine neurons in the ventral tegmental area (VTA) that project to the nucleus accumbens (NAc) in the ventral striatum constitute the core of this "reward" circuit (see Wise 1998; Kelley 2004).

Several lines of evidence suggest that this mesolimbic dopamine circuit can engage pain-modulating circuits. For example, the NAc projects to the hypothalamus and amygdala, both of which could relay input to the PAG and RVM (see Altier and Stewart 1999 for review). Pharmacological studies also support a role for the mesolimbic dopamine pathway in pain modulation. Morphine, psychostimulants, nicotine, and alcohol, which all have analgesic effects, can produce reward through increasing dopamine release in the NAc (Altier and Stewart 1999; DiChiara et al. 2004). Consistent with this, animals can be trained to press a lever to deliver either morphine or alcohol via an implanted cannula directly into their VTA and psychostimulants into their NAc. These manipulations have in common that they raise dopamine levels in the NAc. Furthermore, both morphine given in the VTA and psychostimulants in the NAc have robust antinociceptive actions that are abolished by dopamine blockade (Franklin 1998; Altier and Stewart 1999). These findings led to the proposal that firing of VTA dopaminergic neurons produces an analgesic effect (Altier and Stewart 1999). Although this idea may be premature, there does appear to be a close link between activity in the mesolimbic dopamine pathway and inhibition of behavioral responses to noxious stimulation.

OPIOIDS AND DOPAMINE IN THE NUCLEUS ACCUMBENS: REWARD AND ANALGESIA

Recent studies of NAc opioid regulation of feeding may shed further light on the neurobiology of the decision process. Opioids microinjected into the NAc elicit robust feeding and inhibit nociceptor-elicited behaviors (Manning et al. 1994; Schmidt et al. 2002; Kelley 2004). Both of these actions require the VTA and are blocked by dopamine antagonists injected into the NAc (Gear et al. 1999; Ragnauth et al. 2000). Although the feeding and antinociceptive effect may result from opioid actions on independently functioning subpopulations of NAc neurons, a more intriguing possibility is that a single population of dopamine-modulated NAc neurons both enhances feeding and inhibits nociceptive responses (Yun et al. 2004b).

Some hints about how this process might happen can be gleaned from studies of the VTA-to-NAc circuit in awake, behaving animals. Reward-predictive cues activate putative dopamine neurons in the VTA and elicit release of dopamine in the NAc (Fiorillo et al. 2003; Roitman et al. 2004). We have found that in rats trained to respond to a cue that predicts reward (sucrose), inactivation of the VTA or dopamine antagonists in the NAc block the behavioral response to the cue. Using the same paradigm, we discovered a population of NAc neurons that respond to these same reward-predictive cues (Nicola et al. 2004). Both the neuronal and the behavioral responses to the cue are eliminated when the VTA is inactivated, suggesting that a dopamine action on NAc neurons mediates the behavioral response (Yun et al. 2004a). Subsequent studies revealed a population of NAc neurons that encode the palatability of an ingested food according to its sucrose concentration (Taha and Fields 2005). Higher concentrations of sucrose were associated with greater firing of these neurons as well as longer feeding bouts. Since intra-NAc opioids enhance palatability and produce analgesia, an intriguing possibility is that the firing of these palatability-encoding neurons is enhanced by opioids and has an antinociceptive action. Further experiments are required to test this hypothesis. However, if this idea is confirmed, it would explain why expectancy or consumption of reward is tightly coupled to inhibition of responses to pain; activity in the same neurons produces both effects concurrently.

IS THERE EVIDENCE THAT A DECISION PROCESS PRECEDES THE EXPERIENCE OF PAIN?

If this decision hypothesis is correct, the brain regions involved must have access to information relating to current motivations, imminent rewards (benefits), and punishments (costs). Since the salient cost under consideration here is potential tissue damage, the decision circuitry must have access to early information about noxious stimulation. In fact, the rodent NAc receives direct input from putative nociceptive neurons in the spinal cord dorsal horn (Cliffer et al. 1991). I suggest that this projection provides input used in the decision process but does not directly lead to conscious perception of pain.

It is obviously quite difficult to confirm the proposal that a complex decision process precedes the conscious experience of pain. It is particularly difficult to do so in human subjects, who provide the only portal to subjective experience. On the other hand, the idea of an early, possibly preconscious, decision process receives some support from human functional imaging studies. Becerra and colleagues (2001) have made an important contribution in this area using functional magnetic resonance imaging (fMRI) in humans during repeated application of noxious stimulation. They divided the period following noxious thermal stimulation into an early and late phase. While the temporal resolution of the fMRI signal is relatively poor, they reported very robust early activations in the midbrain tegmentum and ventral striatum (areas which include the VTA and NAc, respectively). Importantly, there was concurrent activation in the region of the midbrain PAG. In the late phase, these activations were not seen; rather, the pattern was of consistent activation in "classical" afferent pain circuitry, including the thalamus and the anterior cingulate, insular, and somatosensory cortices. While these findings need to be replicated, they indicate that these so-called "reward" areas are activated by noxious stimuli and by reward-predictive stimuli. Perhaps they should be more accurately described as "decision circuitry."

SUMMARY AND CONCLUSIONS

In this chapter I have presented a motivation/decision model of pain. This approach broadens our understanding of a large body of psychophysical data including the powerful effect of expectancy on pain perception. I believe this model provides a global explanation for the biological function of pain-modulatory pathways, in particular their role in resolving motivational conflict. This approach also informs our understanding of pharmacological studies, implicating both dopamine and opioids in analgesia and reward.

ACKNOWLEDGMENTS

The author thanks Sharif Taha, Greg Hjelmstad and Saleem Nicola for useful discussions of this paper. Research was supported by the USPHS DA01949, NS21445, the Wheeler Center for the Neurobiology of Addiction at the University of California San Francisco, and the Alcohol and Addiction Research Program of the State of California.

REFERENCES

Altier N, Stewart J. The role of dopamine in the nucleus accumbens in analgesia. *Life Sci* 1999; 65:2269–2287.

Becerra L, Breiter HC, Wise R, Gonzalez RG, Borsook D. Reward circuitry activation by noxious thermal stimuli. *Neuron* 2001; 32:927–946.

Bellgowan PS, Helmstetter FJ. The role of mu and kappa opioid receptors within the periaqueductal gray in the expression of conditional hypoalgesia. *Brain Res* 1998; 791:83–89.

Blass EM, Fitzgerald E. Milk-induced analgesia and comforting in 10-day-old rats: opioid mediation. *Pharmacol Biochem Behav* 1988; 29:9–13.

Cliffer KD, Burstein R, Giesler GJ Jr. Distributions of spinothalamic, spinohypothalamic, and spinotelencephalic fibers revealed by anterograde transport of PHA-L in rats. *J Neurosci* 1991; 11:852–868.

Craig AD. A new view of pain as a homeostatic emotion. *Trends Neurosci* 2003; 26:303–307.

Decker MW, Rueter LE, Bitner RS. Nicotinic acetylcholine receptor agonists: a potential new class of analgesics. *Curr Top Med Chem* 2004;4:369–384.

DiChiara G, Bassareo V, Fenu S, et al. Dopamine and drug addiction: the nucleus accumbens shell connection. *Neuropharmacology* 2004; 47(Suppl 1):227–241.

Dum J, Herz A. Endorphinergic modulation of neural reward systems indicated by behavioral changes. *Pharmacol Biochem Behav* 1984; 21:259–266

Fanselow MS. Conditioned fear-induced opiate analgesia: a competing motivational state theory of stress analgesia. *Ann N Y Acad Sci* 1986; 467:40–54.

Fields H. State-dependent opioid control of pain. *Nat Rev Neurosci* 2004; 5:565–575.

Fields HL, Basbaum AI, Heinricher MM. Central nervous system mechanisms of pain modulation. In: McMahon SB, Koltzenburg M (Eds,) *Wall & Melzack's Textbook of Pain*, 5th ed. Edinburgh: Churchill Livingstone, 2006, pp 125–142.

Fiorillo CD, Tobler PN, Schultz W. Discrete coding of reward probability and uncertainty by dopamine neurons. *Science* 2003; 299:1898–1902.

Foo H, Helmstetter FJ. Hypoalgesia elicited by a conditioned stimulus is blocked by a mu, but not a delta or a kappa, opioid antagonist injected into the rostral ventromedial medulla. *Pain* 1999; 83:427–431.

Franklin KB. Analgesia and abuse potential: an accidental association or a common substrate? *Pharmacol Biochem Behav* 1998; 59:993–1002.

Gear RW, Aley KO, Levine JD. Pain-induced analgesia mediated by mesolimbic reward circuits. *J Neurosci* 1999; 19:7175–7181.

Girdler S, Maixner W, Naftel H, et al. Cigarette smoking, stress-induced analgesia and pain perception in men and women. *Pain* 2005; 114:372–385.

International Association for the Study of Pain. *IASP Pain Terminology.* Available at: www.iasp-pain.org/terms. Accessed December 13, 2005.

Iwamoto ET. Characterization of the antinociception induced by nicotine in the pedunculo-pontine tegmental nucleus and the nucleus raphe magnus. *J Pharmacol Exp Ther* 1991; 257:120–133.

James MFM, Duthrie AM, Duffy BL, McKeag AM, Rice CP. Analgesic effect of ethyl alcohol. *Br J Anaesth* 1978; 50:139–141.

Johansen JP, Fields HL. Glutamatergic activation of anterior cingulate cortex produces an aversive teaching signal. *Nat Neurosci* 2004; 7:398–403.

Julius D, Basbaum AI. Molecular mechanisms of nociception. *Nature* 2001; 413:203–210.

Kelley AE. Memory and addiction: shared neural circuitry and molecular mechanisms. *Neuron* 2004; 44:161–179.

Lorenz J, Casey KL. Imaging of acute versus pathological pain in humans. *Eur J Pain* 2005; 9:163–165.

Manning BH, Morgan MJ, Franklin KB. Morphine analgesia in the formalin test: evidence for forebrain and midbrain sites of action. *Neuroscience* 1994; 63:289–294.

Neubert MJ, Kincaid W, Heinricher MM. Nociceptive facilitating neurons in the rostral ventromedial medulla. *Pain* 2004; 110:158–165.

Nicola SM, Yun I, Wakabayashi KT, Fields HL. Cue-evoked firing of nucleus accumbens neurons encodes motivational significance during a discriminative stimulus task. *J Neurophysiol* 2004; 91:1840–1865.

Ragnauth A, Znamensky V, Moroz M, Bodnar RJ. Analysis of dopamine receptor antagonism upon feeding elicited by mu and delta opioid agonists in the shell region of the nucleus accumbens. *Brain Res* 2000; 877(1):65–72.

Roitman MF, Stuber GD, Phillips PE, Wightman RM, Carelli RM. Dopamine operates as a subsecond modulator of food seeking. *J Neurosci* 2004; 24:1265–1271.

Schmidt BL, Tambeli CH, Levine JD, Gear RW. mu/delta cooperativity and opposing kappa-opioid effects in nucleus accumbens-mediated antinociception in the rat. *Eur J Neurosci* 2002; 15:861–868.

Taha S, Fields HL. Encoding of palatability and appetitive behaviors by distinct neuronal populations in the nucleus accumbens. *J Neuroscience* 2005; 25:1193–202.

Wise RA. Drug-activation of brain reward pathways. *Drug Alcohol Depend* 1998; 51(1–2):13–22.

Yun IA, Wakabayashi KT, Fields HL, Nicola SM. The ventral tegmental area is required for the behavioral and nucleus accumbens neuronal firing responses to incentive cues. *J Neurosci* 2004a; 24:2923–2933.

Yun I, Nicola S, Fields HL. Contrasting effects of dopamine and glutamate receptor antagonist injection in the nucleus accumbens suggest a neural mechanism underlying cue-evoked goal-directed behavior. *Eur J Neurosci* 2004b; 20:249–263.

Correspondence to: Howard L. Fields, MD, PhD, 5858 Horton Avenue, Suite 200, Emeryville, CA 94608, USA. E-mail: hlf@phy.ucsf.edu.

Proceedings of the 11th World Congress on Pain,
edited by Herta Flor, Eija Kalso, and Jonathan O.
Dostrovsky, IASP Press, Seattle, © 2006.

40

Genetic Variation in the Catechol-*O*-Methyl-Transferase Gene Is Associated with Response to Morphine in Cancer Patients

Joy R. Ross,[a,b] Julia Riley,[a] and K.I. Welsh[b]

[a]Department of Palliative Medicine, Royal Marsden Hospital, London, United Kingdom; [b]Department of Clinical Genomics, Imperial College, London, United Kingdom

For patients with cancer, pain is the symptom that is most feared. Ongoing or progressive pain is physically debilitating and has a marked impact on quality of life. Effective treatment of cancer-related pain remains a high priority and an ongoing challenge in clinical practice. Individuals with moderate to severe cancer-related pain require treatment with opioids. Morphine is the opioid of choice for the treatment of moderate to severe cancer pain (World Health Organization 1996), but 10–30% of patients treated with oral morphine do not have successful outcomes because of intolerable adverse effects, inadequate analgesia, or a combination of both (Cherny et al. 2001). For patients who do not receive the desired analgesic effect, or for those who suffer intolerable adverse effects from morphine, significant clinical benefit can be achieved by switching to alternative strong opioids (Riley et al. 2006). Little of the variability in response to opioids can be explained by clinical, hematological, or biochemical variables (Riley et al. 2004). Our group is investigating the impact of genetic variation in candidate genes, which we hypothesise may influence clinical response to morphine in cancer patients (Ross et al. 2005a,b).

The catechol-*O*-methyl-transferase (COMT) gene has been proposed as a candidate gene to explain inter-individual variation in pain. Zubieta et al. (2003) demonstrated a correlation between COMT genotype and μ-opioid receptor neurotransmitter responses to a pain stressor in normal volunteers. COMT is one of the enzymes that metabolizes catecholamines. It is an important modulator of the neurotransmitters dopamine, norepinephrine, and epinephrine. The dopaminergic, adrenergic, and opioid-signaling pathways in the central nervous system interact with one another. The COMT gene is polymorphic, and the most widely studied variant in this gene results in an amino acid substitution (valine/methionine) in the transcribed protein. This variant causes a three- to four-fold decrease in enzyme activity (Lotta et al. 1995).

The COMT gene is located on chromosome 22q11.21 and has six exons. The gene has two promoter regions that control transcription of two separate mRNAs (Tenhunen et al. 1994). These mRNAs are transcribed into a membrane-bound COMT protein (MB-COMT) and a shorter soluble COMT protein (S-COMT). The MB-COMT protein is predominately expressed in neurons in the central nervous system and in peripheral lymphocytes; it has a higher substrate affinity but lower catalytic activity than S-COMT, which is predominately expressed in other tissues including the liver, blood, and kidneys (Tenhunen et al. 1994; Lotta et al. 1995; Chen et al. 2004).

This chapter describes a study we performed to determine whether single-nucleotide polymorphisms (SNPs) in the COMT gene, either singly or in combination, would influence the analgesic response to morphine in cancer patients.

METHODS

We prospectively recruited 186 cancer patients who were receiving morphine treatment for pain. Good clinical benefit, defined by satisfactory analgesia and minimal adverse effects, was achieved by 133 patients, who served as controls in our study, but 53 patients needed to switch to an alternative opioid and were designated "switchers." The full methodology for the clinical study has been described elsewhere (Riley et al. 2006). DNA was extracted and stored for genetic analysis (Salazar et al. 1998). Putative SNPs in the COMT gene were identified from the literature and from SNP databases http://www.ncbi.nlm.nih.gov, http://snpper.chip.org/bio). Assays were developed to determine individual genotypes using sequence-specific primers in a polymerase chain reaction (SSP-PCR) (Bunce 1995; Ross et al. 2005b). Individual SNP associations were examined by comparison of genotype and allele frequencies and allele carriage between switchers and controls. Different SNPs (within a gene or between different genes) may work in combination having additive or opposing influences on outcome. As such, interactions between SNPs were considered and haplotypes of SNPs within genes constructed because they might have functional implications for the resultant protein. Linkage disequilibrium was calculated, and presumed haplotypes were constructed. Identification of rare intra-gene haplotypes can also identify genotype errors, and so samples identified as having rare intra-gene haplotypes were re-genotyped (Ahmad et al. 2003). The database of clinical, laboratory, and genetic data was analyzed using data-mining software and standard statistical software.

RESULTS

Primer sequences were designed and titrated for 15 putative SNPs in the COMT gene (Fig. 1); 13 SNPs, spanning a 29-kilobase region, were polymorphic in this population. The 133 controls were compared with the 53 switchers. Switchers had an increase in the G allele frequency for the SNP –7370 C/G ($\chi^2 = 6.78$, $P = 0.009$), whereas four neighboring SNPs showed weaker associations (–21958 A/G, $P = 0.03$; –7053 A/G, $P = 0.01$; –5051 A/G, $P = 0.03$; –4873 A/G, $P = 0.02$). No significant difference was seen between switchers and controls for the functional SNP 1222 A/G (*Val158Met*). Switchers, compared with controls, were less likely to carry the common ancestral haplotype, which was carried on 21/106 chromosomes in switchers and on 89/266 chromosomes in controls ($\chi^2 = 6.78$, $P = 0.009$; Table I). No association was seen between morphine dose and genotype.

DISCUSSION

Genetic variation in the COMT gene was associated with response to morphine in this cohort. However, the known functional SNP (*Val158Met*) was not associated with response to morphine, but rather intron 1 was found to be the region of interest. This region is proximal to the promoter for the soluble form of COMT and may therefore be important in regulating gene expression via alteration of transcription factor-binding sites. In the center of this region, there is a four-base-pair tandem repeat that cannot be typed using SSP-PCR. Another group has analyzed this region with microsatellite analysis (DeMille et al. 2002). Attempts by our group to conduct a similar analysis have been unsuccessful to date because we have been unable to fully correlate microsatellite and direct sequencing data from patients who are heterozygous for different alleles (J.R. Ross, unpublished data, 2005).

One other pain study has analyzed the influence of the COMT *Val158Met* polymorphism on the efficacy of morphine in a cohort of patients suffering from cancer-related pain (Rakvag et al. 2005). The authors compared morphine doses and serum concentrations of morphine and morphine metabolites between the genotype groups and found a weak association between morphine dose and genotype ($P = 0.025$). This finding was not confirmed in our cohort.

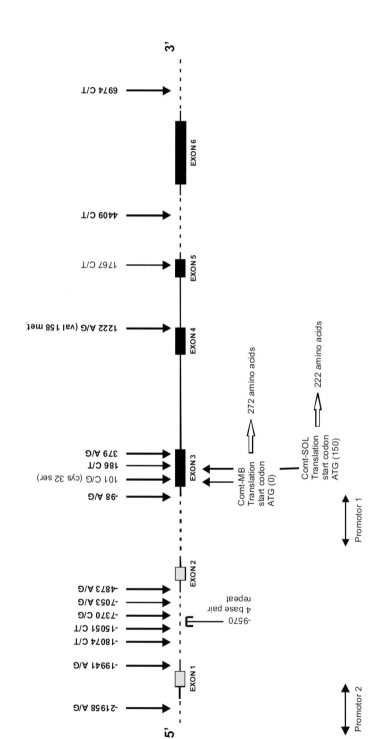

Fig. 1. Schematic diagram of the catechol-*O*-methyl-transferase (COMT) gene. Fifteen single-nucleotide polymorphisms (SNPs) were examined; 13 were polymorphic in this cohort and are shown in boldface type.

Table I
The common ancestral haplotype, constructed from 13 SNPs, spanning a 29 kb
region from the promoter to 3' untranslated region (3'UTR)

Allele at Individual SNP Position (5' to 3')												
SNP 1	SNP 2	SNP 3	SNP 4	SNP 5	SNP 6	SNP 7	SNP 8	SNP 9	SNP 10	SNP 11	SNP 12	SNP 13
-21958 promoter	-1994 intron 1	-18074 intron 1	-15051 intron 1	-7370 intron 1	-7053 intron 1	-4873 intron 1	-98 intron 2	186 exon 3	379 exon 3	1222 exon 4	4409 intron 5	6974 3 UTR
G	A	C	C	C	G	G	A	T	A	A	T	T

The COMT locus is best known for its link to schizophrenia and various mood-related disorders. However, studies correlating the *Val158Met* polymorphism to a variety of clinical diseases have produced conflicting results (reviewed by Palmatier et al. 1999). While differences in study design and population may explain some of these findings, most studies have focused solely on this one SNP, ignoring the potential interaction of other SNPs across the gene. Data from more recent studies indicate that SNPs in the promoter, intron 1, and the 3'UTR region may be more strongly linked to schizophrenia (Shifman et al. 2002; Palmatier et al. 2004) and have highlighted the need to consider haplotype analysis of multiple SNPs across the gene (Handoko et al. 2005).

However, we lack clear data explaining a functional impact of other SNPs. Chen et al. (2004) compared genotype with both mRNA expression, protein levels, and enzyme activity in both post-mortem brain samples and lymphocytes and found that the 158met variant correlated with a decrease in protein level and enzyme activity but did not alter mRNA expression. A small effect of the promoter polymorphism on mRNA expression in lymphocytes was noted, but this effect did not translate into altered protein expression or enzyme activity. No effects were seen from intron 1 or 3'UTR polymorphisms.

A recent study by Diatchenko et al. (2005), looking at six SNPs across the human gene, correlated combinations of SNPs (haplotypes) with high, average, and low pain sensitivity to both experimental pain and the risk of developing temporomandibular joint disorder. However, the SNPs defining the haplotypes covered intron 2 to exon 4 and did not include intron 1 or the promoter regions.

CONCLUSION

This chapter has described a study showing that genetic variation in the COMT gene is associated with clinical response to morphine in cancer patients.

Further work is needed to genotype the four-base-pair tandem repeat in intron 1 and to establish the functional significance of these variants. We hypothesize that the region of interest will relate to production of a splice variant of the soluble COMT protein.

REFERENCES

Ahmad T, Neville M, Marshall SE, et al. Haplotype-specific linkage disequilibrium patterns define the genetic topography of the human MHC. *Hum Mol Genet* 2003; 12:647–656.

Bunce M, O'Neil CM, Barnardo M, et al. Phototyping comprehensive DNA typing for HLA-A, B, C, DRB1, DRB3, DRB4, DRB5, & DQB1 by PCR with 144 primer mixes utilizing sequence-specific primers (PCR-SSP). *Tissue Antigens* 1995; 46:355–367.

Chen J, Lipska BK, Halim N, et al. Functional analysis of genetic variation in catechol-O-methyltransferase (COMT): effects on mRNA, protein, and enzyme activity in postmortem human brain. *Am J Hum Genet* 2004; 75:807–821.

Cherny N, Ripamonti C, Pereira J, et al. Expert Working Group of the European Association of Palliative Care Network. Strategies to manage the adverse effects of oral morphine: an evidence-based report. *J Clin Oncol* 2001; 19:2542–2554.

DeMille MM, Kidd JR, Ruggeri V, et al. Population variation in linkage disequilibrium across the COMT gene considering promoter region and coding region variation. *Hum Genet* 2002; 111:521–537.

Diatchenko L, Slade GD, Nackley AG, et al. Genetic basis for individual variations in pain perception and the development of a chronic pain condition. *Hum Mol Genet* 2005; 14:135–143.

Handoko HY, Nyholt DR, Hayward NK, et al. Separate and interacting effects within the catechol-*O*-methyltransferase (COMT) are associated with schizophrenia. *Mol Psychiatry* 2005; 10:589–597.

Lotta T, Vidgren J, Tilgmann C, et al. Kinetics of human soluble and membrane-bound catechol O-methyltransferase: a revised mechanism and description of the thermolabile variant of the enzyme. *Biochemistry* 1995; 34:4202–4210.

Palmatier MA, Kang AM, Kidd KK. Global variation in the frequencies of functionally different catechol-O-methyltransferase alleles. *Biol Psychiatry* 1999; 46:557–567.

Palmatier MA, Pakstis AJ, Speed W, et al. COMT haplotypes suggest P2 promoter region relevance for schizophrenia. *Mol Psychiatry* 2004; 9:859–870.

Rakvag TT, Klepstad P, Baar C, et al. The *Val158Met* polymorphism of the human catechol-O-methyltransferase (COMT) gene may influence morphine requirements in cancer pain patients. *Pain* 2005; 116:73–78.

Riley J, Ross JR, Rutter D, et al. A retrospective study of the association between haematological and biochemical parameters and morphine intolerance in patients with cancer pain. *Palliat Med* 2004; 18:19–24.

Riley J, Ross JR, Rutter D, et al. No pain relief from morphine? Individual variation in sensitivity to morphine and the need to switch to an alternative opioid. *Support Care Cancer* 2006;14:56–64.

Ross JR, Riley J, Rutter D, et al. Pharmacogenomics of opioids: predicting response to morphine in cancer patients. In: Capasso A (Ed). *Recent Developments in Pain Research*. Kerala: Research Signpost, 2005a.

Ross JR, Rutter D, Welsh K, et al. Clinical response to morphine in cancer patients and genetic variation in candidate genes. *Pharmacogenomics J* 2005b; 5:324–336.

Salazar LA, Hirata MH, Cavalli SA, Machado MO, Hirata RD. Optimized procedure for DNA isolation from fresh and cryopreserved clotted human blood useful in clinical molecular testing. *Clin Chem* 1998; 44:1748–1750.

Shifman S, Bronstein M, Sternfeld M, et al. A highly significant association between a COMT haplotype and schizophrenia. *Am J Hum Genet* 2002; 71:1296–1302.

Tenhunen J, Salminen M, Lundstrom K, et al. Genomic organization of the human catechol *O*-methyltransferase gene and its expression from two distinct promoters. *Eur J Biochem* 1994; 223:1049–1059.

World Health Organization. *Cancer Pain Relief.* Geneva: World Health Organization, 1996.

Zubieta JK, Heitzeg MM, Smith YR, et al. COMT *val158met* genotype affects mu-opioid neurotransmitter responses to a pain stressor. *Science* 2003; 299:1240–1243.

Correspondence to: Joy R. Ross, MBBS, MRCP, Department of Palliative Medicine, Royal Marsden Hospital, London SW3 6JJ, United Kingdom. Email: joy.ross@rmh.nhs.uk.

Proceedings of the 11th World Congress on Pain,
edited by Herta Flor, Eija Kalso, and Jonathan O.
Dostrovsky, IASP Press, Seattle, © 2006.

41

Managing Acute Pain in the Opioid-Dependent Patient

Roman D. Jovey

*Addiction and Concurrent Disorders Centre, Credit Valley Hospital,
and CPM Health Centres, Inc., Mississauga, Ontario, Canada*

Opioids are increasingly being utilized for the treatment of opioid addiction and for the management of patients with chronic cancer and noncancer pain. Patients on long-term opioid therapy for any reason can develop acute pain superimposed on their chronic pain secondary to acute medical illness, trauma, or surgery. Both groups of patients may have developed some degree of opioid tolerance, creating a challenge for adequate pain management. Tolerance can be especially problematic in the patient receiving methadone or buprenorphine maintenance treatment for addiction (known as opioid agonist therapy). Each patient needs to be evaluated and treated individually, but the clinician can follow certain principles in order to optimize the outcome and reduce the risks.

DEFINITIONS OF ADDICTION IN A PATIENT IN PAIN ON OPIOIDS

It is important to know whether pain or addiction is the primary problem, and so it is important for the clinician to understand the definition of addiction in a patient on therapeutic opioids. In 2001, a joint committee of the American Academy of Pain Medicine, The American Pain Society, and the American Society of Addiction Medicine (Liaison Committee on Pain and Addiction) agreed on key definitions related to addiction in the patient with pain on therapeutic opioids. Addiction is defined as: "a primary Chronic neurobiologic disease with genetic, psychosocial, and environmental factors influencing its development and manifestations. It is characterized by behaviors that include one or more of the following: impaired Control of drug use, Compulsive use, Continued use despite harm and Craving" (Savage et al. 2003). These criteria have also been called the "5 Cs" of addiction.

Physical dependence is defined as: "a state of adaptation that is manifested by a drug class specific withdrawal syndrome that can be produced by abrupt cessation, rapid dose reduction, decreasing blood level of the drug, and/or administration of an antagonist" (Savage et al. 2003). Although physical dependence to opioids may be part of an addictive illness, it is not synonymous with addiction. Most patients with cancer pain on long-term opioids are physically dependent but would not usually be considered addicted. Physical dependence is a neuropharmacological phenomenon, while addiction is both a neuropharmacological and behavioral phenomenon.

Tolerance is defined as "a state of adaptation in which exposure to a drug induces changes that result in a diminution of one or more of the drug effects over time" (Savage et al. 2003). The fact that the analgesic effect of a given opioid at a given dose may decrease over time in a given patient does not always equate to tolerance. The key to defining true tolerance in patients on opioids is that all other conditions remain constant. The term "pseudotolerance" refers to a need to increase opioid dosage to treat pain due to other factors, such as underlying disease progression, the onset of a new painful condition, increased physical activity in response to better pain control, lack of compliance with proper dosing, a change in medication, a drug interaction, manifestation of an addictive disorder, or criminal drug diversion. It is fortunate that humans develop tolerance to most of the adverse effects of opioids, because otherwise we would not be able to use them clinically. Clinically significant pharmacodynamic tolerance in a patient with pain whose opioid dosage has been appropriately titrated to effect is generally thought to be uncommon, although we lack data from large prospective studies.

Pseudoaddiction is defined as a misinterpretation of patient behaviors that occurs when a patient with unrelieved chronic pain seeks additional medication, either appropriately or inappropriately. Such a patient may undertake behaviors that would normally be associated with substance abuse or addiction, such as buying opioids from illicit drug dealers. When a pseudoaddicted patient's pain is appropriately managed, this inappropriate behavior ceases.

It can be difficult for the pain clinician to differentiate pseudoaddiction from true addiction. The diagnosis of addiction is made prospectively when a patient repeatedly manifests aberrant drug-related behaviors in spite of rational pharmacotherapy for his or her pain. The diagnosis of pseudoaddiction is usually made retrospectively (D. Gourlay, personal communication, 2005). The patient's behaviors and compliance with the treatment agreement typically normalize with rational pharmacotherapy for the pain (D. Gourlay, personal communication, 2005).

THE ILLNESS OF ADDICTION

Addiction disorders are very common in the general population. It is estimated that approximately 10% of people at any given time will manifest such an illness. Addiction to clinical opioids in the context of pain treatment has been reported to be rare in those patients without a previous history of addictive disorders; however, data are not available to establish the true incidence.

All mammals are born with a reward pathway located in the mesolimbic area of the brain. This common reward pathway mainly involves the ventral tegmental area, the nucleus accumbens, and the prefrontal cortex. The primary neurotransmitter in this circuit is dopamine, with endogenous opioids also playing a modulating role. Certain behaviors associated with survival, such as eating and sex, as well as all of the drugs commonly associated with abuse and addiction, will activate various parts of this reward pathway. In a biogenetically susceptible individual, repeated exposure to a potentially addictive substance can result in changes in brain circuitry that begin with *liking* the substance (the pleasure circuit in the nucleus accumbens), leading to *wanting* the substance (the desire and urge circuit in the basolateral nucleus of the amygdala) and finally to *needing* the substance (the desire and demand circuit in the periaqueductal gray matter of the brainstem) (Robinson and Berridge 2001; Gardner 2004). Opioids can contribute to the development of addiction in a susceptible individual. A psychoactive drug that rapidly achieves a peak blood level, crosses the blood-brain barrier quickly, avidly attaches to receptors in the reward pathways of the brain, and leaves the body quickly is more likely to have addicting properties than a drug that slowly achieves a peak blood level and stays in the body for a long period of time. Heroin is a good example of the former and methadone an example of the latter.

OPTIMIZING OPIOIDS IN CHRONIC PAIN MANAGEMENT

Optimizing the use of opioids in chronic pain management involves titrating the opioid dosage, in a given patient, to produce a steady-state blood level just above the level that reduces pain without severe, persistent adverse effects, thus allowing the patient to achieve functional improvement. Maintaining such steady blood levels reduces the possibility of euphoria and inter-dose withdrawal symptoms. It is much easier pharmacologically to achieve such a steady-state blood level with use of controlled-release or long-acting opioid analgesics.

UNIVERSAL PRECAUTIONS IN PAIN MEDICINE

Observing universal precautions in pain medicine requires utilizing the same assessment process, prescribing protocol, and limit setting in each patient who is treated with long-term opioid therapy (Gourlay et al. 2005). Using this uniform approach in all patients with chronic pain, regardless of the clinician's initial estimate of risk, can reduce stigma, improve patient care, and reduce the overall risks of pain management with opioids, both to the clinician and to society. The key universal precautions are listed in Table I.

Several standardized screening questionnaires for addiction have been validated in clinical populations. The best known example is the four-item CAGE Questionnaire, which asks about Cutting down drinking, being Annoyed by criticism of drinking, Guilt over drinking, and taking an Eye-opener or using alcohol first thing in the morning to compensate for withdrawal or hangover symptoms (Ewing 1984). A score of two out of four positive responses on the CAGE questionnaire results in a sensitivity of 77% to 94% in the diagnosis of alcohol addiction, with a specificity of 79% to 97%. A derivative of the CAGE, called the CAGE-AID, includes the same questions for drugs as well as alcohol (Brown and Rounds 1995). Other screening tools have been reviewed elsewhere (Jovey 1999; Savage 2002).

Routinely providing an addiction assessment in all patients with chronic pain allows the clinician to stratify the management of each patient according to risk level. Group I patients have no previous history of addiction, no active addiction disorder, and no family history of addiction. These patients can be managed by nonspecialist physicians with little concern for the risk of opioid misuse. Group II patients may have a remote past history of appropriately treated addictive disorder. They may have had a past history or a recent history

Table I
Universal precautions in pain medicine

Form a diagnosis with an appropriate differential diagnosis
Provide a psychological assessment, including screening for addictive disorders
Provide informed consent (oral or written and signed)
Document a treatment agreement (oral or written/signed)
Document a pre-trial assessment of pain and function
Provide an appropriate trial of opioid therapy with or without adjuvants
Regularly reassess pain scores and level of function
Assess and document the "Four A's" (analgesia, activity, adverse effects, and ambiguous drug-related behaviors) at follow-up visits
Periodically review the pain diagnosis and comorbid conditions, including the development of addictive disorders
Document clearly

Source: Gourlay (2005).

of a significant psychiatric disorder or may have a strongly positive family history for addiction. These patients are ideally seen in consultation by an addiction specialist or psychiatrist, with closer monitoring of treatment. Group III patients either have an active addictive disorder or an active significant psychiatric disorder. These patients should ideally be co-managed by an addiction specialist or a psychiatrist, or both, and must be monitored very carefully (Gourlay et al. 2005).

There is no one behavior that will reliably differentiate a patient with pain who is using opioids appropriately from an addicted patient. Some characteristics are illustrated in Table II that can help the clinician make this distinction.

One key aspect of universal precautions is the use of urine drug testing—both for illicit substances and for the presence of prescribed medications. Such testing can play a key role in the safe management of a patient on long-term opioid therapy. It helps to confirm the agreed-upon treatment plan and monitor the absence of any illicit drugs, and can help to diagnose relapse or drug misuse as early as possible. Such testing also allows the clinician to advocate for the patient with third parties.

Initial urine drug testing is most commonly done with class-specific immunofluorescence drug panels, which are fast and inexpensive but typically do not identify individual drugs within a class. Greater sensitivity in this regard might be important for checking whether the opioid being prescribed is actually what is found in the urine. For example, patients taking oxycodone would not be expected to have morphine in their urine. A more sensitive assay uses high-performance liquid chromatography, which can typically differentiate individual drugs within a class. This assay can also detect synthetic or semisynthetic opioids, such as methadone, fentanyl, and oxycodone. Confirmation by gas chromatography and mass spectrometry is the most accurate test, but it is typically much more expensive.

Table II
Differences between a chronic pain patient and an addicted patient

Chronic Pain Patient	Addicted Patient
Controls medication use	Cannot control medication use
Quality of life is improved by medication	Quality of life is decreased by medication
Asks to decrease medication if adverse effects occur	Wants to continue or increase medications despite adverse effects
Expresses concerns about addiction potential	Is unaware of, or in denial about, potential addiction
Follows agreed-upon treatment plan	Repeatedly deviates from the agreed-upon treatment plan
Frequently has leftover medication	Often runs out of medication early and always has an excuse

Source: Schnoll and Finch (1994), Heit (2001).

To interpret the results of urine drug testing, clinicians must be aware of the metabolism of opioids and drugs of abuse. For example, heroin is metabolized quickly to 6-monoacetyl morphine and then to morphine. Therefore, if the clinician is planning to use controlled-release morphine to treat chronic pain in a patient with a past history of heroin abuse, the urine drug screen may not be helpful in differentiating therapeutic morphine use from ongoing heroin abuse. Choosing an alternative long-acting opioid, such as methadone, would allow the clinician to be better able to detect a recurrence of heroin abuse using urine drug testing. An excellent monograph is available from the California Academy of Family Physicians detailing the metabolism of clinical opioids as well as the approximate retention time of most drugs of abuse (Gourlay et al. 2003).

ACUTE PAIN IN THE OPIOID-DEPENDENT PATIENT

Opioid-dependent patients can present to the emergency department with acute pain on a background of chronic pain—with or without concurrent addiction. They may have previously been taking opioids on a regular basis, either opioid agonist therapy for addiction or long-term opioids for chronic cancer or noncancer pain. They may have developed some degree of tolerance and may be suffering from inter-dose, withdrawal-mediated pain. Such patients may be taking multiple other medications, such as benzodiazepines, that may further complicate their management.

Patients on opioid agonist therapy for addiction usually have a clearly established addiction history and are typically polysubstance abusers. They are usually taking either methadone or buprenorphine with supervised daily dosing. They can present in various stages of their illness, from healthy recovery to frequent relapses to abuse of various drugs.

Is the problem one of pain or addiction or both? If both problems are involved, which is the primary disorder? Are resources available to treat a combined problem? Is there an addiction physician available to help co-manage complex patients? Is the pain likely to be opioid responsive, and are non-opioid treatment modalities a possibility?

When treating an unfamiliar patient who is on opioid agonist therapy for addiction, caution is recommended in providing the first dose of opioid based on the patient's self-report. Patients who have recently been abusing drugs may exaggerate their reported regular dose. In the case of acute illness or a relapse to addiction, patients may not have been taking their regular dose of opioid in the past few days and may have lost some of their tolerance to opioids. Therefore, it is important to try to confirm the most recent daily dose with the treatment provider, if possible.

When consultation with the treatment provider is not possible, one can split the patient's reported once-daily methadone dosage into three or four smaller doses given every 6 hours and titrated to effect. In such circumstances, one could use 5–10-mg doses of methadone not more than once every 3 hours as needed for breakthrough pain. This regimen allows the clinician to continue to use urine drug screens to assist in the management of the patient. It is also easier to return to once-daily methadone dosing once the acute pain problem has settled. The disadvantage of this approach is that potentially unstable patients may have to be given take-home doses of their methadone. Timely communication with the methadone provider is required when planning patient discharge.

In a patient being treated for addiction with buprenorphine, one can also split the buprenorphine dosage into t.i.d. or q.i.d. doses. As an agent for the treatment of chronic pain, buprenorphine has many good qualities. It is at least 40 times more potent than morphine over a linear range. It has a long duration of action for opioid agonist therapy, but only lasts for 6–8 hours as an analgesic agent. Because of the partial agonist nature of buprenorphine, there is a dose ceiling effect at 6–8 mg per dose, above which no additional analgesia or respiratory depression will occur. This ceiling effect of buprenorphine may limit its usefulness in the treatment of severe pain, but it also makes it a safer drug in the case of overdose. One advantage of using buprenorphine for analgesia in this manner is that urine drug screens remain interpretable (i.e., use of any other opioids will be detectable on urinary testing). Also, the patient can go back on the regular buprenorphine dosing regimen once the acute pain has settled. The high affinity of buprenorphine for the μ-opioid receptor may make the use of other concurrent μ-opioid agonists less effective for pain. Titrated intravenous fentanyl may be a better choice for acute pain management in this case. Also, the addition of buprenorphine for treatment of acute pain in the patient who is already on another opioid chronically for pain or addiction is not recommended. The buprenorphine could displace the other opioid from the μ-opioid receptor, precipitating acute withdrawal.

Another option in the patient on opioid agonist therapy for addiction is to use a different opioid for pain while maintaining the regular opioid for addiction. This option can make the interpretation of urine drug screens more challenging. One could provide immediate-release, short-acting opioids titrated to effect, and taper them as the acute pain settles. An acceptable option in the postoperative setting is to use a patient-controlled analgesia pump with lockouts and frequent monitoring.

In the opioid-dependent patient with acute pain—whether on opioids for pain or addiction—it is important not to accumulate an "opioid debt." Patients on a stable daily dose of an opioid who present to the hospital with acute pain need to have their baseline dose of opioid, or a calculated equianalgesic dose of an alternative opioid, provided as usual. This dose is augmented with the initial use of immediate-release, short-acting opioids every 1–4 hours p.r.n. to treat the acute pain. A useful analogy is the patient with insulin-dependent diabetes who is admitted with some type of acute illness. Such patients typically require their baseline dose of long-acting insulin as well as regular doses of short-acting insulin determined according to capillary blood sugar levels.

With elective surgical procedures, it is important for the clinician in charge of pain management to communicate in advance with the surgeon or anesthesiologist. In patients with previous intravenous abuse of drugs, venous access may be difficult. In those with addictive disorders, there are other analgesic options for postoperative pain. If available, regional and/or multimodal anesthetic techniques should be utilized for surgery and in the immediate postoperative setting (Joshi 2005). For example, there is good evidence for the postoperative effectiveness of regular acetaminophen, 1 g given four times a day, and for the use of nonsteroidal anti-inflammatory drugs (NSAIDs) (Altman 2004). For more severe pain one could consider medication delivery via an indwelling epidural or intrathecal catheter. However, patients previously dependent on systemic opioids may manifest withdrawal symptoms if the sole source of postoperative opioid is via the epidural or intrathecal route. Small, titrated aliquots of intravenous opioid will usually solve this problem.

In the pain patient dependent on opioids, one can use opioid equianalgesic tables preoperatively to calculate an approximate intravenous infusion prior to surgery. Published equianalgesic tables are only guidelines, however. When calculating a starting dose of an alternative opioid, it is safer to switch to half of the calculated dose and then titrate to effect. Opioids can be given postoperatively via a patient-controlled analgesia pump until the acute pain stabilizes. Other alternatives are to utilize the suppository form of controlled-release morphine, where available, during the surgical period and then to switch back to an oral opioid once the patient is taking oral fluids again. Patients who are on transdermal opioids can remain on their usual dose of opioid with the addition of either intravenous or oral immediate-release, short-acting opioids to treat the acute postoperative pain.

Postoperatively, opioid-dependent patients may be more pain sensitive and will therefore require higher doses of opioids given more frequently than in non-opioid-dependent patients. When in doubt, repeated administration of smaller doses titrated every hour orally or every 15–20 minutes intravenously can be provided based on regular monitoring of reported pain, level of consciousness, and respiratory rate.

Prescription of opioids on discharge from hospital for the patient with addiction should be time-limited, with early follow-up and the avoidance of problematic polypharmacy, such as concomitant prescription of benzodiazepines. Addicted patients on opioids in stable recovery should be advised to increase their recovery-oriented activities and be screened more frequently with urine drug testing. Clinicians should reassure patients, however, that inadequate pain relief is a much higher risk trigger for relapse to addiction rather than the availability of too much analgesic.

Other strategies to decrease the risk of misuse include maintaining tight prescribing boundaries; using a formal, written treatment agreement; enlisting the support of a family member; and using only one prescriber and one pharmacy. One can limit the number of opioid doses that high-risk patients have in their possession by using part-fill prescriptions on a frequent basis, where this is allowed by law.

DENTAL AND OBSTETRIC PAIN

When possible, the pain clinician and dental specialist should communicate prior to any major dental procedures in patients dependent on opioids. Acetaminophen and NSAIDs or COX-2 inhibitors are effective for dental pain in patients at low risk for gastropathy or cardiovascular disease (Altman 2004; Barden (2004). The same baseline dosage of daily controlled-release or long-acting opioids should be maintained and immediate-release, short-acting pain medication provided every 4 hours after the procedure as for any other patient.

For obstetrical analgesia in the opioid-dependent patient, communication in advance with both the attending obstetrician and pediatrician is essential. Daily opioids for the mother should be maintained, and regional analgesia techniques are preferred at the time of delivery. In the case of methadone, changes in pharmacokinetics mean that the total daily dose requirements will decrease in the first 1–2 weeks after delivery. Breast feeding is not contraindicated in women on methadone maintenance treatment since the transfer of methadone into human milk is minimal (Philipp et al. 2003).

SUMMARY

Patients dependent on opioid therapy who present with an acute pain problem require assessment to determine the presence or absence of an addictive disorder. This problem does not change our ethical responsibility to treat acute pain in a humane fashion. An acute pain crisis is not the time to "punish" patients for their addiction illness by undertreating pain. It does, however, increase the clinician's responsibility to take some basic precautions and monitor patients closely.

When using opioids to treat acute pain on a background of chronic pain in a patient with a history of addiction, relapse to drug abuse can always be a possibility. However, poorly managed pain is probably a much greater risk for the addicted patient than the rational use of prescribed analgesics with careful monitoring.

ACKNOWLEDGMENTS

The author acknowledges the valuable information provided by Dr. Douglas Gourlay. MD, FRCPC, FASAM, Toronto, Canada, and Dr. Howard A. Heit, MD, FACP, FASAM, Washington, DC, USA. The author is a member of the speakers' bureau and has consulted for the following companies: Purdue Pharma, Janssen Ortho, Pfizer, and Bayer. No remuneration was received for the writing of this paper.

REFERENCES

Altman RD. A rationale for combining acetaminophen and NSAIDs for mild-to-moderate pain. *Clin Exp Rheumatol* 2004; 22(1):110–117.

American Academy of Pain Medicine, American Pain Society, and American Society of Addiction Medicine. *Definitions Related to the Use of Opioids for the Treatment of Pain.* Glenview, IL: American Academy of Pain Medicine, 2001.

Barden J, Edwards JE, McQuay HJ, Wiffen PJ, Moore RA. Relative efficacy of oral analgesics after third molar extraction. *Br Dent J* 2004; 197(7):407–411.

Brown RL, Rounds LA. Conjoint screening questionnaires for alcohol and other drug abuse: criterion validity in a primary care practice. *Wis Med J* 1995; 4(3):135–140.

Ewing JA. Detecting alcoholism: the CAGE questionnaire. *JAMA* 1984; 252:1905–1970.

Gardner E. *Review Course.* Toronto: American Society of Addiction Medicine, 2004.

Gourlay DL, Heit HA, Caplan YH. *Urine Drug Testing in Primary Care: Dispelling the Myths and Designing Strategies.* California Academy of Family Physicians, 2003.

Gourlay DL, Heit HA, Almahrezi A. Universal precautions in pain medicine: a rational approach to the treatment of chronic pain. *Pain Med* 2005; 6(2):107–112.

Heit HA. The truth about pain management: the difference between a pain patient and an addicted patient. *Eur J Pain* 2001; 5(Suppl A):27–29.

Joshi GP. Multimodal analgesia techniques and postoperative rehabilitation. *Anesthesiol Clin North America* 2005; 23(1):185–202.

Jovey RD. Screening for addiction risk in pain patients. In: Max M (Ed). *Pain 1999—An Updated Review: Refresher Course Syllabus.* Seattle: IASP Press, 1999, pp 107–110.

Philipp BL, Merewood A, O'Brien S. Methadone and breastfeeding: new horizons. *Pediatrics* 2003; 111: 1429–1430.

Robinson TE, Berridge KC. Mechanisms of action of addictive stimuli. Incentive-sensitization and addiction. *Addiction* 2001; 96: 103–114.

Savage SR. Assessment for addiction in pain-treatment settings. *Clin J Pain* 2002; 18:S28–S38.

Savage SR, Joranson DE, Covington EC, et al. Definitions related to the medical use of opioids: evolution towards universal agreement. *J Pain Symptom Manage* 2003; 26(1):655–667.

Schnoll SH, Finch J. Medical education for pain and addiction: making progress toward answering a need. *J Law Med Ethics* 1994; 22(3):252–256.

Correspondence to: Roman D. Jovey, MD, 1611 Sherwood Forest Circle, Mississauga, ON, Canada L5K 2G8. Fax: 905-855-7304; email: drjovey@sympatico.ca.

Proceedings of the 11th World Congress on Pain,
edited by Herta Flor, Eija Kalso, and Jonathan O.
Dostrovsky, IASP Press, Seattle, © 2006.

42

Androgen Deficiency in Pain Patients on Long-Term Methadone Therapy

Esam Hamed,[a] William Blau,[b]
and Jeanne Hernandez[b]

*[a]Department of Anesthesiology, Faculty of Medicine, Assiut University,
Assiut, Egypt; [b]Department of Anesthesiology, School of Medicine,
University of North Carolina, Chapel Hill, North Carolina, USA*

Chronic pain is a significant health problem with a profound negative impact on quality of life. It places a heavy economic burden on the health care system. In addition to the physiological response to tissue damage, chronic pain involves psychological, behavioral, and cultural factors, which may account for the lack of a straightforward relationship between the nociceptive component of injury and the extent of suffering observed in chronic pain patients (Raspe and Kohlmann 1994). Recent findings suggest that pain may lead to dysregulation of the hypothalamic-pituitary-end organ system and consequently to other hormonal alterations (Oliver and Taylor 2003). Another study has demonstrated sexual dysfunction and subnormal sex hormone levels in male chronic pain patients using sustained-release opioids (Daniell 2002).

Methadone, a synthetic opioid, has become an important item on the list of opioids used successfully for treatment of chronic pain. Methadone is used by about 45% of the chronic pain patient population at the University of North Carolina pain center (Hamed and Dogra 2004). This chapter describes a study designed to test our hypothesis that the complex sexual alterations experienced by male chronic noncancer pain patients are directly attributable to the effects of long-term methadone therapy prescribed for the management of their pain.

METHODS

After approval by the Institutional Review Board of the University of North Carolina at Chapel Hill, a comparative, cross-sectional, observational study was conducted on 60 male chronic pain patients, divided into two groups of 30 patients each. Both groups were similar with regard to age and diagnosis (Table I). The first group was a control group comprising patients who required continuous use of non-opioid analgesics, and the second group comprised patients on regular methadone therapy.

Inclusion criteria. Patients were included who were 18–55 years old and had suffered from chronic noncancer pain conditions for more than 6 months. Body mass index (BMI) was within the range of 20–30 kg/m². Patients assigned to the methadone group had been taking 15 mg or more of methadone per day for more than 3 months.

Exclusion criteria included a history of orchidectomy, a history or current use of sex hormone replacement therapy, a history of liver or kidney dysfunction, morbid obesity (BMI > 30 kg/m²) or underweight (BMI < 18 kg/m²), or drinking alcohol more than twice a week.

SUBJECTIVE ASSESSMENT

We used an existing 10-point screening tool known as the Androgen Deficiency in Aging Males (ADAM) questionnaire, which was developed and validated

Table I
Patient demographics

	Control Patients	Methadone Patients
Number of patients	30	30
Mean age in years (SD)	40 (8.31)	43 (6.1)
Mean average pain score (SD)	5.3 (1.9)	5.4 (1.88)
Mean maximum pain score (SD)	7.7 (1.9)	7.79 (1.89)
Mean minimum pain score (SD)	2.7 (2)	2.86
Mean body mass index (SD)	27 (3)	26.97 (3.26)
Mean methadone dose (SD), mg/day	0.0	55.5 (27.5)
Mean (SD) period of methadone therapy, in years	0.0	3 (0.7)
Diagnosis	Chronic low back pain (n = 21)	Chronic low back pain (n = 26)
	Shoulder pain (n = 4)	Chronic pancreatitis (n = 1)
	Ankylosing spondylitis (n = 2)	Complex regional pain syndrome (n = 1)
	Ilioinguinal neuralgia (n = 1)	Osteoarthritis in knee (n = 1)
	Osteoarthritis in knee (n = 1)	Shoulder pain (n = 1)
	Multiple sclerosis (n = 1)	

to identify various parameters thought to be related to androgen deficiency in middle-aged and older males. A positive questionnaire result is defined as the affirmative (yes) answer to question 1 (decreased libido) or 7 (decreased erection) or a combination of any three other questions. The ADAM questionnaire has been estimated to have 88% sensitivity and 60% specificity to screen for deficiency of testosterone in male patients (Morley et al. 2000). In another study the sensitivity recorded was 97% (Morley et al. 2006).

We assessed the maximum, minimum, and average pain score experienced by the patients during the week of the study. Pain score was based on an 11-point verbal numeric rating scale.

OBJECTIVE ASSESSMENT

We completed a sex hormone panel including total testosterone, free testosterone, dihydrotestosterone, follicle-stimulating hormone, luteinizing hormone, estradiol, and prolactin. Tests were completed using enzyme-linked immunosorbent assay at the central laboratory of the General Clinical Research Center of University of North Carolina at Chapel Hill.

RESULTS

All 60 patients successfully completed the study. The ADAM questionnaire (Table II) showed highly significant positive questionnaire results in 96.7% of methadone users compared to 66.7% of controls ($P < 0.0001$). Decreased libido was found in 90% of methadone users as contrasted to 30% of controls, a highly

Table II
Percentage of affirmative answers on the ADAM Questionnaire in both groups

Questions		Control Group		Methadone Group		
		Yes	No	Yes	No	P
1	Decreased libido	30	70	90	10	0.000**
2	Lack of energy	33.3	66.7	80	20	0.000**
3	Decreased strength	50	50	83.3	16.7	0.006**
4	Lost height	13.3	86.7	23.3	76.7	0.325
5	Decreased enjoyment	46.7	53.3	76.7	23.3	0.016*
6	Sadness	30	70	66.75	33.25	0.004**
7	Decreased erection strength	30	70	76.7	23.3	0.000**
8	Decreased ability to play	60	40	86.7	13.3	0.019*
9	Falling asleep after dinner	30	70	46.7	53.3	0.190
10	Decreased work performance	43.3	56.7	80	20	0.003**
Overall questionnaire result		66.7	33.3	96.7	3.3	0.000**

significant difference ($P < 0.0001$). Decreased erection strength was experienced in 76.7% of methadone users versus 30% of controls ($P < 0.0001$).

A significantly higher percentage of patients in methadone users experienced lack of energy ($P < 0.0001$), decreased strength ($P = 0.006$), decreased enjoyment ($P = 0.016$), sadness ($P = 0.004$), decreased ability to play ($P = 0.019$), and decreased work performance ($P = 0.003$) in comparison to controls.

Regarding pain parameters, no significant difference was encountered between groups in terms of maximum, minimum, or average pain scores. Regarding the sex hormone panel (Table III), statistically significant lower mean serum levels of total testosterone were measured in methadone users (mean $\pm$ SD = 2.26 $\pm$ 1.65 ng/mL) compared to controls (4.95 $\pm$ 3.47 ng/mL) ($P = 0.002$). Statistically significant lower mean serum levels of dihydrotestosterone were estimated in methadone users (274.98 $\pm$ 153.39 pg/mL) contrasted to controls (467.35 $\pm$ 323.32 pg/mL) ($P = 0.009$).

The comparisons were calculated using General Linear Model statistical software, with adjustment for age and BMI. In methadone users, there was no significant correlation between the results of the ADAM questionnaire and sex hormone serum levels versus the daily dose of methadone.

DISCUSSION AND CONCLUSIONS

The assessment of sexual dysfunction in opioid users has been studied thoroughly in the context of an addiction management protocol using methadone maintenance therapy (Hagman 1995). This study evaluated the sexual

Table III
Comparison of sex hormone levels in both groups

Hormones	Control Group		Methadone Group		
	Mean	SD	Mean	SD	P
Total testosterone (ng/mL)	4.95	3.47	2.26	1.65	0.002**
Free testosterone (pg/mL)	24.22	68.91	4.96	5.01	0.240
Dihydrotestosterone (pg/mL)	467.35	323.32	274.98	153.39	0.009**
Follicle-stimulating hormone (mIU/mL)	10.42	6.75	11.33	15.90	0.816
Luteinizing hormone (mIU/mL)	20.98	22.73	23.14	29.92	0.665
Estradiol (pg/mL)	32.40	32.79	22.02	15.70	0.218
Prolactin (ng/mL)	4.80	2.70	5.72	3.91	0.188

effects of chronic methadone use versus non-opioid use among similar groups of patients with a variety of pain syndromes requiring chronic use of analgesics. In the design of this study we reduced the effect of selection bias by enrolling patients with the same criteria in terms of pain parameters, BMI, and general demographics in both groups. Chronic methadone therapy was the only prominent difference in pain regimen between both groups.

In the pain management literature, sexual dysfunction has been studied in protocols measuring sex hormone serum levels and evaluating sexual performance in chronic pain patients consuming a variety of opioids compared with a group of community-dwelling men without chronic pain. The results of this comparison confirmed significant hypogonadism and poor sexual performance in opioid users (Daniell 2002).

The number of patients in each group was relatively small, and the selection of patients was not randomized. A larger, randomized sample of patients would have strengthened our results. However, these results appear to be in support of our hypothesis regarding the role of methadone in altering sexual performance compared to patients who are not consuming opioids.

Our results are in agreement with the literature reports demonstrating severe hypogonadism in patients treated with opioids intrathecally for control of their chronic pain (Paice et al. 1994; Abs et al. 2000; Roberts et al. 2002). These results warrant further studies to explore the potential causative relationship between methadone and sexual variables and to determine whether these effects are derived solely or primarily from alterations in sex hormones. Prospective studies are planned with extensive psychological evaluation to explore the nature of changes that occur as patients are started on methadone therapy.

This study provides subjective and objective evidence on the sexual dysfunction that may be experienced in chronic pain patients on long-term methadone therapy. The ADAM questionnaire defines a symptom complex associated with the decline in testosterone that may be amenable to therapeutic intervention (Morley et al. 2000). Our findings suggest the necessity for systemic endocrine work-up in older male patients taking long-term opioids to assess the need for substitutive hormonal therapy.

ACKNOWLEDGMENTS

This study was supported in part by a grant (RR00046) from the General Clinical Research Center, program of the Division of Research Resources, National Institutes of Health. Thanks are due to Cherie Price and Sebastian Perretta, our research team members at the University of North Carolina at Chapel Hill, for their outstanding technical help in this study.

REFERENCES

Abs R, Verhelst J, Maeyaert J, et al. Endocrine consequences of long-term intrathecal administration of opioids. *J Clin Endocrinol Metab* 2000; 85:2215–2222.

Daniell HW. Hypogonadism in men consuming sustained-action oral opioids. *J Pain* 2002; 3:377–384.

Hagman G. A psychoanalyst in methadonia. *J Subst Abuse Treat* 1995; 12:167–179.

Hamed EM, Dogra S. "One-year assessment of opioid use and dose adjustments in patients with chronic non-cancer pain." *J Pain* 2004; 5:69.

Morley JE, Charlton E, Patrick P, et al. Validation of a screening questionnaire for androgen deficiency in aging males. *Metabolism* 2000; 49:1239–1242.

Morley JE, Perry HM III, Kevorkian RT, Patrick P. Comparison of screening questionnaires for the diagnosis of hypogonadism. *Maturitas* 2006; 53:424–429.

Oliver RL, Taylor A. Chronic pain and male sexual dysfunction. *Practical Pain Manage* 2003; Sep/Oct. Available at: www.ppmjournal.com.

Paice JA, Penn RD, Ryan WG. Altered sexual function and decreased testosterone in patients receiving intraspinal opioids. *J Pain Symptom Manage* 1994; 9:126–131.

Raspe H, Kohlmann T. Disorders characterized by pain: a methodological review of population surveys. *J Epidemiol Community Health* 1994; 48:531–537.

Roberts LJ, Finch PM, Pullan PT, Bhagat CI, Price LM. Sex hormone suppression by intrathecal opioids: a prospective study. *Clin J Pain* 2002; 18:144–148.

Correspondence to: Esam Hamed MD, MSCA, Department of Anesthesiology, Faculty of Medicine, Assiut University, Assiut 71516, Egypt. Email: ehamed@gmail.com.

Proceedings of the 11th World Congress on Pain,
edited by Herta Flor, Eija Kalso, and Jonathan O.
Dostrovsky, IASP Press, Seattle, © 2006.

43

Do the Analgesic Effects of Opioids and Tricyclic Antidepressants Differ in Subtypes of Patients with Postherpetic Neuralgia?

Prabhav K. Tella,[a] Shefali Agarwal,[a] Brendan Klick,[b] Mitchell B. Max,[c] Jennifer A. Haythornthwaite,[b] and Srinivasa N. Raja[a]

Departments of [a]Anesthesiology and Critical Care Medicine, [b]Psychiatry and Behavioral Science, The Johns Hopkins University, Baltimore, Maryland, USA; [c]Clinical Pain Research Section, National Institute of Dental and Craniofacial Research, National Institutes of Health, Department of Health and Human Services, Bethesda, Maryland, USA

The rising prevalence of metabolic disorders such as diabetes mellitus (Wareham and Forouhi 2005) and the aging of the population have led to an increase in chronic neuropathic disorders such as diabetic neuropathy and postherpetic neuralgia (PHN). PHN is a debilitating chronic neuropathic pain state that is a common sequel to acute herpes zoster in elderly patients (Tenser and Dworkin 2005). Reactivation of the varicella zoster virus during a period of decrease in cell-mediated immunity (Arvin 2005) causes varying degrees of inflammation in the dorsal root ganglion and results in degeneration of primary afferent sensory neurons. Because PHN is easy to diagnose and the pain is generally limited to the dermatomal or peripheral nerve distribution on one side of the body, it has been used as a model to examine the mechanisms of neuropathic pain and to study the efficacy of drug therapies.

The mechanisms of pain and allodynia in PHN have been carefully examined in patients using quantitative sensory tests (Rowbotham and Fields 1996; Pappagallo et al. 2000). Although PHN has been historically classified as a single disease entity, more recent studies suggest that different mechanisms may underlie the generation and maintenance of pain in individual patients (Fields et al. 1998). The diversity of mechanisms contributing to pain has led to the suggestion that the treatment strategy in a given patient with PHN should be based on the underlying mechanism rather than merely on an etiological diagnosis (Woolf 2004). However, practical barriers have hampered the adoption of this strategy. First, translating symptoms and signs into pathophysiological mechanisms in a given patient has been difficult (Jensen and Baron 2003). Second, studies have not examined whether the effects of drugs commonly used in the treatment of neuropathic pain vary in their effectiveness in patients with different underlying pain mechanisms.

In a recent randomized crossover trial, we compared the analgesic effects of opioids and tricyclic antidepressants (TCAs) in patients with PHN (Raja et al. 2002). We observed that both opioids and TCAs were more effective than placebo in decreasing the intensity of pain. In addition, opioids were preferred by a higher percentage of patients than TCAs. However, there was considerable interindividual variability in the magnitude of the effectiveness of opioids and TCA in the study population (Fig. 1). Many patients had little pain relief with opioids at doses at which adverse effects limited further dose escalation. We postulated that differences in pain mechanisms, such as those described earlier (Fields et al. 1998), might explain some of the variation in drug effects. This chapter describes a study in which we investigated whether the analgesic effects of opioids and TCAs differ in subtypes of patients with PHN who have a predominant peripheral versus central mechanism for their pain and allodynia.

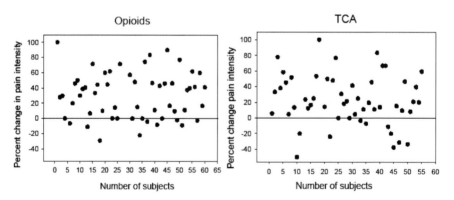

Fig. 1. Percentage change in pain intensity with opioids and tricyclic antidepressants (TCAs) in subjects with postherpetic neuralgia (PHN). Figure shows data from 59 patients who had a trial of opioid treatment and 55 patients treated with TCAs. Note the considerable interindividual variability in response.

METHODS

Sixty-eight adult PHN patients were enrolled into a randomized, double-blinded, clinical trial whose primary aim was to compare the analgesic and cognitive effects of opioids and TCAs. Patients received three separate 8-week treatments with oral opioids, TCAs, and placebo in a cross-over paradigm. The trial methodology and inclusion and exclusion criteria are described in an earlier publication (Raja et al. 2002). Prior to initiation of the drug trial, patients were titrated off their analgesic drugs, and baseline pain scores were obtained. Patients reported pain intensity on a 0–10 numerical rating scale. In addition, we conducted quantitative sensory testing in areas of maximum pain or cutaneous allodynia and at corresponding contralateral sites prior to randomization and titration with study drugs.

Quantitative sensory tests included thermal thresholds for warm detection, cool detection, heat pain, and cold pain with a contact Peltier device (a 2×2 cm thermal probe), using stimuli from a baseline of 30°C increased or decreased at a rate of 1°C/second. Mechanical sensory testing was performed using static stimuli (applied with a thermally neutral brass rod), dynamic stimuli (strokes with a camel hair brush), and punctate stimuli (von Frey filaments). Testing occurred on both the painful side and the same site on the unaffected side.

Thermal sensitivity data along with the presence or absence of allodynia were used to classify patients into two subtypes based on the putative mechanisms underlying the pain. Subjects were classified in the *irritable nociceptor* subtype if they had mechanical allodynia and had a heat pain threshold in the affected region that was normal or reduced by less than 1°C compared to the unaffected contralateral region, indicating intact peripheral nociceptor function. Sensitized peripheral nociceptors were considered to be the predominant generators of pain in this subgroup. The second, *deafferentation,* subtype comprised subjects with or without mechanical allodynia who had a heat pain threshold that was at least 1°C higher in the region of pain than in the unaffected contralateral area. It has been suggested that increased heat pain threshold is indicative of nociceptor deafferentation; central mechanisms are considered to predominate in this group of patients with PHN.

The primary pharmacological agents were morphine during the opioid phase and nortriptyline during the TCA phase. These drugs were replaced by methadone and desipramine, respectively, when alternate agents were required due to intolerable side effects.

The primary outcomes included pain intensity, reported by patients on a numeric rating scale of 0 (no pain) to 10 (most severe pain imaginable), and pain relief, rated as a percentage from 0 (no relief) to 100 (complete relief). Pain intensity and relief scores were collected from subjects during twice-weekly telephone interviews. Subjects with at least 30% reduction in pain intensity were defined as responders (Farrar et al. 2000). We compared the proportion of such responders among the three treatment groups.

Data were analyzed according to mixed-effect models (Laird et al. 1992) using statistical analysis software. Proportional weighting was used to account for subject participation. A P value of 0.05 was considered statistically significant.

RESULTS

Based on the presence or absence of cutaneous allodynia and the distribution of heat pain threshold scores (the difference between affected and unaffected regions), 36 patients were classified under the irritable nociceptor category and 32 were included in the deafferentation subtype. Demographic comparisons between the two subtypes did not reveal any significant differences. In both subtypes of PHN, opioids and TCAs, when compared to placebo, produced statistically significant pain reduction according to the two primary analgesic outcomes that were evaluated.

In the irritable nociceptor subtype, opioid treatment resulted in a significant reduction in pain intensity and pain relief compared to TCAs ($P = 0.04$). In contrast, in the deafferentation subtype, the reduction in pain intensity with opioid treatment was similar to that with TCAs ($P = 0.86$). Similarly, pain relief with opioids did not differ statistically from that of TCAs ($P = 0.35$) in this group of patients with deafferentation pain.

The proportion of responders was significantly greater with opioids and TCAs compared to placebo ($P < 0.02$) in the study population. In the irritable nociceptor subtype, the proportion of responders was statistically greater with opioid treatment than with TCAs ($P = 0.03$) or placebo ($P = 0.0008$). However, in the deafferentation subtype, the proportion of responders with opioids and TCAs did not differ significantly.

DISCUSSION

Our post hoc analyses of data obtained from a controlled clinical trial in subjects with PHN indicates that a subset of patients with intact heat nociception, suggestive of a predominant peripheral mechanism for pain and allodynia (the irritable nociceptor subtype), are more likely to have a beneficial analgesic effect with opioid analgesia compared to TCAs and placebo. In patients with deficits in heat pain threshold (the deafferentation subtype), opioids and TCAs do not differ from each other in their effectiveness in attenuating pain.

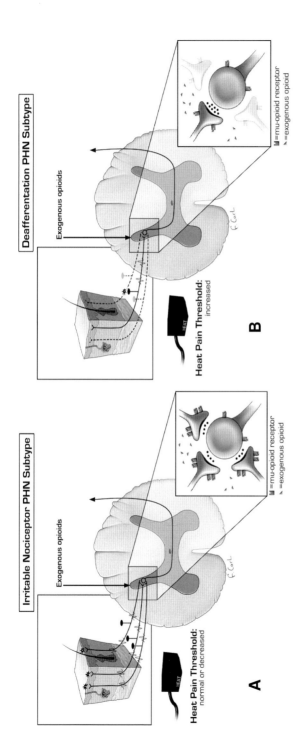

Fig. 2. Hypothesis for how loss of primary afferents in postherpetic neuralgia may reduce opioid analgesic response. (A) In patients with intact primary afferent nociceptors, heat pain threshold in the affected side is normal or decreased compared to the unaffected side. Ongoing pain is signaled by ectopic activity from nociceptive afferents from the injured region. A large part of opioid analgesia is mediated by presynaptic μ-opioid receptors on the central termination of primary afferent fibers. Activation of these presynaptic receptors by opioids decreases the release of nociceptive neurotransmitters. (B) Patients in whom the zoster attack has destroyed most of their peripheral nociceptors lose the opioid-bearing central terminations and have increased heat pain threshold. The ongoing pain may result from ectopic activity in neurons in the dorsal root ganglia or spinal neurons. In addition, peripheral damage may lead to partial loss of postsynaptic opioid receptors on spinal pain projection neurons and a decrease in presynaptic receptors on damaged peripheral neurons that survive. The decrease in presynaptic μ-opioid receptors may result in decreased inhibition and increase in neurotransmitter release from primary afferents.

The concept of variable drug response in individual PHN patients may be related in part to the predominant mechanisms underlying the generation and maintenance of pain (Fig. 2). Subjects in the irritable nociceptor subtype are likely to have intact, or even sensitized, peripheral C-fiber nociceptors. The superior opioid analgesia in this subgroup may be due to the predominance of intact or sensitized primary afferents. An important locus of action of opioids is at presynaptic sites on the central terminals of nociceptors. Activation of presynaptic opioid receptors leads to closure of voltage-gated calcium channels and inhibition of release of the excitatory neurotransmitters glutamate and substance P. Hence, opioids are particularly effective at reducing pain in this subset of patients (Beydoun and Backonja 2003).

The deafferentation subtype most likely comprises PHN patients with reduced peripheral nociceptive input and a predominant central pain-generating mechanism. In this subgroup, loss of primary afferents secondary to zoster-mediated neuronal loss in the dorsal root ganglia may reduce the number of opioid receptors in the dorsal horn of the spinal cord. Recent evidence suggests that approximately half of all spinal dorsal horn opioid receptors are presynaptic (Abbadie et al. 2002). Therefore, it can be hypothesized that a proportional decrease in opioid-mediated analgesia will result from the reduction in presynaptic opioid receptors (Fig. 2).

If our findings of superior analgesia from opioids relative to TCAs in a subset of patients with PHN are reproduced by further studies, quantitative sensory testing may be a useful tool to help characterize patterns of sensory loss in PHN patients and classify patients into subtypes. Complemented with a comprehensive history and physical examination, quantitative sensory testing may help the pain clinician to identify PHN patients with sensory profiles that show normal or greater thermal sensitivity in affected regions. Such patients may then benefit from initial selection of an opioid for a therapeutic trial.

A mechanism-based approach to pain management is a useful paradigm that appears promising. Future investigations should attempt to examine the effectiveness of drugs of different classes, such as anticonvulsants and antidepressants, in PHN subtypes. Such an effort may enhance our ability to make a more rational choice of first-line therapy in a given patient with PHN.

ACKNOWLEDGMENTS

Supported in part by NIH grant NS32386 and GCRC grant RR0052.

REFERENCES

Abbadie C, Lombard MC, Besson JM, Trafton JA, Basbaum AI. Mu and delta opioid receptor-like immunoreactivity in the cervical spinal cord of the rat after dorsal rhizotomy or neonatal capsaicin: an analysis of pre- and postsynaptic receptor distributions. *Brain Res* 2002; 930:150–162.

Arvin A. Aging, immunity, and the varicella-zoster virus. *N Engl J Med* 2005; 352:2266–2267.

Beydoun A, Backonja MM. Mechanistic stratification of antineuralgic agents. *J Pain Symptom Manage* 2003; 25:S18–S30.

Farrar JT, Portenoy RK, Berlin JA, Kinman J, Strom BL. Defining the clinically important difference in pain outcome measures. *Pain* 2000; 88:287–294.

Fields HL, Rowbotham M, Baron R. Postherpetic neuralgia: irritable nociceptors and deafferentation. *Neurobiol Dis* 1998; 5:209–227.

Jensen TS, Baron R. Translation of symptoms and signs into mechanisms in neuropathic pain. *Pain* 2003; 102:1–8.

Kohno T, Ji RR, Ito N, et al. Peripheral axonal injury results in reduced mu opioid receptor pre- and post-synaptic action in the spinal cord. *Pain* 2005; 117:77–87.

Laird NM, Donnelly C, Ware JH. Longitudinal studies with continuous responses. *Stat Methods Med Res* 1992; 1:225–247.

Pappagallo M, Oaklander AL, Quatrano-Piacentini AL, Clark MR, Raja SN. Heterogenous patterns of sensory dysfunction in postherpetic neuralgia suggest multiple pathophysiologic mechanisms. *Anesthesiology* 2000; 92:691–698.

Raja SN, Haythornthwaite JA, Pappagallo M, et al. Opioids versus antidepressants in postherpetic neuralgia: a randomized, placebo-controlled trial. *Neurology* 2002; 59:1015–1021.

Rowbotham MC, Fields HL. The relationship of pain, allodynia and thermal sensation in postherpetic neuralgia. *Brain* 1996; 119(Pt 2):347–354.

Tenser RB, Dworkin RH. Herpes zoster and the prevention of postherpetic neuralgia: beyond antiviral therapy. *Neurology* 2005; 65:349–350.

Wareham NJ, Forouhi NG. Is there really an epidemic of diabetes? *Diabetologia* 2005; 48:1454–1455.

Woolf CJ. Dissecting out mechanisms responsible for peripheral neuropathic pain: implications for diagnosis and therapy. *Life Sci* 2004; 74:2605–2610.

Correspondence to: Srinivasa N. Raja, MD, Division of Pain Medicine, Department of Anesthesiology and Critical Care Medicine, The Johns Hopkins University, 600 N. Wolfe Street, Osler 292, Baltimore, MD 21287, USA. Fax: 410-614-2019; email: sraja@jhmi.edu.

Proceedings of the 11th World Congress on Pain, edited by Herta Flor, Eija Kalso, and Jonathan O. Dostrovsky, IASP Press, Seattle, © 2006.

44

Profile of Opioid Use in Burn Patients One Year or More after Hospital Discharge

Dominique Dion,[a,b] Marie-Christine Taillefer,[b,c] and Manon Choinière[c,d]

aDepartment of Family Medicine, Maisonneuve-Rosemont Hospital, Montreal; bFaculty of Medicine, University of Montreal; cDepartment of Anesthesiology, Montreal Heart Institute, Montreal; dUniversity of Montreal, Montreal, Quebec, Canada

Burn injuries are responsible for intense and sustained pain, which results not only from tissue damage itself but also from therapeutic procedures such as wound dressings, skin grafts, and physical therapy (Choinière 2003; Patterson et al. 2004). In addition, some studies suggest that many burn survivors suffer from chronic pain at the site of their healed wounds (Malenfant et al. 1996; Dauber et al. 2002).

Use of opioids is relatively well accepted by the medical community and by members of the general public for managing moderate to severe acute pain, but its long-term utilization remains controversial for the treatment of many types of chronic nonmalignant pain (Bloodworth 2005; Breivik 2005). Fear of iatrogenic addiction is one of the reasons why clinicians may be uncomfortable with long-term opioid therapy (Morley-Forster et al. 2003; Grahmann et al. 2004).

The profile of opioid use in the years following a burn injury is scarcely documented. Few data, if any, are currently available on the incidence of aberrant drug-taking behaviors that would suggest addiction to opioids in burn survivors. This chapter summarizes a study designed to determine the prevalence and characteristics of chronic burn-related pain 1 year or more post-injury and to document the profile of opioid use and the incidence of potentially aberrant drug-taking behaviors in burn patients who were treated with opioids during their hospitalization. This study also explores whether current and past use of illicit drugs or alcohol are risk factors for problematic use of opioids after hospital discharge.

METHODS

PARTICIPANTS

We conducted a cross-sectional survey among patients treated at the burn center of the Hôtel-Dieu Hospital of the University of Montreal between 1995 and 1999. The study was approved by the institutional research ethics committee. All patients who were eligible to participate had been hospitalized for 5 days or more for acute thermal, chemical, cold, or abrasion burns and were between the ages of 18 and 65 years. Of the 393 eligible patients, 259 were located and were mailed a questionnaire 1–5 years following their hospitalization. The response rate was 76% (197/259).

DATA COLLECTION

Patient questionnaire. Section 1 evaluated the presence of chronic burn-related pain, its frequency, its intensity (measured on a numerical rating scale ranging from 0 = no pain to 10 = unbearable pain), and its perceived interference with normal work in the past 4 weeks (question 8 of the SF-36; Ware et al. 1993). Section 2 asked about opioid use in the past 6 months and the past 4 weeks. Section 3 measured the frequency of potentially aberrant drug-related behaviors regarding opioid use in the past 6 months. As there is no validated tool to measure opioid abuse and addiction, we developed this section based on published literature from experts in addiction medicine (Portenoy 1996; Compton et al. 1998; Passik et al. 2000; Savage 2002). The selected aberrant drug-related behaviors were going to the emergency room or to a walk-in clinic to obtain opioids, running out of opioids, borrowing opioids from others, and using opioids to relieve symptoms other than pain. Sections 4 and 5 gathered data on current and past history (i.e., prior to burn injury) of illicit drug and alcohol use as well as demographic information.

Medical form. We reviewed the patients' hospital records and used the computerized database of the burn center to determine the total area of body surface burned, the length of hospital stay, the daily amount of opioids received (expressed in intravenous morphine equivalents using standard equianalgesic ratios), and the duration of opioid use during hospitalization.

DATA ANALYSIS

Data were analyzed with descriptive and inferential statistics (Student t test and χ^2). A logistic regression analysis was planned to identify whether current and past use of illicit drugs or alcohol were risk factors for problematic use of opioids. A P value < 0.05 was considered statistically significant.

RESULTS

CHARACTERISTICS OF THE SUBJECTS

Our sample was mainly composed of middle-aged men (Table I); of the 197 patients in the sample, 162 (82.2%) were men. The mean percentage of total body surface burned was 17.2%, and patients were hospitalized for an average of about a month. During their hospital stay, patients received a median daily dose of 56.2 mg of i.v. morphine for a median duration of 22 days. When our sample (n = 197) was compared to the nonparticipants (i.e., those who could not be located or did not return the questionnaire; n = 196), the two groups were similar with regard to gender, percentage of total body surface burned, and length of hospitalization. However, they were slightly but significantly different in terms of age (participants were 3.9 years older on average) and time elapsed since burn injury (3.8 years for participants, 4.1 for others).

CHRONIC BURN-RELATED PAIN

A total of 34.5% of patients (68/197) reported chronic burn-related pain 1 year or more after their injury. As shown in Fig. 1, pain severity decreased progressively over time (χ^2 = 11.7, P = 0.02). The occurrence of pain was not significantly related to age, gender, or percentage of total body surface burned. However, the length of hospitalization in patients having chronic burn-related pain was significantly longer than in asymptomatic patients (35.5 ± 30.2 days versus 26.4 ± 23.3 days, P = 0.02).

More than half (56.1%) of the patients who had chronic burn-related pain (37 patients out of the 66 who responded to this question) experienced pain every day or almost every day, while only 10.6% (7/66) had pain less than 1 day a week. Forty-two percent of the patients (28/66) reported moderate to severe

Table I
Patients' demographic and clinical characteristics (n = 197)

Variable	Mean ± SD	Range
Age (years)	45.9 ± 11.3	21–68
Extent of burns (% of body)	17.2 ± 16.1	1–90
Length of hospitalization (days)	29.7 ± 26.1	5–182
Time elapsed since burn injury (years)	3.8 ± 1.5	1–5
	Median	Range
Duration of opioid use during hospitalization (days)	22	2–174
Daily i.v. morphine dose received during hospitalization (mg)	56.2	3.0–1258.4

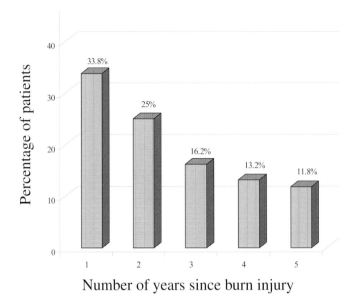

Fig. 1. Percentage of burn survivors who reported chronic burn-related pain according to the length of time elapsed since injury.

pain (greater than or equal to 4 on the 0–10-point scale). Almost half of the patients (49.3%; 33/67) stated that their pain interfered moderately to extremely with their normal work (either at the workplace or at home).

PROFILE OF OPIOID USE

In the 6 months prior to the survey, 15.9% of the patients (31 of the 195 patients who responded to this question) reported using opioids at least once. When asked about their intake in the past 4 weeks, only 9.4% of the patients (18/191) had taken opioids once or more. Almost 90% of them (16/18) used opioids to relieve their burn-related pain, whereas two patients took them to alleviate other types of pain. Half of them (9/18) were taking the medication every day or almost every day. Codeine was most frequently used (55.6%; 10/18), followed by morphine (33.3%; 6/18), hydromorphone (11.1%; 2/18), fentanyl patches (5.6%; 1/18), and oxycodone (5.6%; 1/18).

POTENTIALLY PROBLEMATIC DRUG-TAKING BEHAVIORS

Among the 31 patients who had used opioids in the 6 months prior to the survey, 20 of them (64.5%) reported at least one drug-taking behavior that could be viewed as potentially aberrant (Table II). In 11 of these patients, these behaviors occurred only occasionally (no more than five times in 6 months). Only one patient reported two of these behaviors more than five times in 6 months. No patient reported all four behaviors. Seven patients out of the 30 who responded to the question (23.3%) used opioids to relieve symptoms such as insomnia or mood disorders.

CURRENT AND PAST HISTORY OF ILLICIT DRUG AND ALCOHOL USE

A total of 88.9% (175/197) patients reported that their current alcohol consumption was lower than it was before their burn injury. Close to 20% (38/194) of the patients who responded to this question had used an illicit drug at least once in the past 6 months (cannabis only: 19.2%, 37/193 patients; other illicit drugs with or without cannabis: 4.4%, 8/180 patients). Patients' illicit drug intake during that period was less than their lifetime use. It was not possible to analyze whether a history of drug or alcohol abuse was a significant predictor of problematic use of opioids after hospital discharge because the incidence of potentially aberrant drug-taking behaviors on a sustained basis was very low.

DISCUSSION

The results of this study confirm that chronic burn-related pain is frequent and can be severe enough to interfere with daily living. The prevalence rate in

Table II
Frequency and percentage of potentially aberrant drug-taking behaviors as reported by 31 patients who used opioids in the 6 months preceding the study*

Behaviors	N (%)			
	At least once	1–2 times	3–5 times	>5 times
Going to the emergency room or to a walk-in clinic to obtain opioids	16 (53.4)	9 (30.0)	2 (6.7)	5 (16.7)
Running out of opioids	5 (17.9)	4 (14.3)	0 (0)	1 (3.6)
Borrowing opioids from others†	7 (24.1)	4 (13.8)	2 (6.9)	1 (3.4)
Using opioids to relieve the following symptoms:	7 (23.3)			
Anxiety or stress		2 (6.7)	2 (6.7)	2 (6.7)
Insomnia		1 (3.3)	2 (6.7)	3 (3.3)
Feeling depressed		2 (6.7)	1 (3.3)	1 (3.3)

* The size of the denominator may vary as some patients did not answer all of the questions. The percentage is the number of patients who reported each behavior divided by the total number of patients who used opioids in the past 6 months.
† Codeine was the opioid borrowed in all cases.

this study, 34.5%, compares to those reported in previous studies: 36% (Malenfant et al. 1996) and 52% (Dauber et al. 2002). Less than 5% of the participants in our study were taking opioids on a regular basis to relieve their pain. Patients with chronic burn-related pain might benefit from a therapeutic trial with an opioid, either alone or in combination with other types of medication or treatment modalities.

All patients who were still taking opioids 1 year or more after their burn injury had chronic pain. In the 6 months prior to the survey, at least one potentially problematic drug-taking behavior was reported by almost two-thirds of the patients on opioids. However, most of these behaviors were occasional. Furthermore, behaviors such as running out of opioids and going to the emergency room may also suggest inadequate pain management in some patients. Passik et al. (2000) reported that 10% of cancer patients and 44% of HIV/AIDS patients who were experiencing pain had borrowed opioids from a friend or spouse at least once, and that up to 4% and 28% of cancer and HIV/AIDS patients, respectively, had done so more than three times. The major challenge for clinicians and researchers facing these behaviors is to distinguish those indicative of poor pain control or drug misuse from those associated with drug abuse and addiction. There is currently no validated and widely used tool to assess these issues in patients who are prescribed opioids for chronic pain (Passik et al. 2000; Robinson et al. 2001; Nedeljkovic et al. 2002; Savage 2002).

In our study, about one patient out of five had used opioids at least once to relieve symptoms other than pain (i.e., insomnia or mood disorders). These behaviors, observed in other studies with pain patients (Compton et al. 1998; Passik et al. 2000), emphasize how important it is for physicians to address this issue closely with their patients. Sleep problems and mood disorders are frequent in chronic pain patients and could be left undiagnosed if they are not specifically evaluated.

Taken together, the results of the present survey suggest that inadequate relief of chronic pain is perhaps a bigger problem in burn patients than inappropriate use of opioids. As many experts have pointed out (Passik et al. 2000; Robinson et al. 2001; Nedeljkovic et al. 2002), epidemiological studies are needed to more thoroughly document the incidence of problematic drug-taking behaviors in larger groups of patients receiving long-term opioids for a variety of chronic pain disorders. Such data would also help researchers to develop valid screening instruments for drug abuse or addiction, something eagerly awaited by clinicians.

ACKNOWLEDGMENTS

This work was supported by grants from la Fondation des pompiers du Québec pour les grands brûlés and the Quebec Pain Research Initiative. The authors would like to thank Hélène Lanctôt, research nurse, and the patients involved in the study. At the time this study was carried out, the authors were working at the burn center of the Hôtel-Dieu Hospital of the University of Montreal.

REFERENCES

Bloodworth D. Issues in opioid management. *Am J Phys Med Rehabil* 2005; 84:S42–S55.

Breivik H. Opioids in chronic non-cancer pain, indications and controversies. *Eur J Pain* 2005; 9:127–130.

Choinière M. Pain of burns. In: Melzack R, Wall PD (Eds). *Handbook of Pain Management: A Clinical Companion to Wall and Melzack's Textbook of Pain.* Toronto: Churchill Livingstone, 2003, pp 591–601.

Compton P, Darakjian J, Miotto K. Screening for addiction in patients with chronic pain and "problematic" substance use: evaluation of a pilot assessment tool. *J Pain Symptom Manage* 1998; 16:355–363.

Dauber A, Osgood PF, Breslau AJ, Vernon HL, Carr DB. Chronic persistent pain after severe burns: a survey of 358 burn survivors. *Pain Med* 2002; 3:6–17.

Grahmann PH, Jackson KC, Lipman AG. Clinician beliefs about opioid use and barriers in chronic nonmalignant pain. *J Pain Palliat Care Pharmacother* 2004; 18:7–28.

Malenfant A, Forget R, Papillon J, et al. Prevalence and characteristics of chronic sensory problems in burn patients. *Pain* 1996; 67:493–500.

Morley-Forster PK, Clark AJ, Speechley M, Moulin DE. Attitudes toward opioid use for chronic pain: a Canadian physician survey. *Pain Res Manag* 2003; 8:189–194.

Nedeljkovic SS, Wasan A, Jamison RN. Assessment of efficacy of long-term opioid therapy in pain patients with substance abuse potential. *Clin J Pain* 2002; 18:S39–S51.

Passik SD, Kirsh KL, McDonald MV, et al. A pilot survey of aberrant drug-taking attitudes and behaviors in samples of cancer and AIDS patients. *J Pain Symptom Manage* 2000; 19:274–286.

Patterson DR, Hofland HW, Espey K, Sharar S. Pain management. *Burns* 2004; 30:A10–A15.

Portenoy RK. Opioid therapy for chronic nonmalignant pain: a review of the critical issues. *J Pain Symptom Manage* 1996; 11:203–217.

Robinson RC, Gatchel RJ, Polatin P, et al. Screening for problematic prescription opioid use. *Clin J Pain* 2001; 17:220–228.

Savage SR. Assessment for addiction in pain-treatment settings. *Clin J Pain* 2002; 18:S28–S38.

Ware JE Jr, Snow KK, Kosinski M, Gandek B. *SF-36 Health Survey: Manual and Interpretation Guide.* Boston: Nimrod Press, 1993.

Correspondence to: Manon Choinière, PhD, Montreal Heart Institute, Room R-2231, 5000 Belanger, Montreal, PQ, Canada H1T 1C8. Tel: 1-514-376-3330 ext. 2042; Fax: 1-514-593-2160; email: manon.choiniere@icm-mhi.org.

Proceedings of the 11th World Congress on Pain,
edited by Herta Flor, Eija Kalso, and Jonathan O.
Dostrovsky, IASP Press, Seattle, © 2006.

45

Opioid Side-Effect Profiles: Associations with Analgesic Response and Psychological Factors

Barbara A. Hastie,[a] Joseph L. Riley III,[a] Toni Glover,[a]
Claudia M. Campbell,[b] Roland Staud,[c]
and Roger B. Fillingim[a,d]

*[a]College of Dentistry, Division of Public Health Services and Research,
University of Florida; [b]Department of Clinical and Health Psychology,
University of Florida; [c]Division of Rheumatology, College of Medicine,
University of Florida; [d]Malcom Randall V.A. Medical Center,
Gainesville, Florida, USA*

Opioid-induced side effects are inevitable; they involve multiple systems such as the gastrointestinal tract (i.e., constipation, nausea, and vomiting), the respiratory system, and the central nervous system. Their frequency and severity are characterized by substantial interindividual variability. Importantly, patients may reduce or discontinue their analgesic treatment to mitigate adverse effects (Bowdle 1998; Cherny et al. 2001; Maier et al. 2002; Stamer et al. 2005). Thus, a balance must be struck between the advantages of opioid pain relief and the adverse effects (Edwards et al. 1999; McQuay 1999; Kalso et al. 2004).

Successful pain management with opioids requires that adequate analgesia be achieved without excessive adverse effects. Reviews of clinical trials based on these criteria reveal that a substantial minority of patients treated with oral morphine (10–30%) generally have an unsuccessful outcome because of excessive adverse effects, inadequate analgesia, or both (Edwards et al. 1999; McQuay 1999; Barden et al. 2004). Similar responses have been reported with other opioids. The adverse effects of different opioids vary depending on which receptor each drug activates (Bowdle 1998; Kalso et al. 2004; Meert and Vermeirsch 2005). Despite the clinical importance of the topic, there is a lack of systematic investigation on the determinants of the side effects of opioids.

Consequently, understanding the etiology of side effects, particularly adverse experiences, remains a major clinical challenge.

Psychological processes have a substantial influence on the experience of pain (Gatchel and Turk 1999; Dworkin and Breitbart 2004). However, few studies have examined the potential influence of psychological factors on opioid-induced side effects and analgesia. Moreover, despite the significant interindividual differences in side effects that are often reported clinically, little is known about symptom clusters and their relationship to a particular opioid, to analgesic response, and to psychological factors. This chapter describes a study that evaluated the influences of affective factors, gender, and analgesic response to a μ-opioid receptor agonist (morphine) and a mixed-action opioid (pentazocine) and their associations with side-effect profile.

METHODS

We enrolled 213 healthy subjects, 57.7% of whom were female, with a mean age of 24.4 years (SD = 5.6 years). Subjects completed several psychological instruments, as described below, and underwent psychophysical pain testing prior to and following drug administration. Subjects were randomly assigned to receive an opioid (either morphine 0.08 mg/kg or pentazocine 0.5 mg/kg) or saline intravenously on separate days. All procedures were approved by the Human Subjects Committee at the University of Florida. Written and verbal informed consent was obtained from each participant.

Several measures were utilized to assess side effects, psychological and affective status, and experimental pain. Side-effects measures included the Somatic Side Effects questionnaire (SSE; Davies et al. 1997) and the Cognitive and Affective Side-Effect questionnaire (CASE; Roth-Roemer et al. 1997). The SSE is a 28-item questionnaire that measures a range of common somatic adverse effects associated with opioid use, and the CASE is a 44-item questionnaire that assesses a range of common cognitive and affective side effects that might be experienced as positive or negative effects. For both instruments, items are rated on a 5-point scale (0 = "Not at all" to 5 = "Extremely").

Psychological instruments included the Coping Strategies Questionnaire-Revised (CSQ-R), the Kohn Reactivity Scale (KRS), the Pennebaker Inventory of Limbic Languidness (PILL), and the Positive and Negative Affect Scale (PANAS). The CSQ is a widely used, well-validated instrument to assess coping techniques employed by individuals with chronic pain (Rosenstiel and Keefe 1983). The revised and shortened version, CSQ-R, has been validated in healthy individuals (Hastie et al. 2004). The KRS is a valid, reliable measure consisting of 24 items that assess an individual's level of reactivity or central nervous system arousability (Kohn 1985; Dubreuil and Kohn 1986). It has also been used to measure the construct of hypervigilance (McDermid et al. 1996). PILL assesses the frequency of 54 common physical symptoms and sensations and has been related to the construct of somatization, or the tendency to report increased physical symptoms (Pennebaker 1982). It has also been used to assess hypervigilance in chronic pain patients (McDermid et al. 1996). PILL has high internal consistency ($\alpha = 0.88$) and high test-retest reliability (0.70 over 2 months). Lastly, the PANAS is a 20-item self-report instrument consisting of a 10-item Positive Affect and 10-item Negative Affect scale (Watson et al. 1988).

Thermal pain procedures were assessed with contact heat stimuli delivered to the forearm using a computer-controlled Medoc Thermal Sensory Analyzer, a 30 by 30 mm Peltier element-based stimulator. From a baseline of 32°C, the probe temperature increased at a rate of 0.5°C per second until the subject responded by pressing a button on a handheld device. There were four trials for each heat pain threshold ("when you first feel pain") and heat pain tolerance ("when you no longer feel able to tolerate the pain"). The cutoff temperature to avoid tissue damage was 52°C.

Temporal summation of thermal pain was assessed through brief, repetitive suprathreshold thermal stimuli that were applied to the right forearm to elicit temporal summation of pain. Two intertrial stimulus intensities were used, 39°C and 40°C. The two target temperatures of 49°C and 52°C were delivered for approximately 1 second each, with a 2.5-second interpulse interval. Subjects rated the intensity of each pulse using a 101-point scale. The procedure continued for up to 10 trials, or until the subject provided a rating of 100 or requested that the testing be terminated.

Pressure pain threshold was measured with a handheld pressure algometer. Through the instrument's 1-cm diameter rubber tip, pressure was applied at the constant rate of 1 kg per second. The order of the trials was counterbalanced, and the assessment included three trials, which were delivered at each of three sites—the center of the right upper trapezius, the right masseter, and the right ulna, midway between the wrist and elbow on the dorsolateral midline of the forearm. The average of the trials was calculated for each site.

Ischemic pain was applied through a modified submaximal effort tourniquet test (Moore et al. 1979; Pertovaara et al. 1984). The right arm was exsanguinated by elevating it above heart level for 60 seconds and was then occluded with a standard blood pressure cuff inflated to 240 mm Hg. Subjects then performed 20 hand grip exercises of 2-second duration at 4-second intervals at 50% of their maximum grip strength and continued until the perceived pain was deemed intolerable or for 15 minutes, whichever came first. Each minute, subjects rated the intensity (which assessed the sensory dimension) and unpleasantness (which assessed the affective dimension) of their arm pain using

0–20-point numerical rating scales and verbal descriptor box scales. Times to pain threshold and pain tolerance were used as ratings for ischemic pain (IP) threshold (IPTh) and IP tolerance (IPTo), respectively. Sum scores were computed for pain intensity and pain unpleasantness ratings.

STATISTICAL METHODS

Initially, exploratory factor analysis was conducted to evaluate the distribution of factor loadings for each of the symptom measures (i.e., SSE and CASE). Confirmatory factor analysis with bootstrap sampling was performed to study the distribution of factor loadings. Factor composite scores were calculated and entered into principal components analysis with an Oblimin rotation to test for dimensional overlap. The higher-order symptom factors were then subjected to a hierarchical cluster analysis to assign participants into groups, revealing side-effect profiles. Within-session change scores were calculated from pain measures across experimental pain modalities for predrug baseline to post-analgesia scores. Next, analgesic indices were calculated from these change scores (drug session change scores minus saline session change scores) to account for any influence of placebo effect. Analysis of variance and chi-square analyses were performed for categorical data using factors of opioid, profile group, and gender to test for differences on analgesic indices and psychological measures. Main effects and interaction effects were determined with regression. Significance was set at the 0.05 level.

RESULTS

Side-effect factors. Initial factor analysis revealed seven factors for the SSE and six factors for the CASE. Confirmatory factor analysis demonstrated that the final models of side effects for each drug were identical after elimination of all items with factor loadings less than 0.40. Composite factors scores were generated and submitted to principal components analysis, which revealed three higher-order factors and accounted for 68% of the variance from (1) positive feelings (relaxed, euphoric), (2) confusion or unusual thoughts, and (3) somatic effects (dry mouth, sedation, and tremors).

Cluster analysis: groupings of side-effect profiles. Hierarchical cluster analysis of the factor composite scores showed that agglomeration coefficients were most suitable for a grouping of three profile groups characterized by (1) low side effects (LSE); (2) high positive feelings, mild confusion, and mental dullness (euphoric/mild confusion/mental dullness, EMD); and (3) the highest somatic effects and confusion (HSC). Participants were evenly distributed

across the cluster groups for pentazocine. However, participants were dispropor-
tionately distributed for morphine with more individuals represented in group
3, HSC. The HSC group had a greater proportion of women than men (67%
versus 59%, respectively).

Analgesic response and side-effect profiles. Side-effect profile groups
differed on analgesic response for various experimental indices on experimental pain and also differed by opioid. Analgesic indices were standardized for
comparison and appear in Figs. 1 and 2. Specifically, for morphine on heat pain
and pressure pain responses, the EMD group had the highest analgesic response
for heat pain threshold (HPTh), temporal summation (TS), and pressure pain
(PP) and had median ratings on heat pain tolerance (HPTo). Conversely, the
HSC group had the lowest analgesic response on HPTh, TS, and PP, but the
highest response on HPTo. The LSE cluster had moderate analgesic response
on all measures except HPTo, where they had the lowest response. On ischemic
pain measures with morphine, the EMD group reported the greatest analgesic

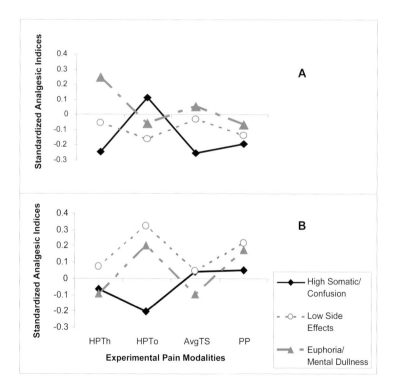

Fig. 1. Side-effect profiles and analgesic indices for heat pain and pressure pain with (A)
morphine and (B) pentazocine. HPTh = heat pain threshold; HPTo = heat pain tolerance;
AvgTS = average temporal summation; PP = pressure pain.

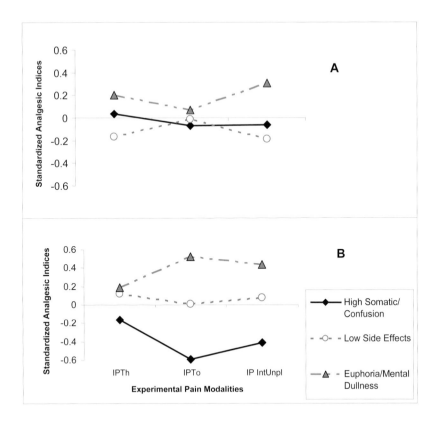

Fig. 2. Side-effect profiles and analgesic indices for ischemic pain with (A) morphine and (B) pentazocine. IPTh = ischemic pain threshold; IPTo = ischemic pain tolerance; IPIntUnpl = ischemic pain intensity and unpleasantness.

response on all measures of ischemic pain threshold (IPTh) ($P = 0.05$), tolerance (IPTo), and intensity/unpleasantness (IPIU) ($P = 0.027$), while the LSE group had the lowest response on IPTh and IPIU, and the HSC group had the worst response on IPTo.

With pentazocine, the EMD group also had the highest analgesic response for all ischemic pain measures. In contrast, the HSC group had the lowest analgesic response on all ischemic pain measures as well as on HPTo and PP, with moderate responses only on HPTh and TS. The LSE profile demonstrated moderate pentazocine analgesic responses on ischemic measures and highest analgesic responses on all heat and pressure pain measures (HPTh, HPTo, TS, and PP). Apart from the influence of opioids, significant interaction effects were found between side-effect profile group and gender on analgesic index only for ischemic pain measures (IPTo, $P = 0.046$; IP intensity/unpleasantness, $P = 0.022$; and IPTh, $P = 0.073$).

Side-effect profiles and psychological factors. Significant main effects were found for side-effect profile cluster on the psychological measures of the KRS ($P < 0.001$), PANAS positive ($P = 0.025$), PILL no pain ($P = 0.041$), CSQ-R coping self-statements (CSS) ($P = 0.010$), and CSQ-R active ($P = 0.013$); it approached significance for PANAS negative ($P = 0.060$). Post hoc comparisons revealed that HSC responders were highest on the KRS, whereas they were lowest on the PANAS positive, CSQ-R CSS, and CSQ-R active domain. EMD responders had the highest scores on PANAS positive, PILL no pain, CSQ CSS, and CSQ-R active domain ($P < 0.05$) (Table I). Further evaluation revealed that gender did not interact with side-effect profile group on any of the outcomes.

DISCUSSION

In this sample of healthy young adults receiving equianalgesic dosing of morphine or pentazocine, hierarchical cluster analysis revealed three distinct side-effect profile groups. The EMD profile group achieved the greatest analgesic response on most experimental pain modalities (HPTh, TS, PP, IPTh, IPTo, and IPIU) for both drugs. The EMD group also reported the lowest KRS scores and the highest PANAS positive, CSQ CSS, and active coping scores, suggesting that a positive psychological profile predicted a more positive side-effect profile. Conversely, the HSC group showed a more negative psychological profile, as reflected in the highest KRS scores, the lowest PANAS positive, CSQ-R CSS, and active coping scores, and comparatively poorer analgesia for both drugs. The LSE profile group had moderate analgesic response for morphine on several pain measures (HPTh, TS, PP, and IPTo) and for pentazocine, they had the highest analgesic response for heat and pressure pain measures and moderate analgesic responses for ischemic pain measures.

These findings highlight the importance of considering interindividual differences in side effects, which may be influenced by pretreatment differences in psychological factors. These intraindividual differences could have important implications for treatment plans and opioid choice and might affect the overall pain experience and analgesic relief in clinical populations. For example, the profile group that was more predisposed to high adverse effects also showed a more negative psychological profile, suggesting a potential target for intervention. Specifically, given the strong and synergistic influence of psychological states on physiological processes, it is conceivable that psychological interventions for improving mood, enhancing coping, or reducing anxiety could potentially reduce the experience of heightened adverse events associated with opioid therapy, and might influence analgesic response as well. Conversely, clinically addressing the beneficial attributes of positive affective states has

Table I
Side-effect profiles across psychological measures

Psychological Measure	Cluster Profile 1: Low Side Effects (LSE)	Cluster Profile 2: Euphoria, Mild Confusion, and Mental Dullness (EMD)	Cluster Profile 3: High Somatic Effects and Confusion (HSC)	Overall Significance	Post Hoc Comparisons
Kohn Reactivity Scale	63.59	62.29	72.05*	$P < 0.001$	HSC > LSE; $P < 0.001$ HSC > EMD; $P < 0.001$
PANAS: Positive	37.04	37.69	34.80*	$P = 0.025$	HSC < LSE; $P = 0.019$ HSC < EMD; $P = 0.013$
PANAS: Negative	15.86†	17.77	16.85	$P = 0.060$	LSE < EMD; $P = 0.019$ HSC < EMD; $P = 0.056$
PILL: No Pain	57.58‡	61.33	59.95	$P = 0.041$	LSE < HSC; $P = 0.106$ LSE < EMD; $P = 0.016$
CSQ-R: Coping Self-Statements	3.64	3.96	3.15*	$P = 0.010$	HSC < LSE; $P = 0.027$ HSC < EMD; $P = 0.003$
CSQ-R: Active Domain	2.51	2.76	2.17*	$P = 0.013$	HSC < LSE; $P = 0.039$ HSC < EMD; $P = 0.004$

Abbreviations: CSQ-R = Coping Strategies Questionnaire-Revised; PANAS = Positive and Negative Affect Scale; PILL = Pennebaker Inventory of Limbic Languidness.

* HSC is significantly different from LSE and EMD, but LSE and EMD do not differ from each other.

† LSE is significantly different from EMD.

‡ LSE is significantly different from EMD but not different from HSC.

the potential to further improve treatment outcomes and create better side-effect profiles. While this possibility remains highly speculative, evidence from disparate studies suggests that side effects may be mediated by multiple factors including genetic, pharmacokinetic, and pharmacodynamic influences as well as emotional, cognitive, and psychosocial factors. This study lends initial support to the associations between analgesic responses and psychological factors.

ACKNOWLEDGMENTS

This material is the result of work supported with resources and the use of facilities at the Malcom Randall VA Medical Center, Gainesville, Florida. This work was supported by NIH grant NS41670 and General Clinical Research Center Grant RR00082. B.A. Hastie is also supported as a Health Disparities Scholar of the NIH National Center on Minority Health and Health Disparities.

REFERENCES

Barden J, Edwards JE, Mason L, McQuay HJ, Moore RA. Outcomes in acute pain trials: systematic review of what was reported? *Pain* 2004; 109:351–356.

Bowdle TA. Adverse effects of opioid agonists and agonist-antagonists in anaesthesia. *Drug Safety* 1998; 19:173–189.

Cherny N, Ripamonti C, Pereira J, et al. Strategies to manage the adverse effects of oral morphine: an evidence-based report. *J Clin Oncol* 2001; 19:2542–2554.

Davies PS, Roth-Roemer S, Coda B, et al. Somatic side effects of morphine and hydromorphone during sustained equianalgesic infusions. *Proc Am Pain Soc* 1997; 16:120.

Dubreuil DL, Kohn PM. Reactivity and response to pain. *Pers Individ Dif* 1986; 7:907–909.

Dworkin RH, Breitbart WS (Eds). *Psychosocial Aspects of Pain: A Handbook for Health Care Providers,* Progress in Pain Research and Management, Vol. 27. Seattle: IASP Press, 2004.

Edwards JE, McQuay HJ, Moore RA, Collins SL. Reporting of adverse effects in clinical trials should be improved: lessons from acute postoperative pain. *J Pain Symptom Manage* 1999; 18:427–437.

Gatchel RJ, Turk DC. *Psychosocial Factors in Pain*. New York: Guilford Press, 1999.

Hastie BA, Riley JL III, Fillingim RB. Ethnic differences in pain coping: factor structure of the coping strategies questionnaire and CSQ-revised. *J Pain* 2004; 5:304–316.

Kalso E, Edwards JE, Moore RA, McQuay HJ. Opioids in chronic non-cancer pain: systematic review of efficacy and safety. *Pain* 2004; 112:372–380.

Kohn PM. Sensation-seeking, augmenting-reducing, and strength of the nervous system. In: Spence JT, Izard DE (Eds). *Motivation, Emotion, and Personality*. Amsterdam: Elsevier, 1985, pp 167–173.

Maier C, Hildebrandt J, Klinger R, Henrich-Eberl C, Lindena G. Morphine responsiveness, efficacy and tolerability in patients with chronic non-tumor associated pain—results of a double-blind placebo-controlled trial (MONTAS). *Pain* 2002; 97:223–233.

McDermid AJ, Rollman GB, McCain GA. Generalized hypervigilance in fibromyalgia: evidence of perceptual amplification. *Pain* 1996; 66:133–144.

McQuay H. Opioids in pain management. *Lancet* 1999; 353:2229–2232.

Meert TF, Vermeirsch HA. A preclinical comparison between different opioids: antinociceptive versus adverse effects. *Pharmacol Biochem Behav* 2005; 80:309–326.

Moore PA, Duncan GH, Scott DS, Gregg JM, Ghia JN. The submaximal effort tourniquet test: its use in evaluating experimental and chronic pain. *Pain* 1979; 6:375–382.

Pennebaker JW. *The Psychology of Physical Symptoms.* New York: Springer-Verlag, 1982.

Pertovaara A, Nurmikko T, Pontinen PJ. Two separate components of pain produced by the sub-maximal effort tourniquet test. *Pain* 1984; 20:53–58.

Rosenstiel AK, Keefe FJ. The use of coping strategies in chronic low back pain patients: relationship to patient characteristics and current adjustment. *Pain* 1983; 17:33–44.

Roth-Roemer S, Coda B, Davies PS, et al. Cognitive and psychomotor side effects of morphine and hydromorphone during sustained equianalgesic infusions. *Proc Am Pain Soc* 1997; 16:120.

Stamer UM, Bayerer B, Stuber F. Genetics and variability in opioid response. *Eur J Pain* 2005; 9:101–104.

Watson D, Clark LA, Tellegen A. Development and validation of brief measures of positive and negative affect: the PANAS scales. *J Pers Soc Psychol* 1988; 54:1063–1070.

Correspondence to: Barbara A. Hastie, PhD, University of Florida College of Dentistry, Department of Community Dentistry and Behavioral Science, 1329 SW 16th Street, Suite 5180, P.O. Box 103628, Gainesville, FL 32610-3628, USA. Tel: 352-273-5964; Fax: 352-273-5985; email: bhastie@dental.ufl.edu.

Part VI

Psychological and Psychosocial Factors, Gender Issues, and Epidemiology of Pain

Proceedings of the 11th World Congress on Pain, edited by Herta Flor, Eija Kalso, and Jonathan O. Dostrovsky, IASP Press, Seattle, © 2006.

46

Hypervigilance and Attention to Pain: Experimental and Clinical Evidence

Geert Crombez

Department of Experimental Clinical Psychology and Health Psychology, Ghent University, Ghent, Belgium

Many chronic pain patients experience persistent, distressing, and overwhelming pain. They often complain of cognitive problems such as difficulties in concentrating and in focusing attention (Jamison 1988). Many also report a diversity of somatic complaints that cannot easily be explained by observable biomedical phenomena. Growing in popularity are explanations based on the idea of dysfunctional attentional processes. Patients are thought to pay excessive attention to pain and pain-associated information at the expense of other aspects of their lives. This chapter reviews experimental and clinical evidence regarding the role of attention and hypervigilance in the experience of pain. I will focus in particular on recent work on dysfunctional attention to threatening information, and on the different attentional components involved. I suggest that selective attention to pain may occur in two different ways, and I present conceptual definitions of and evidence for both. Central to my theory is the assumption that the attentional selection of pain at the expense of other demands in the environment is an evolutionary valuable process in normal situations. I argue, however, that the same mechanisms may result in persistent and dysfunctional disruption of attention and behavior when the situation is abnormal—when the pain is chronic and cannot be escaped or avoided. The chapter concludes with some theoretical and clinical implications of this view.

TWO FORMS OF ATTENTION TO PAIN

In order to understand attentional processes in the experience of pain, we can consider models of attention in other domains. Within cognitive psychology, Allport (1989) has provided one of the most detailed functional accounts of attention, working primarily through the example of visual attention. Accepting the basic axiom that attention involves the selection of certain information at the expense of other information, he discussed attention within the context of the need of the organism to behave in a purposeful and coherent way. He argued that an efficient attentional system serves two apparently contradictory needs. On the one hand, it is important that the current behavior and attentional focus are maintained and protected from less important demands. On the other hand, in an unpredictable and potentially dangerous environment, it is necessary that attentional engagement or ongoing behavior can be interrupted by new, more important, demands such as threat.

In line with this reasoning, pain may become the focus of attention in two different ways. First, it may have immediate relevance for the current goals or concerns of the individual. For example, in a laboratory study, participants may be instructed by the experimenter to report when the nociceptive stimulus becomes painful. Patients may be fearfully anticipating the worsening of pain during an activity. They may worry about the ineffectiveness of previous medical interventions and continue to search for other ways to manage their pain (Aldrich et al. 2000). Although these examples are phenomenologically different, they have in common that the current goal of the individual is related to pain. In these situations, vigilance or hypervigilance to pain or pain-related information emerges (see Klinger 1996). Second, pain is an archetypical signal of physical threat, and it is meant to interrupt attention, even in situations when the current concern of the individual is not related to pain at all. The attentional selection of pain is then goal-independent and reflects its interruptive quality. Our distinction between these two forms of attention to pain in terms of goal-dependency is not new. It is similar to the distinction between active and passive attention (Graham and Hackley 1991) and between top-down and bottom-up aspects of attention (Sarter et al. 2001).

INTERRUPTION OF ATTENTION BY PAIN

Eccleston and Crombez (1999) have developed a cognitive-affective model of the interruptive function of pain. Following the core ideas of Allport (1989), they argued that pain imposes an overriding priority for attentional engagement by activating a primitive defensive system that urges escape from somatic threat. Indeed, pain seems designed to interrupt attention, even in situations when the current concern of the individual is not related to pain. It is a signal of physical threat that enables an organism to respond promptly to the perceived source of threat (Wall 1994). In the model it is proposed that the interruptive quality of pain is not mediated by its sensory characteristics, but by its affective-motivational characteristics, otherwise stated as its threat value. Thus, Eccleston and

I stressed that pain is an experience that activates an inclination to act and to escape. A further core idea of the model is that the interruptive quality of pain is not a passive process, but depends upon a dynamic interaction between the characteristics of pain and the characteristics of the context in which pain may emerge.

Although intuitively it makes sense that pain has an interruptive quality and demands attention, systematic research on this topic started only recently. In 1994 a primary task paradigm was developed that allowed the experimental investigation of the variables that affect the interruptive quality of pain (Crombez et al. 1994; Eccleston 1994). The rationale of the paradigm is that the selection of pain in favor of other demands will result in decreased attention to other task demands. In this paradigm, participants are asked to perform a task that demands attention (e.g., a detection or discrimination task). During the task, a painful stimulus is administered, and participants are instructed to ignore it. The deterioration of task performance during pain, in terms of speed and accuracy, is used to measure the interruption of attention by pain. Psychophysiological methods have also been applied to assess the interruptive quality of pain. In particular, evoked potentials have proven useful (Zaslansky et al. 1996; Lorenz and Bromm 1997; Legrain et al. 2004). We review below the available studies that have investigated pain characteristics and environmental characteristics that moderate the interruptive function of pain.

PAIN CHARACTERISTICS

Several variables that amplify the interruption of attention by pain in healthy volunteers and clinical populations have been identified.

Intensity of chronic pain. Since pain is meant to interrupt behavior, chronic pain of high intensity will also interrupt task performance in patients. Indeed, while pain can be considered a "false alarm," it remains an ontogenetic and phylogenetic cue of bodily threat and cannot be switched off. Chronic pain of high intensity will therefore remain interruptive and keep interfering with cognitive functioning. This idea was confirmed by Eccleston (1994, 1995). He found that, in samples of chronic pain patients, those patients with high-intensity pain showed significant decrements in the performance of a highly demanding task compared to those with low-intensity pain and pain-free controls. Lorenz et al. (1997) also showed that the attentional demand of chronic pain is diminished by analgesia induced by morphine.

Unpredictability and novelty. In pain-free students, a painful heat stimulus of which none of the participants had prior experience resulted in significant task interference; this interference was more pronounced at the beginning compared to the end of the pain stimulus (Crombez et al. 1994). Research using evoked potentials has revealed that when attention is not focused on pain, an unexpected and rare pain stimulus evokes an involuntary attentional shift to pain (Legrain et al. 2004).

Threat value of pain. In line with the idea that the affective characteristics are of particular importance for interruption, Crombez et al. (1999) found that patients experiencing high-intensity pain and a high fear of pain show the largest decrements in task performance. This finding is preliminary evidence that in chronic pain situations, the interruptive function of pain is mediated by its threat value.

ENVIRONMENTAL CHARACTERISTICS

In the cognitive-affective model of pain (Eccleston and Crombez 1999), pain interrupts current behavior due to the selection of pain-related information at the expense of other demands in the environment. Attentional interruption by pain is therefore always the result of a dynamic interaction between the characteristics of the painful event and the characteristics of the other demands of the environment. It follows that pain will interrupt more in environments with fewer competing demands. In the context of symptom reporting, Pennebaker (1982) described the principle of cue competition, which states that individuals are most likely to notice physical sensations when there is a lack of external cues to compete with internal cues. This premise may be particularly true in monotonous and unrewarding environments. For example, joggers run faster and become less fatigued in an interesting cross-country run in comparison with repetitive running of laps (Pennebaker and Lightner 1980). Furthermore, in environments that lack stimulation, participants cough more (Pennebaker 1980), experience more extreme emotions (Pennebaker 1982), and are more aware of feelings of fatigue (Pennebaker and Brittingham 1982).

However, little is known about how and when this principle applies to the more aversive experience of pain. Studies investigating the mechanisms underlying distraction from pain have been inconclusive (McCaul et al. 1992; Johnson et al. 1998). Leventhal (1992) proposed emotional significance as the most important aspect of environmental demands. Evidence in support of this hypothesis remains, however, inconclusive in humans (Stevens et al. 1989), although it is well illustrated by the phenomenon of stress-induced analgesia (Bolles and Fanselow 1980). For example, when confronted with a rival or predator, rats become less sensitive to pain (Bolles and Fanselow 1980). An often cited example in humans has to do with the reduced complaints of pain and fewer requests for analgesia seen in soldiers with extensive injuries after combat (Beecher 1956). Beecher emphasized that in the battlefield environment, the threat to one's life is more important than the threat of pain. However, only in exceptional situations such as a threat to one's life does pain lose its demanding character.

SUMMARY

Pain demands attention and interrupts ongoing behavior even in situations when the current concern of the individual is not related to pain. Whether pain will interrupt behavior is the result of both pain-related characteristics (the intensity, novelty, and threat value of pain) and characteristics of other demands in the environment. According to the cognitive-affective model of pain, the threat value of pain is considered to be the key mediating pain-related variable.

VIGILANCE AND HYPERVIGILANCE TO PAIN

VIGILANCE

Systematic research about vigilance started in 1950 with Mackworth's work on naval recruits. He explored the phenomenon that many enemy submarines that were on the radar screen remained undetected by radar operators. In his studies, participants were instructed to watch the hand of a clock for 2 hours. Whenever the hand of the clock jumped 2 seconds instead of 1 second, the participant had to report it. Typically, vigilance experiments are employed to investigate the extent to which participants are able to sustain alertness in order to respond to weak external signals (such as visual or auditory stimuli). In this respect vigilance is dependent upon a currently activated goal (i.e., it is goal dependent) and involves the conscious and intentional alertness to respond to task-relevant targets.

VIGILANCE TO PAIN

Pain may also become the focus of attention because of its immediate relevance for the current goals or concerns of the individual. Individuals may then become vigilant for pain. So far, no studies have been done to test a paradigm in which participants would be instructed to sustain attention to detect painful stimuli or changes in pain experience in a monotonous environment. Many studies have, however, examined the immediate relevance of pain or pain-related information by giving explicit instructions (for review see Bushnell et al. 2004; Van Damme et al. 2004b). Miron et al. (1989) instructed healthy volunteers to detect as quickly as possible any subtle change in experimental pain or light intensity. Trials in which a change could occur were correctly cued (40%), not cued (50%), or erroneously cued (10%). Results indicated a better performance in terms of accuracy and speed when trials were correctly signaled. Self-reports of pain intensity and unpleasantness indicated the distraction of attention. When participants were cued for a change in light intensity, the pain stimulus was rated as less intense and unpleasant in comparison with trials in which changes were not cued. Expecting and paying attention to a change in pain intensity had no effect upon perceived pain intensity and unpleasantness. In a cross-modal cueing paradigm, Van Damme et al. (2002) instructed healthy volunteers to detect as quickly as possible a pain or auditory stimulus. Trials were cued with the words "pain" or "tone" or a series of X's. Although there was no contingency between the type of cue and the type of stimulus, participants believed cues to be predictive of stimuli. As hypothesized, stimulus detection was fastest with the congruent cue, and slowest with the incongruent cue. Particularly intriguing was the finding that participants had difficulty disengaging attention from the pain cue when they were cued for a pain stimulus, and an auditory stimulus appeared instead. In summary, these vigilance studies indicate that pain processing was prioritized over processing information in other modalities by means of a conscious intention to do so. Overall, the findings are in line with research in other perceptual modalities (Spence and Driver 1997). A conscious and intentional alertness to detect pain leads to a faster identification and a more accurate discrimination of pain information.

HYPERVIGILANCE TO PAIN

The helpfulness of the above vigilance studies for understanding hypervigilance is debatable for two reasons. First, hypervigilance emerges when a person's goal or concern is related to avoidance or escape from pain. Second, hypervigilance is primarily thought to be automatic and not intentionally controlled (McNally 1995). In order to understand hypervigilance to pain, we must take into account these two qualifications.

Hypervigilance is related to threat. The idea that hypervigilance is related to threat is straightforward. Chapman (1978), one of the first to apply this construct to pain, thought of hypervigilance as an emergent property of the threat value of pain. Individuals who use bodily sensation to evaluate danger were thought to be more likely to develop a habit of scanning the body for threatening sensations. Chapman's view is similar to that of Watson and Pennebaker (1989), who defined hypervigilance to bodily sensations as the increased likelihood of noticing and attending to normal bodily sensations and pains because they are fraught with anxiety and uncertainty. It comes as no surprise, then, that several models of hypervigilance can be found in the fear and anxiety literature (Eysenk 1992; Mogg and Bradley 1998). In several of these models, attention to threat plays a critical role in the etiology and maintenance of anxiety disorders.

Eysenck (1992) has provided one of the most elaborate accounts of hypervigilance. In contrast to Chapman (1978) and Watson and Pennebaker (1989), Eysenck did not restrict hypervigilance to an attentional scanning mechanism, but suggested that hypervigilance may be manifest in a variety of ways. Most importantly, these manifestations depend upon the temporal imminence of threat. The following example may clarify this idea. Imagine a man with a fear of spiders who goes to retrieve a bottle of wine from the cellar. The thought of descending the cellar stairs will be sufficient to make him fearful. This thought may also allow him to be distracted by several irrelevant stimuli in the environment (general hypervigilance). From the moment he descends the stairs, with the possibility of being confronted with a spider, he begins to scan the environment for the presence of spiders (broad attentional field and scanning). This behavior will result in the rapid detection of a spider. Attention will automatically be drawn to the spider (specific hypervigilance), and once it is detected, the man will have serious difficulties disengaging his attention from the spider and directing his focus to other stimuli, such as the labels on the wine bottles (narrowing of attention).

An application of this model in the area of pain is the body scanning paradigm of Peters et al. (2000). Patients suffering from fibromyalgia and pain-free volunteers were required to perform several tasks. One task was the detection of visual stimuli, and a second task was the detection of somatosensory stimuli. In the first two phases, both tasks were performed separately. Peters et al. hypothesized that there would be no difference in the detection of the somatosensory stimuli between the patient and the control groups. They reasoned that all participants were paying close attention to the somatosensory stimuli and to the visual stimuli. Results confirmed that there were indeed no differences between tasks. In a subsequent phase, both tasks were performed simultaneously. This phase was a critical test of the hypothesis that fibromyalgia patients are hypervigilant to somatosensory information, and the authors reasoned that the tendency to scan for somatic information would result in faster detection of somatosensory information. Counter to expectations, there was no evidence for scanning and specific hypervigilance to somatosensory information in the fibromyalgia patients. Of importance seemed to be the threat value of the somatosensory information independent of group membership. All participants with pain-related fear were quicker to detect somatosensory information. This finding is in line with a recent questionnaire study that revealed that hypervigilance to pain is not a unique and abnormal characteristic of fibromyalgia but is dependent upon the threat value of pain (Crombez et al. 2004). In summary, hypervigilance to pain can usefully be considered to be one particular example of hypervigilance to threat. Hypervigilance to threat is a dynamic process that consists of diverse components depending upon the imminence of threat, such as distractibility, selective attention, scanning, and difficulty disengaging. Scanning is only one possible attentional component of hypervigilance. Studies indicate that hypervigilance is not an abnormal and unique characteristic of patients, but emerges in everyone when the threat value of pain is high.

Hypervigilance is related to automatic processes. The qualification that hypervigilance is related to automatic processes is less obvious and requires clarification. In contrast to the reported vigilance studies, we propose that hypervigilance is not under conscious control (controlled processes), but is largely the result of automatic processes. Given that controlled processes have been characterized as intentional, controllable, effortful, and conscious, it is tempting to attribute the opposite features to the processes underlying hypervigilance: unintentional, uncontrollable, efficient, and occurring outside awareness. However, current views of automaticity have abandoned such dualistic views (Bargh 1994; Moors and De Houwer, in press). Cognitive processes are not exclusively automatic or exclusively controlled, but often involve features of each. It is therefore of paramount importance to identify those features that characterize the automatic nature of hypervigilance.

Recent experiments suggest that hypervigilance is unintentional. A prime characteristic of most experiments regarding hypervigilance is that the processing of pain or pain-related information is irrelevant, or sometimes counterproductive for the task at hand. In the primary task paradigm, for example, participants must perform as quickly as possible an auditory discrimination task in the presence of painful distracters (Crombez et al. 1998b). Despite the fact that the processing of pain-related information is irrelevant and not instrumental for immediate escape and avoidance, clear attentional effects may be found. These effects were more pronounced when the threat value of pain was high. A low-intensity stimulus produced marked interference with the performance of an auditory discrimination task in participants who were threatened by the possibility of high-intensity pain (Crombez et al. 1998a). This is especially the case when participants have catastrophic thoughts about pain (Crombez et al. 1998b). In particular, participants with catastrophic thoughts about pain have difficulty in disengaging attention from pain-related information (Van Damme et al. 2004a). Other studies substantiate that these attentional effects are threat-related and are not unique to pain (Koster et al. 2004).

Although the above effects are unintentional, we presume that they are, to a certain extent, controllable. In fact, all participants in our experiments were able to switch their attention back to the task and to complete it. In this sense attention is a controllable process. We argue, however, that this control is far from optimal and may hamper the efficacy of attentional coping strategies, in particular distraction. For example, individuals who catastrophize about imminent pain have difficulty performing distraction tasks. Goubert et al. (2004) studied patients with chronic low back pain who were required to lift a bag while performing a cognitive distraction task. The task consisted of responding as quickly as possible to a random series of tones. Those who experienced catastrophic thoughts about pain during the lifting task reported paying more attention to pain while lifting and, as expected, performed worse on the distraction task than those who experienced less catastrophic thoughts about pain. Evidence also indicates that those who catastrophize about pain experience less analgesia from distraction (Heyneman et al. 1990; Hadjistavoupoulos et al. 2000). Hadjistavropoulos et al. (2000) found that distraction from pain only works for patients who are not anxious about their health.

Because hypervigilance is an efficient process, control of hypervigilance has both limitations and costs. First, the attentional effects occur quickly (within a time window of 250 milliseconds), making it almost impossible to prevent or control them. Second, activation of the fear system that drives hypervigilance is not easily stopped. In some exceptional situations, the goal to escape and avoid pain may be displaced by a goal of higher priority (usually an even more threatening priority). In many situations, however, attempts to suppress fear and anxiety may prove futile or may even lead to a paradoxical increase of anxious thoughts once attempts to suppress fear are stopped (Sullivan et al. 1997; Koster et al. 2003). Koster et al. (2003) informed students who volunteered for their study that a painful but tolerable electrocutaneous stimulus would be applied. During the anticipation period, half of the students were instructed to suppress thoughts about the electrocutaneous stimulus (suppression group). The other half were allowed to think about anything (non-suppression group). The suppression group experienced a rebound once attempts to suppress the thoughts were halted: these students experienced more thoughts about the electrocutaneous stimulus and also reported more anxiety than the non-suppression group. Attempting to stop the fear system has costs.

As with the experience of fear, individuals may become conscious of the experience of hypervigilance and may thus report it. A corollary of this is that hypervigilance may be assessed in patients by using self-report instruments. Two types of self-report instruments may be considered. One type of questionnaire assesses the consequences of hypervigilance, i.e., to what extent persons are aware of particular bodily sensations, such as the Pennebaker Inventory of Limbic Languidness (Pennebaker 1982) or the Modified Somatic Perceptions Questionnaire (Main 1983). It is apparent that this type of instrument may be problematic because alternative interpretations for the presence of bodily sensations are not accounted for. Also, one should be aware of potential confusion between the item content of these questionnaires and the diagnostic criteria of syndromes. For instance, the diagnostic criteria for fibromyalgia and chronic fatigue include multiple somatic complaints. The second, and more useful, type of questionnaire assesses more directly the experience of hypervigilance. For example, the Pain Vigilance and Awareness Questionnaire (McCracken 1997) assesses vigilance for pain sensations using 16 items (e.g., "I am quick to notice changes in pain intensity"); respondents are asked to indicate how frequently each item was experienced during the past 2 weeks.

SUMMARY

Vigilance is a conscious and intentional alertness characterized by a readiness to respond to environmental changes. To my knowledge, no study has used the prototypical vigilance paradigm in which participants are instructed to sustain attention to detect painful stimuli or changes in pain experience in a monotonous environment. However, many experiments have manipulated the immediate relevance of pain or pain-related information by giving explicit instructions. Overall, the results of these studies indicate that vigilance to pain leads to a faster identification and a more accurate discrimination of pain information. In contrast to vigilance, hypervigilance is an unintentional and efficient process that emerges when the threat value of pain is high, the fear system is activated, and the individual's current concern is to escape and avoid pain. Hypervigilance can be controlled, but not without costs.

IMPLICATIONS

Our analysis of interruption and hypervigilance has several theoretical and clinical implications. From an evolutionary perspective, pain is meant to interrupt attention and ongoing behavior. The experience of chronic pain is therefore the chronic interruption of attention. Cognitive complaints about memory and concentration in patients suffering from chronic pain may be related to this interruptive function. Of importance is that attention to pain does not seem to result from abnormal characteristics of the individual. Available evidence suggests that attention to pain emerges as a normal cognitive mechanism in abnormal situations. Optimal use of pain medication should be a priority, but other techniques to lower the threat value of pain also may have value.

Interruption of attention by pain is dependent upon environmental characteristics. Although we know of no study that has investigated the natural environments in which chronic pain patients live, it is plausible that many patients have a restricted and monotonous life that lacks external stimulation. It will be a challenge to identify those environments or activities that may compete with pain in a natural and spontaneous way.

Hypervigilance is primarily a goal-dependent attentional process, and it should not be confused with other central mechanisms that account for hyperalgesia, allodynia, and hyperresponsivity. Hypervigilance cannot easily be studied in paradigms that instruct all participants to attend to pain. For these reasons, the standard assessment of pain threshold or pain tolerance should be considered inadequate when used as an indicator of hypervigilance. Hypervigilance may be better studied in situations with competing attentional demands. Most useful are those paradigms in which attention is directed away from pain, or in which attention to pain is irrelevant for the task at hand.

Because hypervigilance is unintentional and efficient, it may undermine distraction strategies. Pain is designed to demand attention, and especially when one is fearful about it, pain is easily detected and difficult to disengage from. There may be merit in attentional training strategies that teach patients to use attention in a flexible way and to disengage their attention from pain once it is detected (Morley et al. 2003). Hypervigilance facilitates the detection of pain and pain-related information and is probably strongly related to action tendencies to escape or avoid. More research is needed to corroborate the idea that the interruptive quality of pain and hypervigilance is intrinsically related to action and motor control mechanisms.

Whether hypervigilance directly amplifies the sensory experience of pain (Barsky and Klerman 1983) is still a matter of debate, and empirical research needs to be carried out in both healthy volunteers and pain patients. In line with this idea are the findings that pain expectancies in clinical samples do not amplify pain intensity, but intensify escape or avoidance tendencies (Crombez et al. 1996). I propose that the so-called "amplification of pain" is the consequence of a failure to successfully distract oneself from pain. However, other explanations should also be considered. It is possible that pain evokes a more intense defensive and fearful response in those hypervigilant to pain and amplifies the affective qualities of pain instead of its sensory qualities. The clinical impression that hypervigilance may cause more intense pain is based upon correlational data, and therefore no conclusive inference may be made about its causal status. It is equally possible that the experience of high-intensity pain creates fear of pain and hypervigilance.

Because hypervigilance emerges when the threat value of pain is high, it is not unique to a particular syndrome such as low back pain or fibromyalgia. Every pain syndrome may contain subgroups of patients displaying hypervigilance to pain. Hypervigilance may be a characteristic of both medically explained and medically unexplained pain.

Because both the interruptive quality of pain and hypervigilance are dependent upon the threat value of pain, a valuable treatment option is to target its threat value. This goal may be accomplished by a diversity of therapeutic techniques. It is possible both to challenge erroneous beliefs about pain (Vlaeyen and Linton 2000) and to learn to accept that a meaningful life is possible despite pain (McCracken et al. 2004).

REFERENCES

Aldrich S, Eccleston C, Crombez G. Worrying about chronic pain: vigilance to threat and misdirected problem solving. *Behav Res Ther* 2000; 38:457–470.

Allport A. Visual attention. In: Posner MI (Ed). *Foundation of Cognitive Science*. Cambridge, MA: MIT Press, 1989, pp 631–682.

Bargh JA. The four horsemen of automaticity: awareness, intention, efficiency, and control in social cognition. In: Wyer RS, Srull TK (Eds). *Basic Processes*, Handbook of Social Cognition, Vol. 1. Hillsdale NJ: Lawrence Erlbaum, 1994, pp 1–40.

Barsky AJ, Klerman GL. Overview: hypochondriasis, bodily complaints, and somatic styles. *Am J Psychiatry* 1983; 140:273–283.

Beecher HK. Relationship of significance of wound to pain experienced. *JAMA* 1956; 161:1609–1613.

Bolles RC, Fanselow MS. A perceptual-defensive-recuperative model of fear and pain. *Behav Brain Sci* 1980; 3:291–323.

Bushnell MC, Villemure C, Duncan GH. Psychophysical and neurophysical studies of pain modulation by attention. In: Price DD, Bushnell MC (Eds). *Psychological Methods of Pain Control: Basic Science and Clinical Perspective.* Seattle: IASP Press, 2004, pp 99–116.

Chapman CR. Pain: the perception of noxious events. In: Sternbach RA (Ed). *The Psychology of Pain.* New York: Raven Press, 1978, pp 169–202.

Crombez G, Baeyens F, Eelen P. Sensory and temporal information about impending pain: the influence of predictability on pain. *Behav Res Ther* 1994; 32:611–622.

Crombez G, Vervaet L, Baeyens F, Lysens R, Eelen P. Do pain expectancies cause pain in chronic low back pain patients? A clinical investigation. *Behav Res Ther* 1996; 34:919–925.

Crombez G, Eccleston C, Baeyens F, Eelen P. Attentional disruption is enhanced by the threat of pain. *Behav Res Ther* 1998a; 36:195–204.

Crombez G, Eccleston C, Baeyens F, Eelen P. When somatic information threatens, catastrophic thinking enhances attentional interference. *Pain* 1998b; 75:187–198.

Crombez G, Eccleston C, Baeyens F, Van Houdenhove B, Van den Broeck A. Attention to chronic pain is dependent upon pain-related fear. *J Psychosom Res* 1999; 47:403–410.

Crombez G, Eccleston C, Van den Broeck A, Goubert L, Van Houdenhove B. Hypervigilance to pain in fibromyalgia: the mediating role of pain intensity and catastrophic thinking about pain. *Clin J Pain* 2004: 20:103–110.

Eccleston C. Chronic pain and attention: a cognitive approach. *Br J Clin Psychol* 1994; 33:535–547.

Eccleston C. Chronic pain and distraction: an experimental investigation into the role of sustained and shifting attention in the processing of chronic persistent pain. *Behav Res Ther* 1995; 33:391–405.

Eccleston C, Crombez G. Pain demands attention: a cognitive-affective model on the interruptive function of pain. *Psychol Bull* 1999; 125:356–366.

Eysenck MW. *Anxiety: The Cognitive Perspective.* Hillsdale, NJ: Lawrence Erlbaum, 1992.

Goubert L, Crombez G, Eccleston C, Devulder J. Distraction from chronic pain during a pain-inducing activity is associated with greater post-activity pain. *Pain* 2004; 110:220–227.

Graham FK, Hackley SA. Passive and active attention to input. In: Jennings JR, Coles MGH (Eds). *Handbook of Cognitive Psychophysiology: Central and Autonomic Nervous System Approaches.* Chichester: John Wiley & Sons, 1991, pp 251–356.

Hadjistavropoulos HD, Hadjistavropoulos T, Quine A. Health anxiety moderates the effects of distraction versus attention to pain. *Behav Res Ther* 2000; 38:425–438.

Heyneman NE, Fremouw WJ, Gano D, Kirkland F, Heiden L. Individual differences and the effectiveness of different coping strategies for pain. *Cogn Ther Res* 1990; 14:63–77.

Jamison RN, Sbrocco T, Paris WCV. The influence of problems with concentration and memory on emotional distress and daily activities in chronic pain patients. *Int J Psychiatry Med* 1988; 18:183–191.

Johnson MH, Breakwell G, Douglas W, Humphries S. The effects of imagery and sensory detection distractors on different measures of pain: how does distraction works? *Br J Clin Psychol* 1998; 37:141–154.

Klinger E. The contents of thoughts: interference as the downside of adaptive normal mechanisms in thought flow. In: Sarason IG, Pierce GR, Sarason BR (Eds). *Cognitive Interference: Theories, Methods and Findings.* Mahwah, NJ: Lawrence Erlbaum, 1996.

Koster EHW, Crombez G, Van Damme S, Verschuere B, De Houwer J. Does imminent threat capture and hold attention? *Emotion 2004*;4: 312-317.

Koster EHW, Rassin E, Crombez G, Naring GWB. The paradoxical effects of suppressing anxious thoughts during imminent threat. *Behav Res Ther* 2003; 41:1113–1120.

Legrain V, Bruyer R, Guerit JM, Plaghki L. Nociceptive processing in the human brain of infrequent task-relevant and task-irrelevant noxious stimuli. A study with event-related potentials evoked by CO_2 laser radiant heat stimuli. *Pain* 2004; 103:237–248.

Leventhal H. I know distraction works even though it doesn't. *Health Psychol* 1992; 11:208–209.

Lorenz J, Bromm B. Event-related potential correlates of interference between cognitive performance and tonic experimental pain. *Psychophysiology* 1997; 34:436–445.

Lorenz J, Beck H, Bromm B. Cognitive performance, mood and experimental pain before and during morphine-induced analgesia in patients with chronic non-malignant pain. *Pain* 1997; 73:369–375.

Mackworth NH. *Researches in the Measurement of Human Performance.* Medical Research Council Special Report Series 268, 1950.

Main CJ. The Modified Somatic Perception Questionnaire (MSPQ). *J Psychosom Res* 1983; 2:503–514.

McCaul KD, Monson N, Maki RH. Does distraction reduce pain-produced distress among college students? *Health Psychol* 1992; 11:210–217.

McCracken LM. Attention to pain in persons with chronic pain: a behavioural approach. *Behav Res Ther* 1997; 28:271–284.

McCracken LM, Carson JW, Eccleston C, Keefe FJ. Acceptance and change in the context of chronic pain. *Pain* 2004; 109:4–7.

McNally RC. Automaticity and the anxiety disorders. *Behav Res Ther* 1995; 33:747–754.

Miron D, Duncan GB, Bushnell MC. Effects of attention on the intensity and unpleasantness of thermal pain. *Pain* 1989; 39:345–352.

Mogg K, Bradley BP. A cognitive-motivational analysis of anxiety. *Behav Res Ther* 1998; 36:809–848.

Moors A, De Houwer J. Automaticity: a theoretical and conceptual analysis. *Psychol Bull,* in press.

Morley S, Shapiro DA, Biggs J. Developing a treatment manual for attention management in chronic pain. *Cogn Behav Ther* 2003; 32:1–12.

Pennebaker JW. Perceptual and environmental determinants of coughing. *Basic Appl Soc Psych* 1980;1:83–91.

Pennebaker JW. *The Psychology of Physical Symptoms.* New York: Springer-Verlag, 1982.

Pennebaker JW, Lightner JM. Competition of internal and external information in an exercise setting. *J Pers Soc Psychol* 1980; 39:165–174.

Pennebaker JW, Brittingham GL. Environmental and sensory cues affecting the perception of physical symptoms. In: Baum A, Singer J (Eds). *Advances in Environmental Psychology,* Vol. 4. Hillsdale, NJ: Erlbaum, 1982.

Peters ML, Vlaeyen JWS, van Drunen. Do fibromyalgia patients display hypervigilance for innocuous somatosensory stimuli? Application of a body scanning reaction time paradigm. *Pain* 2000; 86:283–292.

Sarter M, Givens B, Bruno JP. The cognitive neuroscience of sustained attention: where top-down meets bottom-up. *Brain Res Rev* 2001; 35:146–160.

Spence C, Driver J. On measuring selective attention to an expected sensory modality. *Percept Psychophys* 1997; 59:389–403.

Stevens MJ, Heise RA, Pfost KS. Consumption of attention versus affect elicited by cognitions in modifying acute pain. *Psychol Rep* 1989; 64:284–286.

Sullivan MJL, Rouse D, Bishop S, Johnston S. Thought suppression, catastrophizing, and pain. *Cogn Ther Res* 1997; 21:555–568.

Van Damme S, Crombez G, Eccleston C. Retarded disengagement from pain cues: the effects of pain catastrophizing and pain expectancy. *Pain* 2002; 100:111–118.

Van Damme S, Crombez G, Eccleston C. The anticipation of pain modulates spatial attention: evidence for pain-specificity in high-pain catastrophizers. *Pain* 2004a; 111:392–399.

Van Damme S, Crombez G, Eccleston C, Roelofs J. The role of hypervigilance in the experience of pain. In: Asmundson GJG, Vlaeyen JWS, Crombez G (Eds). *Understanding and Treating Fear of Pain.* Oxford University Press, 2004b, pp 71–94.

Vlaeyen JWS, Linton SJ. Fear-avoidance and its consequences in chronic musculoskeletal pain: a state of the art. *Pain* 2000; 85:317–332.

Wall PD. Introduction to the edition after this one. In: Wall PD, Melzack R (Eds). *The Textbook of Pain,* 3rd ed. Edinburgh: Churchill Livingstone, 1994, pp 1–7.

Watson D, Pennebaker JW. Health complaints, stress, and distress: exploring the central role of negative affectivity. *Psychol Rev* 1989; 96:234–254.

Zaslansky R, Sprecher E, Tenke CE, Hemli JA, Yarnitsky D. The P300 in pain evoked potentials. *Pain* 1996; 66:39–49.

Correspondence to: Geert Crombez, PhD, Professor of Health Psychology, Department of Experimental Clinical Psychology and Health Psychology, Ghent University, Henri Dunantlaan 2, 9000 Ghent, Belgium. Email: geert.crombez@ugent.be.

Proceedings of the 11th World Congress on Pain, edited by Herta Flor, Eija Kalso, and Jonathan O. Dostrovsky, IASP Press, Seattle, © 2006.

47

Who Will Develop Chronic Pain and Why? The Epidemiological Evidence

Gary J. Macfarlane

Epidemiology Group, Department of Public Health, Medical School, University of Aberdeen, Aberdeen, United Kingdom

In this chapter I will review the epidemiological data on who develops pain, particularly chronic pain. I will focus on low back pain because it is the most common regional pain syndrome and one that exhibits epidemiological features that are fairly typical of other regional pain syndromes (Macfarlane 1999). The chapter will be divided into four sections. The first two are concerned with the burden (prevalence) and the causes (etiology) of back pain. Epidemiology is at its most useful with respect to pain syndromes when the information from such studies influences and optimizes management, and therefore the third section will focus briefly on influences on secondary prevention and pain management. Finally, in the fourth section, I will give some personal thoughts on possible future areas for useful investigation by epidemiological study.

BURDEN (PREVALENCE)

One of the first issues in the study of low back pain is definition. What should we ask participants about in a study? How does one define the low back? Should one leave it to the respondent to decide whether the pain he or she is experiencing is in the low back, or should one provide a reference area or definition? What time period should be considered—any low back pain or pain that has been experienced for a minimum period of time? It is unlikely that *any* low back pain would be of interest, since such an experience is almost universal and in most cases will have little implication for the individual or for health services. But how long should the pain last before it becomes "significant"? Finally, should there be some measure of severity, and if so, how should this be defined—perhaps in terms of pain rating or functional ability? The lack of a standard definition hampers, as exemplified later, comparison between studies and evaluation of prevalence over time. In one study conducted in children in the North-West of England, in response to the question "Have you experienced low back pain lasting at least 24 hours during the past month," 27% of participants responded positively (Jones et al. 2003). When asked the same question but referred to a picture of the area as shown in Fig. 1 rather than using the words "low back," 33% responded positively. Finally, when asked to indicate any pain experienced in the last month lasting at least 24 hours on a blank diagram, 46% shaded at least some pain in the area shown in Fig. 1 (G.T. Jones, personal communication). This example demonstrates the important influence of the manner in which patients are asked to report pain. A recent working group (de Vet et al. 2002) proposed some standard definitions of episodes of low back pain for use in epidemiological research (Table I). These definitions, used in combination with a drawing similar to Fig. 1, are not necessarily better than other possible definitions, but their use in epidemiological research will aid comparability between studies.

Low back pain has a high prevalence, even in young adults. A study in Lübeck, Germany, found a prevalence of "back pain today" above 20% among adults in their twenties, and prevalence increased throughout adult years until approximately the age of 60 (Raspe and Kohlmann 1994; Raspe 2001) (Fig. 2). This observed pattern of prevalence by age has often been used to support the effect of cumulative exposures, particularly in the workplace. Several studies have suggested that prevalence may decrease after the age of 60, and a recent study conducted in the Midlands region of England confirmed that at older ages, low back pain becomes less common (Thomas et al. 2004). Further, a study

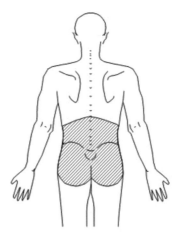

Fig 1. A body diagram that can be used to define the low back area.

Table I
Definitions of an episode of low back pain

Low Back Pain Episode: Period of pain in the lower back lasting for more than 24 hours preceded and followed by a period of at least 1 month without low back pain.

Episode of Care: Consultation(s) preceded and followed by a period of at least 3 months without consultation for low back pain.

Episode of Work Absence: A period of work absence due to low back pain preceded and followed by a period of at least 1 day at work.

Source: From de Vet et al. (2002).

of U.S. veterans found that among persons aged 100 years or older, back pain prevalence was less than half of that among those aged 85–99 years (Selim et al. 2005). The reasons for the decrease in back pain at older ages could include (1) increased mortality amongst persons reporting back pain, (2) a decreasing risk factor load, (3) the presence of comorbidities lessening the perceived importance or troublesomeness of back pain, or (4) the expectation of pain at older ages reducing the likelihood of it being reported. There is no evidence for hypothesis 1 (Heliövaara et al. 1995), although the number of studies conducted is small, and data from the previously mentioned study in the Midlands, the North Staffordshire Osteoarthritis Project (Thomas et al. 2004), suggest that pain reported at older ages is just as severe and disabling, if not more so, than at younger ages, making hypotheses 3 and 4 unlikely. The understanding of why back pain, in addition to several other regional pains, becomes less common

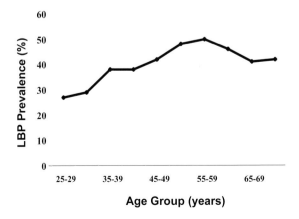

Fig. 2. The population prevalence of low back pain in Lübeck, Germany. Based on data from from Raspe and Kohlmann (1994).

with older age is an interesting and important area for future research (Gibson and Weiner 2005).

The observed pattern of an increased prevalence through adult ages until approximately the seventh decade and a decrease at older ages is evident in both males and females, but at all ages the prevalence is higher in females than males. The reasons for this difference in pain prevalence between males and females is discussed in detail in this volume in the chapter "Gender, Sex, and Clinical Pain" by LeResche.

For reasons of definition mentioned previously, it is difficult to compare prevalence rates among studies to determine whether there are between-country or within-country regional differences. A study conducted in the United Kingdom assessed the prevalence of back pain in different regions using the same definition ("back pain that had lasted for 24 hours or longer during the previous 12 months" in the area shown in Fig. 1) and found very similar rates (Palmer et al. 2000). In all areas, with the exception of the South-East (mainly Greater London), with a prevalence of 60%, regional rates varied between 52% and 56%. Similarly, in studies conducted in other European countries, any variations observed could easily be accounted for by variations in definition, although there is some evidence from studies conducted in more than one country that differences in prevalence may exist (Raspe et al. 2004). Studies are under way using consistent definitions across several countries that will allow the examination of this issue in more detail.

Have rates of back pain changed over time? Media headlines may convince us that we are experiencing a pain epidemic, and certainly if one uses surrogate measures such as health care spending, one may believe that this premise is supported (Waddell 2004). The best data over time on back pain prevalence comes from Finland, where data have been collected annually from 1979 to 1992 (Fig. 3), using a consistent definition (Leino et al. 1994). This study found no substantial increase in back pain prevalence over time, a finding that is generally, but not universally (e.g., Palmer et al. 2000), supported by other data.

CAUSES (ETIOLOGY)

I will consider potential risk factors under two broad categories: environmental and individual factors. The prevalence of low back pain varies with social class. In a United Kingdom study, prevalence was lowest amongst professional grades and generally increased as class decreased, being highest in unskilled manual workers (Palmer et al. 2000). This observation suggests that factors associated with social class may influence risk. The first likely candidate is lifestyle: obesity is a predictor (either a risk factor or risk marker) of developing low back pain (Leboeuf-Yde 2000; Dunn and Croft 2004), and there is some evidence relating a lack of exercise to an increased risk of onset of low back pain and poor outcome (Hildebrandt et al. 2000). Further, and independently, those who smoke cigarettes are also at increased risk (Skovron 1992). Whether the added risk is due to mechanical effects of coughing amongst smokers or due to vascular effects is not clear. These lifestyles are more common among low social classes and will therefore at least partly explain the increased prevalence of back pain in this group. The second obvious influence on persons of lower social class (who by definition are more likely to be manual workers) is work-place mechanical injury. A review by the National Institute for Occupational Safety and Heath (1999) has identified four such factors with strong evidence relating them to back pain: mechanical load (lifting), forceful load movement (such as pushing and pulling), awkward posture, and whole-body vibration. For each factor, most studies examining the relationship had found an association, and there was a dose-risk relationship in terms of the amount of time spent carrying out the activity. Taken together, these exposures were associated with important increased risks and are activities that are relatively common in the population. In a prospective population study conducted in Manchester, in the North-West of England, which followed prospectively 7,699 subjects to moni-tor the onset of low back pain, two of the five factors that best predicted which subjects would develop back pain were workplace mechanical factors (lifting heavy weights and prolonged periods of standing). The population attributable

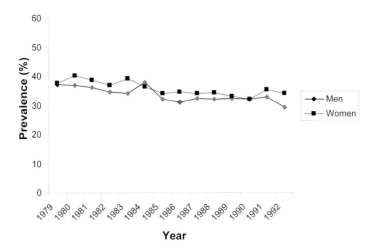

Fig. 3. Population prevalence time trends in back pain in Finland between 1979 and 1992. The definition of back pain was changed between 1984 and 1985. Adapted from Leino et al. (1994).

risk (i.e., the proportion of episodes related to these chapters) was approximately 10% (Thomas 1999).

PSYCHOSOCIAL FACTORS

An area that has been a topic of particular interest during the past decade is the role of psychosocial factors in the workplace on pain, including low back pain. In a comprehensive review, Bongers et al. (1993) concluded that "even though the overall picture is unclear, an association has been seen between low back pain and several psychosocial job variables ... but many of the studies suffer from methodological shortcomings." One of these shortcomings was related to the fact that many studies were cross-sectional, and it is generally not possible to determine from such studies whether the adverse psychosocial factor (e.g., lack of job satisfaction) preceded the onset of back pain and therefore may be a risk factor or at least a risk marker, or whether persons who developed back pain found it more difficult to carry out their job and therefore felt under pressure because of suboptimal performance and thus had lower job satisfaction. The only way to disentangle this effect is to conduct prospective cohort studies among persons free of low back pain, measuring potential risk factors at the beginning of the study. A follow-up survey should determine which persons go on to develop low back pain and then determine whether this pain onset is predicted by the previously measured factors. Hartvigsen et al. (2004) recently conducted a review of workplace psychosocial factors using information only from prospective studies. They examined perception of work, organizational aspects, support, and stress. The results showed that for each of these areas, only around one in five studies reported a relationship with low back pain; the results were only marginally stronger among studies rated as high quality (Table II). Therefore, at present there is a lack of consistent evidence from high-quality studies that specific adverse psychosocial factors are related to the onset of low

Table II
Psychosocial factors predicting low back pain: a systematic review
of data from prospective studies

	No. Studies (High Quality)	
Psychosocial Factor	Total	Demonstrated Positive Association
Perception of work	9 (4)	2 (1)
Organizational aspects of work	9 (3)	2 (1)
Social support at work	9 (3)	2 (0)
Stress at work	5 (2)	1 (1)

Source: Data from Hartvigsen et al. (2004).

back pain. However, evidence continues to accumulate from individual studies that at least some psychosocial factors increase the future risk of low back pain onset. One study conducted among a cohort of newly employed workers (primarily entering their first occupation) aimed to identify factors that pertained around the time of recruitment as predictors of low back pain during the next two years. Some of the most important factors were psychosocial, namely high demands (stressful or hectic work), low demands (monotonous work, seldom learning new things), and dissatisfaction with support from colleagues (Harkness et al. 2003). In contrast to the inconsistent data on work-related psychosocial factors, individual psychological factors are important; increasing levels of psychological distress in those free of low back pain increases the risk of a new episode (Croft et al. 1995).

PATHOLOGY

With respect to individual factors, disease pathology such as tumor or infection is a very uncommon cause of low back pain. Spinal degeneration is only weakly related to low back pain. Genetic factors have been related to degenerative conditions of the spine (Manek and MacGregor 2005) rather than to the reporting of low back pain or pain perception generally (MacGregor et al. 1997).

BIOLOGICAL FACTORS

The data above are presented assuming that a given risk factor or risk factor load will have the same effect on all individuals. However, casual observation, combined with data available from epidemiological studies, demonstrates that some persons develop pain with a low risk factor load, while many do not develop pain despite having multiple risk factors. We hypothesized that there would be some biological factors that would importantly modify the risk of pain onset among those evaluated at high risk of developing symptoms. We examined the role of the hypothalamic-pituitary-adrenal (HPA) axis, which is responsible for the stress response. We identified, from a population study of 11,000 subjects, people who were at risk of developing chronic widespread pain based on psychosocial factors, past symptom history, and aspects of illness behavior. We then evaluated aspects of HPA function by measuring morning and evening salivary cortisol, as well as serum cortisol after administration of low-dose dexamethasone and a after a tender point examination (as a marker of physical stress). On multivariate analysis we found that older age (more than 50 years), serum cortisol in the middle or highest tertile post-dexamethasone and high evening salivary cortisol predicted development of chronic widespread pain in this at-risk group. Among this at-risk group, none of the participants who did not have any of the three risk factors listed developed chronic widespread pain, while among those with all three risk factors the new onset rate was just below 30% (McBeth et al. 2005). It is not known whether the same results would hold for a regional pain syndrome such as low back pain, and this possibility will need to be tested in future studies. However, the data suggest that biological factors can be important modifiers of environmental influences on disease.

SECONDARY PREVENTION AND MANAGEMENT

Epidemiological studies of back pain will partly be judged on their success at informing successful pain management. In order to design potential intervention strategies, it is important to understand the predictors of outcome of a consulting episode of back pain. In a population of 1,000 persons, around 30 individuals will experience an episode of back pain during the course of a year. However, only approximately one in five (i.e., six individuals) will consult a primary care physician with these symptoms. Of these six persons, three will have symptoms that will resolve in the short term, while three will continue to have pain and disability. What are the factors that distinguish those persons whose symptoms will improve from those whose symptoms will persist? The South Manchester Low Back Pain Study identified 180 consulters to primary care, measured potential predictive factors, and then followed them over the subsequent 6 months. Six factors of three types (demographic, clinical, and psychosocial) identified those at high risk of developing symptoms (Fig. 4) (Thomas et al. 1999). A recent review has also highlighted the important role of psychological factors in predicting outcome (Pincus et al. 2002). There was strong evidence linking poor outcome to psychological distress and depressive mood, moderate evidence in relation to somatization, and weak evidence in relation to style of coping.

Given that it is possible to identify which persons consulting with back pain are at high risk of persistent symptoms, it is instructive to review the results of three major randomized clinical trials of back pain management that were recently published. The first study, the UK BEAM trial, was an evaluation of "best care" alone—principally encouragement to return to normal activities and provision of a copy of *The Back Book* along with information and advice about back pain (Burton et al. 1999)—in comparison with best care plus exercise classes, manipulation, or both. The exercise component comprised initial individual assessment followed by group exercise classes incorporating cognitive-behavioral principles. Up to 10 people took part in each group, which comprised eight 60-minute sessions. Participants who were randomized to manipulation were

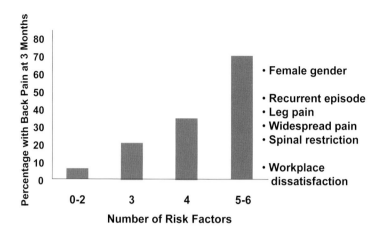

Fig. 4. Predicting the persistence of back pain. Based on data from the South Manchester Low Back Pain Study (Thomas et al. 1999).

invited to receive eight 20-minute sessions over 12 weeks. Where subjects were randomized to manipulation and exercise, they received manipulation first. All groups had improved over 12 months, but for exercise alone there was no significant improvement over best care on the Roland and Morris Disability Scale, whereas for manipulation the improvement was 1.0 (95% CI= 0.2–1.8), and for both interventions the improvement was 1.3 (0.5–1.2). These improvements in disability for the intervention are very modest (UK BEAM Trial Team 2004).

The second study was a comparison of physical treatment versus a brief pain management program amongst persons consulting primary care physicians for treatment of back pain (so-called "hands-on" versus "hands-off" physiotherapy). The hands-on physiotherapy was orientated toward spinal manual-therapy techniques and was designed to be consistent with best current manual therapy in the United Kingdom. The brief pain management program was designed to identify and address psychosocial risk factors for persistent or recurrent disability relating to back pain. Both interventions consisted of one 40-minute assessment and treatment session and six 20-minute treatment sessions. Outcome was almost identical at 12 months in the hands-on and hands-off physiotherapy groups: 68% and 67% were completely or much better, respectively, and the degree of satisfaction was 93 mm (on a 0–100-mm scale) with both interventions. It is not known if either of the interventions would have been superior to "best care" because there was no such arm in this study (Hay et al. 2005).

The final study, from the Netherlands, and also in primary care, examined the effect of trained general practitioners identifying and discussing any potential psychosocial barriers to recovery in a special 20-minute consultation session. The particular issues addressed were the patient's idea of cause, fear avoidance beliefs, worries about pain, catastrophizing, pain behavior, reactions from family, and physical and physical or psychological work factors. Participants who were not randomized to this intervention received usual care. There was no significant difference in outcome over 12 months on any of the outcome measures used (Jellema et al. 2005).

These results, when considered together, are important because two of the studies were identifying either mechanical treatments (exercise or manipulation) or psychosocial interventions which a priori were expected to deliver better outcomes. The benefits observed, if any, were very small. The Hay study showed no difference between two alternative management strategies, but whether they were better than "best care" is unknown.

Thus, the current phase of intervention studies, partly designed on data from epidemiological studies of onset and outcome, are failing to deliver important improvements in outcome. There are several possible reasons. Perhaps these interventions are not effective, or if they are, perhaps they are not being properly delivered (e.g., the training and monitoring may not be sufficient to ensure delivery of the intervention package, or the patients may not be receiving the intended messages). Future studies and refinements of clinical trials will be necessary in order to understand why these interventions may not be effective.

FUTURE DIRECTIONS

What, then, does the future hold for epidemiological investigations? Some have suggested that there is little point in conducting future epidemiological studies of onset and outcome and have questioned the use to which the results of such studies would be put. If future studies are conducted to measure the burden of symptoms, they will only be useful if they use standard definitions allowing direct comparison with other studies.

Given that the improvements observed in functional outcome with low back pain have been at best modest with current intervention studies, the challenge for future epidemiological studies will be to ensure that their results are relevant for informing studies examining management. What are the options for future study? Some might argue that there is a need to re-examine the role of etiology. If this approach is taken, we will need some novel hypotheses with respect to etiology. What might these be? One area for investigation is the role of early life factors. Evidence from retrospective studies indicates that early life events (or the perception of such events) may be important in the experience of pain in adulthood. Further, prospective studies of functional disorders such as abdominal pain have shown that early life events are important determinants of future health, although not necessarily of abdominal symptoms themselves (Hotopf et al. 1998). Such factors may influence the response to management strategies. This chapter has presented data on the possible modification of the effect of certain psychological factors by the function of the HPA axis. There may be other biological determinants of risk factor effects, including the response of such systems to the effects of stressors and the sensory processing of information. I have not considered genetic factors in this chapter because the available evidence is inconsistent on their importance. However, large-scale studies are being set up to examine the influence of genetic and environmental factors on health in some countries, and they may also provide an opportunity to collect information on pain and examine how genetic factors may further refine the identification of persons at risk for developing regional and widespread pain syndromes. Some might argue that we need to further refine our measure of some risk factors for onset and persistence of such syndromes. This suggestion applies particularly to psychosocial factors because the available information suggests that they may be important, but the data are inconsistent, and we do not fully understand how some of these factors might operate.

There are challenges on how therapeutic interventions might result in a better functional outcome for patients. At present, trials of primary care most often offer a standard intervention to which participants may or may not be assigned. It may be that in the next generation of studies the interventions will need to be more closely related to the risk factor profile of the patients. A further area of interest centers around patient preference for treatment, which may provide useful information relevant to improving patient outcome.

Despite the hope that these future avenues of research may allow us to further understand the epidemiology and outcome of low back pain and other pain syndromes, it is unlikely that a single treatment or series of targeted managements will result in a greatly improved outcome in comparison to those offered currently. Given that low back pain and other regional pains are very common and have a multifactorial etiology, we may have to rethink our expectations and consider that new interventions are likely to provide at most modest improvements over current best care. Such improvements, particularly if they are achieved at reasonable cost, are worthwhile. The challenge to those conducting epidemiological studies of pain in the future is to ensure that they design their studies so as to provide information that will contribute to these new programs of management.

ACKNOWLEDGMENTS

I would like to acknowledge the contribution to the work on back pain of my colleagues at The University of Manchester. Alan J. Silman has been co-principal investigator on the program of work undertaken. Peter R. Croft was co-principal investigator on the South Manchester Low Back Pain Study, and Elaine Thomas undertook much of the analysis of this study; both are now at The University of Keele. All have made important intellectual contributions to the work on back pain. I would like to thank also Drs. John McBeth and Gareth T. Jones, who latterly have been responsible for running the research programs within my group at the University of Manchester.

REFERENCES

Bongers PM, de Winter CR, Kompier MA, Hildebrandt VH. Psychosocial factors at work and musculoskeletal disease. *Scand J Work Environ Health* 1993; 19:297–312.

Burton AK, Waddell G, Tillotson KM, Summerton N. Information and advice to patients with back pain can have a positive effect. A randomized controlled trial of a novel educational booklet in primary care. *Spine* 1999; 24:2482–2491.

Croft PR, Papageorgiou AC, Ferry S, et al. Psychologic distress and low back pain. Evidence from a prospective study in the general population. *Spine* 1995; 20:2731–2737.

de Vet HC, Heymans MW, Dunn KM, et al. Episodes of low back pain: a proposal for uniform definitions to be used in research. *Spine* 2002; 27:2409–2416.

Dunn KM, Croft PR. Epidemiology and natural history of low back pain. *Eura Medicophys* 2004; 40:9–13.

Gibson SJ, Weiner DK. *Pain in Older Persons,* Progress in Pain Research and Management, Vol. 35. Seattle: IASP Press, 2005.

Harkness EF, Macfarlane GJ, Nahit ES, Silman AJ, McBeth J. Risk factors for new-onset low back pain amongst cohorts of newly employed workers. *Rheumatology* 2003; 42:959–968.

Hartvigsen J, Lings S, Leboeuf-Yde C, Bakketeig L. Psychological factors at work in relation to low back pain and consequences of low back pain; a systematic, critical review of prospective cohort studies. *Occup Environ Med* 2004; 61:e2.

Hay EM, Mullis R, Lewis M, et al. Comparison of physical treatments versus a brief pain-management programme for back pain in primary care: a randomised clinical trial in physiotherapy practice. *Lancet* 2005; 365:2024–2030.

Heliövaara M, Mäkelä M, Aromaa A, et al. Low back pain and subsequent cardiovascular mortality. *Spine* 1995; 20:2109–2111.

Hildebrandt VH, Bongers PM, Dul J, van Dijk FJ, Kemper HC. The relationship between leisure time, physical activities and musculoskeletal symptoms and disability in worker populations. *Int Arch Occup Environ Health* 2000; 73:507–518.

Hotopf M, Carr S, Mayou R, Wadsworth M, Wessely S. Why do children have chronic abdominal pain, and what happens to them when they grow up? Population based cohort study. *BMJ* 1998; 18:316:1196–1200.

Jellema P, van der Windt DA, van der Horst HE, et al. Should treatment of (sub) acute low back pain be aimed at psychosocial prognostic factors? Cluster randomised clinical trial in general practice. *BMJ* 2005; 331:84–?.

Jones GT, Watson KD, Silman AJ, Symmons DP, Macfarlane GJ. Predictors of low back pain in British schoolchildren: a population-based prospective cohort study. *Pediatrics* 2003; 8:922–928.

Leboeuf-Yde C. Body weight and low back pain. A systematic literature review of 56 journal articles reporting on 65 epidemiologic studies. *Spine* 2000; 25:226–237.

Leino PI, Berg MA, Puska P. Is back pain increasing? Results from national surveys in Finland during 1978/9–1992. *Scand J Rheumatol* 1994; 23:269–276.

Macfarlane GJ. Generalized pain, fibromyalgia and regional pain: an epidemiological view. *Baillieres Best Pract Res Clin Rheumatol* 1999; 13:403–414.

MacGregor AJ, Griffiths GO, Baker J, Sector TD. Determinants of pressure pain threshold in adult twins: evidence that shared environmental influences predominate. *Pain* 1997; 73:253–257.

Manek NJ, MacGregor AJ. Epidemiology of back disorders: prevalence, risk factors, and prognosis. *Curr Opin Rheumatol* 2005; 17:134–140.

McBeth J, Silman AJ, Gupta A, et al. Altered hypothalamic pituitary adrenal (HPA) stress axis function influences the risk of new onset chronic widespread body pain (CWP): a population based prospective study. In: *Abstracts: 11th World Congress on Pain.* Seattle: IASP Press, 2005, p 447.

Palmer KT, Walsh K, Bendall H, Cooper C, Coggon D. Back pain in Britain: comparison of two prevalence surveys at an interval of 10 years. *BMJ* 2000; 320:1577–1578.

Pincus T, Burton AK, Vogel S, Field AP. A systematic review of psychological factors as predictors of chronicity/disability in prospective cohorts of low back pain. *Spine* 2002; 27:e109–120.

Raspe H. Back pain. In: Silman AJ, Hochberg MC (Eds). *Epidemiology of the Rheumatic Diseases,* 2nd ed. Oxford: Oxford University Press, 2001.

Raspe HH, Kohlmann T. Die aktuelle Rückenschmerzepidemic [The present back pain epidemic]. *Ther Umsch* 1994; 51:367.

Raspe H, Matthis C, Croft P, O'Neill T. Variation in back pain between countries: the example of Britain and Germany. *Spine* 2004; 29:1017–1021.

Selim AJ, Fincke G, Berlowitz DR, et al. Comprehensive health status assessment of centenarians: results from the 1999 large health survey of veteran enrollees. *J Gerontol A Biol Sci Med Sci* 2005; 60:515–519.

Skovron ML. Epidemiology of low back pain. *Baillieres Clin Rheumatol* 1992; 6:559–573.

Thomas E. *The Epidemiology of Back Pain.* PhD Thesis. Manchester: University of Manchester, 1999.

Thomas E, Silman AJ, Croft PR, et al. Predicting who develops chronic low back pain in primary care: a prospective study. *BMJ* 1999; 318:1662–1667.

Thomas E, Peat G, Harris L, et al. The prevalence of pain and pain interference in a general population of older adults: cross-sectional findings from the North Staffordshire Osteoarthritis Project (NorStOP). *Pain* 2004; 110:361–368.

UK BEAM Trial Team. United Kingdom back pain exercise and manipulation (UK BEAM) randomised trial: effectiveness of physical treatments for back pain in primary care. *BMJ* 2004; 329:13771381.

Waddell G. *The Back Pain Revolution,* 2nd ed. Edinburgh: Churchill Livingstone, 2004.

Correspondence to: Prof. Gary J. Macfarlane, PhD, Epidemiology Group, Department of Public Health, University of Aberdeen, The Medical School, Foresterhill, Aberdeen AB25 2ZD, Scotland, United Kingdom. Email: g.j.macfarlane@abdn.ac.uk.

Proceedings of the 11th World Congress on Pain,
edited by Herta Flor, Eija Kalso, and Jonathan O.
Dostrovsky, IASP Press, Seattle, © 2006.

48

Sex, Gender, and Clinical Pain

Linda LeResche

Department of Oral Medicine, University of Washington,
Seattle, Washington, USA

This chapter addresses the relationships of sex and gender to clinical pain, particularly the most common pain conditions, which are typically chronic or recurrent. Gender differences in responses to experimental pain have been reviewed elsewhere (Rollman et al. 2000). Issues concerning how the experience of clinical pain differs in men and women relate both to sex and to gender. The term "sex" is used when discussing biological aspects of identity, i.e., whether an individual has two X chromosomes or one X and one Y, whereas "gender" refers to societal influences and a person's self-expression as masculine or feminine.

In assessing sex and gender differences in pain, the first fundamental question is whether there are differences in the rates of occurrence (i.e., prevalence) and experience of clinical pain conditions in men and women. An earlier comprehensive review (Unruh 1996) documented gender variation in the prevalence of common recurrent pain conditions, pain due to common health care procedures and disease, and pain-related stress, depression, disability, coping and health care utilization. From an epidemiologic perspective, it is important to consider age as well as gender when examining possible differences in pain prevalence and pain experience in men and women. For example, pain conditions that increase in prevalence with age and those that decrease in prevalence with age are likely to be associated with different risk factors. The age- and gender-specific prevalence patterns of a wide range of common pain conditions have been reviewed elsewhere (LeResche 1999). This chapter will look at prevalence patterns of a selected set of pain conditions and some factors that affect sex and gender differences in prevalence and pain experience.

PREVALENCE PATTERNS OF SELECTED
CLINICAL PAIN CONDITIONS

When conducting population-based studies, epidemiologists routinely calculate rates of diseases or symptoms by age and gender. Thus, existing epidemiologic studies can provide a great deal of information about the age and gender distribution of pain conditions in populations, even if these studies were originally designed to investigate other questions. Although there is little research on the incidence (rates of onset) of common recurrent pain conditions, a number of studies report the prevalence of pain—the proportion of the population with a specific pain condition during a particular period of time.

Age- and sex-specific prevalence patterns are not the same for all common chronic pain conditions. Some pain conditions, for example neck and shoulder pain, are more prevalent in women and increase in prevalence with age. In a large population-based study conducted in 20- to 56-year-olds in Tromsø, Norway, Hasvold and Johnson (1993) found that approximately 10% more women than men reported neck or shoulder pain in the prior week. This pattern was similar for each age group. The prevalence rose fairly steadily from 10.8% to 26.9% in men and from 19% to 36.3% in women between age 20 and age 56. Pain in various joints also shows a pattern of increasing prevalence with age in both sexes, with a higher prevalence in women than in men beginning at about age 45 (Lawrence et al. 1966).

Abdominal pain (i.e., gastrointestinal pain, excluding menstrual pain) is more prevalent in women than in men, but decreases in prevalence with age across the adult life span (Agréus et al. 1994; Kay et al. 1994; Adelman et al. 1995). For example, a population-based study in Östhammer, Sweden (Agréus et al. 1994) found that the prevalence of mid-abdominal pain dropped from 24.2% in 20- to 34-year-old men to 8.9% in men between 65 and 79 years old. In women, 35.3% of the 20- to 34-year-olds experienced this pain problem, compared with only 17.3% of the women in the oldest age group. At all ages, rates were 7–10% higher in women than in men.

Tension-type headache is also more prevalent in women than in men and appears to decline in prevalence with age, although the decline is steeper for women than for men (Rasmussen et al. 1991; Scher et al. 1999).

Migraine headache, however, shows a large female predominance in the middle years, with a bell-shaped curve over the adult life span (see Fig. 1; Scher et al. 1999). Data from children indicate that the prevalence of migraine is similar in girls and boys before puberty, or may be somewhat higher in boys than in girls (Unruh and Campbell 1999). Temporomandibular disorder (TMD) pain is a musculoskeletal pain in the region of the jaw joint and the associated facial muscles. The overall prevalence pattern is fairly similar to that of

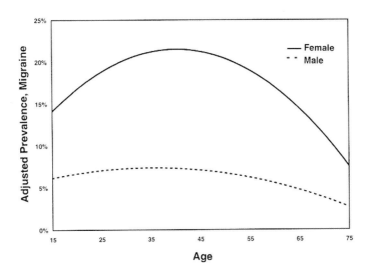

Fig. 1. Gender- and age-specific estimates of migraine prevalence (North America) based on 18 population studies that used International Headache Society diagnostic criteria. From Scher et al. (1999).

migraine. The peak prevalence is in the 25–44-year-old age group, and TMD pain is about twice as common in women as in men across the adult life span (LeResche 1997).

Finally, it is frequently reported that women are at higher risk than men for experiencing multiple pain conditions (Berkley 1997). Data from one population-based study of adults indicate that women between 18 and 44 years old were more than twice as likely as men in the same age group to experience at least three of the five pain conditions studied. However, the gender difference was not so dramatic in the 45–64-year-olds, and there was no difference in the prevalence of multiple pain conditions between women and men aged 65 or older (Von Korff et al. 1988; LeResche 2000).

This brief summary suggests that women are more likely to experience most common clinical pain conditions than are men. Back pain, which may be influenced by a range of occupational exposures that differ in men and women, does not show such a clear female predominance in prevalence rates. Young and middle-aged women also appear to be at greater risk than men for experiencing multiple pain conditions at the same time. However, the age- and sex-specific prevalence patterns differ for different pain conditions. These age differences in prevalence patterns are important because they may provide clues to the factors that influence the rates of onset or persistence of these pain conditions in women and men.

FACTORS INFLUENCING SEX AND GENDER DIFFERENCES IN PAIN EXPERIENCE

To what could these prevalence differences be attributable, and specifically, how might not only the presence of pain, but also the experience of pain differ for males and females? As numerous authors (e.g., Loeser 1991; Dworkin et al. 1992) have pointed out, the experience of pain is complex and multidimensional. Differences in pain experience could be due to differences in the biological substrates that transmit and modulate pain signals, in the organism's ability to detect and discriminate between stimuli, or in pain appraisal, i.e., the cognitive and emotional response to pain, including how one copes with a pain condition. Gender differences may occur in pain-related behaviors, including pain report, nonverbal expressiveness, and use of medications and health care. Finally, men and women with pain may assume or be expected to assume different social roles. The remainder of this section presents a brief review of the evidence for differences in each of these domains of pain. More complete information on specific factors is included in the IASP Press volume, *Sex, Gender, and Pain* (Fillingim 2000) and in recent reviews (Myers et al. 2003; Rollman 2003).

NOCICEPTION

Studies of nociceptive and pain modulation mechanisms are most easily accomplished in animal models, where these systems can be directly manipulated. However, variability in patterns of sex differences, found even across strains of laboratory mice (e.g., Kest et al. 1999), suggests that direct extrapolation from animal studies should be undertaken very cautiously. In humans, brain-imaging studies, which can be conducted in the presence and absence of clinical pain in the same subjects, offer great promise, although few clear findings have emerged to date (e.g., Derbyshire et al. 2002). Finally, studies of differential response to analgesics (Holdcroft 2002; Fillingim and Gear 2004) may provide clues concerning underlying nociceptive and pain modulation mechanisms that may differ in men and women.

PAIN PERCEPTION

What do we know about sex differences in pain perception? Certainly, such differences might be expected, since women have lower thresholds for a number of different sensory modalities (Aloisi 2000). However, in human laboratory studies of pain perception, the mean differences between men and women are frequently not large, and may depend on whether the stimulus is heat, cold, or mechanical pressure (Fillingim and Maixner 1995; Berkley 1997; Derbyshire et al. 2002). Another issue with laboratory studies is that the majority have been conducted with young adults in North America or Europe. Thus, there is a very real possibility that the observed differences in pain report may relate at least somewhat to the gender role expectations in these particular cultures (LeResche 1995).

PAIN APPRAISAL

Women report a greater number of symptoms, more frequent symptoms and more intense symptoms of all kinds than men (Barsky et al. 2001). Pain follows this general pattern as well. Unruh et al. (1999) examined coping strategies in a community sample of adults with pain. Women used a broader range of coping strategies than did men, reporting significantly more problem solving, more positive self-statements, and more palliative behaviors. Women experiencing pain also sought more social support than men. Thus, more people in the social network are likely to be aware and available to provide support for women than for men who are experiencing pain. There is some evidence that women may also be more likely than men to use dysfunctional coping strategies. In a study of elderly arthritis patients (Keefe et al. 2000), women reported higher pain levels and greater pain-related disability than did men. However, women in this sample were more likely to cope with pain by catastrophizing, and when the investigators controlled for catastrophizing statistically, the gender differences in pain and disability disappeared.

PAIN BEHAVIOR

In Western culture, it is generally believed that women are more willing to report pain than men. Surveys of nonclinical populations support this cultural belief (Robinson et al. 2001). It is also widely reported that women seek more health care for pain than men (Unruh 1996). Perhaps women seek more care because they experience greater levels of pain. In one of the only studies examining this question (Von Korff et al. 1991), men and women in the community who reported a particular level of pain sought care at a similar rate. Individuals who report the most severe pain are those most likely to seek care. Thus, while we may find a larger number of women than men in clinical care settings, the pain levels of the patients in those settings may be very similar. Thus, clinics may not be the best settings in which to examine certain questions concerning gender differences in pain experience.

PAIN AND SOCIAL ROLES

U.S. national data indicate that headache and back pain are major causes not only of absenteeism, but also of lost productivity when a person is present in the work setting. Overall lost productive time does not differ by gender. However, women are more likely to lose productive time specifically because of headache (Stewart et al. 2003). Among men and women with disabling musculoskeletal injuries associated with back pain, women wait longer to return to work than men, often because the need for women to fulfill their other roles as mothers and housekeepers can take precedence. However, once women return to work, their probability of staying at work is higher than for men (Crook and Moldofsky 1994).

Some (e.g., Derbyshire 1997) have speculated that women who occupy more social roles such as partner, mother, worker, student, or family caregiver are under greater stress and, consequently, possibly at greater risk for developing clinical pain conditions. A recent survey of three generations of Australian women (Lee and Powers 2002) suggests that the relationship between the number of social roles a woman occupies and her risk of pain is not simple. Among young women between 18 and 23 years old, those with four or five out of the five possible roles investigated had the highest risk for headaches, whereas no relationship was observed between headache and number of roles in middle-aged women between 40 and 45 years old and elderly women between 70 and 75 years old. For back pain, young women with three of five roles were at greatest risk, whereas middle-aged and elderly women who occupied none of the social roles had the highest risk. Thus, there is not an obvious direct relationship between number of roles and pain. Based on this single study, the relationship between pain and social roles appears to differ at different ages and for different pain conditions. Additional research is clearly needed in this area.

HORMONAL FACTORS AND CLINICAL PAIN

Both psychosocial and biological changes take place throughout the life cycle. These changes include assuming and abandoning various occupational, social, and family roles, as well as physical maturation and hormonal changes (e.g., pubertal development for both sexes and menopause in women). Considering the prevalence pattern of a pain condition by age and sex in relation to the biological and psychosocial changes occurring at specific life stages may provide clues to etiological factors or factors that predict persistence of pain in men and women.

Our own work on hormonal factors in TMD and other pain conditions provides an example of this approach. As previously mentioned, the general pattern of the age- and sex-specific prevalence curve for TMD is similar to that for migraine headache (see Fig. 1), although the overall gender difference in TMD prevalence is not quite as dramatic as for migraine. TMD pain prevalence rises steeply in early adulthood and then drops relatively steeply in late middle age. Thus, prevalence peaks during the reproductive years. Because hormonal factors are known to influence migraine, which has a similar prevalence pattern, we began to investigate the possibility of hormonal influences in TMD. In our first study assessing this possibility (LeResche et al. 1997), we used case-control methodology to examine the natural experiment of use versus nonuse of hormone replacement therapy (HRT) among postmenopausal women. We hypothesized that those women using HRT would have a hormonal profile more like younger women, and would consequently be at greater risk for TMD. That study indeed found an increased risk of TMD among postmenopausal women using HRT. Interestingly, the risk of TMD increased with increasing exposure to estrogen over the year prior to referral for TMD care, with women using the equivalent of 220 mg or more of estradiol having a risk almost double that of women using no estrogen.

Although the findings of this initial study were intriguing, the decision to use exogenous hormones such as HRT and oral contraceptives may be influenced by a number of factors including age, education, and the presence of symptoms. Thus, we began to investigate whether exposure to a woman's own endogenous hormones might be a risk factor for TMD and other pain conditions. We approached this question using two entirely different study designs. The first investigation was an epidemiologic study of pain in adolescents (LeResche et al. 2005). The steep rise in estradiol levels occurring in girls between the ages of 11 and 14 years presents a major opportunity to study the relationship between endogenous hormonal changes and pain. Although variability in timing of development is wide among individuals, for the majority of girls, these ages capture the period surrounding the start of menstrual periods (menarche) as estrogen levels rise sharply and then plateau. Thus, we speculated that there would be a relationship between pubertal development and the rates of occurrence of TMD pain and other pain conditions.

We conducted a cross-sectional telephone survey of 3,101 children and adolescents between 11 and 17 years old, selected from the membership of a not-for-profit, pre-paid health plan in Seattle. Respondents were asked whether they had experienced back pain, headache, facial pain, and/or stomach pain in the past 3 months. They were asked to report only pains lasting a whole day or more, or pains that recurred several times. In addition, information was gathered on demographic variables, on an index of pubertal development, and on levels of depressive and somatic symptoms.

We found that the prevalence of all four pain conditions rose with increasing pubertal development in girls. For boys, the picture was mixed, with different pain conditions showing different patterns. Specifically, in boys, back pain and facial pain prevalence increased, the prevalence of stomach pain declined, and headache prevalence was virtually unchanged.

For both boys and girls, the probability of experiencing at least one pain condition rose significantly with progressing puberty. For both sexes, the percentage that experienced two or more pain problems also rose with increasing development, but the rise was only statistically significant for girls. The percentage of girls who experienced high levels of depressive symptoms and the percentage that experienced high levels of non-pain somatic symptoms also increased with increasing pubertal development. Again, for boys, the increase in risk of experiencing these symptoms was not dramatic. For both boys and girls, in multivariate models, puberty was a much better predictor of pain and symptoms than was age. Thus it appears that the combination of being female and becoming sexually mature puts adolescent girls at higher risk of all kinds of symptoms, both physical and psychological.

A second approach to assessing possible relationships between hormones and TMD pain involves examining changes in pain with changes in hormonal status within individual women. We initially investigated whether TMD pain levels vary in a cyclic pattern across the menstrual cycle (LeResche et al. 2003). The subjects in this study were three groups of TMD patients, all of whom met research diagnostic criteria for both facial muscle and temporomandibular joint pain disorders: normally cycling women, women using oral contraceptives, and men.

Subjects completed daily diaries over the course of three menstrual cycles or over 3 months in men, reporting daily levels of average and worst TMD pain. Women also recorded whether they were having their menstrual period each day, and we used biological measures to identify time of ovulation and to confirm that ovulation did, in fact, occur. In order to examine menstrual cycle-related changes, we controlled for the overall trend in pain over the 3-month time period for each subject.

Estradiol (the predominant form of estrogen) peaks just before ovulation in the middle of the menstrual cycle. In the middle of the second half of the cycle, there is a secondary peak of estradiol, as well as a peak in progesterone. We found that TMD pain was highest for all women during the menstrual period and that there was a pattern of rising pain towards the end of the cycle, a time of dropping estradiol for naturally cycling women and a time of withdrawal of synthetic estrogen for women taking oral contraceptives. Interestingly, we also found a peak in TMD pain intensity around the time of ovulation for normally

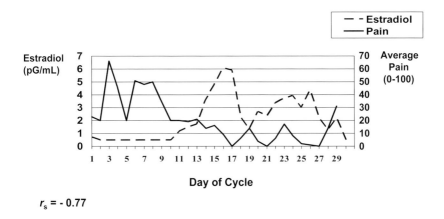

$r_s = -0.77$

Fig. 2. Relationship of ratings of temporomandibular disorder pain and salivary estradiol levels across the menstrual cycle. Data are from a single female subject with normal menstrual cycles.

cycling women: again, a time of rapid fluctuation in estradiol. There was no mid-cycle peak for the women on oral contraceptives, who do not have estradiol peaks mid-cycle and usually do not ovulate. There was no discernible pattern for men.

One hypothesis to explain the observed pattern of pain is that estradiol may be a pain modulator in women, as it is in some strains of mice (Mogil et al. 1993). If this were the case, we would expect highest levels of pain when estradiol is low and lowest levels of pain when estradiol is high. Fig. 2 shows pilot data from one woman with TMD pain that lends support to this hypothesis. The pain pattern is almost a mirror image of the salivary estradiol pattern, showing higher levels of pain when estradiol is low and lower levels of pain when estradiol is high. After about Day 13 of the cycle, pain almost always rises when estradiol drops and drops when estradiol rises. These data come from only a single subject and should be interpreted with caution. Studies are currently under way investigating whether this relationship will be apparent in a larger sample of women.

We also found a similar pattern of pain/hormone relationship with clinical TMD pain during pregnancy, i.e., lower pain during the later months of pregnancy, when estradiol (and progesterone) levels are high, with pain levels rising again 1 year postpartum when these hormone levels drop (LeResche et al. 2005). Again, there was a negative correlation between levels of salivary estradiol and levels of TMD pain intensity within each woman over time.

SUMMARY AND WORKING HYPOTHESES

The data reviewed in this chapter suggest a number of working hypotheses: (1) Gender-related factors (e.g., social role expectations, coping) likely influence the report of pain in clinical and epidemiologic studies, contributing to the observed higher prevalence of many pain conditions in women. (2) Hormonal factors appear to influence women's experience of TMD, and possibly other pain conditions. (3) It appears likely that withdrawal or fluctuation (rather than the mere presence) of estrogen is associated with increased pain in women. These data also present a number of opportunities for pain researchers of all disciplines. Research is definitely needed to assess the relationship between gender-related factors—such as social role expectations and coping—and pain in non-Western cultures. Further studies are needed to confirm the estrogen/pain relationships found by our research group. If our initial findings are confirmed, research into the mechanisms by which estrogen and other hormones influence TMD and possibly other pain conditions could eventually lead to new treatments tailored specifically for either women or men.

Finally, this chapter has focused on the differences in pain phenomena between men and women. Future research should also examine whether different pain mechanisms may be operating in men and women, even if pain outcomes appear similar.

ACKNOWLEDGMENTS

The author's research was supported by Grant Nos. P01 DE 08773, R01 DE 12470, and R01 DE 016212 from the National Institute of Dental and Craniofacial Research and the NIH Office of Research on Women's Health, USA. Numerous colleagues contributed to the work described here. Primary contributors include Drs. Samuel F. Dworkin, Michael Von Korff, Lloyd Mancl, Mark T. Drangsholt, Jeffrey J. Sherman, Ms. Kimberly Huggins, and Ms. Kathleen Saunders.

REFERENCES

Adelman AM, Revicki DA, Magaziner J, Hebel R. Abdominal pain in an HMO. *Fam Med* 1995; 27:321–325.

Agréus L, Svardsudd K, Nyren O, Tibblin G. The epidemiology of abdominal symptoms: Prevalence and demographic characteristics in a Swedish adult population. *Scand J Gastroenterol* 1994; 29:102–109.

Aloisi AM. Sensory effects of gonadal hormones. In: Fillingim RB (Ed). *Sex, Gender and Pain, Progress in Pain Research and Management*, Vol. 17. Seattle: IASP Press, 2000, pp 7–24.

Barsky AJ, Peekna HM, Borus JF. Somatic symptom reporting in women and men. *J Gen Intern Med* 2001; 16:266–275.

Berkley KJ. Sex differences in pain. *Behav Brain Sci* 1997; 20:371–380.

Crook J, Moldofsky H. The probability of recovery and return to work from work disability as a function of time. *Qual Life Res* 1994; 3:S97–S103.

Derbyshire SWG. Sources of variation in assessing male and female responses to pain. *New Ideas Psychology* 1997; 15:83–95.

Derbyshire SWG, Nichols TE, Firestone L, Townsend DW, Jones AKP. Gender differences in patterns of cerebral activation during equal experience of painful laser stimulation. *J Pain* 2002; 3:401–411.

Dworkin SF, Von Korff M, LeResche L. Epidemiologic studies of chronic pain: A dynamic-ecologic perspective. *Ann Behav Med* 1992; 14:3–11.

Fillingim RB (Ed). *Sex, Gender and Pain*, Progress in Pain Research and Management, Vol. 17. Seattle: IASP Press, 2000.

Fillingim RB, Gear RW. Sex differences in opioid analgesia: clinical and experimental findings. *Eur J Pain* 2004; 8:413–425.

Fillingim RB, Maixner W. Gender differences in the responses to noxious stimuli. *Pain Forum* 1995; 4:209–221.

Hasvold T, Johnsen R. Headache and neck or shoulder pain—frequent and disabling complaints in the general population. *Scand J Prim Health Care* 1993; 11:219–224.

Holdcroft A. Sex differences and analgesics. *Eur J Anesthesiol* 2002; 19(Suppl 26).

Kay L, Jorgensen T, Jensen KH. Epidemiology of abdominal symptoms in a random population: prevalence, incidence, and natural history. *Eur J Epidemiol* 1994; 10:559–566.

Keefe FJ, Lefebvre JC, Egert JR, et al. Relationship of gender to pain, pain behavior, and disability in osteoarthritis patients: the role of catastrophizing. *Pain* 2000; 87:325–334.

Kest B, Wilson SG, Mogil JS. Sex differences in supraspinal morphine analgesia are dependent on genotype. *J Pharmacol Exp Ther* 1999; 289:1370–1375.

Lawrence JS, Bremner JM, Bier F. Osteo-arthrosis prevalence in the population and relationship between symptoms and x-ray changes. *Ann Rheum Dis* 1966; 25:1–23.

Lee C, Powers JR. Number of social roles, health, and well-being in three generations of Australian women. *Int J Behav Med* 2002; 9:195–215.

LeResche L. Gender differences in pain: epidemiologic perspectives. *Pain Forum* 1995; 4:228–230.

LeResche L. Epidemiology of temporomandibular disorders: implications for the investigation of etiologic factors. *Crit Rev Oral Biol Med* 1997; 8:291–305.

LeResche L. Gender considerations in the epidemiology of chronic pain. In: Crombie IK, Croft PR, Linton SJ, LeResche L, Von Korff M (Eds). *Epidemiology of Pain*. Seattle: IASP Press, 1999, pp 43–52.

LeResche L. Epidemiologic perspectives on sex differences in pain. In: Fillingim RB (Ed). *Sex, Gender and Pain*, Progress in Pain Research and Management, Vol. 17. Seattle: IASP Press, 2000, pp 233–249.

LeResche L, Saunders K, Von Korff M, Barlow W, Dworkin SF. Use of exogenous hormones and risk of temporomandibular disorder pain. *Pain* 1997; 69:153–160.

LeResche L, Mancl L, Sherman JJ, Gandara B, Dworkin SF. Changes in temporomandibular pain and other symptoms across the menstrual cycle. *Pain* 2003; 106:253–261.

LeResche L, Sherman JJ, Huggins KH, et al. Musculoskeletal orofacial pain and other signs and symptoms of temporomandibular disorders during pregnancy: a prospective study. *J Orofac Pain* 2005; 19:193–201.

LeResche L, Mancl LA, Drangsholt MT, Saunders K, Von Korff M. Relationship of pain and symptoms to pubertal development in adolescents. *Pain* 2005; 118:201–209.

Loeser JD. What is chronic pain? *Theor Med* 1991; 12:213–225.

Myers CD, Riley JL, Robinson ME. Psychosocial contributions to sex-correlated differences in pain. *Clin J Pain* 2003; 19:225–232.

Mogil JS, Sternberg WF, Kest B, Marek P, Liebeskind JC. Sex differences in the antagonism of swim stress-induced analgesia: effects of gonadectomy and estrogen replacement. *Pain* 1993; 53:17–25.

Rasmussen BK, Jensen R, Schroll M, Olesen J. Epidemiology of headache in a general population—a prevalence study. *J Clin Epidemiol* 1991; 44:1147–1157.

Robinson ME, Riley JL III, Myers CD, et al. Gender role expectations of pain: relationship to sex differences in pain. *J Pain* 2001; 2:251–257.

Rollman GB. Sex makes a difference: experimental and clinical pain responses. *Clin J Pain* 2003; 19:204–207.

Rollman GB, Lautenbacher S, Jones KS. Sex and gender differences in responses to experimental pain in humans. In: Fillingim RB (Ed). *Sex, Gender and Pain,* Progress in Pain Research and Management, Vol. 17. Seattle: IASP Press, 2000, pp 165–190.

Scher AI, Stewart WF, Lipton RB. Migraine and headache: a meta-analytic approach. In: Crombie IK, Croft PR, Linton SJ, LeResche L, Von Korff M (Eds). *Epidemiology of Pain.* Seattle: IASP Press, 1999, pp 159–170.

Stewart WF, Ricci JA, Chee E, Morganstein D, Lipton R. Lost productive time and cost due to common pain conditions in the UW workforce. *JAMA* 2003; 290:2443–2454.

Unruh AM. Gender variations in clinical pain experience. *Pain* 1996; 65:123–167.

Unruh AM, Campbell MA. Gender variation in children's pain experiences. In: McGrath PJ, Finley GA (Eds). *Chronic and Recurrent Pain in Children and Adolescents,* Progress in Pain Research and Management, Vol. 13. Seattle: IASP Press, 1999, pp 199–241.

Unruh AM, Ritchie J, Merskey H. Does gender affect appraisal of pain and pain coping strategies? *Clin J Pain* 1999; 15:31–40.

Von Korff M, Dworkin SF, LeResche L, Kruger A. An epidemiologic comparison of pain complaints. *Pain* 1988; 32:173–183.

Von Korff M, Wagner EH, Dworkin SF, Saunders KW. Chronic pain and use of ambulatory health care. *Psychosom Med* 1991; 53:61–79.

Correspondence to: Linda LeResche, ScD, Department of Oral Medicine, Box 356370, University of Washington, Seattle, WA 98195, USA. Email: leresche@u.washington.edu.

Proceedings of the 11th World Congress on Pain,
edited by Herta Flor, Eija Kalso, and Jonathan O.
Dostrovsky, IASP Press, Seattle, © 2006.

49

Motivational Issues in Pain Self-Management

Robert D. Kerns,[a] Mark P. Jensen,[b]
and Warren R. Nielson[c]

*[a]Departments of Psychiatry, Neurology, and Psychology, Yale University, VA
Central Office, and Psychology Service, VA Connecticut Healthcare System,
West Haven, Connecticut, USA; [b]Department of Rehabilitation Medicine,
University of Washington, Seattle, Washington, USA; Department of Medicine
(Rheumatology), University of Western Ontario and St. Joseph's Health Care,
London, Ontario, Canada*

Because the ability of patients to manage chronic pain depends much more
on what they do than on what is done to them, motivation can be viewed as a
primary issue in pain self-management. In cognitive-behavioral and multidisciplinary pain treatment, for example, patients are asked to make significant
changes in their behavior (Turk et al. 1983; Bradley 1996; Loeser and Turk
2001), and it is the change in patient responses to pain that is thought to lead to
improvement. A significant effort on the part of the patient is required to make
and maintain such changes.

In this chapter we describe a motivational model of pain self-management and discuss its potential relevance in clinical situations. We also describe
methods for assessing motivation and readiness to adopt a self-management
approach to chronic pain, methods for promoting motivation for pain treatment
and for learning and implementing adaptive pain-coping skills, and strategies
for tailoring pain treatment to patient preferences, interests, and expectations
for treatment.

MODELS OF MOTIVATION AND A MOTIVATIONAL MODEL OF PAIN SELF-MANAGEMENT

Theories of motivation attempt to explain the initiation, direction, persistence, intensity, and termination of a particular behavior (Landy and Becker 1987). Motivation can thus be viewed as a process that involves all of the factors that influence behavior. Most theories and models of human behavior, including a motivational model we are developing for understanding pain self-management, assume that behavioral change is influenced primarily by two factors: (1) the perceived importance of behavior change and (2) the patient's belief that behavior change is possible (i.e., self-efficacy) (Jensen et al. 2003). In fact, because of the high degree of overlap among the models, as well as the fact that it is often possible to explain changes in motivation or behavior from the viewpoint of any one of the models, finding unequivocal support for one model over the others is quite difficult (Weinstein 1993).

The great deal of overlap among motivational models may be used to form a foundation for a general model of motivation for pain self-management. An initial version of such a model, the motivational model for pain self-management, is presented in Fig. 1. The primary outcome variable in this model is pain self-management coping behavior, which may be defined by a set of behaviors and cognitions that are thought to reflect "adaptive" pain management and by avoidance of behaviors or cognitions that are thought to reflect "maladaptive" pain management. The specific self-management coping behaviors listed in Fig. 1 were drawn from the coping responses that clinicians and researchers have most closely associated with improved function and with positive outcomes in pain treatment (Jensen et al. 1994; Loeser and Turk 2001; Nielson et al. 2001), but the list is by no means exhaustive.

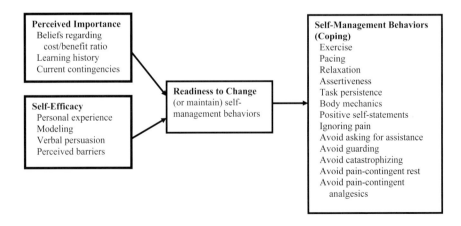

Fig. 1. Preliminary motivational model of pain self-management.

Self-management behavior that is adaptive for one condition may, however, be ineffective or even harmful for another condition. For example, while patients with low back pain may benefit from maintaining a program of regular aerobic exercise, the same exercises might cause further joint damage in patients with knee or hip arthritis. As more is learned about the relative importance of specific coping behaviors and cognitions and about the conditions under which these are adaptive, maladaptive, or neutral, the operational definition of pain self-management listed in Fig. 1 should be updated.

The concept of readiness to self-manage pain (Prochaska and DiClemente 1984; Kerns et al. 1997) is central to the motivational model for pain self-management because it defines motivation. The model hypothesizes that patients will engage in specific pain self-management strategies depending on their readiness, or motivation, to use these strategies. In the model, motivation is influenced by the two primary variables already mentioned—beliefs about the importance of engaging versus not engaging in pain self-management behaviors ("outcome expectancies," "value," "importance") and beliefs about one's ability to engage in pain self-management behaviors ("self-efficacy," "confidence"). Perceived importance is influenced by the value of expected outcomes, such as pain reduction, increased strength and activity tolerance, and increased cognitive abilities, versus the perceived costs of pain self-management. The outcome expectancies are in turn affected by the patient's learning history, since a history of reinforcers or punishers for certain pain self-management behaviors will respectively increase or decrease the value placed on pain self-management.

Similarly, a number of factors can contribute to a patient's confidence in his or her ability to engage in a specific behavioral response. These include a history of successfully engaging in that response while undergoing treatments that elicit new behavioral responses to pain (Fordyce et al. 1968; Fordyce 1976), modeling of behavior by others (Bandura 1986), effective persuasion (Miller and Rollnick 2002), and the removal of perceived barriers.

Although the motivational model for pain self-management may appear static, with its final endpoint determined by the effects of perceived importance and self-efficacy on readiness to self-manage pain, we view the model as dynamic because of the many factors described above that influence motivation. The model provides what we hope is a frame of reference for understanding patient motivation for self-management, and, more importantly, for identifying ways to improve this motivation.

MEASUREMENT OF MOTIVATION IN PAIN SELF-MANAGEMENT

PAIN STAGES OF CHANGE QUESTIONNAIRE

Demonstrations of the efficacy and cost-effectiveness of self-management approaches to chronic pain have encouraged clinical investigators to consider strategies for promoting motivation, particularly engagement and active participation, in these treatments. Informed by a cognitive-behavioral perspective on chronic pain (Turk et al. 1983) and by the transtheoretical model of behavior change (Prochaska and DiClemente 1984), Kerns and his colleagues (Kerns et al. 1997; Kerns and Habib 2004) have developed a model of readiness to change in order to measure this capacity in patients participating in self-management treatments for chronic pain. According to the model, individuals vary in their degree of readiness to adopt a self-management approach to chronic pain. Those who believe that their pain condition is a physical one that requires medical attention are defined as being in "precontemplation," while those who believe that there are limits to the utility of a medical approach and that learning self-management approaches may be useful are in "contemplation." Within the model, the active learning of self-management strategies takes place in the "action" stage, while persons who have already incorporated self-management into their overall approach to chronic pain are in the "maintenance" stage.

The Pain Stages of Change Questionnaire (PSOCQ; Kerns et al. 1997) was developed to provide a reliable measure of motivation or readiness to adopt a self-management approach to chronic pain and to assess the validity and utility of the pain readiness to change model. Published data largely support the reliability, factor structure, and criterion-related validity of the PSOCQ (Kerns et al. 1997; Biller et al. 2000; Jensen et al. 2000, 2004; Maurischat et al. 2002). Four scales of the PSOCQ have been identified that are consistent with the four stages of the change process described above, examples of which are presented in Table I.

Evidence is growing of the predictive validity of the PSOCQ. Kerns and Rosenberg (2000) demonstrated that pretreatment scores on the PSOCQ reliably discriminated persons who completed a 10-session program of cognitive-behavioral therapy for chronic pain. Furthermore, these investigators found that increased action and maintenance scale scores, inferred as evidence of "forward stage movement," i.e., enhanced motivation and commitment to a self-management approach, were correlated with improved outcomes on several key variables. These results have generally been confirmed (Jensen et al. 2004; Kerns et al. 2005), although concerns have arisen about the sensitivity and specificity of the PSOCQ in predicting treatment engagement and participation (Biller et al. 2000), as well as about the validity of the measure (e.g., Strong et al. 2002; Habib et al. 2003). Most recently, Burns and his colleagues have demonstrated

Table I
Examples of items from the Pain Stages of Change Questionnaire

Precontemplation
1. My pain is a medical problem, and I should be dealing with physicians about it.
2. All of this talk about how to cope is a waste of my time.

Contemplation
1. I have been thinking that the way that I cope with my pain could improve.
2. I have been thinking that doctors can only help so much in managing my pain and that the rest is up to me.

Action
1. I am developing new ways to cope with my pain.
2. I am learning new ways to help myself control my pain without doctors.

Maintenance
1. I have made a lot of progress in coping with my pain.
2. I am currently using suggestions that people have made about how to live with my pain problem.

Source: Kerns et al. (1997).

that early treatment increases in readiness predict subsequent improvements in outcomes, providing the strongest evidence to date of a role of enhanced motivation or readiness as a mediator of improved outcomes associated with self-management treatments (Glenn and Burns 2003; Burns et al. 2005).

MULTIDIMENSIONAL PAIN READINESS TO CHANGE QUESTIONNAIRE

Nielson et al. (2003) initially developed the Multidimensional Pain Readiness to Change Questionnaire (MPRCQ) based on the notion that readiness to change pain management behaviors may not be a unitary phenomenon. In other words, rather than having the same level of motivation to learn and apply all of the coping strategies taught in multidisciplinary pain programs, an individual is likely to have a greater readiness to adopt some strategies than others. For example, at a given point in time a patient may be more motivated to learn and utilize physical exercises than cognitive restructuring or activity pacing techniques. Unlike the one-dimensional PSOCQ, the MPRCQ was designed to detect this type of variation.

The MPRCQ items were based on the self-management behaviors depicted in our motivational model of pain self-management (Fig. 1). As item development proceeded, 10 primary scales as well as five cognitive control content scales were identified (Table II). One scale, "avoid guarding," was subsequently dropped because of insufficient internal consistency. The scales on the resulting 46-item questionnaire had adequate internal reliability ($\alpha = 0.70$ to 0.93) and were essentially unaffected by social desirability. Moderate correlations with the PSOCQ, a pain coping measure (Chronic Pain Coping Inventory; Jensen et al. 1995), and attitudes about pain management (Survey of Pain Attitudes; Jensen et al. 1994) suggest good concurrent validity. Although these data were encouraging, we sought to refine the MPRCQ further in a number of areas. Some items had apparent double negatives that made them difficult for patients to understand, and we wanted to alter the response options so that they reflected a readiness to change continuum rather than discrete stages of change. In the broader literature on changes in health behavior, the concept of discrete stages has been challenged because divisions between such stages seem arbitrary, the definition of a stage contains multiple constructs (i.e., time, past attempts to change, and intent), and the focus only on conscious decisional processes is overly simplistic (e.g., West 2005). Although some evidence suggests that in pain patients, forward stage movement is associated with improved treatment outcomes (e.g., Burns et al. 2005), it is not clear whether it is helpful to classify patients according to discrete stages versus using scores based on a continuum of readiness to change in predicting outcomes (e.g., Biller et al. 2000). Moreover, difficulties have emerged in identifying consistent stages of change among pain patients (e.g., Jensen et al. 2000).

In revising the MPRCQ, we divided items into two categories: one for behaviors that would be increased (e.g., exercise) and one for behaviors that would be reduced (e.g., contingent rest) to improve coping. For greater clarity, separate sets of instructions and response options were provided for these two sets of items. Thus for the former category, the following options were available:

1) I am not doing this now, and am not interested in ever doing it.

2) I might do this someday but I have made no plans to do it.

3) I will probably start doing this sometime (in the next 6 months).

4) I have made plans to start doing this soon (within the next month).

5) I have recently started doing this (within the past month).

6) I have been doing this for a while (more than a month but less than 6 months).

7) I have been doing this for a long time (at least 6 months).

In contrast, for the items in which a decrease in the behavior would be expected to be adaptive, respondents were asked to rate their intention to stop using each of the methods of coping with or managing their pain (see Table II) using a scale that ranged from 1, "I am doing this now and am not interested in ever stopping," to 7, "I have not done this for a long time (at least 6 months)." Each response option for both "use" and "stop using" categories contains both an intent/usage and a timeframe component.

Our hope is that this revision of the MPRCQ, which we expect to make available within the next year, will provide researchers with a valid, reliable

Table II
Multidimensional Pain Readiness to Change Questionnaire
scales and sample questions

Exercise	"Exercise for at least 30 minutes three times a week or more"
Task persistence	"Keep on doing what I need to despite pain"
Relaxation	"Use slow, deep breathing to relax"
Cognitive control:	
Divert attention	"Pay attention to something else when I hurt"
Make self-statements	"Remind myself that I will feel better in the future"
Reinterpret sensations	"Think about the pain differently so that it hurts less"
Avoid catastrophizing	"Tell myself I can't go on with this pain"*
Ignore pain	"Ignore the pain"
Activity pacing	"Pace myself so I can keep working slowly and steadily"
Avoid contingent rest	"Rest when I hurt"*
Avoid asking for assistance	"Ask for help with chores when I hurt"*
Assertive communication	"Tell people I am close to what is on my mind"
Proper body mechanics	"Stand straight when I carry something heavy"
Avoid guarding	"Keep a body part still when it hurts"*

* Examples of "stop using" items.

tool with which they can study motivational processes associated with adoption of—or failure to adopt—pain self-management strategies. Clinicians working in programs that teach such skills are keenly aware of the importance of motivation and the wide variation in the extent to which patients are willing to adopt and benefit from learning these strategies. An improved understanding of the motivational processes that influence these outcomes is perhaps long overdue.

The ability of the MPRCQ to predict treatment outcomes is not yet established, but as research in this area progresses, the measure may be used to identify appropriate treatments or to suggest targets for motivational interviewing of patients. Research will also establish whether a multidimensional measure such as the MPRCQ represents an improvement over a more widely used evaluation of motivation such as the PSOCQ and determine whether stage assignment versus simple scoring offers any predictive advantage. Finally, because it reflects the specific behavioral targets within our motivational model of pain self-management, the MPRCQ is perhaps ideally suited for future efforts to evaluate that model.

CLINICAL AND RESEARCH IMPLICATIONS

MOTIVATIONAL INTERVIEWING

As indicated previously, we view motivation for pain self-management as a state that can be altered by a number of factors, many of which can be influenced by clinician responses to patient behaviors. To enhance patient perceptions of the importance of pain self-management, clinicians can encourage positive outcome expectancies and outline the costs of not engaging in self-management strategies. They can help patients identify and incorporate into their lives positive contingencies (reinforcers) for self-management coping behaviors, and they can praise patients for making gradual changes in the direction of pain self-management (i.e., "shaping"). To increase self-efficacy, the clinician can encourage the patient to practice self-management strategies; provide the patient with opportunities to observe other patients engaging in pain self-management strategies; gently challenge "distorted" cognitions, providing directed active listening to encourage and support self-efficacy beliefs; and help the patient develop a plan to address any perceived or real barriers to pain self-management.

Many of these suggestions have been incorporated into a set of therapeutic strategies called motivational interviewing (Miller and Rollnick 2002), which was designed specifically to increase motivation for positive change. Motivational interviewing is both a general approach and a set of specific therapeutic strategies designed to address ambivalence about adaptive change (e.g., adaptive pain management and return to work).

In terms of the general approach, motivational interviewing is patient centered (Douaihy et al. 2005), so that what the patient says and does during a motivational interaction guides clinician responses. Motivational clinicians should seek to assess and address the patient's worries and concerns, build and enhance rapport and a collaborative relationship, provide information that the clinician knows or believes the patient is truly ready to hear, alter the focus of interventions from making treatment recommendations (the expert model) to supporting and enhancing patient self-care practices (the coaching model), and foster greater control of decision making and responsibility for self-care. To help facilitate an atmosphere of positive change and to build rapport, the single most important clinician response is listening to the patient, especially in a reflective way, rephrasing the thoughts and feelings that the patient is trying to communicate.

While skilled reflective listening might be considered the foundation of motivational interviewing, other specific responses are involved, including developing discrepancy, avoiding argumentation, rolling with resistance, and supporting self-efficacy (Miller and Rollnick 2002). Clinicians help patients see discrepancies by encouraging them to talk about the problem, listening specifically for discrepancies between their goals and their behaviors, and then reflecting back those discrepancies that are consistent with adaptive pain management. Arguments with patients are to be avoided because they could provide patients with an opportunity to talk themselves out of positive change. The concept of rolling with resistance refers to a strategy of avoiding confrontation, and in fact seeking to identify and reflect some adaptive component of any resistant comments a patient might make. Supporting self-efficacy refers to a set of clinician responses that elicit and reinforce positive patient statements about their capabilities.

When applied to pain self-management, the goal of motivational interviewing is to increase the probability that patients will make adaptive decisions concerning their response to chronic pain (Jensen 2002). In our motivational model for pain self-management, motivational interviewing can specifically target self-efficacy beliefs and the perceived importance of change, so as to alter a patient's readiness or motivation to change or maintain self-management behavior, leading to subsequent changes in these behaviors.

IMPLICATIONS FOR REFINEMENTS OF SELF-MANAGEMENT TREATMENTS

Overall, findings from research on the pain readiness to change model provide preliminary support for its utility and encourage future research on the role of motivation and pain readiness to change in increasing the effectiveness of self-management treatment approaches. For example, the model may be useful in suggesting refinements in referral and engagement in self-management approaches, improvements in the treatments themselves to enhance motivation and forward stage movement, and development and implementation of stage-matched treatments. In one recent study, primary care providers were trained to utilize motivational interviewing and patient-centered counseling in an effort to increase the likelihood that patients would accept a referral to a multidisciplinary pain treatment program (Heapy et al., in press). In this study, pretreatment PSOCQ scores on the contemplation scale significantly predicted adherence to the therapist's recommendations for inter-session practice of pain-coping skills (e.g., relaxation, activity pacing). Furthermore, inter-session adherence was correlated with forward stage movement and behavioral goal accomplishment.

In a study in progress at the VA Connecticut Healthcare System, we are evaluating the efficacy of a modified cognitive-behavioral therapy approach that explicitly incorporates patient preferences, perceived importance, and expectancies of effectiveness for learning specific pain-coping skills, using a modified version of the MPRCQ and motivational interviewing in an effort to enhance forward stage movement and adherence. The treatment, labeled "tailored cognitive-behavioral therapy," is informed by the motivational model of pain self-management and by observations of the inherent flexibility in cognitive-behavioral therapy that allows for prescriptive treatment planning. The model also encourages the development of alternative strategies that attempt to match patients' apparent degree of readiness to change with specific interventions.

REFERENCES

Bandura A. *Social Foundations of Thought and Action: A Social Cognitive Theory.* Englewood Cliffs, NJ: Prentice Hall, 1986.

Biller N, Arnstein P, Caudill M, Federman C, Guberman C. Predicting completion of cognitive-behavioral pain management program by initial measurement of chronic pain patients' readiness to change. *Clin J Pain* 2000; 16:352–359.

Bradley L. Cognitive-behavioral therapy for chronic pain. In: Gatchel R, Turk D (Eds). *Psychological Approaches to Pain Management: A Practitioner's Handbook.* New York: Guilford Press, 1996, pp 131–147.

Burns JW, Glenn B, Lofland K, Bruehl S, Harden RN. Stages of change in readiness to adopt a self-management approach to chronic pain: the moderating role of early-treatment stage progression in predicting outcome. *Pain* 2005; 115:322–331.

Douaihy A, Jensen MP, Jou RJ. Motivating behavior change in persons with chronic pain. In: McCarberg B, Passik S (Eds). *Expert Guide to Pain Management.* Philadelphia: American College of Physicians, 2005.

Fordyce W. *Behavioral Methods for Chronic Pain and Illness.* Saint Louis: Mosby, 1976.

Fordyce W, Fowler R, DeLateur B. An application of behavior modification technique to a problem of chronic pain. *Behav Res Ther* 1968; 6:105–107.

Glenn B, Burns JW. Pain self-management in the process and outcome of multidisciplinary treatment of chronic pain: evaluation of a stage of change model. *J Behav Med* 2003; 26:417–433.

Habib S, Morrisey SA, Helmes E. Readiness to adopt a self-management approach to pain: evaluation of the pain stage of change model in a non-clinic sample. *Pain* 2003; 22:283–290.

Heapy A, Otis J, Marcus KS, et al. Intersession coping skill practice mediates the relationship between readiness for self-management treatment and treatment outcome. *Pain*; in press.

Jensen MP. Enhancing motivation to change in pain treatment. In: Turk DC, Gatchel RJ (Eds). *Psychological Treatment for Pain: A Practitioner's Handbook,* 2nd ed. New York: Guilford Publications, 2002, pp 71–93.

Jensen MP, Turner JA, Romano JM, Lawler BK. Relationship of pain-specific beliefs to chronic pain adjustment. *Pain* 1994; 57:301–309.

Jensen MP, Turner JA, Romano JM, Strom SE. The Chronic Pain Coping Inventory: development and preliminary evaluation. *Pain* 1995; 60:203–216.

Jensen MP, Nielson WR, Romano JM, Hill ML, Turner JA. Further evaluation of the pain stages of change questionnaire: is the transtheoretical model of change useful for patients with chronic pain? *Pain* 2000; 86:255–264.

Jensen MP, Nielson WR, Kerns RD. Toward the development of a motivational model of pain self-management. *J Pain* 2003; 4:477–492.

Jensen MP, Nielson WR, Turner JA, Romano JM, Hill ML. Changes in readiness to self-manage pain are associated with improvement in multidisciplinary pain treatment and pain coping. *Pain* 2004; 111:84–95.

Kerns RD, Habib S. A critical review of the pain readiness to change model. *Pain* 2004; 5:357–367.

Kerns R, Rosenberg R. Predicting responses to self-management treatments for chronic pain: application of the pain stages of change model. *Pain* 2000; 84:49–55.

Kerns R, Rosenberg R, Jamison R, Caudill M, Haythornthwaite J. Readiness to adopt a self-management approach to chronic pain: the Pain Stages of Change Questionnaire (PSOCQ). *Pain* 1997; 72:227–234.

Kerns R, Wagner J, Rosenberg R, Haythornthwaite J, Caudill-Slosberg M. Identification of subgroups of persons with chronic pain based on profiles on the pain stages of change questionnaire. *Pain* 2005; 116:302–310.

Landy F, Becker W. Motivation theory reconsidered. *Res Org Behav* 1987; 9:1–38.

Loeser J, Turk D. Multidisciplinary pain management. In: Loeser J, Batler S, Chapman C, Turk D (Eds). *Bonica's Management of Pain*. Philadelphia: Lippincott Williams & Wilkins, 2001, pp 2069–2079.

Maurischat C, Harter M, Ayclair P, Kerns RD, Bengel J. Preliminary validation of a German version of the pain stages of change questionnaire. *Eur J Pain* 2002; 6:43–48.

Miller W, Rollnick S. *Motivational Interviewing: Preparing People to Change,* 2nd ed. New York: Guilford Press, 2002.

Nielson WR, Jensen MP, Hill ML. An activity pacing subscale for the Chronic Pain Coping Inventory: development in a sample of patients with fibromyalgia syndrome. *Pain* 2001; 89:111–115.

Nielson WR, Jensen MP, Kerns RD. The Multidimensional Pain Readiness to Change Questionnaire (MPRCQ): initial development and validation. *J Pain* 2003; 4:149–159.

Prochaska J, DiClemente C. *The Transtheoretical Approach: Crossing Traditional Boundaries of Therapy.* Homewood, IL: Dow Jones Irwin, 1984.

Strong J, Westbury K, Smith G, Mckenzie I, Ryan W. Treatment outcome in individuals with chronic pain: is the Pain Stages of Change Questionnaire (PSOCQ) a useful tool? *Pain* 2002; 97:65–73.

Turk D, Meichenbaum D, Genest M. *Pain and Behavioral Medicine: A Cognitive-Behavioral Perspective*. New York: Guilford Press, 1983.

Weinstein N. Testing four competing theories of health-protective behavior. *Health Psychol* 1993; 12:324–333.

West R. Time for a change: putting the Transtheoretical (Stages of Change) model to rest. *Addiction* 2005; 100:1036–1039.

Correspondence to: Robert D. Kerns, PhD, Psychology Service (116B), VA Connecticut Healthcare System, West Haven, CT 06516, USA. Fax: 203-937-4951; email: robert.kerns@med.va.gov.

Proceedings of the 11th World Congress on Pain,
edited by Herta Flor, Eija Kalso, and Jonathan O.
Dostrovsky, IASP Press, Seattle, © 2006.

50

Multidimensional Associations with Health Care Use for Pain in the Community

Rebecca K. Papas,[a] Joseph L. Riley III,[b]
and Michael E. Robinson[c]

[a]Yale University School of Medicine, VA Connecticut Healthcare System,
New Haven, Connecticut, USA; [b]Department of Operative Dentistry
and [c]Department of Clinical and Health Psychology, University of Florida,
Gainesville, Florida, USA

Pain complaints are the leading reason for health care use, producing exorbitant annual costs. Although several studies have linked pain and the use of health care resources (e.g., Rekola et al. 1993), they studies have typically used prevalence as the operational definition for pain. Yet the pain experience has been defined as multidimensional (International Association for the Study of Pain 2006), incorporating the influence of learning history, beliefs, appraisals, coping strategies, and emotions on the maintenance, exacerbation, or attenuation of pain perception or related experience.

Evidence supports a multidimensional approach to the study of health care use for pain, with some epidemiological and clinical studies demonstrating the value of negative emotion, pain symptoms, and attitudes in predicting health care use (Andersson et al. 1999; Riley et al. 1999). A model developed by Andersen and colleagues conceptualizes health care use as a health behavior, subject to psychosocial influences as well as potential and realized access to services (Andersen and Newman 1973; Andersen 1995). The model posits individual characteristics in three domains that influence health care use: predisposing variables, need variables, and enabling variables. Predisposing variables include social and demographic characteristics, as well as beliefs and attitudes about health care, health care professionals, and disease. Need variables describe the extent to which individuals need a given service and include signs or symptoms as perceived by an individual or as interpreted by a health care professional. Enabling variables include factors that may influence access to services. The model has been employed in studies predicting health care use for all causes of morbidity (Fernandez-Mayoralas et al. 2000) and provides a useful heuristic for categorizing potential causal variables in the study of health care use for pain.

Despite evidence for the multidimensionality of the pain experience, most studies examining health care use examine prevalence of use for clinical pain symptoms with little emphasis on examining predictors of use. Contributions to increased health care use for pain are not limited to increased pain symptoms, but also extend to predisposing attitudes toward health care, social support, and other need-associated variables reflecting pain-related impact such as disability and emotional distress, as well as enabling variables.

Given the financial resources committed annually to health care for pain, examining multidimensional variables that influence patterns of health care use would be beneficial to both public health and health services researchers. Understanding predictive variables in predisposing and need domains, in particular, could lead to targeted public health interventions that could reduce health care costs. This chapter describes a correlational study employing a multidimensional prediction model of health care use for pain consistent with Andersen's domains in a sample of community-dwelling adults. We hypothesized that attitudes and pain-related impact variables would be more strongly associated than pain ratings with the decision to seek health care or to continue care-seeking for pain.

METHODS

To be eligible, the participants were required to be 18 years of age or older, to be English-speaking, to have been a state resident for the previous 6 months, and to have experienced nonmalignant pain with a duration of 5 days or longer in the past 6 months. The participants were recruited from the county drivers' license bureau in an urban, southeastern U.S. city. After giving verbal consent to participate in the study in accordance with university review board requirements, participants were interviewed briefly by the examiner to determine whether inclusion/exclusion criteria were met. If criteria were met, the examiner gained additional information through a brief interview. Each participant was then given a clipboard with a written self-administered survey, which required approximately 15 minutes to complete. The 66-item questionnaire requested information about recent health care visits for pain, demographics, access to care, responses and thoughts about pain, pain-related interference, pain ratings, social support, and health care attitudes and expectations. Data collection was conducted randomly during three different time slots—morning (8–9:30 a.m.), lunchtime (12–1:30 p.m.), and late afternoon (4:30–6 p.m.)—so as to ensure adequate representation of the sample.

Health care use was the self-report, dependent variable. It was measured in two ways: (1) as a dichotomous item assessing whether participants had sought health care for pain in the past 6 months and (2) as a continuous item assessing the number of visits for pain in the past 6 months. The 6-month interval was chosen to ensure that an adequate proportion of participants had made a health care visit, based on previous pain prevalence estimates (Von Korff et al. 1991), and has been associated with better memory recall of health care visits than a 12-month period (Jobe et al. 1990).

Eight independent variables measuring predisposing and need characteristics were employed in this study. In the predisposing domain, variables were early intervention attitudes, attitudes toward health care providers, expectations for an improved pain condition, and social support. In the need domain, variables were pain, disability, pain-related emotions and cognitions, and sleep interference.

The sampling methods and questionnaire employed in this study were piloted in a sample of 135 individuals recruited at the same site. Most of the items in the pilot questionnaire were adapted from well-known measures in the chronic pain literature with excellent psychometric properties including the Coping Strategies Questionnaire (Rosenstiel and Keefe 1983), the Pain Disability Index (Tait et al. 1990), and numeric ratings scales of pain intensity and unpleasantness (Price and Harkins 1992). Psychometric properties of items in the pilot questionnaire were evaluated based on results of a 7-day test-rest reliability study, a concurrent validity study, and a factor analysis (Papas et al. 2000, 2001). Items were retained or modified in the final questionnaire based on results of these studies.

STATISTICAL ANALYSES

A factor analysis was performed on questionnaire items intended to be independent variables in subsequent regression analyses. Principle Axis Factoring was chosen because it eliminates error variance across items and increases reliability, and a Varimax rotation was selected to minimize collinearity among predictors in the multiple regression analyses. A seven-factor solution resulted. The early intervention attitudes variable did not form a factor, but provided conceptual validity for the model. A composite variable was formed using a significantly correlated pair of these items. Eight independent variables were regressed onto the variables measuring health care use. Significance level was set to $P = 0.05$.

Two models were tested. First, a logistic regression model was tested in the entire sample, predicting having made at least one visit to a health care provider for pain in the past 6 months. Variables measuring age, access to health care, and socioeconomic status as well as the eight independent variables, were entered into the model. Second, a hierarchical linear regression model was tested among those who had reported having made at least one health care visit for pain in the past 6 months. In this model, age, access to health care, and socioeconomic status were entered in the first step. In the second step, the eight independent variables were entered (see Fig. 1).

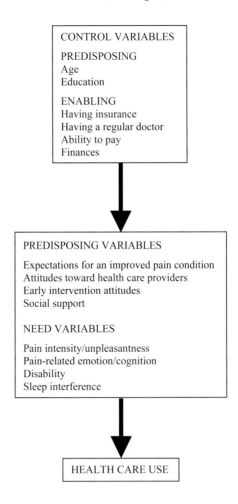

Fig. 1. Regression models of health care use employing the Andersen domains described in the text.

RESULTS

The sample consisted of 410 participants with a mean age of 40 years (SD = 14.3) and a range of 18–84 years. Median education was "some college." Fifty percent of the sample were women. Fifty-six percent of the sample were non-Hispanic white, 32% were non-Hispanic black, 8% were Hispanic, and 4% were identified as other race/ethnicity. The most common pain sites reported were the neck/back and leg/foot.

Table I presents results of the logistic regression model conducted in the entire sample. With age socioeconomic status, and access to health care controlled in the model, pain-related emotion/cognition, sleep interference, expectations for an improved pain condition, and early intervention attitudes toward health concerns were associated with having made at least one visit to a health care provider for pain in the past 6 months.

Table II presents results of the hierarchical linear regression model conducted among those who had made at least one health care visit in the past 6 months. After we controlled for age and access to health care, pain-related emotion/cognition and early intervention attitudes toward health concerns were significantly associated with number of visits during the 6-month period. The model explained 13% of the variance.

DISCUSSION

This chapter has described a study employing a multidimensional prediction model of health care use for pain. We found that attitudes and pain-related impact variables, but not pain ratings of intensity and unpleasantness, were significantly associated with health care use. Emotional and catastrophic variables demonstrated a significant association with health care initiation and continued care-seeking. The findings are consistent with literature showing that clinical populations report strong catastrophic responses to chronic pain (Harkapaa 1991). Our study included a range of emotional responses to pain (anger, fear, frustration, depression, and anxiety) and hence may have been more effective than the measurement of any single emotion at capturing the relationship between emotion and pain. Among those with strong catastrophic and emotional responses to pain, seeking health care may represent an effort to disconfirm negative thoughts and relieve distress.

Results also demonstrated a significant association between health care attitudes and expectations and health care use for pain. An expectation for an improved pain condition was associated with the initiation of care during the study period, but this variable was not associated with continued care-seeking.

Table I
Logistic regression model for predictors of having made at least one health
care visit for pain in the past 6 months ($N = 410$)

Variable	Slope	SE	Odds Ratio (95% CI)	Wald Statistic
Age (years)				13.98*
18–29			1.0 (Referent)	
30–39	1.03	0.36	2.81 (1.40–5.66)	8.40**
40–49	0.96	0.33	2.61 (1.36–5.01)	8.36**
50–59	0.61	0.37	1.85 (0.90–3.80)	2.79
60–69	0.47	0.51	1.60 (0.59–4.31)	0.86
70 and older	1.60	0.75	4.97 (1.15–21.46)	4.62*
Education				9.78
Less than high school			1.0 (Referent)	
High school graduate	0.58	0.44	1.78 (0.76–4.21)	1.74
Some college	1.12	0.43	3.07 (1.33–7.09)	6.85**
College graduate and beyond	1.28	0.46	3.59 (1.47–8.77)	7.84**
Having a regular doctor	0.87	0.29	2.39 (1.34–4.25)	8.76**
Having insurance	0.08	0.30	1.08 (0.60–1.96)	0.06
Financial difficulty	−0.82	0.07	0.92 (0.80–1.06)	1.41
Ability to pay	0.09	0.19	1.09 (0.75–1.59)	0.20
Early intervention attitudes	0.22	0.09	1.25 (1.05–1.49)	6.01*
Sleep interference	0.55	0.13	1.73 (1.33–2.25)	16.79***
Pain-related emotion/cognition	0.58	0.15	1.79 (1.34–2.39)	15.30***
Disability	0.21	0.14	1.24 (0.94–1.63)	2.36
Expectations for improved condition	0.38	0.13	1.46 (1.12–1.89)	8.05**
Attitudes toward health care provider	0.18	0.15	1.20 (0.89–1.61)	1.46
Pain ratings	0.13	0.13	1.14 (0.88–1.48)	0.93
Social support	0.22	0.17	1.24 (0.88–1.74)	1.55
Constant	−3.20	0.87	0.41	13.52***

* $P < 0.05$, ** $P < 0.01$, *** $P < 0.001$.

This finding suggests that the goal for improvement for pain became less important or was seen as less realistic following contact with the health care system. In both prediction models, proactive attitudes toward taking care of health problems were associated with use of health care. As delays in care-seeking can result in pain chronicity, unnecessary lost work days, and unnecessary hospitalizations (Kendall 1999; Foster et al. 2002; American Pain Society 2005), these data can inform the design of public health promotion campaigns, which target attitudes as the mediators of behavior change (e.g., Mastro and Atkin 2002).

Finally, our results showed that sleep interference was significantly associated with initiation of care, but not with continued care-seeking. Our findings

Table II
Hierarchical linear regression model for predictors of number of health care visits for pain among those who had made at least one visit in the past 6 months (n = 224)*

	Slope	SE	β	t	P
Model (13.4% of variance)†					
Step 1					
Control variables (6.4% of variance):					
Age	–0.04	0.02	–0.12	–1.76	0.080
Education	0.15	0.36	0.03	0.40	0.686
Finances	–0.03	0.17	–0.01	–0.17	0.868
Insurance	–2.24	0.83	–0.21	–2.71	0.007
Ability to pay	0.51	0.51	0.08	1.02	0.311
Regular doctor	1.56	0.86	0.14	1.81	0.071
Step 2					
Predictors (7% of variance):					
Early intervention attitudes	0.59	0.21	0.23	2.87	0.005
Sleep interference	0.07	0.38	0.01	0.18	0.861
Pain-related emotion/cognition	0.95	0.39	0.18	2.42	0.016
Disability	0.39	0.35	0.08	1.14	0.257
Expectations for improved condition	0.08	0.42	0.01	0.20	0.844
Attitudes toward health care provider	0.41	0.45	0.07	0.91	0.365
Pain ratings	0.05	0.36	0.01	0.13	0.897
Social support	–0.33	0.45	–0.05	–0.74	0.462
Constant	2.04	2.82		0.72	0.470

* SE = standard error, slope = unstandardized regression coefficient, β = standardized regression weight, t = t-statistic.
† F = 2.32, degrees of freedom = 14, 224, P = 0.005.

suggest that insomnia associated with pain provides an impetus for care-seeking, even with mood and pain variables controlled in the model, but not with continued care-seeking. More research is needed to understand the important relationships between sleep, pain and health care use.

Together, these findings provide validity for a multidimensional focus in public health inquiries of pain in order to develop more effective community interventions. Additional studies are needed to replicate our findings.

ACKNOWLEDGMENT

This study was supported by a U.S. NIMH Individual Training Fellowship, Grant F31-MH12880-02.

REFERENCES

American Pain Society. Former HHS Secretary Louis Sullivan, former Surgeon General David Satcher announce new educational tool to fight 'epidemic' of untreated pain. Available at: www.ampainsoc.org/decadeofpain/news/090803.htm. Accessed January 3, 2005,

Andersen RM, Newman JF. Societal and individual determinants of medical care utilization in the United States. *Milbank Mem Fund Q Health Soc* 1973; 51:95–124.

Andersen RM. Revisiting the behavioral model and access to medical care: does it matter? *J Health Soc Behav* 1995; 36:1–10.

Andersson HI, Ejlertsson G, Leden I, Schersten B. Impact of chronic pain on health care seeking, self care, and medication. Results from a population-based Swedish study. *J Epidemiol Community Health* 1999; 53:503–509.

Fernandez-Mayoralas G, Rodriguez V, Rojo F. Health services accessibility among Spanish elderly. *Soc Sci Med* 2000; 50:17–26.

Foster NE, Pincus T, Underwood M, et al. Treatment and the process of care in musculoskeletal conditions. A multidisciplinary perspective and integration. *Orthop Clin North Am* 2002; 34:239–244.

Harkapaa K. Relationships of psychological distress and health locus of control beliefs with the use of cognitive and behavioral coping strategies in low back pain patients. *Clin J Pain* 1991; 7:275–282.

International Association for the Study of Pain. *IASP Pain Terminology*. Available at: www.iasp-pain.org/terms-p.html. Accessed February 2006.

Jobe JB, White AA, Kelley CL, Mingay DJ, Loftus EF. Recall strategies and memory for health-care visits. *Milbank Mem Fund Q* 1990; 68.

Kendall NA. Psychosocial approaches to the prevention of back pain chronicity paradigm. *Baillieres Best Pract Res Clin Rheumatol* 1999; 13:545–554.

Mastro DE, Atkin C. Exposure to billboards and beliefs and attitudes toward drinking among Mexican Americans. *Howard J Communication* 2002; 13:129–151.

Papas RK, Riley JL III, Robinson ME, Myers CD. Multidimensional prediction models of health care utilization. Poster presented at the American Pain Society Annual Meeting, Atlanta, 2000.

Papas RK, Riley JL III, Robinson ME, Myers CD, Waxenberg LB. Sex-differentiated predictors of health care utilization. Poster presented at the Society for Behavioral Medicine Annual Meeting, Seattle, 2001.

Price DD, Harkins SW. Psychophysical approaches to pain measurement and assessment. In: Turk DC, Melzack R (Eds). *Handbook of Pain Assessment*. New York: Guilford Press, 1992.

Rekola KE, Keinanen-Kiukaanniemi S, Takala J. Use of primary health services in sparsely populated country districts by patients with musculoskeletal symptoms: consultations with a physician. *J Epidemiol Community Health* 1993; 47:153–157.

Riley JL III, Gilbert GH, Heft MW. Health care utilization by older adults in response to painful orofacial symptoms. *Pain* 1999; 81:67–75.

Rosenstiel AK, Keefe FJ. The use of coping strategies in chronic low back pain patients: relationship to patient characteristics and current adjustment. *Pain* 1983; 17:33–44.

Tait RC, Chibnall JT, Krause S. The Pain Disability Index: psychometric properties. *Pain* 1990; 40:171–182.

Von Korff M, Wagner EH, Dworkin SF, Saunders KW. Chronic pain and use of ambulatory health care. *Psychosom Med* 1991; 53:61–79.

Correspondence to: Rebecca K. Papas, PhD, Yale University School of Medicine, VA Connecticut Healthcare System, 950 Campbell Avenue, 11-ACSLG, West Haven, CT 06516, USA. Fax: 203-937-4926; email: rebecca.papas@yale.edu.

Proceedings of the 11th World Congress on Pain,
edited by Herta Flor, Eija Kalso, and Jonathan O.
Dostrovsky, IASP Press, Seattle, © 2006.

51

Psychosocial Factors in Back Pain: A Comparison of Factors Listed by Health Care Providers with the Evidence

Thomas Overmeer,[a,b] Katja Boersma,[a,c]
and Steven J. Linton[a,c]

*[a]Department of Occupational and Environmental Medicine, University Hospital
Örebro, Örebro, Sweden; [b]Departments of Clinical Medicine and [c]Behavioral,
Social and Legal Sciences, Örebro University, Örebro, Sweden*

During the last decade, researchers have clearly recognized the importance of psychosocial factors in back pain (Nachemson and Jonsson 2000). Evidence indicates that psychosocial factors are associated with the onset of back pain and that they are linked to the transition from acute to chronic disability (Nachemson and Jonsson 2000). In fact, psychosocial variables generally have more impact on back pain disability than biomedical or biomechanical factors (Burton and Erg 1997; Turk 1997; Nachemson and Jonsson 2000). Specific factors such as depression, fear avoidance, stress, anxiety, catastrophizing, and job dissatisfaction have been put forward as some of the main predictors of chronic back pain and disability (Waddell et al. 2003; Burton et al. 2004). However, even though these risk factors are widely recognized within the research community, little is known about how much clinicians know about them or whether they implement knowledge about them in their clinical practice.

The implementation of evidence regarding psychosocial factors in back pain is problematic. For example, national guidelines, based on systematic reviews, recommend that practitioners both *assess* and *treat* psychosocial factors (Nachemson and Jonsson 2000; Burton et al. 2004). However, a comparison of 11 different national evidence-based guidelines on low back pain showed that these guidelines gave no clear advice about which factors to take into consideration, when to assess them, or how to screen for them (Koes et al. 2001). Specific information on which factors to take into consideration may be of crucial importance given the myriad of psychosocial issues patients may present in a clinical contact. Clinicians may be able to modify a number of psychological factors, such as fear avoidance, catastrophizing, and distress, within the scope of the available treatments. Therefore, it is important to gain more knowledge about whether clinicians know about these specific factors.

There is reason to believe that many practitioners lack up-to-date knowledge about these specific psychosocial factors. For example, a recent study shows that despite great efforts to distribute evidence-based guidelines in Sweden, approximately half of the clinicians in primary care were unfamiliar with their content (Overmeer et al. 2005). Moreover, a study of physiotherapists in Great Britain and Australia showed that physiotherapists ranked research results last in importance as a basis for treatment choice (Turner and Whitfield 1997). Treatment techniques they learned during their initial training, their experience with treatment effects in their own patients, and information gained in practice-related courses were instead primary reasons for choosing one treatment over another. Such attitudes may prevent practitioners from incorporating recent evidence on psychosocial factors into their clinical practice.

This chapter describes a study whose aim was to list, categorize, and compare health care providers' spontaneous listings of specific psychosocial factors with those established in evidence-based reviews. This study was part of a larger study on implementation of back pain guidelines that has been reported in detail elsewhere (Overmeer et al. 2005).

METHODS

We performed a qualitative and descriptive study using an open question to investigate health care providers' notions of psychosocial factors in the context of back pain.

PARTICIPANTS

In March 2003, a questionnaire was sent to all physicians and physiotherapists ($N = 235$) working in primary health care settings in Örebro County, Sweden. A reminder was sent to nonresponders 2 weeks later. One hundred and fifty-seven physicians and physiotherapists completed the questionnaire (a response rate of 67%). The response rate for physicians was 58% (51 men and 37 women, mean age = 48 years, SD = 8.7 years). For physiotherapists, the response rate was 83% (19 men and 47 women, mean age = 35 years, SD = 10.6 years). The ethics committee of the Örebro University Hospital approved the study.

QUESTIONNAIRE

Health care providers received a back pain questionnaire dealing with different aspects of back pain as well as the implementation of guidelines for back pain management. In order to allow the physicians and physiotherapists to describe specific psychosocial factors, we used the open-ended question: "When psychosocial factors are mentioned, which factors do you think of?" This question appeared at the beginning of the questionnaire in order to minimize biased responses.

ANALYSIS

The results were analyzed in three steps. First, all factors that were mentioned by the health care providers were listed, and identical items were combined, yielding a list of 936 separate psychosocial factors. Second, one of the authors performed an initial categorization by grouping together items that had similar content or meaning, and the other two authors checked the categorization for reliability. This first categorization step resulted in 34 categories incorporating items with similar content or meaning. For example, the items "economy," "economic factors," "economic standard," and "economic position" were considered to have similar content that could be captured under the category heading "economy." We then grouped the newly formed categories into eight higher-order categories according to their content. For example, the categories "family," "social support," "economy," "interpersonal," and "environment" were all grouped under the heading "social and environmental factors." The categorization process was supervised by two independent researchers who were not involved in the project. Disagreements about categorization were discussed, and agreement was reached through consensus.

CATEGORIZATION OF RESPONSES

Table I gives an overview of psychosocial factors that were mentioned by health care providers when answering the open-ended question: "When psychosocial factors are mentioned, which factors do you think of?" A total of 936 different factors were indicated. Included in the table are the categories and themes under which these answers are grouped. Most prevalent (mentioned 340 out of 936 times) were factors grouped under the theme "social and environmental factors." This higher-order category included categories such as "family" (e.g., family, family situations, familial circumstances), "social support" (e.g., marital status, loneliness, social network), and "economy" (e.g., economy,

Table I

Psychosocial factors mentioned by health care providers as relevant to patients with back pain; factors directly related to pain are italicized

Category (No. Mentions)	Psychosocial Factors (No. Mentions)
Social and Environmental Factors (340)	
Family (122)	Family (50), family situations (29), familial circumstances (17), family conflicts (8), familial well-being (1), children with social problems (1), home (4), home circumstances (4), home situation (6), relatives (1), alcohol abuse by husband (1)
Social support (74)	Civil status (4), loneliness (5), single (4), interconnected with others (1), social network (29), friends (17), support (5), social belonging (9)
Economy (52)	Economy (38), economic factors (12), economic standard (1), economic position (1)
Interpersonal (24)	Relationships characterized by conflict (1), relationships (9), relationships to people close by (2), relationships in leisure time (3), intimate relationships (2), divorce (7)
Environment (22)	Living conditions (5), place of residence (2), housing (3), homelessness (1), housing conditions (6), environment (4), surroundings (1)
Social status (21)	Social status (2), education (19)
Abuse and trauma (15)	Abuse (1), mobbing (3), crisis and trauma experiences (10), social trauma (1)
Other (10)	Parents receiving a disability pension (1), criminality (2), problems at home or work (1), social problems (1), social situation (4), social anamnesis (1)
Psychological Factors (208)	
Emotion (57)	Depression (7), emotional factors (3), sense of coherence (1), worry (9), fear (2), inability to relax(1), aggression (1), stress (17), stress level (4), tension (1), apathy (1), anxiety (8), *anxiety/worry about pain (2)*
Personal interests (37)	Interests (4), leisure time (16), leisure time interests (4), leisure time activities (13)
Cognitions (26)	Attitudes (2), destructive thoughts (1), own view of health (1), too high a demand on self and others (1), crushed expectations (1), expectations (2), cognitive factors (1), demands (2), ideology (1), view of health and illness (2), view of own role and function (1), knowledge (1), *view on pain: normal vs. alarm (1), causal theory about pain (1), catastrophizing (1), own thoughts about illness (1), thoughts about prognosis (1), knowledge about illness/problem (1), fear-avoidance (3), differences between patient's view and health care provider's view (1)*

Table continues on next page

Table I (Continued)

Category (No. Mentions)	Psychosocial Factors (No. Mentions)
Coping (22)	Coping (14), possibilities of leisure time for self (2), capacity to set boundaries (1), strategies to solve conflicts (1), control possibilities at work and in free time (1), life strategies (1), *pain coping (2)*
Self-esteem (18)	Invisibility (1), self-efficacy (8), inadequacy (1), self-confidence at work (1), self-confidence (3), self-image (3), view of self together with others (1)
Personality (17)	Autonomy (1), loss of initiative (1), personality (10), personality resources (1), vulnerability (1), hyperactivity (1), psychological profile (1), current vulnerability (1)
Psychological status (11)	Mental load (1), mental problem (2), mental status (2), mental illness (5), contact with mental health and social services (1)
Motivation (11)	Indifference (1), motivation (2), drive (2), attitude to work/sick listing (1), learned norm system (1), illness gain (4)
Other (6)	Behavior (1), body awareness (1), time for recovery (1), conflicts—internal and external (2), social maturity (1)
Sexuality (3)	Sexuality (1), sex and personal relationships (1), sex life and romantic experiences (1)
Work Factors (195)	
Work, general (105)	Work (70), profession (9), work situation (19), work environment problem (1), work problem (3), sick listing (3)
Unemployment (28)	Unemployment (27), unemployed husband (1)
Interpersonal at work (17)	Work relations (12), relational problem at work (4), lack of support from colleagues/employer (1)
Intrapersonal at work (24)	Job satisfaction (20), job stress (4)
Work characteristics (21)	Work environment (11), workload (5), work tasks (1), demands for flexibility at work (1), heavy work (1), work hours (2)
Substance Abuse (66)	
Substance abuse (66)	Use of stimulating substances (1), tobacco (10), own alcohol consumption (2), relation to alcohol and tobacco (1), substance abuse (52)
General Health and Health Behavior (49)	
Comorbidity (19)	Life with illness (1), illness/disease, own or of relative (6), somatic illness/disease history (2), handicap (1), comorbidity (1), picture of the illness/disease (1), previous illness/disease and load (7)

Table continues on next page

Table I (Continued)

Category (No. Mentions)	Psychosocial Factors (No. Mentions)
Lifestyle (16)	Diet and exercise (1), learned life habits (1), lifestyle (4), food and beverage habits (1), how the patient chooses to live (1), exercise (7), obesity (1)
Psychosomatic symptoms (9)	Muscle pain (1), psychosomatic symptoms (1), tension headache (2), sleep (2), sleep difficulties (1), fatigue (1), feebleness (1)
Other (5)	Care of one's health (1), health (2), complex pain syndrome (1), pain problem (1)
Other (42)	
Life in general (22)	Quality of life (1), problem/problem-free (1), satisfaction (5), all parts of a person's life (1), general poorness (1), internal and external factors (1), well-being (3), hurt in life (1), experience of current life situation (1), phase in life (1), life situation (5), life events (1)
Other (20)	Age (2), season (1), nothing (12), religion (1), service (1), women (1), gender (2)
History Factors (37)	
Ethnicity (22)	Ethnicity (2), refugee problems (1), immigrant background (3), cultural factors (9), nationality (1), language (2), born outside the country (1), origin (2)
Background (7)	Background (4), psychosocial behavior pattern transferred from parents (1), social background (2)
Childhood (5)	Childhood (3), conditions the person grew up under (2)
Heredity (3)	Heredity (1), heredity for certain illnesses (1), heredity of attitudes about illness (1)

economic factors). Second-most prevalent were factors grouped under the theme "psychological factors" (mentioned 208 out of 936 times), including categories such as "emotion" (e.g., depression, stress, anxiety), "personal interests" (e.g., leisure-time activities, leisure time), and "cognitions" (e.g., attitudes, destructive thoughts, expectations). The third-most prevalent higher-order category was "work factors" (mentioned 195 out of 936 times), including categories such as "work" (e.g., work, work situation, profession), "unemployment," and "interpersonal issues at work."

Health care providers mentioned a large variety of factors that typically were broad and general terms, such as "work," "family," and "economy." In fact, specific psychosocial factors directly related to pain such as pain-specific cognitions, emotions, and behaviors were mentioned only 16 times.

Table II presents a list of 13 factors that have moderate to strong support in the literature as psychosocial predictors of chronic pain and disability (Waddell et al. 2003). Included in the table is a column indicating how often these factors were mentioned by the health care providers in the study. Because the wording of the factors was quite nonspecific, we relaxed the criteria so that all factors that might be interpreted as similar to the evidence-based factors were included. Of the evidence-based factors, psychological distress, employment status, and job dissatisfaction were the factors that were mentioned most often (47, 27, and 20 out of 936 times, respectively). However, even these most popular factors were mentioned so infrequently that only 16% (147 out of 936) of the factors mentioned overall could be regarded as evidence-based.

Table II
A comparison of evidence-based psychosocial factors and the number of times they were mentioned by the health care providers in the study

Predictor of Chronic Pain/Disability*	No. Mentions by Health Care Providers†
Age	2
Pain intensity, functional disability	0
Poor perceptions of general health	3 (including own view of health, view on health and illness)
Psychological distress	47 (including emotional factors, worry, fear, inability to relax, stress, stress level, tension, anxiety, and anxiety/worry about pain)
Depression	7
Fear avoidance	9 (including view on pain: normal vs. alarm, causal theory about pain, own thoughts about illness, knowledge about illness/problem, fear-avoidance, attitudes)
Catastrophizing	3 (including catastrophizing, destructive thoughts, cognitive factors)
Pain behavior	17 (including behavior, coping, and pain coping)
Job (dis)satisfaction and worker's dissatisfaction	20
Duration of sickness absence	3 (including sick listing)
Employment status (not employed)	27
Expectations about return to work	4 (including crushed expectations, expectations, thoughts about prognosis)
Financial incentives	4 (including illness gain)

* Factors are listed that have moderate to strong support in the literature as psychosocial predictors of chronic pain and disability (Waddell et al. 2003).
† Verbatim factors are mentioned when they were somewhat dissimilar in wording compared to the evidence-based factors.

DISCUSSION

Health care providers listed a large variety of variables when asked about their notion of psychosocial factors in the context of back pain. In total, 936 different factors were listed. Over 80% of these factors were not evidence-based. This finding underscores a mismatch in communication between the research community and clinical practice. Further, it raises concerns about the assessment and treatment of psychosocial features in patients with back pain.

Because the factors that the clinicians indicated were typically broad and general such as "family" or "social support," they may be difficult or impossible to influence within the scope of available treatments. However, other data from the same sample showed that more than 70% of the clinicians in this study indicated that they "know how to" and "do" assess psychosocial factors (Overmeer et al. 2005). Perhaps clinicians meant that they discuss broad and general life concerns that may arise in the clinical context such as family problems, housing issues, or loneliness. This possibility leads to concerns about the implementation of evidence-based psychosocial factors in clinical practice, particularly since only 16% of the factors listed by clinicians were evidence-based. In fact, fear-based avoidance, one of the most prominent psychosocial factors reported in the research literature, was mentioned a mere 9 out of 936 times.

The results of this study indicate a mismatch in communication between clinicians and researchers. It seems that health care providers may have different conceptions of the relationships between psychosocial factors and back pain disability than those currently proposed in the literature. A recent study showed that practitioners are very aware of the importance of psychosocial factors and have a favorable attitude toward paying attention to them (Overmeer et al. 2004). However, perhaps they are focusing on the *wrong* factors. This possibility is not surprising, given that evidence-based guidelines give no clear advice about *which* factors to take into consideration but simply recommend that practitioners should both *assess* and *treat* psychosocial factors (Koes et al. 2001).

The results reviewed in this chapter have implications for the implementation of research findings on psychosocial factors. To date, the traditional model of disseminating research findings has involved publication in peer-reviewed journals. This model assumes that clinicians have the time, energy, and skills to appraise research and the ability to introduce new methods into their clinical practice. However, the clinicians in this study seem to have failed to translate research findings on psychosocial factors into practice. Incorporating psychosocial factors in clinical practice requires not only favorable attitudes but also up-to-date knowledge and skills (Cabana et al. 1999).

This study is a first attempt at tapping into clinicians' notions about psychosocial factors that affect treatment outcomes for patients with back pain. More research from different perspectives is needed. It would, for example, be of great value to study clinicians' actual practice behavior in dealing with psychosocial factors. Such research is crucial for improving our understanding of the obstacles against putting research results into clinical practice.

One possible weakness of this study is the assessment method employed. We used a question that did not ask for specific factors, and we did not ask separately for psychological and social factors. We chose this wording so as to avoid introducing phrases that might point to a particular factor. Nevertheless, it is still surprising that only about 16% of the indicated factors were evidence-based.

In summary, this study shows that health care providers may lack adequate knowledge on evidence-based psychosocial factors in the context of back pain. The respondents in this study indicated a wide range of psychosocial factors, of which only 16% had evidence to show they were predictors of chronic pain and disability. Most of the listed factors mirror various life difficulties that patients may describe in a clinical context, such as family problems or lack of social support. These factors are broad and general and are difficult for clinicians to modify within the scope of their treatment possibilities. In summary, health care providers seem to have different conceptions of the relationships between psychosocial factors and back pain disability than those currently proposed in the literature, and they appear to lack knowledge on specific, modifiable, and evidence-based factors.

REFERENCES

Burton AK, Erg E. Back injury and work loss. Biomechanical and psychosocial influences. *Spine* 1997; 22:2575–2580.

Burton AK, Eriksen HR, Leclerc A, et al. *European Guidelines for Prevention in Low Back Pain.* 2004. Available at: www.backpaineurope.org/web/files/WG3_Guidelines.pdf.

Cabana MD, Rand CS, Powe NR, et al. Why don't physicians follow clinical practice guidelines? A framework for improvement. *JAMA* 1999; 282:1458–1465.

Koes B, van Tulder M, Ostelo R, Burton K, Waddell G. Clinical guidelines for the management of low back pain in primary care. *Spine* 2001; 26:2504–2514.

Nachemson A, Jonsson E (Eds). *Neck and Back Pain, The Scientific Evidence of Causes, Diagnosis, and Treatment.* Philadelphia: Lippincott Williams & Wilkins, 2000.

Overmeer T, Linton S, Boersma K. Do physical therapists recognise established risk factors? Swedish physical therapists' evaluation in comparison to guidelines. *Physiotherapy* 2004; 90:35–41.

Overmeer T, Linton SJ, Holmquist L, Eriksson M, Engfeldt P. Do evidence-based guidelines have an impact in primary care? A cross-sectional study of Swedish physicians and physiotherapists. *Spine* 2005; 30:146–151.

Turk DC. The role of demographic and psychosocial factors in transition from acute to chronic pain. In: Jensen TS, Turner JA, Wiesenfeld-Hallin Z (Eds). *Proceedings of the 8th World Congress on Pain,* Progress in Pain Research and Management, Vol. 8. Seattle: IASP Press, 1997, pp 185–213.

Turner P, Whitfield TA. Physiotherapists' use of evidence based practice: a cross-national study. *Physiother Res Int* 1997; 2:17–29.

Waddell G, Burton K, Main C. *Screening to Identify People at Risk of Long-Term Incapacity of Work: A Conceptual and Scientific Review.* London: Royal Society of Medicine Press, 2003.

Correspondence to: Thomas Overmeer, MSc, Department of Occupational and Environmental Medicine, University Hospital Örebro, SE 701 85 Örebro, Sweden. Email: thomas.overmeer@orebroll.se.

Proceedings of the 11th World Congress on Pain,
edited by Herta Flor, Eija Kalso, and Jonathan O.
Dostrovsky, IASP Press, Seattle, © 2006.

52

Overuse as a Risk Factor for Pain Disability: Cognitive-Behavioral Models and Interventions

Johan W.S. Vlaeyen,[a] Warren R. Nielson,[b] and Boudewijn van Houdenhove[c]

[a]Department of Medical, Clinical and Experimental Psychology, Maastricht University, Maastricht, The Netherlands; [b]Arthritis Institute, St. Joseph's Health Care, London, Ontario, Canada; [c]Department of Liaison Psychiatry, Gasthuisberg University Hospital, Leuven, Belgium

In patients with chronic pain, the level of pain disability has long been assumed to have a one-to-one relationship with pain severity because individuals with more pain tend to show poorer performance in tasks of daily living than those with less pain. In the last decade this view has been questioned, and cognitive-behavioral mechanisms associated with pain are now considered to be more important than the severity of pain. In particular, the fear/avoidance model has become influential as an explanation for the transition from acute to chronic pain disability, particularly in the case of low back pain. The model predicts that those who catastrophize about pain become fearful and that this fear is associated with impaired physical performance and increased self-reported disability because of self-imposed protective behaviors such as escape or avoidance of activities and selective attention to bodily sensations (Vlaeyen and Linton 2000). Although accumulating evidence supports the fear/avoidance model as a predictor of disability in patients with back and neck pain, there are unresolved issues that merit further scientific attention. Firstly, several anomalous findings in the current literature cannot be explained by the fear/avoidance model. For example, van den Hout et al. (2001) observed better performance after experimentally inducing a negative mood in participants who were asked to perform a lifting task for "as long as possible." Similarly, in a cold pressor study in which healthy volunteers were requested to immerse their hands for "as long as possible," Severeijns et al. (2005) found longer tolerance times in those participants who were given threatening instructions that increased negative mood. Some prospective studies reveal that self-efficacy beliefs or more general negative affect are more important determinants of disability than fear/avoidance beliefs in primary health care patients with musculoskeletal pain (Denison et al. 2004; Sieben et al. 2005). These inconsistent but intriguing results suggest pathways to disability other than fear/avoidance behavior. Second, it is difficult to apply the model to musculoskeletal pain syndromes associated with task persistence rather than avoidance. Some patients with chronic pain (such as work-related upper extremity pain) tend to persist in, rather than escape or avoid, physical activity (Arntz and Peters 1995), although research is scarce. In some cases, task persistence is so excessive that it may take the form of ergomania (excessive devotion to work), a relatively stable condition that might be considered a predisposing factor for chronic pain. Many cognitive-behavioral management programs would assist such patients by introducing pacing techniques to teach them to find a balance between rest and activity. Finally, novel theoretical models are emerging in which variability in task performance is considered a function of the interaction between certain "stop-rules" and current mood. To date, however, few studies have considered cognitive-behavioral mechanisms behind the seemingly paradoxical relationship between task persistence and chronic pain. In this chapter, we provide a critical overview of what is known about task persistence, ergomania, pacing techniques, and the role of "stop-rules," and current mood in chronic pain. It should be noted that given the scarcity of empirical studies in this area, we will probably raise more questions than provide answers.

TASK PERSISTENCE AS AN ADAPTIVE STRATEGY

Cognitive-behavioral models of chronic pain emphasize the importance of an individual's attempts to cope with pain and pain-related issues or problems. Coping responses can be considered adaptive or maladaptive, depending on the usual outcome of the coping behavior, cognition, or emotion. Certain coping responses, such as task persistence, have been associated with better physical and psychological functioning among individuals with chronic pain, whereas others, such as pain-contingent resting and guarding, have been correlated with impaired function. However, the recent literature seems inconsistent as to the validity of task persistence as an adaptive coping strategy. For example, the task persistence subscale of the Chronic Pain Coping Inventory was found to be positively associated with general activity level and negatively associated with depression, functional disability, and interference of pain in situations of daily life (Jensen et al. 1995; Tan et al. 2005). One subscale of the relatively new Work Style Questionnaire that conceptually shows great overlap with task persistence is "working through pain" (Feuerstein et al. 2005). Interestingly, another pattern of correlations emerges. Working through pain appears to be positively associated with pain severity and functional limitations and negatively associated with a measure of physical and mental health. A closer look at the items of both measures may lead to a possible explanation. Items of the Chronic Pain Coping Inventory task persistence scale imply "despite pain, I continue my activity," which reflects active approach behavior. Items of the Work Style Questionnaire's working through pain scale are worded differently; they take the form of "I continue to prevent problems," reflecting active avoidance behavior such that continuing to work avoids the consequences of aversive behavior. A typical item is: "I continue to work with pain and discomfort so that the quality of my work won't suffer." These intriguing data reflect the controversy about the validity of the coping concept (Tunks and Bellissimo 1988), and force us to critically rethink our theoretical models of task persistence in chronic pain.

ERGOMANIA AS A VULNERABILITY FACTOR

Patients suffering from chronic pain and chronic fatigue frequently report premorbid tendencies toward physical and mental overachievement, as well as perfectionistic or self-effacing behavior. We refer to these features using the term "ergomania": from the Greek roots "ergon" and "mania," meaning "excessive desire for work." It could also be described as "workaholism" or as a "hyperactive" or "overactive" lifestyle. In many patients, preexisting ergomania often persists after the onset of an illness and may lead patients to exceed their physical or mental limits, exacerbating pain and symptoms. Consequently, persisting ergomanic tendencies may impede successful adaptation to chronic pain and fatigue and constitute an important illness-maintaining factor. However, despite the potential pathogenetic role of ergomania in chronic pain and fatigue, research interest in this topic has been rather minimal until recently, with a few exceptions (Van Houdenhove 1986; Van Houdenhove et al. 1987, 1995; Alfici et al. 1989; Gamsa and Vikis-Freibergs 1991; Van Houdenhove et al. 2005). For example, in one descriptive study, patients with fibromyalgia and chronic fatigue syndrome as well as healthy controls were requested to complete a measure of "action prone-ness," including items such as "I have always been an active and busy person," "I do not like to postpone things," and "I love making a supreme effort." Because patients' self-descriptions might have been biased by retrospective idealization, significant others were invited to complete a slightly modified version of the same questionnaire, replacing "I" by "he/she." Again, significant others rated patients as more action-prone as compared to the significant others' ratings of the healthy controls (Van Houdenhove et al., 2001). Despite these attempts, ergomania remains a vague concept. Many questions concerning its precise definition, delineation, and determination remain unanswered. For example, could ergomania be quantitatively defined and expressed in terms of number of working hours, or are qualitative factors such as work style, decision latitude, and perception of control more important? Although the matter is still quite speculative, ergomania is suggested to play a perpetuating role in chronic pain and fatigue via interacting physical and psychological mechanisms, such as stress to the body from physical overuse and sleep deprivation, which can lead to a dysregulation of neuroendocrine, immunological, and central pain-processing systems (van der Hulst 2003; Glass et al. 2004). Additionally, tendencies toward ergomania that persist after the onset of an illness may also make it more difficult for patients to accept their illness (Viane et al. 2003), to take full account of their functional limitations, and to carefully pace their daily activities (Van Houdenhove and Egle 2004).

THERAPEUTIC AND RESEARCH IMPLICATIONS

Although the concept of ergomania is still speculative, clinicians should be aware that this tendency might negatively interfere with pain and symptom management and thus compromise a patient's long-term prognosis. Some preliminary evidence indicates that a multidisciplinary program of cognitive-behavioral therapy, including pacing techniques, could help fibromyalgia patients change their ergomania-related attitudes and tendencies in order to find a new equilibrium (Nielson et al., 1992). One of the key aspects of such a cognitive-behavioral intervention is the use of pacing techniques. Patients with a tendency to be overactive work toward limiting their involvements and learn to allow themselves contrasting activities (such as relaxation) to interrupt the habitual task persistence.

ACTIVITY PACING: THEORETICAL BASIS AND CURRENT STATUS

DEFINITIONAL PROBLEMS

Activity pacing is a common but imprecisely and inconsistently defined element of many treatment programs for chronic musculoskeletal pain. It appears to have developed along two quite distinct lines: within behavioral treatment programs for pain, and as a self-management strategy for patients with chronic illnesses such as rheumatoid arthritis. Behavioral treatment programs for chronic pain have, from the beginning, recognized that some patients tend to seek relief from pain by engaging in activities. Fordyce (1976, pp 181–183) referred to patients who use activity rather than rest to reduce pain as "pacers" and recommended elimination of excessive activity via contingency management procedures that set quotas for "uninterrupted periods of reclining or sitting" plus relaxation training techniques. It is worth noting that the term "pace" in this context meant to walk back and forth rather than the rate of behavior. Some later behavioral approaches (e.g., Gil et al. 1988) used the latter meaning of the term and included activity-rest cycling as an important element of behavioral treatment in a manner entirely consistent with Fordyce's recommendations. This approach assumes that the delay in pain that occurs following overactivity reduces its inhibitory effect on activity and that the pain-relieving effect of activity is a strong reinforcer. Increasing intervals of positively reinforced *moderate* activity interspersed with time-contingent rest produce a gradual improvement in both activity level and pain. Activity-rest cycling is also an approach taken in physical therapy to increase strength and mobility. The therapist sets the length of the activity and rest periods so that during the active phase the patient learns to "pace his/her physical output carefully" (Fey and Fordyce 1983).

In contrast to its use within behavioral approaches to pain, activity pacing as a self-management strategy for patients with chronic illnesses appears to have arisen along with the concept of energy conservation. For example, patients with rheumatic diseases are encouraged to remain active but to "listen to their bodies" and to take regular breaks rather than to "work through" pain. They are asked to alternate periods of rest and activity as a coping strategy that will reduce stress on their joints and minimize their symptoms (Gerber et al. 1987). While limited evidence suggests that activity pacing may increase physical activity, others have found that it is associated with worse physical functioning (e.g., Chorus et al. 2001; Boonen et al. 2004).

MEASUREMENT OF ACTIVITY PACING

Three questionnaires have been developed to measure activity pacing. Van Lankveld et al. (1993) created a "coping with rheumatic stressors" questionnaire, which includes some items relevant to pacing oneself in order to cope with limitations. Pacing behaviors are described as avoidant coping and are associated with decreased physical functioning, but not with pain. However, in this correlational study, the use of activity pacing may have been influenced by pain and functional limitations. Different results might also have been obtained if the content of the pacing items assessed coping with pain rather than coping with physical limitations. In contrast, Nielson et al (2001) conceptualized activity pacing as an active, adaptive strategy for coping with pain. They developed a brief therapeutic scale, which included taking breaks, going more slowly, maintaining a steady pace, and breaking tasks into smaller pieces. More recently, Cane et al. (2004) began development of a Pain Patterns of Activity Questionnaire that includes an activity pacing scale. Initial results indicate that among a heterogeneous sample of chronic pain patients completing a multi-disciplinary pain program, the use of activity pacing was lower than expected (40% said they used this strategy "somewhat" or "not at all"). Women were less likely to use it than men, and it was associated with lower rates of depression and fear of re-injury, but not with pain intensity, disability, or activity level (Cane et al. 2004). An advantage of the Pain Patterns of Activity Questionnaire is that it allows categorization of pacing according to inactive/avoidant and overactive/underactive patterns.

ACTIVITY PACING AND TREATMENT
OF FIBROMYALGIA SYNDROME

Activity pacing has been included in cognitive-behavioral treatment programs for fibromyalgia syndrome for about 15 years (Nielson et al. 1992). A common pattern of behavior among fibromyalgia patients is that when they have lower pain levels, they "make up for lost time" by becoming overactive, which, in turn, leads to an increase in pain and fatigue. Activity pacing in such patients includes not only having them set quotas for themselves, but also ensuring that they do not overdo activities on days when they feel better (Turk and Sherman 2002). Fibromyalgia patients in general may have a tendency to push themselves beyond their tolerance levels and may experience a greater amount of exercise-induced muscle ischemia than healthy individuals (Elvin et al. 2006). Some authors have even suggested that it may be inappropriate to have patients with fibromyalgia exercise to tolerance (e.g., Clark et al. 2001). Cognitive-behavioral treatment programs for chronic pain often include pacing both as a skill designed to prevent overuse (Turk and Monarch 2002) and as part of a quota-based approach to increase activity (Turk and Sherman 2002). Although such treatment programs are effective for most types of chronic pain and often include a pacing component (Morley et al. 1999), few randomized controlled trials have assessed their efficacy for patients with fibromyalgia syndrome and even fewer have included activity pacing as a component (Williams et al. 2002). Thus the clinical utility of activity pacing alone or in conjunction with other interventions for fibromyalgia and other chronic pain conditions has yet to be clearly established. And, as noted above, pacing as a self-management strategy is similarly unproven and in need of empirical evaluation. Understanding which strategies would most effectively help patients moderate overactivity and who would benefit from this approach represents an unexplored avenue for future research.

STOP-RULES, MOOD, AND PHYSICAL PERFORMANCE

THE "MOOD-AS-INPUT" MODEL

The fear/avoidance and the ergomania model both share a basic assumption that main affects determine task performance. In contrast, more complex models suggest that behavioral performance should be approached in the context of affect regulation processes, in which interactions rather than main affects are more accurate predictors of performance. The mood-as-input model (Martin et al. 1993) is one of these emerging paradigms. Mood-as-input uses the effects of mood in a certain context, rather than the mood itself, to predict whether participants will persist at a certain task. It also assumes that individuals implicitly or explicitly use "stop-rules" that guide them in persisting with or terminating a given task. The "As-Many-As-[You]-Can" stop-rule is used when the individual persists until reaching satisfaction about dealing with the task. In contrast, when individuals adopt the "Feel-Like-Discontinuing" stop-rule, they terminate activities when they are not enjoying the task anymore. The basic tenet of the mood-as-input model is that task performance is a function of the interaction between mood and the stop-rule used. When individuals use an As-Many-As-Can stop-rule, negative mood will facilitate task persistence, while positive mood will inhibit task performance. The negative mood signals to the individual that progress on the task has been insufficient and facilitates continuation with the task. Using the Feel-Like-Discontinuing stop-rule, the opposite pattern is found. A negative mood here signals that continuing with the task is no longer appropriate, leading to disengagement from the task. Thus, with different stop-rules, the same mood can have different motivational effects. Evidence of this kind of reversal is provided by a number of experiments in which subjects are placed in either positive or negative moods by having them watch video clips with positive or negative valence. They subsequently are asked to perform an impression-formation task: reading a number of behaviors with the goal to form an impression of the person described by these behaviors. Half of the subjects were instructed to go on with the task until they felt having enough information to form the impression (As-Many-As-Can). The remaining subjects were instructed to continue until they were not enjoying the task anymore (Feel-Like-Discontinuing). The results were consistent with the mood-as-input predictions. When given the "enough" instruction, subjects in the positive mood stopped sooner than did those in the negative mood. The opposite pattern was found in the "enjoy" condition. In fact, the stop-rule instructions directed the subjects to a different interpretation of their moods, resulting in a different type of processing (Martin et al., 1993)

In the area of chronic pain, mood-as-input may provide a new theoretical model that is likely to produce new assessment and treatment approaches

(Vlaeyen and Morley 2004). A particular strength is that it provides predictions, including those based on the existing models. Indeed, back pain patients who are convinced that certain movements are harmful may use the Feel-Like-Discontinuing stop-rule when dealing with a task that consists of these movements. Consistent with the fear/avoidance model, such patients will quickly terminate the task when in a negative mood. However, if they are instructed to perform as much as possible (As-Many-As-Can stop-rule), they will tend to persist longer with the task. This theoretically predicted effect could account for the findings reported by Van den Hout and colleagues (2001) as noted above. The mood-as-input model further predicts that there are four cognitive-behavioral pathways to linking mood, stop-rules, and task performance. Fig. 1 illustrates the two pathways that occur in the context of a negative mood state (possibly fueled by pain, or by failure in achieving one's goals). In this context, the Feel-Like-Discontinuing rule (e.g., when the patient considers the task as threatening and has a negative outcome expectancy) will lead to task avoidance, resulting in disuse, in accordance with the fear/acceptance model. In the same context, the As-Many-As-Can stop-rule will result in task persistence (e.g., when the patient considers the task to be meaningful and goal-directed and has a positive outcome expectancy), with overuse possibly causing tissue damage (Barr and Barbe 2002) as a potential risk. Although positive mood generally is considered to be much more beneficial (Aspinwall 1998), the process may be reversed. For example, the use of the Feel-Like-Discontinuing stop-rule in a positive mood may also lead to overuse. As such, the model also may explain fluctuations in activity levels typical of pain patients.

In individuals who habitually adopt a certain stop-rule, fluctuating moods parallel changes in the level of task performance, or alternatively, when a certain

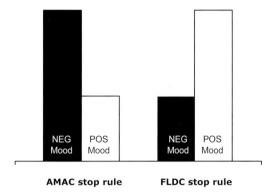

Fig. 1. Graphic presentation of the predictions in task performance based on "mood-as-input" model (from Martin et al. 1993, in Vlaeyen and Morley 2004). AMAC = "As Many as [You] Can"; FLDC = "Feel Like Discontinuing."

mood predominates, fluctuations in task performance occur as a function of changing stop-rules. While the mood-as-input model may help to identify mechanisms of risks of overuse or disuse, there is complementary and compelling evidence that an accommodating style of "flexible goal pursuit" may protect against disability (Schmitz et al. 1996; McCracken and Eccleston 2003).

CLINICAL IMPLICATIONS

A final question is whether stop-rules are modifiable. The mood-as-input model may provide a single framework for helping chronic pain patients to adopt stop-rules in a flexible way, including both exposure to feared activities (encouraging As-Many-As-Can stop-rules; Vlaeyen et al. 2002) and pacing techniques (encouraging Feel-Like-Discontinuing stop-rules; Nielson et al. 2001). More insight into the interplay between mood, stop-rules, and physical performance is likely to enhance our understanding of disability in chronic musculoskeletal pain. Certainly, a sound theoretical framework and successful novel interventions in this area are badly needed.

CONCLUSIONS

This chapter offers a critical review of cognitive-behavioral mechanisms that may lead to an overactive lifestyle in patients with chronic pain. Given the scarcity of empirical studies in this area, we have raised more questions than we have provided answers. The main issues can be summarized as follows:

1) Task persistence can be understood as active approach or active avoidance behavior. The evidence so far suggests that task persistence, as an active approach behavior, tends to be associated with beneficial outcomes, whereas task persistence as an avoidance strategy is often associated with dysfunctional outcomes. However, it also appears that task persistence can be maladaptive, and hence further clarification is needed.

2) Further research is needed to clarify the multidimensional character of the ergomania concept, its multiple determinants, and its relevance for the pathogenesis and therapy of chronic pain and fatigue. One of the problems with the concept of ergomania is that it is difficult to measure for the purposes of experimental investigation.

3) Broadly speaking, activity pacing can be defined as any intervention designed to moderate overactivity. However, more work needs to be done to determine the most effective clinical strategies to accomplish this goal and to understand who will benefit from such approaches.

4) The mood-as-input model presents a number of challenges concerning the transfer and generalization of the model to the real-world setting of chronic

pain. Although it is an attractive model, both theoretically and clinically, research examining the causal relationship between stop-rules, mood and behavior in patients with chronic pain is badly needed.

5) A final issue is how the concepts reviewed in this chapter can contribute to a better understanding of persistence rather than avoidance or escape from physical activity as a cause of chronic disability in individuals with chronic pain.

We hope that this brief review will encourage further research to find answers to these questions and provide insight into overuse as a risk factor for pain disability, with the ultimate goal of allowing clinicians to refine and customize their interventions for patients with chronic pain (Vlaeyen and Morley 2005).

ACKNOWLEDGMENTS

We are grateful to Stephen Morley, Madelon Peters, and Marielle Goossens for inspiring discussions during the preparation of the workshop. Work related to this paper was, in part, supported by the innovational grant no. 453-04-003 of the Netherlands Organization for Scientific Research (NWO-MAGW) to Johan W.S. Vlaeyen.

REFERENCES

Alfici S, Sigal M, Landau M. Primary fibromyalgia syndrome—a variant of depressive disorder? *Psychother Psychosom* 1989; 51:156–161.

Arntz A, Peters M. Chronic low back pain and inaccurate predictions of pain: is being too tough a risk factor for the development and maintenance of chronic pain? *Behav Res Ther* 1995; 33:49–53.

Aspinwall L. Rethinking the role of positive affect in self-regulation. *Motivation Emotion* 1998; 22:1–32.

Barr AE, Barbe MF. Pathophysiological tissue changes associated with repetitive movement: a review of the evidence. *Phys Ther* 2002; 82:173–187.

Boonen A, Van Der Heijde D, Landewe R, et al. Is avoidant coping independent of disease status and stable over time in patients with ankylosing spondylitis? *Ann Rheum Dis* 2004; 63:1264–1268.

Cane D, McCarthy M, Lynch ME. Prevalence of pacing in patients attending a multidisciplinary pain treatment program. *Pain Res Manage* 2005.

Chorus AM, Miedema HS, Wevers CW, van der Linden S. Work factors and behavioural coping in relation to withdrawal from the labour force in patients with rheumatoid arthritis. *Ann Rheum Dis* 2001; 60:1025–1032.

Clark SR, Jones KD, Burckhardt CS, Bennett RM. Exercise for patients with fibromyalgia: risks versus benefits. *Curr Rheumatol Rep* 2001; 3:135–140.

Denison E, Asenlof P, Lindberg P. Self-efficacy, fear avoidance, and pain intensity as predictors of disability in subacute and chronic musculoskeletal pain patients in primary health care. *Pain* 2004; 111:245–252.

Elvin A, Siosteen A-K, Nilsson A, Kosek E. Decreased muscle blood flow in fibromyalgia patients during standardised muscle exercise: a contrast media enhanced colour Doppler study. *Eur J Pain* 2006; 10:137–144.

Feuerstein M, Nicholas RA, Huang GD, et al. Workstyle: development of a measure of response to work in those with upper extremity pain. *J Occup Rehabil* 2005; 15:87–104.

Fey SG, Fordyce WE. Behavioral rehabilitation of the chronic pain patient. *Annu Rev Rehabil* 1983; 3:32–63.

Fordyce WE. *Behavioral Methods for Chronic Pain and Illness*. St. Louis: Mosby, 1976.

Gamsa A, Vikis-Freibergs V. Psychological events are both risk factors in, and consequences of, chronic pain. *Pain* 1991; 44:271–277.

Gerber L, Furst G, Shulman B, et al. Patient education program to teach energy conservation behaviors to patients with rheumatoid arthritis: a pilot study. *Arch Phys Med Rehabil* 1987; 68:442–445.

Gil KM, Ross SL, Keefe FJ. Behavioral treatment of chronic pain: Four pain management protocols. In: France RD, Krishnan KRR (Eds). *Chronic Pain*. Washington, DC: American Psychiatric Press, 1988.

Glass JM, Lyden AK, Petzke F, et al. The effect of brief exercise cessation on pain, fatigue, and mood symptom development in healthy, fit individuals. *J Psychosom Res* 2004; 57:391–398.

Jensen MP, Turner JA, Romano JM, Strom SE. The Chronic Pain Coping Inventory: development and preliminary validation. *Pain* 1995; 60:203–216.

Martin LL, Ward DW, Achee JW, Wyer RS. Mood as input: people have to interpret the motivational implications of their moods. *J Pers Soc Psychol* 1993; 64:317–326.

McCracken LM, Eccleston C. Coping or acceptance: what to do about chronic pain? *Pain* 2003; 105:197–204.

Morley S, Eccleston C, Williams AC. Systematic review and meta-analysis of randomized controlled trials of cognitive behaviour therapy and behaviour therapy for chronic pain in adults, excluding headache. *Pain* 1999; 80:1–13.

Nielson WR, Walker C, McCain GA. Cognitive behavioral treatment of fibromyalgia syndrome: preliminary findings. *J Rheumatol* 1992; 19:98–103.

Nielson WR, Jensen MP, Hill ML. An activity pacing scale for the chronic pain coping inventory: development in a sample of patients with fibromyalgia syndrome. *Pain* 2001; 89:111–115.

Schmitz U, Saile H, Nilges P. Coping with chronic pain: flexible goal adjustment as an interactive buffer against pain-related distress. *Pain* 1996; 67:41–51.

Severeijns R, van den Hout MA, Vlaeyen JW. The causal status of pain catastrophizing: an experimental test with healthy participants. *Eur J Pain* 2005; 9:257–265.

Sieben JM, Vlaeyen JW, Portegijs PJ, et al. A longitudinal study on the predictive validity of the fear-avoidance model in low back pain. *Pain* 2005; 117:162–170.

Tan G, Nguyen Q, Anderson KO, Jensen M, Thornby J. Further validation of the chronic pain coping inventory. *J Pain* 2005; 6:29–40.

Tunks E, Bellissimo A. Coping with the coping concept: a brief comment. *Pain* 1988; 34:171–174.

Turk DC, Monarch ES. A biopsychosocial perspective on chronic pain. In: Turk DC, Gatchel RJ (Eds). *Psychological Approaches to Pain Management: A Practitioner's Handbook,* 2nd ed. New York: Guilford, 2002, pp 3–29.

Turk DC, Sherman JJ. Treatment of patients with fibromyalgia syndrome. In: Turk DC, Gatchel RJ (Eds). *Psychological Approaches to Pain Management: A Practitioner's Handbook,* 2nd ed. New York: Guilford, 2002, pp 390–416.

van den Hout JH, Vlaeyen JW, Houben RM, Soeters AP, Peters ML. The effects of failure feedback and pain-related fear on pain report, pain tolerance, and pain avoidance in chronic low back pain patients. *Pain* 2001; 92:247–257.

van der Hulst M. Long workhours and health. *Scand J Work Environ Health* 2003; 29:171–188.

Van Houdenhove B. Prevalence and psychodynamic interpretation of premorbid hyperactivity in patients with chronic pain. *Psychother Psychosom* 1986; 45:195–200.

Van Houdenhove B, Egle UT. Fibromyalgia: a stress disorder? Piecing the biopsychosocial puzzle together. *Psychother Psychosom* 2004; 73:267–275.

Van Houdenhove B, Stans L, Verstraeten D. Is there a link between 'pain-proneness' and 'action-proneness'? *Pain* 1987; 29:113–117.

Van Houdenhove B, Onghena P, Neerinckx E, Hellin J. Does high 'action-proneness' make people more vulnerable to chronic fatigue syndrome? A controlled psychometric study. *J Psychosom Res* 1995; 39:633–640.

Van Houdenhove B, Neerinckx E, Onghena P, Lysens R, Vertommen, H. Premorbid "overactive" lifestyle in chronic fatigue syndrome and fibromyalgia. An etiological factor or proof of good citizenship? *J Psychosom Res* 2001; 51:571–576.

Van Houdenhove B, Egle U, Luyten P. The role of life stress in fibromyalgia. *Curr Rheumatol Rep* 2005; 7:365–370.

van Lankveld W, Naring G, van der Staak C, van't Pad Bosch P, van de Putte L. Stress caused by rheumatoid arthritis: relation among subjective stressors of the disease, disease status, and well-being. *J Behav Med* 1993; 16:309–321.

van Rijswijk K, Bekker MH, Rutte CG, Croon MA. The relationships among part-time work, work-family interference, and well-being. *J Occup Health Psychol* 2004; 9:286–295.

Viane I, Crombez G, Eccleston C, et al. Acceptance of pain is an independent predictor of mental well-being in patients with chronic pain: empirical evidence and reappraisal. *Pain* 2003; 106:65–72.

Vlaeyen JWS, Linton SJ. Fear-avoidance and its consequences in chronic musculoskeletal pain: a state of the art. *Pain* 2000; 85:317–332.

Vlaeyen JW, Morley S. Active despite pain: the putative role of stop-rules and current mood. *Pain* 2004; 110:512–516.

Vlaeyen JW, Morley S. Cognitive-behavioral treatments for chronic pain: what works for whom? *Clin J Pain* 2005; 21:1–8.

Vlaeyen JW, De Jong J, Geilen M, Heuts PH, Van Breukelen G. The treatment of fear of movement/(re)injury in chronic low back pain: further evidence on the effectiveness of exposure in vivo. *Clin J Pain* 2002; 18:251–261.

Williams DA, Meredith CA, Groner KH, et al. Improving physical functional status in patients with fibromyalgia: a brief cognitive behavioural intervention. *J Rheum* 2002; 29:1280–1286.

Correspondence to: Johan Vlaeyen, PhD, Professor of Behavioral Medicine. Department of Medical, Clinical and Experimental Psychology, Maastricht University, P.O. Box 616, 6200 MD Maastricht, The Netherlands. Email: j.vlaeyen@dep.unimaas.nl.

Proceedings of the 11th World Congress on Pain,
edited by Herta Flor, Eija Kalso, and Jonathan O.
Dostrovsky, IASP Press, Seattle, © 2006.

53

Maternal and Child Emotional Regulation in Pediatric Chronic Pain

Sophia Franks,[a] Marie Joyce,[b] and George Chalkiadis[a]

[a]Department of Anaesthesia and Pain Management, Royal Children's Hospital, Parkville, Victoria, Australia; [b]Psychology Department, Australian Catholic University, Fitzroy, Victoria, Australia

Cicchetti and Rogosch (1997) define emotional regulation as the ability to redirect, control, and modify emotionally arousing situations. Emotional regulation has recently received attention regarding its role in child development. Regulation of emotional arousal has been associated with both internalizing and externalizing of problems (Eisenberg et al. 2001). Contributions from developmental theory, psychoanalysis, and attachment theory demonstrate that difficulty in regulating affect is an important risk factor for developing psychological and physical disease, somatoform disorder, eating disorders, substance abuse, and perhaps persistent pain (Taylor et al. 1997). Research has identified a multitude of factors that can contribute to both the distress and disability associated with persistent pain, but as yet little has been done to examine the role of emotional regulation in chronic pain patients (McGrath and Finch 2003).

Empirical studies have linked emotional regulation to the functioning of the autonomic nervous system and to somatic disorders. Flor at al. (1997) proposed that the association of stressful situations and the overactivation of the autonomic nervous system generate and perpetuate chronic pain through increased perceptual sensitivity and a reduced pain threshold. Grunau (2000) proposed that high levels of arousal in an infant or a child may produce physiological dysregulation and affect the threshold of emotional reactivity and pain. Caregiver interactions may influence the development of emotional regulation in children. However, there is little research investigating how these interactions shape the functional outcomes of children and adolescents with persisting pain.

A large body of literature describes the early parent-child relationship and the level of responsiveness and attunement of mothers to their children

(Fonagy 2001). Mothers who are sensitive to their children's distress or other emotional cues help the children to maintain an optimal level of arousal. The capacity to regulate one's own emotions develops from early relationships in which parents regulate the infant's emotional state; if development proceeds well, children are able to internalize this process and develop their own capacity to regulate emotional affect. If the primary caregiver has not regulated the child's emotional states, increased physiological arousal may lead the child to interpret somatic sensations as something to fear and to avoid. Difficulties with early parenting experiences, life stressors, physical and psychological illness in the family, and a tendency to dissociate the connection between physical and psychological experience have been reported as risk factors for somatization (the conversion of psychological distress into somatic symptoms) in childhood (Craig et al. 2002).

PARENTAL FACTORS AND PAIN

Strong evidence indicates that parental behavior influences illness behavior and disability in young persons with persistent pain. There is less literature investigating the role of emotional factors in pediatric pain. The emphasis on social learning theory has led to a focus on the more observable aspects of the parent-child relationship, as opposed to the internal psychological processes within the parent and the child. Research by Walker and colleagues (2002) has shown that psychosocial factors do not operate in isolation but are moderated by children's psychological factors (such as self-worth and academic competence). Findings also suggest a link between mothers' emotional distress and children's symptoms. Walker and Greene (1989) found strong support for a positive relationship between levels of maternal anxiety, depression, and somatization and recurrent abdominal pain in their children. The transmission of maternal anxiety and somatic symptoms to their children is poorly explained by modeling and reinforcement (Craig et al. 2004). Fonagy (2001) proposes reflective functioning as a new theory in the transgenerational consistencies of emotional regulation and somatic symptoms. Reflective functioning refers to the ability to understand the feelings, beliefs, and intentions of others, as well as in one's self. It is the parent's understanding of the child's mind and emotions, the accurate reading of the child's mental state, and the parent's ability to cope with the child's distress that lead to the child's symbolization (mental representation) of affective experience. Thus, reflective functioning in parents has been associated with attachment and affect regulation in children.

MATERNAL EMOTIONAL AWARENESS

Parents have the primary responsibility for recognizing their children's emotions, assessing the significance and severity of their pain symptoms, and determining the best course of action. Parents need to distinguish expressions of pain from other emotional states and reflect on the child's internal state rather than his or her overt pain behavior. Some parents respond so strongly to their child's distress that they do not allow themselves the opportunity to stop and assess just what the distress means for the child. Some parents may not be able to tolerate their child's display of emotion, yet they are able to respond as a soothing parent when the child complains of pain.

No empirical studies in pediatric chronic pain have investigated reflective functioning in mothers whose children have developed persisting pain. Both the Reflective Functioning Scale and the Meta-Emotion Interview are strong predictors of affect regulation in parents and their children. Hoover et al. (1995) devised the Meta-Emotion Interview to study parents' awareness, acceptance, and regulation of emotions and their coaching of these emotions in their children. The authors proposed that meta-emotion directly affects children's physiology, which in turn affects children's ability to regulate emotions. Research findings indicate that meta-emotion is directly and significantly related to the child's achievement level, relationship with peers, and health, and suggest that parents may be able to influence a child's physiology. This chapter describes our research on the emotional regulation component of the Meta-Emotion Interview and its relationship with children's functional outcomes in a sample of young persons experiencing persisting pain.

MATERNAL DISTRESS

One of the challenges for parents seeing their child in pain is for these parents to manage their own level of distress. Parents who have difficulties regulating their emotions are more likely to experience high levels of emotional distress. In general, the mother is the primary caregiver who attends to the child's medical appointments, and usually the mother is the decision maker regarding the child's attendance at appointments. Thus mothers were chosen to participate in the study. Garber (1990) found that distressed mothers tended to report more emotional and somatic complaints in their children. Maternal emotional distress may interfere with a mother's ability to be sensitive to the child's internal state. Distressed mothers are more likely to read ambiguous cues in their child as reflecting distress. It is helpful if parents can distinguish between their own feelings of distress and those of their child. Increased closeness around health issues has been observed in families with somatic symptoms (Craig et al. 2004). Some findings are starting to emerge regarding maternal emotional distress and emotional involvement in children's pain. Investigating the relationship between parental distress and physical functioning, Eccleston et al. (2002) concluded that disability in adolescents with chronic pain was accounted for by the adolescents' high pain intensity, by their low mood, and by high levels of parental distress. Findings suggest that mothers of poorly coping adolescents tend to discourage coping behavior and generally intrude more (Dunn-Geier at al. 1986). The role of the mother in pain promotion was also demonstrated in a laboratory-based experimental study of school-aged children's pain experience (Chambers et al. 2002).

While some findings are emerging regarding maternal interactions and pain, the lack of knowledge about maternal regulation and children's persisting pain led to the study described in this chapter. The theoretical framework of this study emphasizes the significance of maternal emotional distress and emotional involvement in the context of empathic reactions to others. Maternal emotional distress was a variable we used to assess maternal empathy, emotional distress, and emotional involvement of a mother with her child. It is argued that empathic reactions toward another that lead to personal distress are a reflection of low emotional regulation and may suggest a lack of differentiation between mother and child (Eisenberg 2000). Wood et al. (2000) also considers affect dysregulation at the individual level and the interactional effects between family members that may activate pathological processes via the autonomic nervous system, such as maternal emotional involvement and distress.

HYPOTHESES

We proposed that children of mothers who demonstrate poor emotional regulation would show higher levels of anxiety, depression, and somatization. Further, children who themselves have difficulty regulating their emotions will have higher levels of anxiety, depression, and somatization. Finally, maternal emotional distress will increase children's somatic symptoms and emotional distress and reduce their physical functioning.

METHODS

Sixty-two children and adolescents referred to the Children's Pain Management Clinic at the Royal Children's Hospital and their mothers participated in the study. Mothers were interviewed separately using the semi-structured

Meta-Emotion Interview (1999) regarding their awareness, acceptance, and emotional regulation of their own and their child's emotions, specifically, sadness, anger, and fear. In addition, mothers and children completed self-report questionnaires as described below. Maternal emotional distress was assessed using a composite variable defined as the sum of the mean of scores on the Pediatric Inventory for Parents, Family Emotional Involvement and Criticism Scale, and Interpersonal Reactivity Index. Path modeling, which enables the estimation of relationships between observed variables, was used to test the proposed relationships. Path analysis can be viewed as an extension of multiple regression in which there is more than one dependent variable.

Child variables measured were somatization (Children's Somatization Inventory, Walker and Greene 1989), emotional regulation (Bar-On Emotional Quotient Inventory, Youth Version, Bar-On and Parker 2000), depression (Children's Depression Inventory, Kovacs 1992), and anxiety (Revised Children's Manifest Anxiety Scale, Reynolds and Richmond 2000).

Maternal variables measured were maternal emotional regulation (Meta-Emotion Interview, Katz and Gottman 1999), maternal emotional distress (Pediatric Inventory for Parents, Streisand et al. 2001; Interpersonal Reactivity Index, Davis 1983; and Family Emotional Involvement and Criticism Scale, Shields et al. 1992), perceptions of child physical functioning (Pediatric Orthopedic Society of North America), and child somatization (Children's Somatization Inventory, Walker and Greene 1989).

RESULTS

Table I shows the pain presentation of the participants. Many of the children and adolescents experienced multiple pain problems, with chronic daily headaches and complex regional pain syndrome being the most prevalent. The mean age of the children was 13 years (standard deviation = 2.52 years); 29% were male and 71% female. Table I also illustrates the psychosocial issues of the participants in the study. Most subjects reported multiple psychosocial issues, and only three subjects did not report overt psychosocial issues.

These young people do not appear to be reporting significant levels of anxiety (mean score = 48.02) or depression (mean score = 49.39). However, the global functioning scale indicated that this group of young people experiencing chronic pain are four standard deviations below the normative mean (mean score = 9.87).

Table I
Pain presentations of participants

	N	Additional Pain Problems
Diagnosis		
Chronic daily headache/migraine	20	5
Complex regional pain syndrome	13	5
Conversion disorder	5	5
Patella dislocation/subluxation	7	0
Somatoform pain disorder	4	4
Abdominal pain	6	2
Hip pain	1	0
Back pain	4	2
Widespread musculoskeletal pain	2	2
Psychosocial Issues		
Sleep problems	14	
School problems	18	
Death of a grandparent	6	
Anxiety	8	
Maternal anxiety/depression	20	
Maternal trauma	5	
Marital discord/conflict	10	
Identity/self-esteem problems	5	
Bullying/difficulty with friendships	14	
High expectations/overdoing things	12	
Maternal chronic pain	7	
Enmeshed relationships/dependency	9	

MATERNAL EMOTIONAL REGULATION AND CHILD OUTCOMES

Path analysis results showed significant pathways between maternal emotional regulation and child depression (–0.45), anxiety (0.34), and somatization (0.25) (as assessed by parent report).

CHILD EMOTIONAL REGULATION AND CHILD OUTCOMES

Children's emotional regulation was found to be negatively associated with anxiety and depression. Maternal emotional regulation, but not child emotional regulation, was significantly related to child somatization (see Fig. 1). There was no correlation between maternal and child reports of child emotional regulation. The arrows represent hypothesized effects. The numbers next to the arrows are standardized path coefficients, which are the estimates of the size of the effect if the model is correct. Standardized path coefficients are on the same scale as Pearson product-moment correlations.

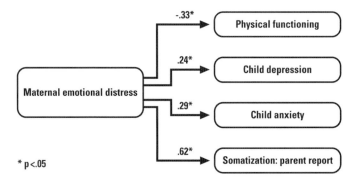

Fig. 1. Paths showing the relationship between child reports of emotional regulation and child anxiety, depression, and somatization.

MATERNAL DISTRESS AND CHILD OUTCOMES

Results show a significant relationship between maternal emotional distress and all child variables, i.e., anxiety, depression, somatization, and physical functioning (see Fig. 2). This relationship was demonstrated differentially for parent and child report of somatization: maternal emotional distress was more strongly associated ($r = 0.62$) with maternal perceived child somatization, whereas the relationship was significant but weaker ($r = 0.42$) with children's reporting of their own somatization (see Fig. 2).

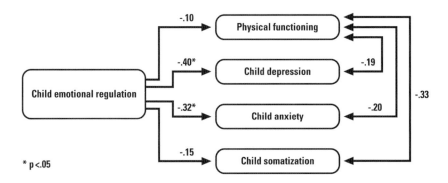

Fig. 2. Paths showing the relationship between maternal emotional distress and child outcomes.

DISCUSSION

Findings supported all three hypotheses, demonstrating the importance of maternal and child emotional regulation in this sample of children with chronic pain. Affect regulation of mothers and children was negatively associated with child depression and anxiety scores, although only maternal emotional regulation was negatively associated with child somatization. Increasing levels of maternal emotional distress were associated with increased perceived child somatization, increased child anxiety and depression, and reduced physical functioning in the child. These results are consistent with earlier studies that reported higher levels of maternal anxiety in children with recurrent abdominal pain and documented the negative impact of maternal distress on children's functioning (Walker and Greene 1989; Eccleston et al. 2002). Despite the high number of associated psychosocial issues identified, these issues were not the primary reason for seeking treatment; the primary reason was the presenting pain complaint.

Thus, it can be postulated that mothers with poor emotional regulation are less likely to be attuned to their children's emotional needs and that failure to respond to these needs may contribute to pain as a presenting complaint. Autonomic arousal and the perception of pain as a threat can lead to hypervigilance of somatic complaints, manifesting as pain and disability and distracting attention from other contributing psychosocial factors. Young people with these complaints do not appear to be reporting clinically significant levels of anxiety and depression, yet they often exhibit functional disability, a finding that has been observed previously by others (Chalkiadis 2001; Breuner 2005).

CONCLUSION

One of the challenges for parents seeing their child in pain is to manage their own level of arousal in response to the child's emotional distress. In order for the mother to contain her child's level of arousal, she needs to be able to monitor and distinguish her own emotional state from her child's. The findings of this study have relevance for the treatment of children experiencing chronic pain. Rather than focusing just on the child's emotional processes, clinicians treating children with persistent pain should also explore the interactional effects between mothers and children. An important component of this interaction has been demonstrated to be maternal emotional involvement, empathy, and distress and the role this involvement plays in a mother's response to her child's pain. Furthermore, perhaps these families are unable to recognize the links between psychosocial stressors in their lives and their child's pain. These findings suggest a link between maternal emotional regulation and children's symptomatology and highlight the importance of working not only with children experiencing chronic pain but also with their parents.

REFERENCES

Breuner CC, Smith MS, Womack WM. Factors related to school absenteeism in adolescents with recurrent headache. *Headache* 2005; 45:127–131.

Bar-On R, Parker JD. *Bar-On Emotional Quotient Inventory: Youth Version: Technical Manual.* New York: Multi-Health Systems, 2000.

Chalkiadis G. Management of chronic pain in children. *Med J Aust* 2001; 175:476–479.

Chambers CT, Craig KD, Bennett S. The impact of maternal behaviour on children's pain experiences: an experimental analysis. *J Pediatr Psychol* 2002; 27:293–301.

Cicchetti D, Rogosch FA. The role of self-organisation in the promotion of resilience in maltreated children. *Dev Psychopathol* 1997; 9:797–815.

Craig TK, Cox, AD, Klein K. Intergenerational transmission of somatisation behaviour: a study of chronic somatisers and their children. *Psychol Med* 2002; 32:805–816.

Craig TK, Hodson BS, Cox AD. Intergenerational transmission of somatisation behaviour: 2. Observation of joint attention and bids for attention. *Psychol Med* 2004; 34:199–209.

Davis MH. Measuring individual differences in empathy. Evidence for a multi-dimensional approach. *J Pers Soc Psychol* 1983; 44:113–126.

Dunn-Geier BJ, McGrath P, Rourke BP, Latter J, D'Astous J. Adolescent chronic pain: the ability to cope. *Pain* 1986; 26:23–32.

Eccleston C, McCracken L, Crombez G. Pain, mood and parental distress predict functional disability in adolescents with chronic pain. *Abstracts: 10th World Congress on Pain.* Seattle: IASP Press, 2002, p 83.

Eisenberg N. Empathy and sympathy. In: Lewis ML, Haviland-Jones JM (Eds). *Handbook of Emotions.* London: Guilford Press, 2000, pp 677–791.

Eisenberg N, Cumberland AJ, Spinrad TL, et al. The relations of regulation and emotionality to children's externalising and internalising problem behaviour. *Child Dev* 2001; 72:1112–1134.

Flor H, Knost B, Birbaumer N. Processing of pain-and body-related verbal material in chronic pain patients: central and peripheral correlates. *Pain* 1997; 73:413–421.

Fonagy P. *Attachment Theory and Psychoanalysis.* New York: Other Press, 2001.

Garber J, Zeman J, Walker LS. Recurrent abdominal pain in children: psychiatric diagnoses and parental psychopathology. *J Am Acad Child Adolesc Psychiatry* 1990; 29:648–656.

Grunau R. Long-term consequences of pain in human neonates. In: Anand KS, Stevens BJ, McGrath P (Eds). *Pain in Neonates,* Pain Research and Clinical Management, Vol. 10. Amsterdam: Elsevier, 2000, pp 55–76.

Hoover C, Gottman JM, Katz LF. Parental meta-emotion structure predicts family and child outcomes. *Cognition Emotion* 1995; 9:229–264.

Katz LF, Gottman JM. *The Meta-Emotion Interview.* Seattle: University of Washington, 1991.

Kovacs M. *Children's Depression Inventory (CDI) Manual.* Canada: Multi-Health Systems, 1992.

McGrath P, Finch AJ. *Pediatric Pain: Biological and Social Context,* Progress in Pain Research and Management, Vol. 26. Seattle: IASP Press, 2003.

Reynolds CR, Richmond BO. *Revised Children's Manifest Anxiety Scale (RCMAS) Manual.* Los Angeles: Western Psychological Services, 2000.

Taylor GJ, Bagby RM, Parker JD. *Disorders of Affect Regulation: Alexithymia and Psychiatric Illness.* Cambridge: Cambridge University Press, 1997.

Shields, Franks P, Harp JJ, McDaniel SH, Campbell TL. Development of the Family Emotional Involvement and Criticism Scale (FEICS). A self-report scale to measure expressed emotion. *J Marital Fam Ther* 1992; 18:395–407.

Streisand R, Braniecki S, Tercyak K. Childhood illness related parenting stress: the pediatric inventory for parents. *J Pediatr Psychol* 2001; 26:155–162.

Walker L, Greene JW. Children with recurrent abdominal pain and their families: more somatic complaints, anxiety and depression than other patient families. *J Pediatr Psychol* 1989; 14:231–243.

Walker L, Claar RL, Garger J. Social consequences of children's pain: when do they encourage symptom maintenance. *J Pediatr Psychol* 2002; 27:689–698.

Wood BL, Klebba KB, Miller BD. Evolving the biobehavioural family model: the fit of attachment. *Fam Process* 2000; 39:319–340.

Correspondence to: Sophia Franks, MPsy, Anaesthesia and Pain Management, Royal Children's Hospital, Flemington Road, Parkville, VIC 3052, Australia. Email: sophia.franks@rch.org.au.

Part VII

Specific Clinical Syndromes and Symptoms

Proceedings of the 11th World Congress on Pain,
edited by Herta Flor, Eija Kalso, and Jonathan O.
Dostrovsky, IASP Press, Seattle, © 2006.

54

Obstetric Pain: New Understanding of Physiology and Treatment

James C. Eisenach

Department of Anesthesiology and Center for the Study of Pharmacologic Plasticity in the Presence of Pain, Wake Forest University School of Medicine, Winston-Salem, North Carolina, USA

Despite being the most common cause of severe pain in young adults, the pain of labor and delivery has historically received little attention. Indeed, analgesia during labor was until recently considered inappropriate, and availability of effective treatment of labor pain remains to this day inconsistent, even in sophisticated medical environments. Research regarding the neurophysiological basis of labor pain and its consequences is scant, with a primary focus on minor variations in clinical practice of epidural or spinal injections. The purpose of this chapter is to review the anatomy, neurophysiology, and consequences of obstetric pain, with a focus on recent developments and important gaps in our knowledge.

ANATOMY

Pain arising from the first stage of labor is carried through afferents that course through the paracervical plexus and hypogastric nerve, commingle with sympathetic efferents along the paravertebral sympathetic chain, and enter the spinal cord at the T10 to L1 dermatomes. Near the end of the first stage and during the remaining phases of labor, input also comes from somatic efferents in the pudendal nerve that innervate the vaginal surface of the cervix, the vagina, and the perineum. Analgesia can be accomplished during the first stage of labor by paracervical, paravertebral, or lumbar epidural administration of local anesthetics.

It is widely stated that uterine innervation underlies the pain of uterine contractions during labor. Uterine afferents clearly respond to distension, can be sensitized by inflammatory mediators and irritant chemicals, and may play an important role in chronic pelvic pain. Yet they are unlikely to play a significant role in obstetric pain, since afferents that innervate the myometrium regress in pregnancy. In a rat model, the density of substance P immunostaining in the myometrium decreased by over 70% in the days preceding the onset of labor (Schmidt et al. 2003). Additionally, Bonica and Chadwick (1989) failed to mimic the pain of labor in women by vigorous manual palpation of the uterine body during cesarean section under field block anesthesia. These anecdotal observations argue that it is not the uterine corpus which signals obstetric pain.

In contrast to myometrial afferents, those which innervate the lower uterine segment and cervix sprout near the end of pregnancy, with a massive increase in neuronal fiber staining in the day preceding the onset of labor in the rat (Yellon et al. 2003). Cervical afferents are conceivably stimulated during the first stage of labor by uterine contractions, resulting in increased deformation and tension on cervical tissue. Experimental cervical distension is painful in nonpregnant women, with pain referred to low thoracic dermatomes (Bajaj et al. 2002). The pain is similar to that of labor and is consistent with a role for these afferents in signaling obstetric pain. Bonica and Chadwick (1989) also noted that manual distension of the uterine cervix in women undergoing cesarean section with field block anesthesia reproduced the pain of labor.

Little is known regarding the phenotype of uterine cervical afferents, or how these may be altered by female sex hormones or pregnancy itself. Low lumbar and upper sacral dorsal root ganglion (DRG) neurons express estrogen receptors (Papka and Storey-Workley 2002), and pregnancy or estrogen exposure increases expression of calcitonin gene-related peptide (CGRP) and substance P by these afferents, as well as immunostaining for these fibers in the spinal cord (Mowa et al. 2003a,b). The relevance of these observations to obstetric pain are, however, uncertain, since these studies did not specifically identify DRG neurons that innervated the cervix and focused on DRG neurons in the pelvic rather than hypogastric nerve distribution. To address these issues, we recently have started a series of studies in which cervical afferents are fluorescently labeled and low thoracic/upper lumbar DRG sections immunostained for various receptors and peptides. Preliminary results suggest that cervical afferent DRG neurons are exclusively of small diameter, consistent with electrophysiological studies indicating that hypogastric afferents responding to uterine cervical distension are exclusively C fibers (Liu et al. 2005). A high proportion of cervically traced DRG neurons appear to express CGRP, with fewer expressing the excitatory purinergic receptor, $P2X_3$. Some cervical afferents express the capsaicin receptor TRPV1, consistent with neurophysiological responses of cervical afferents in the hypogastric nerve to noxious heat (Liu et al. 2005). Once this characterization is complete, we will examine the role of female sex hormones and pregnancy on uterine cervical afferent expression of transducing ion channels and receptors as well as neuropeptide content and inhibitory receptors.

NEUROPHYSIOLOGY

PSYCHOPHYSICS

In humans, experimental visceral pain by distension of the esophagus results in a wider area of referred pain to the body surface than does experimental somatic pain from noxious heat applied to the skin to an equivalent level of pain report (Strigo et al. 2002). This broader, more diffuse representation of visceral pain has been recognized for many years and is thought to reflect the considerable rostrocaudal and deep arborization of visceral afferent input into the spinal cord dorsal horn compared to somatic afferent input. Cessation of noxious stimulation of the skin results in a rapid disappearance of pain, whereas considerably longer is required for pain report to fall to zero after cessation of noxious stimulation of the esophagus. Additionally, experimental noxious visceral stimuli result in greater responses in the emotional and unpleasantness dimensions of pain than do noxious somatic stimuli, and this difference in psychophysical response is paralleled by differences in brain activation in the rostral anterior cingulate cortex in humans (Strigo et al. 2003).

The small amount of human psychophysical literature on pain from uterine cervical distension in humans generally reflects these observations of pain from other visceral organs. As such, distension of the cervix in nonpregnant women results in an increase in pain report that is dependent on the increase in cross-sectional area of the distending device (Bajaj et al. 2002). Pain from experimental uterine cervical distension is referred to the low thoracic dermatomes, similar to the pain of labor, and there is a slow return of pain report to zero following abrupt cessation of distension. Finally, words chosen on the McGill pain questionnaire to describe pain from experimental uterine cervical distension overlap those used to describe labor pain (Bajaj et al. 2002).

AFFERENT PHYSIOLOGY AND REFLEX RESPONSES

Berkley et al. (1987) described the neurophysiological characteristics of uterine afferents in vitro and in vivo nearly 20 years ago, with focus on afferents with responses to uterine body distension. Berkley et al. (1990) observed that hypogastric afferents innervating the uterus were mechanosensitive, some with high and others with low threshold, and that they were polymodal, responding to heat, bradykinin, and lowered pH. We recently extended these observations with a focus on hypogastric afferents innervating the cervix, noting that these were exclusively C fibers, were a mixture of low- and high-threshold mechano-sensitive units, and were responsive to bradykinin and heat (Sandner-Kiesling et al. 2002; Liu et al. 2005).

As with other abdominal visceral nociceptive stimuli, uterine cervical distension results in activation of spinal cord dorsal horn neurons, not only in the superficial laminae, but also in deep laminae and surrounding the central canal. This activation, as measured by expression of the neuronal marker for activation, c-Fos, occurs in lower thoracic and upper lumbar dermatomes in a manner dependent on stimulus duration after uterine cervical distension; it is blocked by instillation of lidocaine into the cervix prior to distension (Tong et al. 2003). The location and pattern of spinal cord c-Fos expression after experimental uterine cervical distension is similar to that observed following labor and delivery in the rat (Lombard et al. 1999), consistent with uterine cervical afferent activation during labor in this species.

As with other abdominal visceral nociceptive stimuli, uterine cervical distension results in nocifensive reflexes in the lightly anesthetized rat, with contraction of the abdominal wall musculature (guarding reflex) and increases in blood pressure (Sandner-Kiesling et al. 2002). Changes in heart rate are more variable, with both increases and decreases observed in individual animals, particularly at moderate distension forces. The stimulus-response relationships for hypogastric nerve single-unit responses, strength of rectus abdominus muscle contraction, and spinal cord c-Fos expression from uterine cervical distension overlie each other, consistent with a nociceptive stimulus (Sandner-Kiesling et al. 2002).

Behavior in the conscious animal represents the clearest indication that a stimulus is noxious. Uterine body distension results in cessation of exploratory behavior in a stimulus-dependent manner (Bradshaw et al. 1999), but lack of a device capable of distending the noncompliant and small uterine cervix in the nonpregnant rat has precluded investigation of behaviors elicited by this stimulus. Labor, however, results in cessation of exploratory movements and in postures of lumbar kyphosis, associated with uterine contractions (Ronca and Alberts 2000). These same behaviors occur following implantation of a ureteral mass to mimic the pain of kidney stone passage (Giamberardino et al. 1997).

PHARMACOLOGY

We have utilized responses elicited by uterine cervical distension in the lightly anesthetized rat to probe the pharmacology of analgesia to this stimulus. Opioids reduce abdominal muscle activity following uterine cervical distension in a dose-dependent manner and with dose responses similar to those which reduce responses to noxious heat on the skin (Sandner-Kiesling et al. 2002;

Sandner-Kiesling and Eisenach 2002a,b). Ligands of κ-opioid receptors, but not of μ-opioid receptors, reduce responses of single units in the hypogastric nerve to uterine cervical distension (Sandner-Kiesling et al. 2002), consistent with the presence of κ-opioid receptors on these visceral afferents, as has been observed pharmacologically in other viscera (Sengupta et al. 1996). Whereas the arylacetamide compound used in those studies has subsequently been shown to act in part via sodium channel blockade (Su et al. 2002; Joshi et al. 2003), preliminary studies indicating similar efficacy of peptide κ-opioid receptor agonists to reduce responses to uterine cervical distension are consistent with peripheral actions on these receptors.

In contrast, reduction in response to uterine cervical distension to μ-opioid receptor agonists results from actions within the central nervous system. As such, intrathecal morphine is highly potent in blocking the abdominal muscle reflex induced by uterine cervical distension (Shin and Eisenach 2003). The antinociceptive activity of systemic morphine in uterine cervical distension is blocked by naloxone, which crosses the blood-brain barrier, but not by methylnaloxone, which does not (Sandner-Kiesling and Eisenach 2002a).

SENSITIZATION

Braxton Hicks contractions, which occur with increasing regularity as pregnancy progresses to full term, are similar in intensity to those during the first stage of labor, but they are typically not perceived as painful. Yet nearly one-third of women in early labor experience severe pain with uterine contractions. We have speculated that sensitization of uterine cervical afferents just prior to and during labor results in this discrepancy in pain report between Braxton Hicks contractions and those during labor. It has long been recognized that sensitization occurs during labor, as indicated by hyperalgesia to mechanical stimuli to the skin of the lower abdomen, whose afferents converge on those receiving input from the uterine cervix (Cleland 1933).

Prior to the onset of labor, there is an increase in estrogen signaling in the stromal cells of the uterine cervix, resulting in nuclear factor κB signaling and production of multiple cytokines (Yellon et al. 2003; Molloy et al. 2004). The resultant inflammatory response, enhanced by recruitment of circulating immune cells, results in cyclooxygenase, nitric oxide synthase, and metalloproteinase induction and activation in the cervix. These molecules result in turn in disorganization of the collagen matrix, transforming the cervix from a thick, noncompliant structure to the supple and distensible structure that allows dilatation to occur. Prostaglandins play key roles in this "ripening" of the cervix, which can also be achieved by application of prostaglandins to the term uterine cervix.

Thus, beginning approximately 1 day before the onset of labor, a state of inflammation of the uterine cervix is established. Inflammation progresses as part of the process described above, exacerbated by intermittent ischemia during contractions and frank injury to tissue late in the first stage of labor. Inflammatory mediators are known to sensitize nociceptors in the skin and the colon, and it would be surprising if they did not sensitize nociceptors in the uterine cervix during this process. Nonetheless, there has been no systematic examination of the effect of inflammatory mediators on cervical afferents, either in the nonpregnant or full-term pregnant state.

Estrogen could also conceivably sensitize uterine cervical afferents, since, as noted above, estrogen signaling increases just prior to the onset of labor. For example, afferents innervating the temporomandibular joint are sensitized by estrogen as well as by inflammatory mediators, with each of these sensitizing agents enhancing the other (Flake et al. 2005). We recently observed an increase in spontaneous activity of single hypogastric units innervating the uterine cervix in ovariectomized rats receiving estrogen in a dose that produced physiological concentrations observed in the nonpregnant animal (Liu et al. 2005). Interestingly, estrogen treatment sensitized the response to uterine cervical distension in high-threshold, but not low-threshold, mechanosensitive units, consistent with sensitization to nociceptive input.

There may be pharmacological consequences of estrogen-induced sensitization as well. Some chronic pain states are more prevalent in women than men, and women report more pain to some experimental noxious stimuli than men (Fillingim et al. 1999). Although the mechanisms for this sexual dimorphism are uncertain, estrogen-induced sensitization could play a role. Additionally, estrogen reduces the efficacy of opioids in some studies in women (Fillingim et al. 1999). Intravenous morphine reduces abdominal muscle reflex contraction to uterine cervical distension in ovariectomized rats, but its effect is greatly reduced during estrogen supplementation (Sandner-Kiesling and Eisenach 2002b). As noted above, morphine and other μ-opioid receptor agonists are antinociceptive to uterine cervical distension by actions in the central nervous system. Interestingly, intrathecal morphine also reduces abdominal muscle responses to uterine cervical distension, and this effect is not reduced by estrogen supplementation (Shin and Eisenach 2003), suggesting that the reduction in efficacy from intravenous morphine by estrogen reflects estrogen modulation of opioid action at supraspinal rather than spinal sites.

In contrast to μ-opioid receptor agonists, women experience greater analgesia from κ-opioid receptor agonists than men (Gear et al. 1996). The reasons for this sexual dimorphism are also uncertain, but they may reflect an anti-analgesic effect of κ-opioid-receptor agonists in men (Gear et al. 2000). Intravenous κ-opioid-receptor agonists reduce hypogastric single-unit afferent responses and abdominal muscle reflex contraction in ovariectomized rats, and, in contrast to μ-opioid-receptor agonists, these agents are unaffected by estrogen supplementation regarding their analgesic efficacy (Sandner-Kiesling and Eisenach 2002b).

CONSEQUENCES OF OBSTETRIC PAIN

PROGRESS OF LABOR

Delivery requires the sequential activation of two processes—cervical ripening to allow dilatation, and regular, coordinated, strong contractions of the myometrium. Most work regarding the normal physiological mechanisms regulating these processes has focused on maternal or maternal-fetal hormonal causes. The role of uterine innervation has received much less attention. Regression of sympathetic efferents and sensory afferents to the myometrium during pregnancy has been suggested to maintain uterine quiescence by eliminating catecholamine and neuropeptide uterine stimulation from these fibers, respectively. Re-innervation of the myometrium does not occur until several days following delivery, arguing against a role of these fibers in the progress of labor.

Uterine cervical afferents, in contrast, sprout in the days preceding the onset of labor (Yellon et al. 2003). Although such sprouting could conceivably increase the sensation of pain during labor, normal innervation of the cervix is quite capable of transducing pain from distension, since uterine cervical dilatation is painful in the nonpregnant state. As such, this sprouting is unlikely to serve an important role for sensation. Denervation of the cervix, but not of the uterus, produces difficult delivery in rats (Higuchi et al. 1987), but the mechanisms by which these nerves participate in the process of labor have not been investigated.

Uterine cervical afferents express substance P and CGRP, and the expression of these neuropeptides increases in lumbar DRG in the last days of pregnancy, coinciding with the time of onset of cervical ripening (Collins et al. 2002; Mowa et al. 2003a,b). Similarly, neurokinin-1 (NK1) receptor expression increases in cervical tissue at this same time, and administration of substance P or CGRP induces extravasation in the cervix at this time (Collins et al. 2002; Mowa et al. 2003a,b). Vascular endothelial growth factor is also expressed in cervical tissue and increases prior to and during the ripening process, most likely increasing access of circulating immune cells to the cervical stroma. Denervation of the cervix prevents this increase in vascular endothelial growth factor (Mowa et al. 2004). These data suggest that uterine cervical afferents may participate in cervical ripening and in the birth process by depolarization-induced release of vasoactive neuropeptides.

Afferent function is altered, at least as regards nociceptive neurotransmission, by spinal or epidural administration of analgesics, and these may affect the progress of labor. Spinal administration of lipophilic opioids provides analgesia during the first stage of labor (Leighton et al. 1989), primarily by actions on afferent terminals in the spinal cord, whereas epidural administration of local anesthetics provides analgesia primarily by axonal blockade of spinal nerve roots. These differing mechanisms of action could presumably alter axon reflex depolarization in different ways, and hence differentially alter neuropeptide release in the cervix. This distinction may explain the considerably more rapid progress of labor observed with intrathecal opioid administration compared with epidural local anesthetic injection (Tsen et al. 1999) or compared with systemic opioid administration (Wong et al. 2005).

CHRONIC PAIN AFTER DELIVERY

Over the past decade, there has been a growing awareness that chronic pain syndromes may result from trauma, including surgery (Crombie et al. 1998). Chronic pain after surgery has been reported to be common after amputation (Flor 2002), cardiac surgery with sternotomy (Ho et al. 2002), thoracic surgery (Sihoe et al. 2004), inguinal hernia surgery (Poobalan et al. 2003), and mastectomy (Rothemund et al. 2004). Almeida et al. (2002) reported an increased incidence of a history of cesarean section in women presenting for treatment of chronic pelvic pain versus those presenting for other surgical procedures. This indirect, retrospective suggestion of an association of chronic pain with cesarean section has been supported by a prospective study from Denmark reporting a 12% incidence of long-term pain after cesarean section (Nikolajsen et al. 2004). Cesarean section may be the most common major surgical procedure performed in the world, and the incidence of this procedure is rising steadily in both the developed and developing world for a variety of reasons, including concerns about both maternal and fetal outcome. Any chronic disability or pain resulting from this procedure would thus be of significant public health importance.

There are also questions as to whether vaginal delivery, or perhaps pregnancy itself, might lead to a chronic pain syndrome in some women. Thompson et al. (2002) reported that 12% of women who had undergone assisted vaginal delivery (vacuum or forceps) still had perineal pain at 6 months, compared to 3% of women who had undergone spontaneous vaginal delivery and 1% of women who were delivered by cesarean section.

Although the incidence of chronic pain following cesarean or vaginal delivery is probably quite small, the large proportion of the population at potential risk suggests that delivery may not be an inconsequential cause of chronic pain in women.

In summary, research and treatment of obstetric pain have been largely neglected until recently. This common cause of severe visceral pain appears to reflect a unique set of afferents with hormonal responsiveness and differing neuropeptide and excitatory channel expression compared to other visceral afferents. Estrogen receptor signaling, which is thought to increase shortly prior to the onset of labor, induces spontaneous activity in afferents innervating the uterine cervix, sensitizes their response to distension, and reduces their inhibition by μ-opioid receptor agonists. Uterine cervical afferents may play an important role in the cervical ripening and birth process. Finally, some women develop chronic pain following cesarean or vaginal delivery, and research into the incidence, risk factors, and prevention of such chronic pain has just begun.

ACKNOWLEDGMENTS

Supported in part by NIH grants NS48065 and NS41386.

REFERENCES

Almeida ECS, Nogueira AA, Candido dos Reis FJ, Rosa e Silva JC. Cesarean section as a cause of chronic pelvic pain. *Int J Gynaecol Obstet* 2002; 79:101–104.

Bajaj P, Drewes AM, Gregersen H, et al. Controlled dilatation of the uterine cervix—an experimental visceral pain model. *Pain* 2002; 99:433–442.

Berkley KJ, Robbins A, Sato Y. Uterine afferent fibers in the rat. In: Schmidt RF, Schaible H-G, Vahle-Hinz C (Eds). *Fine Afferent Nerve Fibers and Pain.* Weinheim: VCH, 1987, pp 28–136.

Berkley KJ, Hotta H, Robbins A, Sato Y. Functional properties of afferent fibers supplying reproductive and other pelvic organs in pelvic nerve of female rat. *J Neurophysiol* 1990; 63:256–272.

Bonica JJ, Chadwick HS. Labour pain. In: Wall PD, Melzack R (Eds). *Textbook of Pain.* New York: Churchill Livingstone, 1989, pp 482–499.

Bradshaw HB, Temple JL, Wood E, Berkley KJ. Estrous variations in behavioral responses to vaginal and uterine distention in the rat. *Pain* 1999; 82:187–197.

Cleland JGP. Paravertebral anaesthesia in obstetrics. *Surg Gynaecol Obstet* 1933; 57:51–62.

Collins JJ, Usip S, McCarson KE, Papka RE. Sensory nerves and neuropeptides in uterine cervical ripening. *Peptides* 2002; 23:167–183.

Crombie IK, Davies HT, Macrae WA. Cut and thrust: antecedent surgery and trauma among patients attending a chronic pain clinic. *Pain* 1998; 76:167–171.

Fillingim RB, Edwards RR, Powell T. The relationship of sex and clinical pain to experimental pain responses. *Pain* 1999; 83:419–425.

Flake NM, Bonebreak DB, Gold MS. Estrogen and inflammation increase the excitability of rat temporomandibular joint afferent neurons. *J Neurophysiol* 2005; 93:1585–1597.

Flor H. Phantom-limb pain: characteristics, causes, and treatment. *Lancet Neurol* 2002; 1:182–189.

Gear RW, Miaskowski C, Gordon NC, et al. Kappa-opioids produce significantly greater analgesia in women than in men. *Nature Med* 1996; 2:1248–1250.

Gear RW, Miaskowski C, Gordon NC, et al. Action of naloxone on gender-dependent analgesic and antianalgesic effects of nalbuphine in humans. *J Pain* 2000; 1:122–127.

Giamberardino MA, Affaitati G, Valente R, Iezzi S, Vecchiet L. Changes in visceral pain reactivity as a function of estrous cycle in female rats with artificial ureteral calculosis. *Brain Res* 1997; 774:234–238.

Higuchi T, Uchide K, Honda K, Negoro H. Pelvic neurectomy abolishes the fetus-expulsion reflex and induces dystocia in the rat. *Exp Neurol* 1987; 96:443–455.

Ho SC, Royse CF, Royse AG, Penberthy A, McRae R. Persistent pain after cardiac surgery: an audit of high thoracic epidural and primary opioid analgesia therapies. *Anesth Analg* 2002; 95:820–823.

Joshi SK, Lamb K, Bielefeldt K, Gebhart GF. Arylacetamide kappa-opioid receptor agonists produce a tonic- and use-dependent block of tetrodotoxin-sensitive and -resistant sodium currents in colon sensory neurons. *J Pharmacol Exp Ther* 2003; 307:367–372.

Leighton BL, DeSimone CA, Norris MC, Ben-David B. Intrathecal narcotics for labor revisited: the combination of fentanyl and morphine intrathecally provides rapid onset of profound, prolonged analgesia. *Anesth Analg* 1989; 69:122–125.

Liu B, Eisenach JC, Tong C. Chronic estrogen sensitizes a subset of mechanosensitive afferents innervating the uterine cervix. *J Neurophysiol* 2005; 93:2167–2173.

Lombard M-C, Touquet B, Morain F, Besson J-M. Parturition-induced neuronal c-fos expression in the spinal cord of primipare and multipare female rats. *Abstracts: 9th World Congress on Pain.* Seattle: IASP Press, 1999, p 395.

Molloy EJ, O'Neill AJ, Grantham JJ, et al. Labor induces a maternal inflammatory response syndrome. *Am J Obstet Gynecol* 2004; 190:448–455.

Mowa CN, Usip S, Collins J, et al. The effects of pregnancy and estrogen on the expression of calcitonin gene-related peptide (CGRP) in the uterine cervix, dorsal root ganglia and spinal cord. *Peptides* 2003a; 24:1163–1174.

Mowa CN, Usip S, Storey-Workley M, Amann R, Papka R. Substance P in the uterine cervix, dorsal root ganglia and spinal cord during pregnancy and the effect of estrogen on SP synthesis. *Peptides* 2003b; 24:761–771.

Mowa CN, Jesmin S, Sakuma I, et al. Characterization of vascular endothelial growth factor (VEGF) in the uterine cervix over pregnancy: effects of denervation and implications for cervical ripening. *J Histochem Cytochem* 2004; 52:1665–1674.

Nikolajsen L, Sorensen HC, Jensen TS, Kehlet H. Chronic pain following Caesarean section. *Acta Anaesth Scand* 2004; 48:111–116.

Papka RE, Storey-Workley M. Estrogen receptor-α and -β coexist in a subpopulation of sensory neurons of female rat dorsal root ganglia. *Neurosci Lett* 2002; 319:71–74.

Poobalan AS, Bruce J, Smith WC, et al. A review of chronic pain after inguinal herniorrhaphy. *Clin J Pain* 2003; 19:48–54.

Ronca AE, Alberts JR. Effects of spaceflight during pregnancy on labor and birth at 1 G. *J Appl Physiol* 2000; 89:849–854.

Rothemund Y, Grusser SM, Liebeskind U, Schlag PM, Flor H. Phantom phenomena in mastectomized patients and their relation to chronic and acute pre-mastectomy pain. *Pain* 2004; 107:140–146.

Sandner-Kiesling A, Eisenach JC. Pharmacology of opioid inhibition to noxious uterine cervical distension. *Anesthesiology* 2002a; 97:966–971.

Sandner-Kiesling A, Eisenach JC. Estrogen reduces efficacy of μ- but not κ-opioid agonist inhibition in response to uterine cervical distension. *Anesthesiology* 2002b; 96:375–379.

Sandner-Kiesling A, Pan HL, Chen SR, et al. Effect of kappa opioid agonists on visceral nociception induced by uterine cervical distension in rats. *Pain* 2002; 96:13–22.

Schmidt C, Lobos E, Spanel-Borowski K. Pregnancy-induced changes in substance P and neurokinin 1 receptor (NK1-R) expression in the rat uterus. *Reproduction* 2003; 126:451–458.

Sengupta JN, Su X, Gebhart GF. Kappa, but not μ or δ, opioids attenuate responses to distention of afferent fibers innervating the rat colon. *Gastroenterology* 1996; 111:968–980.

Shin SW, Eisenach JC. Intrathecal morphine reduces visceromotor response to acute uterine cervical distension in an estrogen-independent manner. *Anesthesiology* 2003; 98:1467–1471.

Sihoe AD, Au SS, Cheung ML, et al. Incidence of chest wall paresthesia after video-assisted thoracic surgery for primary spontaneous pneumothorax. *Eur J Cardiothorac Surg* 2004; 25:1054–1058.

Strigo IA, Bushnell MC, Boivin M, Duncan GH. Psychophysical analysis of visceral and cutaneous pain in human subjects. *Pain* 2002; 97:235–246.

Strigo IA, Duncan GH, Boivin M, Bushnell MC. Differentiation of visceral and cutaneous pain in the human brain. *J Neurophysiol* 2003; 89:3294–3303.

Su X, Joshi SK, Kardos S, Gebhart GF. Sodium channel blocking actions of the kappa-opioid receptor agonist U50,488 contribute to its visceral antinociceptive effects. *J Neurophysiol* 2002; 87:1271–1279.

Thompson JF, Roberts CL, Currie M, Ellwood DA. Prevalence and persistence of health problems after childbirth: associations with parity and method of birth. *Birth* 2002; 29:83–94.

Tong C, Ma W, Shin SW, James RL, Eisenach JC. Uterine cervical distension induces cFos expression in deep dorsal horn neurons of the rat spinal cord. *Anesthesiology* 2003; 99:205–211.

Tsen LC, Thue B, Datta S, Segal S. Is combined spinal-epidural analgesia associated with more rapid cervical dilation in nulliparous patients when compared with conventional epidural analgesia? *Anesthesiology* 1999; 91:920–925.

Wong CA, Scavone BM, Peaceman AM, et al. The risk of cesarean delivery with neuraxial analgesia given early versus late in labor. *N Engl J Med* 2005; 352:655–665.

Yellon SM, Mackler AM, Kirby MA. The role of leukocyte traffic and activation in parturition. *J Soc Gynecol Investig* 2003; 10:323–338.

Correspondence to: Prof. James C. Eisenach, MD, Department of Anesthesiology, Wake Forest University School of Medicine, Winston-Salem, NC 27104, USA. Tel: 336-716-4182; Fax: 336-716-0288; email: jim@eisenach.us.

Proceedings of the 11th World Congress on Pain,
edited by Herta Flor, Eija Kalso, and Jonathan O.
Dostrovsky, IASP Press, Seattle, © 2006.

55

Pain Following Spinal Cord Injury

Philip J. Siddall

*Pain Management Research Institute, University of Sydney,
Royal North Shore Hospital, Sydney, Australia*

THE SCOPE OF THE PROBLEM

Spinal cord injury (SCI) results in pain that not only is distressing but has a major impact on patients regarding their quality of life and their ability to achieve optimal functional goals (Widerström-Noga et al. 1999). The prevalence of pain following SCI is high, with most studies indicating a prevalence of around 60–70% (New et al. 1997; Widerström-Noga et al. 1999; Ravenscroft et al. 2000; Siddall et al. 2003). Most of these studies also reveal that around one-third of SCI pain patients report their pain as being severe.

CLASSIFICATION OF SPINAL CORD INJURY PAIN

Various types of pain are commonly seen following SCI, and attempts have been made to classify these different pain types into a taxonomy or classification system. A taxonomy was recently developed by the Spinal Cord Injury Pain Task Force of the International Association for the Study of Pain (IASP) and was published as a proposed model, as shown in Table I (Siddall et al. 2002). This taxonomy proposes a tiered classification in which pain types are firstly divided into nociceptive (musculoskeletal or visceral) and neuropathic (above-level, at-level, and below-level). A final tier aims to identify a pain type based on specific structures and pathology, when possible. The features of each of these types of pain are described below.

MUSCULOSKELETAL PAIN

Traumatic SCI is usually accompanied by major damage to the vertebral column and its supporting structures. Such trauma results in acute nociceptive

Table I
Proposed classification of pain related to spinal cord injury

Broad Type (Tier One)	Broad System (Tier Two)	Specific Structures/Pathology (Tier Three)
Nociceptive	Musculoskeletal	Bone, joint, muscle trauma or inflammation Mechanical instability Muscle spasm Secondary overuse syndromes
	Visceral	Renal calculus, bowel, sphincter dysfunction, etc. Dysreflexic headache
Neuropathic	Above-level	Compressive mononeuropathies Complex regional pain syndromes
	At-level	Nerve root compression (including cauda equina) Syringomyelia Spinal cord trauma/ischemia (transitional zone, etc.) Dual-level cord and root trauma (double lesion syndrome)
	Below-level	Spinal cord trauma/ischemia

Source: Modified from Siddall et al. (2002, p. 21).

pain arising from damage to structures such as bones, ligaments, muscles, intervertebral disks, and facet joints. Some acute musculoskeletal pain is also related to structural spinal damage and instability. This type of pain is related to activity or position, and although not radicular, it may radiate into the trunk or extremities. Muscle spasm pain is also a common problem in patients with incomplete injuries; it usually occurs well after the injury following resolution of spinal shock.

Chronic musculoskeletal pain is the most common type of pain seen in those with established SCI (Siddall et al. 2003). The pain commonly occurs in normally innervated regions rostral to the level of the SCI. Chronic musculo-skeletal pain can also occur with overuse or "abnormal" use of structures such as the arm and shoulder. The pain is described as aching and is worse with use of involved joints or pressure on the painful area. It is typically seen in the shoulders of those who use wheelchairs, and as many as 72% of paraplegics have evidence of shoulder joint degenerative changes (Lal 1998).

VISCERAL PAIN

SCI may increase the likelihood of pathology affecting visceral structures. For example, it increases the risk of bowel impaction and urinary tract infection. These conditions will give rise to visceral pain, although the level of injury will affect the quality of the pain. Visceral pain is located in the abdomen and is characteristically dull, poorly localized, and described as bloating or cramping.

However, diagnosis is often difficult in the person with SCI, and repeated investigations may fail to find definitive evidence of pathology. If this is the case, and if treatments directed at visceral pathology do not relieve the pain, then consideration must be given to classifying the pain as neuropathic rather than visceral.

ABOVE-LEVEL NEUROPATHIC PAIN

Neuropathic pain can occur above the level of injury. Some "above-level" pains are not specific to SCI, including pain due to peripheral nerve compression and complex regional pain syndromes. Individuals with SCI may be more susceptible to some of these pains because of the extra burden placed on the upper limbs during wheelchair use and transfers.

AT-LEVEL NEUROPATHIC PAIN

At-level neuropathic pain is classically described as electric, shooting, or burning pain in a segmental or dermatomal pattern within two segments above or below the level of injury. Because of the characteristic distribution of this type of pain, it is also referred to as radicular, segmental, transitional zone, border zone, end zone, and girdle pain. It is often associated with allodynia or hyperesthesia of the affected dermatomes.

At-level neuropathic pain may be due to damage either to nerve roots (including the cauda equina) or to the spinal cord itself. Pain arising from nerve root damage is usually unilateral and may be suggested by features such as increased pain in relation to spinal movement. The pain may be due to direct damage to the nerve root during the initial trauma, or it may be secondary to spinal column instability and impingement by facet or disk material.

However, at-level neuropathic pain may also occur in the absence of nerve root damage and may be due to spinal cord rather than nerve root pathology. The only distinguishing feature of at-level neuropathic pain arising from spinal cord damage appears to be that the pain is usually bilateral in distribution. Although this type of pain may be difficult to distinguish from nerve root pain on the basis of descriptors, it is important to make the distinction because the underlying mechanisms and therefore the most appropriate treatment may be different.

The possibility of syringomyelia must always be considered in the patient who has delayed onset of segmental pain, especially where there is a rising level of sensory loss. The loss of pain and temperature sensation is typical, but both sensory and motor functions may be affected. People with this type of pain describe it as a constant, burning pain. It may be associated with allodynia or hyperalgesia.

BELOW-LEVEL NEUROPATHIC PAIN

Below-level neuropathic pain is also referred to as central dysesthesia syndrome, central pain, phantom pain, or deafferentation pain (Beric et al. 1988). It consists of spontaneous or evoked pain, or both, in a diffuse distribution caudal to the level of SCI. It is characterized by sensations of burning, aching, stabbing, or electric shocks that can be triggered by sudden noises or jarring movements, and it often develops some time after the initial injury. The pain is constant, but it may fluctuate with mood, infections, or other factors and is not usually related to position or activity.

Below-level neuropathic pain is the most likely to be described as severe or excruciating and is the most difficult type of SCI pain to treat successfully. It occurs in about one-third of SCI patients who complain of persistent pain. Many of them develop this type of pain months and even years after their initial injury. Unfortunately, those who experience neuropathic pain in the first 3–6 months are likely to continue to experience ongoing pain 3–5 years following injury (Siddall et al. 2003).

FACTORS RELATED TO PAIN

The various factors that are involved in the development of SCI pain are unclear. Studies that have sought to identify physical factors that are more likely to be associated with pain are varied and sometimes contradictory. Some studies have correlated pain with injury at specific levels of the spinal cord, including cervical, thoracolumbar, conus medullaris, and cauda equina levels. However, a number of other studies have failed to find a significant relationship between the presence or severity of pain and the level of injury (Richards et al. 1980; Summers et al. 1991).

It is often stated that pain is more common in patients with incomplete injuries. However, this assumption is in conflict with a survey finding that completeness of injury was significantly related to the presence of pain (Ravenscroft et al. 2000) and with other studies finding no relationship between the extent of injury and the presence of pain (Richards et al. 1980; Summers et al. 1991). Although completeness may not directly relate to the presence of pain, the nature of the injury may be an important factor, with several studies indicating a strong link between damage to the spinothalamic tracts and the development of neuropathic pain (Eide et al. 1996; Defrin et al. 2001).

A link is also apparent between psychosocial factors and the presence or severity of pain following SCI (Richards et al. 1980; Summers et al. 1991). It is difficult to make definitive conclusions on the causal relationship between pain and psychological factors. However, it is clear that pain has a major impact on a patient's ability to participate in daily activities (Ravenscroft et al. 2000) and may have a stronger influence than the extent of SCI on quality of life (West-gren and Levi 1998; Rintala et al. 1999).

Spinal cord injury may result in significant psychological disruption. Persis-tent pain following SCI is associated with more depressive symptoms and more perceived stress (Rintala et al. 1999). There is also a strong relationship between pain, spasticity, "abnormal nonpainful sensations," and sadness (Widerström-Noga et al. 1999). However, the prevalence and severity of disruption are not as high as many would clinicians predict. Many patients who exhibit psychological morbidity return to normal limits within the first year following injury.

Psychological issues have tremendous importance in the experience and expression of any pain condition, and SCI itself may also have an impact on psychological status and quality of life (Rintala et al. 1999). Some authors have included psychological or psychogenic pain as types of pain that occur follow-ing SCI. However, applying a psychological label to the pain and considering "psychogenic pain" as an entity in its own right may not be helpful. Rather, psychological factors should be considered as contributors in any person re-porting pain.

MECHANISMS OF SPINAL CORD INJURY PAIN

As expected, the different types of pain observed following SCI have a range of possible generators and contributing factors. The underlying mecha-nisms responsible for musculoskeletal and visceral pain are similar, if not identi-cal, to those seen in other populations, although the injury may have an impact on presentation and features. Neuropathic pain following SCI may similarly share some of the mechanisms demonstrated in peripheral neuropathic pain conditions. However, even neuropathic SCI pain is not a single entity and may present in different ways that may reflect different underlying pathophysiologi-cal processes. The focus of this chapter will be on the mechanisms that may be responsible for the development of neuropathic SCI pain and in particular at-level and below-level neuropathic pain. As with other types of pain, pain may be due to abnormal processes at peripheral, spinal, and supraspinal levels and it may be helpful to consider pathophysiological mechanisms using this broad framework.

PERIPHERAL GENERATOR

Damage to spinal structures may result in impingement of nerve roots entering the spinal cord. This may lead to the generation of impulses within primary afferents and the production of radicular at-level neuropathic pain. The mechanisms responsible for this type of pain are similar, if not identical, to the mechanisms underlying other conditions in which peripheral neuropathic pain occurs following trauma to nerve roots.

SPINAL GENERATOR

However, neuropathic pain may also be dependent on the presence of a spinal generator or amplifier. Several case reports of spinal local anesthetic blockade in patients with SCI pain describe complete (although temporary) abolition of pain with sensory block up to and above the level of injury. Furthermore, most patients with evidence of spinal canal obstruction, in whom a sensory block could not be achieved above the level of the SCI, had little or no change in their pain. This ability of spinal local anesthetic blockade to relieve neuropathic pain following SCI led to the proposition that there may be an "irritated focus" or "neural pain generator" at the distal end of the proximal segment of the spinal cord. This proposal was supported by a case report in which electrophysiological recordings demonstrated abnormal spontaneous neuronal activity in cells just above the level of injury in a man with an upper lumbar SCI (Loeser et al. 1968).

These clinical observations have, to some extent, been supported by subsequent investigations using animal models of SCI pain. Briefly, these models demonstrate greater neuronal responsiveness to peripheral stimuli, an increase in the level of background neuronal activity, and the occurrence of neuronal afterdischarges following cessation of a stimulus (Hao et al. 1992; Yezierski and Park 1993; Christensen et al. 1996; Hoheisel et al. 2003). These changes in neuronal function occur in spinal dorsal horn neurons close to the site of injury. This increase in neuronal excitability may occur as a result of increased excitation through activation of N-methyl-D-aspartate (NMDA), non-NMDA, and metabotropic glutamate receptors (Mills et al. 2002) and upregulation of sodium channels (Hains et al. 2003). Alternatively, it might be mediated by a reduction in normal GABAergic (Zhang et al. 1994; Drew et al. 2004), opioidergic (Xu et al. 1994), or serotonergic (Hains et al. 2002) and noradrenergic (Hao et al. 1996) inhibition. Thus, neuropathic pain, at least in some patients, may be due to a spinal rather than a peripheral generator.

SUPRASPINAL GENERATOR

The evidence from clinical and animal studies is strong to support the concept of a spinal generator that may underlie neuropathic SCI pain. However, several observations have raised the question of whether changes at more rostral levels may also be important. Spinal local anesthetic blockade does not always relieve pain, despite a demonstrated sensory block above the level of injury (Loubser and Donovan 1991). Notably, Melzack and Loeser (1978) described a group of patients who continued to experience neuropathic SCI pain despite peripheral, sympathetic, and spinal blockade and even surgical removal of cord segments above the level of injury. These findings suggested the possibility that neuropathic pain in some patients might be due to a pain generator in supraspinal structures.

Electrophysiological studies in SCI patients with pain have demonstrated that thalamic neurons that have no discernible receptive field, and therefore have lost their inputs, have abnormal patterns of activity including high rates of spontaneous bursting (Lenz et al. 1989), although thalamic neuronal bursting alone may not be sufficient for pain to occur (Radhakrishnan et al. 1999). Further evidence includes the demonstration of abnormal spontaneous and evoked activity of thalamic neurons, both in a contusion SCI pain model (Gerke et al. 2003) and in patients with neuropathic SCI pain (Llinas et al. 1999).

The extent to which these supraspinal changes are dependent on ongoing abnormal ascending inputs is unclear. In a clinical study, patients with below-level neuropathic SCI pain had significantly more sensory hypersensitivity in dermatomes at the level of injury than pain-free SCI patients (Finnerup et al. 2003). It was therefore suggested that below-level neuropathic pain may be a result of a combined effect of supraspinal neuroplastic changes in response to a spinothalamic lesion together with increased inputs due to neuronal hyperexcitability at the rostral end of the injury. Whatever the role of different regions, increasing evidence shows that pathophysiological changes occur at peripheral, spinal, and supraspinal levels. Changes at all levels may contribute in varying degrees to the development of neuropathic SCI pain.

MANAGEMENT OF SPINAL CORD INJURY PAIN

Although a number of studies point to the underlying mechanisms of neuropathic SCI pain, translation from the laboratory to the clinic has been slow to reap rewards in terms of improved patient outcomes. Many treatments are used for symptom relief, but they are often used with little evidence of efficacy and sometimes in the face of evidence of lack of efficacy. An overview of different treatments used in the management of neuropathic SCI pain is presented below.

SURGICAL APPROACHES

Surgical approaches are often designed to relieve pain by reversing any structural problems giving rise to pain. For example, nerve root or peripheral nerve compression may require surgical decompression, and a syrinx may require drainage and shunting. A detethering procedure may relieve pain caused by scarring around nerve roots.

If it is not possible to address a structural problem, surgical approaches attempt to deal with the pain by destroying the site of abnormal activity or disconnecting it from the brain. This is the simplest conceptual approach to dealing with the pain, and in some cases it does resolve the pain. For example, dorsal root entry zone lesions, which destroy nerve cells in the dorsal horn close to the level of injury, can be effective in providing relief of neuropathic pain, with best results in those with at-level neuropathic pain. However, surgical approaches are relatively invasive, may cause additional neurological deficits and may fail to address supraspinal changes and therefore provide only temporary or incomplete relief.

PHARMACOLOGICAL APPROACHES

Clinicians often rely upon pharmacological approaches to provide pain relief. Unfortunately, few controlled trials have specifically examined the efficacy of pharmaceutical agents in the treatment of at-level and below-level neuropathic SCI pain. The number of patients included was often small, and therefore the conclusions may not be reliable. Evidence-based treatment is therefore sometimes dependent on extrapolation from other neuropathic pain conditions.

Pharmacological approaches attempt to deal more specifically with neurotransmitter and receptor changes that may occur as a result of the injury, leading to increased spontaneous and evoked neuronal activity. As described above, these changes are multiple and complex, but those that have been demonstrated fall broadly into two categories. These are (1) increased excitation, with alterations in glutamate-receptor and sodium channel function, and (2) decreased inhibition, with alterations in GABA, serotonin (5HT), norepinephrine, and opioid systems.

There is evidence that drugs that target increased excitation by blocking NMDA-receptor and sodium channel function may be effective. In the acute, in-patient setting, systemic administration of the NMDA-receptor antagonist ketamine (Eide et al. 1995) and of the sodium channel blocker lidocaine (Attal et al. 2000) both provided effective relief of neuropathic pain. Although Cahana and colleagues (2004) have reported long-term effectiveness with the use of lidocaine, systemic administration is generally not practical for chronic administration, and oral agents with a similar action, such as mexiletine, have not been demonstrated to be effective (Chiou Tan et al. 1996).

A large number of agents target inhibitory mechanisms with varying degrees of success including opioids, antidepressants, and anticonvulsants. Randomized controlled trials demonstrate the effectiveness of opioids including morphine (Attal et al. 2002) and alfentanil (Eide et al. 1995) and of other agents such as propofol (Canavero et al. 1995). However, in these studies, the agents were administered systemically, and there is little direct evidence regarding efficacy with oral opioids. Opioid analgesics such as oxycodone, methadone, and morphine may provide relief, but adverse effects, tolerance, and dependence are issues that need to be considered. If opioids are used, controlled-release preparations provide more stable analgesia and are preferred for long-term use. Tramadol may be less sedating and less constipating, and because of its additional serotonergic and noradrenergic effects, it may be effective in some people with neuropathic pain. Therefore, it may be a useful first step if opioid agents are being considered.

Antidepressants, and in particular tricyclic antidepressants, are widely used in the management of neuropathic pain conditions, although there is little direct evidence for their effectiveness in neuropathic SCI pain. In fact, one randomized controlled study suggests that amitriptyline is ineffective in people with pain following SCI (Cardenas et al. 2002). Nevertheless, given the lack of effective agents and supportive evidence from other neuropathic pain conditions, a trial of tricyclic antidepressants is often part of clinical practice. Newer antidepressants such as the mixed serotonin-norepinephrine reuptake inhibitors may be effective. However, either controlled studies are nonexistent, or in the case of the selective serotonin reuptake inhibitor, trazodone, they indicate a lack of group effect when compared with placebo (Davidoff et al. 1987).

The next large group of drugs is the anticonvulsants. Once again, these agents are widely used in the treatment of neuropathic pain conditions. Although many anticonvulsants have an effect on inhibitory processes, their range of actions is broad. Some enhance GABAergic inhibition, but some also have a sodium-channel-blocking effect, reduce glutamate release, and act on calcium channels. Thus, anticonvulsants may target both excitatory and inhibitory mechanisms, and it is this broad mixture of effects that may be partly responsible for their effectiveness. Several studies indicate that gabapentin (Tai et al. 2002; To et al. 2002) is effective in treating neuropathic SCI pain, and it is regarded by many as a first-line agent in the treatment of this condition. Unpublished evidence from a randomized controlled trial also indicates the effectiveness of pregabalin (Siddall et al. 2005). Other anticonvulsants such as sodium valproate (Drewes et al. 1994), lamotrigine (Finnerup et al. 2002), and topiramate (Dinoff et al. 2003) are effective in some individuals, but there is limited or negative evidence in controlled trials.

Combinations of anticonvulsants and tricyclic antidepressants may be more effective than either class of drugs administered alone. Therefore, if a single agent is ineffective, a combination of an anticonvulsant with either a tricyclic antidepressant or an opioid may produce some relief.

If oral administration of agents fails, spinal administration can be considered, although the invasiveness of such procedures may be a concern to the patient. Spinal administration of drugs such as morphine and clonidine has been found to be effective in some individuals. A positive outcome was found with intrathecal baclofen in a randomized controlled trial (Herman et al. 1992), but other reports have been less supportive (Loubser and Akman 1996). Combinations of morphine or clonidine with baclofen in those with spasms may confer additional benefit (Middleton et al. 1996). In a controlled study, intrathecal administration of a mixture of morphine and clonidine was found to be effective in a group of people with chronic at-level and below-level neuropathic SCI pain (Siddall et al. 2000).

STIMULATION TECHNIQUES

Stimulation techniques such as transcutaneous electrical nerve stimulation and acupuncture may be effective for some patients with neuropathic pain; these modalities may work by activating inhibitory mechanisms. Spinal cord stimulation may also provide relief, with greater effect in those with at-level neuropathic pain and incomplete lesions (Lang 1997). Other available treatments are very invasive, with limited evidence of efficacy. These include deep brain stimulation and motor cortex stimulation.

PSYCHOLOGICAL APPROACHES

Persons with SCI undergo a huge adjustment in relationships, lifestyle, vocation, and self-image, and those with a severe SCI usually have significant psychological distress (Summers et al. 1991). Chronic pain may be an additional factor that prevents expected rehabilitation and return to employment and activities of daily living (Lundqvist et al. 1991; Westgren and Levi 1998; Rintala et al. 1999; Widerström-Noga et al. 2002). Anxiety and depression are both normal responses to injury; they often improve over time. Many patients can develop their inherent coping skills to overcome these problems. Formal intervention may not be required, except for the minority of patients who experience severe or chronic mood dysfunction that has an impact on their ability to function and contributes to their pain. Various approaches for dealing with mood dysfunction include the use of anxiolytic and antidepressant medications and cognitive-behavioral treatment.

In summary, several types of pain commonly occur following SCI that have a major impact on the life of the patient. The mechanisms underlying neuropathic pain are poorly understood, and there are few treatments that provide consistent and substantial pain relief. Recent progress in our understanding of the pathophysiology of this condition and the development of new treatment strategies should lead to greater success in the management of this difficult problem.

ACKNOWLEDGMENTS

I would like to thank Professors Michael Cousins and Arthur Duggan for their enthusiasm, advice, and support for this work and acknowledge the contributions of Dr. Kevin Keay, Dr. Geoff Drew, Dr. Michelle Gerke, Dr. Haydn Allbutt, Ms. Ling Xu, and Ms. Joan McClelland of the Pain Management Research Institute, Royal North Shore Hospital, Sydney, and Drs. Sue Rutkowksi and James Middleton of the Spinal Injury Units at Royal North Shore Hospital and Royal Rehabilitation Centre, Sydney. The work is supported by the National Health and Medical Research Council and by the NSW Government Spinal Cord Injury and Other Neurological Conditions Research Grants Program.

REFERENCES

Attal N, Gaudé V, Brasseur L, et al. Intravenous lidocaine in central pain: a double-blind, placebo-controlled, psychophysical study. *Neurology* 2000; 54:564–574.

Attal N, Guirimand F, Brasseur L, et al. Effects of IV morphine in central pain—a randomized placebo-controlled study. *Neurology* 2002; 58:554–563.

Beric A, Dimitrijevic MR, Lindblom U. Central dysesthesia syndrome in spinal cord injury patients. *Pain* 1988; 34:109–116.

Cahana A, Carota A, Montadon ML, Annoni JM. The long-term effect of repeated intravenous lidocaine on central pain and possible correlation in positron emission tomography measurements. *Anesth Analg* 2004; 98:1581–1584.

Canavero S, Bonicalzi V, Pagni CA, et al. Propofol analgesia in central pain—preliminary clinical observations. *J Neurol* 1995; 242:561–567.

Cardenas DD, Warms CA, Turner JA, et al. Efficacy of amitriptyline for relief of pain in spinal cord injury: results of a randomized controlled trial. *Pain* 2002; 96:365–373.

Chiou Tan FY, Tuel SM, Johnson JC, et al. Effect of mexiletine on spinal cord injury dysesthetic pain. *Am J Phys Med Rehabil* 1996; 75:84–87.

Christensen MD, Everhart AW, Pickelman JT, Hulsebosch CE. Mechanical and thermal allodynia in chronic central pain following spinal cord injury. *Pain* 1996; 68:97–107.

Davidoff G, Guarracini M, Roth E, Sliwa J, Yarkony G. Trazodone hydrochloride in the treatment of dysesthetic pain in traumatic myelopathy: a randomized, double-blind, placebo-controlled study. *Pain* 1987; 29:151–161.

Defrin R, Ovry A, Blumen N, Urca G. Characterization of chronic pain and somatosensory function in spinal cord injury subjects. *Pain* 2001; 89:253–263.

Dinoff BL, Richards JS, Ness TJ. Use of topiramate for spinal cord injury-related pain. *J Spinal Cord Med* 2003; 26:401–403.

Drew GM, Siddall PJ, Duggan AW. Mechanical allodynia following contusion injury of the rat spinal cord is associated with loss of GABAergic inhibition in the dorsal horn. *Pain* 2004; 109:379–388.

Drewes AM, Andreasen A, Poulsen LH. Valproate for treatment of chronic central pain after spinal cord injury. A double-blind cross-over study. *Paraplegia* 1994; 32:565–569.

Eide PK, Stubhaug A, Stenehjem AE. Central dysesthesia pain after traumatic spinal cord injury is dependent on *N*-methyl-D-aspartate receptor activation. *Neurosurgery* 1995; 37:1080–1087.

Eide PK, Jorum E, Stenehjem E. Somatosensory findings in patients with spinal cord injury and central dysaesthesia pain. *J Neurol Neurosurg Psychiatry* 1996; 60:411–415.

Finnerup NB, Sindrup SH, Flemming WB, Johannesen IL, Jensen TS. Lamotrigine in spinal cord injury pain: a randomized controlled trial. *Pain* 2002; 96:375–383.

Finnerup NB, Johannesen IL, Fuglsang-Frederiksen A, Bach FW, Jensen TS. Sensory function in spinal cord injury patients with and without central pain. *Brain* 2003; 126:57–70.

Gerke MB, Duggan AW, Xu L, Siddall PJ. Thalamic neuronal activity in rats with mechanical allodynia following contusive spinal cord injury. *Neuroscience* 2003; 117:715–722.

Hains BC, Everhart AE, Fullwood SD, Hulsebosch CE. Changes in serotonin, serotonin transporter expression and serotonin denervation supersensitivity: involvement in chronic central pain after spinal hemisection in the rat. *Exp Neurol* 2002; 175:347–362.

Hains BC, Klein JP, Saab CY, et al. Upregulation of sodium channel $Na_v1.3$ and functional involvement in neuronal hyperexcitability associated with central neuropathic pain after spinal cord injury. *J Neurosci* 2003; 23:8881–8892.

Hao JX, Xu XJ, Yu YX, Seiger A, Wiesenfeld-Hallin Z. Transient spinal cord ischaemia induces temporary hypersensitivity of dorsal horn wide dynamic range neurons to myelinated, but not unmyelinated, fiber input. *J Neurophysiol* 1992; 68:384–391.

Hao JX, Yu W, Xu XJ, Wiesenfeld-Hallin Z. Effects of intrathecal vs. systemic clonidine in treating chronic allodynia-like response in spinally injured rats. *Brain Res* 1996; 736:28–34.

Herman RM, D'Luzansky SC, Ippolito R. Intrathecal baclofen suppresses central pain in patients with spinal lesions: a pilot study. *Clin J Pain* 1992; 8:338–345.

Hoheisel U, Scheifer C, Trudrung P, Unger T, Mense S. Pathophysiological activity in rat dorsal horn neurones in segments rostral to a chronic spinal cord injury. *Brain Res* 2003; 974:134–145.

Lal S. Premature degenerative shoulder changes in spinal cord injury patients. *Spinal Cord* 1998; 36:186–189.

Lang P. The treatment of chronic pain by epidural spinal cord stimulation. *Axone* 1997; 18:71–73.

Lenz FA, Kwan HC, Dostrovsky JO, Tasker RR. Characteristics of the bursting pattern of action potentials that occurs in the thalamus of patients with central pain. *Brain Res* 1989; 496:357–360.

Llinas RR, Ribary U, Jeanmonod D, Kronberg E, Mitra PP. Thalamocortical dysrhythmia: a neurological and neuropsychiatric syndrome characterized by magnetoencephalography. *Proc Natl Acad Sci USA* 1999; 96:15222–15227.

Loeser JD, Ward AA, White LE. Chronic deafferentation of human spinal cord neurons. *J Neurosurg* 1968; 29:48–50.

Loubser PG, Akman NM. Effects of intrathecal baclofen on chronic spinal cord injury pain. *J Pain Symptom Manage* 1996; 12:241–247.

Loubser PG, Donovan WH. Diagnostic spinal anaesthesia in chronic spinal cord injury pain. *Paraplegia* 1991; 29:25–36.

Lundqvist C, Siosteen A, Blomstrand C, Lind B, Sullivan M. Spinal cord injuries: clinical, functional, and emotional status. *Spine* 1991; 16:78–83.

Melzack R, Loeser JD. Phantom body pain in paraplegics: evidence for a central "pattern generating mechanism" for pain. *Pain* 1978; 4:195–210.

Middleton JW, Siddall PJ, Walker S, Molloy AR, Rutkowski SB. Intrathecal clonidine and baclofen in the management of spasticity and neuropathic pain following spinal cord injury: a case study. *Arch Phys Med Rehabil* 1996; 77:824–826.

Mills CD, Johnson KM, Hulsebosch CE. Group I metabotropic glutamate receptors in spinal cord injury: roles in neuroprotection and the development of chronic central pain. *J Neurotrauma* 2002; 19:23–42.

New P, Lim TC, Hill ST, Brown DJ. A survey of pain during rehabilitation after acute spinal cord injury. *Spinal Cord* 1997; 35:658–663.

Radhakrishnan V, Tsoukatos J, Davis KD, et al. A comparison of the burst activity of lateral thalamic neurons in chronic pain and non-pain patients. *Pain* 1999; 80:567–575.

Ravenscroft A, Ahmed YS, Burnside IG. Chronic pain after SCI. A patient survey. *Spinal Cord* 2000; 38:611–614.

Richards JS, Meredith RL, Nepomuceno C, Fine PR, Bennett G. Psychosocial aspects of chronic pain in spinal cord injury. *Pain* 1980; 8:355–366.

Rintala D, Loubser PG, Castro J, Hart KA, Fuhrer MJ. Chronic pain in a community-based sample of men with spinal cord injury: prevalence, severity, and relationship with impairment, disability, handicap, and subjective well-being. *Arch Phys Med Rehabil* 1999; 79:604–614.

Siddall PJ, Molloy AR, Walker S, et al. Efficacy of intrathecal morphine and clonidine in the treatment of neuropathic pain following spinal cord injury. *Anesth Analg* 2000; 91:1493–1498.

Siddall PJ, Yezierski RP, Loeser JD. Taxonomy and epidemiology of spinal cord injury pain. In: Burchiel KJ, Yezierski RP (Eds). *Spinal Cord Injury Pain: Assessment, Mechanisms, Management, Progress in Pain Research and Management,* Vol. 23. Seattle: IASP Press, 2002, pp 9–24.

Siddall PJ, McClelland JM, Rutkowski SB, Cousins MJ. A longitudinal study of the prevalence and characteristics of pain in the first 5 years following spinal cord injury. *Pain* 2003; 103:249–257.

Siddall P, Cousins M, Otte A, Phillips K, Griesing T. Pregabalin safely and effectively treats chronic central neuropathic pain after spinal cord injury. *Abstracts: 11th World Congress on Pain.* Seattle: IASP Press, 2005, p 232.

Summers JD, Rapoff MA, Varghese G, Porter K, Palmer RE. Psychosocial factors in chronic spinal cord injury pain. *Pain* 1991; 47:183–189.

Tai Q, Kirshblum S, Chen B, et al. Gabapentin in the treatment of neuropathic pain after spinal cord injury: a prospective, randomized, double-blind, crossover trial. *J Spinal Cord Med* 2002; 25:100–105.

To TP, Lim TC, Hill ST, et al. Gabapentin for neuropathic pain following spinal cord injury. *Spinal Cord* 2002; 40:282–285.

Westgren N, Levi R. Quality of life and traumatic spinal cord injury. *Arch Phys Med Rehabil* 1998; 79:1433–1439.

Widerström-Noga EG, Felipe-Cuervo E, Broton JG, Duncan RC, Yezierski RP. Perceived difficulty in dealing with consequences of spinal cord injury. *Arch Phys Med Rehabil* 1999; 80:580–586.

Widerström-Noga EG, Duncan R, Felipe-Cuervo E, Turk DC. Assessment of the impact of pain and impairments associated with spinal cord injuries. *Arch Phys Med Rehabil* 2002; 83:395–404.

Xu XJ, Hao JX, Seiger A, et al. Chronic pain-related behaviors in spinally injured rats—evidence for functional alterations of the endogenous cholecystokinin and opioid systems. *Pain* 1994; 56:271–277.

Yezierski RP, Park SH. The mechanosensitivity of spinal sensory neurons following intraspinal injections of quisqualic acid in the rat. *Neurosci Lett* 1993; 157:115–119.

Zhang AL, Hao JX, Seiger A, et al. Decreased GABA immunoreactivity in spinal cord dorsal horn neurons after transient spinal cord ischaemia in the rat. *Brain Res* 1994; 656:187–190.

Correspondence to: Philip Siddall, MB BS PhD, Pain Management Research Institute, Royal North Shore Hospital, St Leonards, NSW 2065, Australia. Tel: 61-2-9926-6387; Fax: 61-2-9926-6548; email: phils@med.usyd.edu.au.

Proceedings of the 11th World Congress on Pain,
edited by Herta Flor, Eija Kalso, and Jonathan O.
Dostrovsky, IASP Press, Seattle, © 2006.

56

Headache: Clinical and Basic Science Advances Relevant to Practice

Peter J. Goadsby

*Institute of Neurology, The National Hospital for Neurology
and Neurosurgery, London, United Kingdom*

Headache dominates neurology outpatient appointments (Carson et al. 2000) and is one of the most common disorders presenting to doctors. On a day-to-day basis, severe migraine is considered by the World Health Organization to be as disabling as quadriplegia (Menken et al. 2000). Pain is a major part of the presentation of headache syndromes, so physicians interested in pain must be well versed in headache disorders. A significant incentive for clinicians to learn the state of the art of headache treatment is that it offers a considerable opportunity to make many patients much better. This chapter highlights some of the recent advances in a field that now commands a breadth that can only be addressed by textbooks. Interested readers are referred to recent monographs for more detailed accounts of headache disorders and their management (Lance and Goadsby 2005; Olesen et al. 2005).

CLASSIFICATION OF HEADACHE

The development and promulgation of the International Headache Society (IHS) diagnostic criteria in 1988 (Headache Classification Committee of the International Headache Society 1988) was perhaps one of the great advances of the late 20th century for headache. The criteria made it possible to differentiate clear and homogenous populations that formed the basis of all the important studies in the 1990s. They did not suffer from the vagueness of the 1962 classification (Ad Hoc Committee on Classification of Headache of the NIH 1962), but in this research strength the classification has its clinical Achilles' heel. While it is essential to define clear populations for research, this emphasis can force artificial distinctions in clinical practice. Many phenomena in biology are on a continuous distribution. One might expect headache presentations to be on some clinical continuum, and thus it can be difficult to make diagnoses and define appropriate management. In this light, it is not surprising that patients attending headache clinics have sometimes not fit into the system (Sanin et al. 1994; Raieli et al. 1996), although for most patients it does work very well.

The second edition of the classification (Headache Classification Committee of the International Headache Society 2004) has seen fine-tuning of the migraine classification and the inclusion of some important headache types not previously dealt with at all. The classification of migraine has been modified for pediatric populations by allowing headaches with fewer features. In addition, some further thought has been given to the childhood periodic syndromes: cyclical vomiting, abdominal migraine, and benign paroxysmal vertigo of childhood, which so often portend migraine in adolescence and adulthood.

Section three of the classification, on cluster and related headaches, has been altered to accommodate the range of phenotypes of what have been termed the *trigeminal autonomic cephalalgias* (TACs) (Goadsby and Lipton 1997). These syndromes share the pathophysiological feature of pronounced activation of the cranial parasympathetic autonomic outflow in association with pain (May and Goadsby 1999). The terminology in section three has been standardized, such that "chronic" implies the form of the disorder that does not have breaks of at least 1 month, and "episodic" is the form that has breaks of a month or more. It is now recognized that both cluster headache and paroxysmal hemicrania have episodic forms. Short-lasting unilateral neuralgiform headache attacks with conjunctival injection and tearing (SUNCT) has been included (Goadsby 2005d,e).

Other headaches not previously recognized in the 1988 classification include hemicrania continua (Sjaastad and Spierings 1984), hypnic headache (Raskin 1988), and primary thunderclap headache (Dodick et al. 1999). These are important because the first two respond well to therapy; hemicrania continua is very sensitive to indomethacin (Matharu et al. 2003), and hypnic headache usually responds to lithium (Dodick et al. 1998).

Chronic daily headache. The most controversial issue in headache classification, and indeed in some respects in clinical practice, is how to deal with the problem of frequent, daily or near-daily headache (Manzoni et al. 1995; Olesen and Rasmussen 1996). Some 5% of North Americans and Western Europeans have headache on 15 days or more a month for, on average, 4 or more hours a day. If one includes shorter-lasting headaches, then *chronic daily headache* is simply a syndrome defined by frequent headache (Welch and Goadsby 2002) and is not just tension-type headache. Chronic daily headache may be associated with medication overuse. It is often incorrectly equated with the concept of *transformed migraine,* which is operationally defined (Silberstein et al. 1996) and is a subset of chronic daily headache (Table I). Similarly, although IHS has narrowly defined *new daily persistent headache* in a restricted way (Headache Classification Committee of the International Headache Society 2004), an understanding of this term in the syndromic sense (Goadsby and Boes 2002) will help clinicians to remember to look for the important secondary causes (Table II). The concept that migraine sufferers may have a less severe daily headache is not new at all, being recognized by luminaries of the 19th century including Gowers (1888). The revised IHS criteria have adopted the term *chronic migraine* for patients who have 15 days or more a month on which they experience migraine without aura. This seems a biologically implausible dichotomy. Moreover, the committee has not been explicit in its reasoning for excluding probable migraine patients from the umbrella of chronic migraine, nor is there any evidence that it should be considered a complication of migraine in the medical sense. One might use the term *transformed migraine,* as Silberstein

Table I
Classification of chronic daily headache

Primary		Secondary*
More than 4 Hours Daily	Less than 4 Hours Daily	
Chronic migraine, transformed migraine†	Chronic cluster headache§	Post-traumatic (head injury, iatrogenic, post-infectious)
Chronic tension-type headache	Chronic paroxysmal hemicrania	Inflammatory (giant cell arteritis, sarcoidosis, Behcet's syndrome
Hemicrania continua	SUNCT¶	Chronic infection of the central nervous system
New daily persistent headache‡	Hypnic headache	Medication overuse

Note: Headache on 15 days or more a month that may be due to a range of underlying mechanisms and may be complicated by *or* caused by medication overuse.
* The secondary headache list is not exhaustive but illustrative.
† Chronic migraine is a term from the ICHD-II (Headache Classification Committee of the International Headache Society 2004). In essence, it is migraine without aura for 15 days or more a month. Transformed migraine is a useful term in clinical practice; a current working definition is included in Table III.
‡ This term is used by ICHD-II, but the more generic approach of Table II is more clinically practical.
§ Chronic cluster headache patients may have more than 4 hours per day of headache. The inclusion of the syndrome here is to emphasise that, by and large, the attacks themselves last less than 4 hours.
¶ Short-lasting unilateral neuralgiform headache attacks with conjunctival injection and tearing.

and Lipton have evolved the concept (Table III), to indicate 15 days or more a month of migraine or probable migraine. This concept seems to make more biological sense as we see similarities, for example, in functional brain imaging in episodic migraine (Bahra et al. 2001; Afridi et al. 2005a,b) and chronic migraine (Matharu et al. 2004). It is a healthy field that carefully examines its systems or views. Headache research and treatment is a very healthy field.

GENETICS OF HEADACHE

For the moment, the genetics of headache is the genetics of migraine. It seems logical to suppose that all the primary headaches have a predisposition that is in some way activated by physiological and other life events, such as puberty. Clinically, cluster headache (Leone et al. 2001; El Amrani et al. 2002; Goadsby 2002), paroxysmal hemicrania (Cohen et al. 2006) and SUNCT (Gantenbein and Goadsby 2005) can all be seen to run in families. Overall, the concept of genetic predisposition seems a good way to understand primary headache.

For migraine, the description of missense mutations in the $Ca_V2.1$ subunit of the P/Q voltage-gated Ca^{2+} channel gene (Ertel et al. 2000) on chromosome 19 in families with familial hemiplegic migraine (FHM, Ophoff et al. 1996) was a milestone in the field (Ferrari et al. 2003). This effort was further boosted by the description of mutations in *ATP1A2*, the gene that encodes the α_2 subunit of the Na^+/K^+ pump (De Fusco et al. 2003), and by the most recent description of mutations in the neuronal voltage-gated sodium channel *SCN1A* (Dichgans et al. 2005). Both types of mutation seem causal in FHM. In some families with more routine forms of migraine, the headache can be linked to chromosome 19 (May et al. 1995; Nyholt et al. 1998b; Jones et al. 2001), and in some it can be linked to the X chromosome (Nyholt et al. 1998a). Migraine is part of the phenotype of mitochondrial cytopathies (DiMauro and Schon 2004). However, the

Table II
Differential diagnosis of new daily persistent headache

Primary (Phenotype)	Secondary (Cause)
Migrainous-type Featureless (no sensory sensitivity*)	Subarachnoid hemorrhage Low cerebrospinal fluid (CSF) volume headache Raised CSF pressure headache Post-traumatic headache† Chronic meningitis

* No sensitivity to light, sound, smells, or head movement; no throbbing component to the headache.
† Indicates trauma in the broad sense of insult to cranial structures, such as blunt trauma or postinfective triggers.

Table III
Transformed migraine

A)	Headache frequency of at least 15 days/month for 3 months
B)	Average headache duration of at least 4 hours/day (if untreated)
C)	Headache fulfilling IHS criteria for 1.1 *Migraine without aura*, 1.2 *Migraine with aura*, or 1.6 *Probable migraine*, on at least 50% of the headache days
D)	Does not meet criteria for IHS chronic tension-type headache (2.3), hypnic headache (4.5), hemicrania continua (4.7), or new daily persistent headache (4.8)
E)	Is not attributed to another disorder

Source: Modified International Headache Society (IHS) criteria from Silberstein et al. (1996).
Notes: Headache may fulfil any combination of 1.1, 1.2, and 1.6 on 50% or more of total headache days per month. It is important to detect patients with medication overuse (use of an acute attack treatment for more than 10 days per month) because this problem needs to be addressed if treatment with a preventive agent is to be successful.

genotype-phenotype correlations, even in FHM, remain disappointing (Ducros et al. 2001). There will clearly come a point when the known syndromes can be checked by DNA analysis of apparently affected patients. Ultimately, this approach may even guide therapy.

PATHOPHYSIOLOGY OF HEADACHE

Classical neurology, as promulgated by Gowers (1888), sought to provide anatomical answers to clinical questions. In many ways, Sherrington changed this point of view by seeking a physiological approach. The anatomical approach has been very successful, but the problems of primary headache will need a *physiological approach to clinical neurology* (Lance and McLeod 1981). To some extent, human functional imaging begins to offer physiological insights into headache pathophysiology. In the 1960s and 1970s migraine was considered a vascular phenomenon, and is still often referred to incorrectly as a *vascular headache*. Wolff (1948) summarized in his classical book the referral patterns of intracranial pain-producing structures, taking a view that migraine aura was due to vasoconstriction and the subsequent headache due to a reactive vasodilatation. Olesen and colleagues (1981) debunked this link. The spreading depression theory (Lauritzen 1994) points out that the flow changes follow metabolic demand and introduces the concept of *vasoneuronal coupling*. Considering features of the attack, such as nausea, photophobia, and phonophobia, which do not occur in all cases, or of the premonitory phase, such as yawning or diuresis (Giffin et al. 2003), the vascular hypothesis seems unattractive. Looking at the totality of the attack, one might suggest that the brain, and perhaps the brainstem or diencephalon, are likely to be the sites of the disturbance or physiological lesion (Goadsby et al. 1991) (Fig. 1).

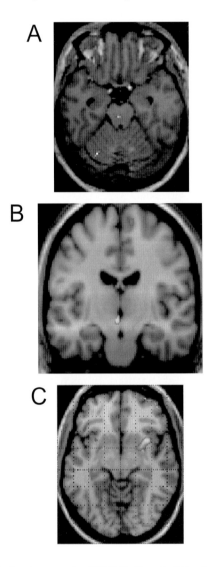

Fig. 1. Positron emission tomography (PET) findings in (A) migraine (Bahra et al. 2001), (B) cluster headache (May et al. 1998a), and (C) experimental head pain (May et al. 1998b). Activation of rostral brainstem structures in migraine and of posterior hypothalamic gray matter in cluster headache seems relatively specific for the syndromes, as neither are seen in experimental ophthalmic division head pain. The findings support the view that primary neurovascular headaches, migraine and cluster headache, are fundamentally disorders of the nervous system.

BRAIN IMAGING AND MIGRAINE

Positron emission tomography (PET) scanning in acute migraine has demonstrated activations in the rostral brainstem that persist after successful treatment of the attack but are not present interictally (Weiller et al. 1995). These changes are not seen in secondary headache, such as experimentally induced ophthalmic division pain (May et al. 1998b) or headache associated with nitroglycerin administration (Iversen et al. 1989; Afridi et al. 2005b). Indeed, these changes are not seen in other headache syndromes in which pain is also a primary symptom, such as cluster headache (May et al. 1998a), paroxysmal hemicrania (Matharu et al. 2006), or SUNCT (May et al. 1999a; Cohen et al. 2004). We observed a patient experiencing a bout of cluster headache who had a phenotypic migraine in the PET scanner and had brainstem changes consistent with migraine and not with cluster headache (Bahra et al. 2001). According to the findings from imaging of either spontaneous attacks (Afridi et al. 2005a) or nitroglycerin-triggered attacks (Afridi et al. 2005b), the dorsal rostral pons seems a crucial area activated consistently in migraine. In chronic migraine, defined as migraine without aura on 15 days or more a month for more than 6 months (Headache Classification Committee of the International Headache Society 2004), the same area of the dorsolateral pons is activated on PET (Matharu et al. 2004), suggesting that infrequent and frequent migraine are the same problem. Blood-oxygen-level-dependent (BOLD) contrast functional magnetic resonance imaging holds the promise of studying single patients and determining the site of abnormal activation (May et al. 1999a). Moreover, magnetic resonance angiography has allowed the demonstration that blood flow changes seen in migraine (Bahra et al. 2001) and cluster headache (May et al. 1998a) are simply a result of ophthalmic division pain (May et al. 1999b, 2001), rather than a cause of the syndrome.

Another recent finding with neuroimaging that further supports the importance of the brainstem, particularly the dorsolateral pons, in migraine is the demonstration that the changes lateralize with the attack. Studies of attacks of typical migraine triggered by nitroglycerin have shown that patients with left-sided attacks have left-sided brain activation and patients with right-sided attacks have right-sided activation, while patients with bilateral pain have bilateral activation (Afridi et al. 2005b). These data suggest that the dorsolateral pons is pivotal in the phenotypic expression of migraine as a lateralized syndrome. These changes persist after resolution of the pain with a triptan, are not present interictally, and were not seen in a control group scanned with the same design but in whom migraine did not develop. Understanding the candidate areas in the pons, such as the locus ceruleus—the major noradrenergic nucleus of the brain (Amaral and Sinnamon 1977)—may provide insights into the disorder and offer directions for preventive management.

HEADACHE PAIN AND CENTRAL SENSITIZATION

Central sensitization (Woolf 1983) as a neurophysiological explanation for allodynia, and thus for many aspects of chronic pain, is not a topic limited to headache (Woolf and Salter 2000). The issue has recently been widely addressed in the headache field because allodynia is a common feature of migraine (Selby and Lance 1960) and indeed of each of the trigeminal autonomic cephalalgias (Lance and Goadsby 2005). Allodynia in headache has been suggested to predict the outcome from acute treatment (Burstein et al. 2004). What has been done in the headache field in this area? A more comprehensive account is already available (Goadsby 2005b), and here I will limit the discussion to the central issue: is allodynia in primary headache due to classical nociceptive input, or is it more dependent on dysfunction of brain modulation of nociception?

Allodynia and the trigeminocervical complex. Studies employing a model of trigeminovascular nociceptive activation by application of an inflammatory "soup" containing bradykinin, serotonin, and substance P have been used to study mechanisms of sensitization in the trigeminal nucleus caudalis (Burstein et al. 1998). The sensitization thus produced is robust and difficult to terminate after 30 minutes or so, but it can be prevented with early use of triptans (Burstein and Jakubowski 2004). Studies have shown that triptans (Kaube et al. 1993a; Cumberbatch et al. 1997) and ergot derivatives, such as dihydroergotamine (Hoskin et al. 1996) and ergometrine (Lambert et al. 1992; Storer and Goadsby 1997), can inhibit second-order neuronal traffic in the trigeminocervical complex. Similarly, triptans disrupt second-order communication after a dural inflammatory stimulus (Levy et al. 2004). Interestingly, dihydroergotamine (Pozo-Rosich and Oshinsky 2005) and the mixed cyclooxygenase 1 and 2 inhibitor ketorolac can reverse the sensitization process associated with dural inflammation (Jakubowski et al. 2005), while sumatriptan alone cannot (Burstein and Jakubowski 2004). Both ketorolac and acetylsalicylic acid inhibit trigeminocervical nociceptive afferents by a mechanism that is naloxone-independent (Kaube et al. 1993b). While it seems clear that treatments of acute attacks may work at the level of the trigeminocervical complex, would that be a sufficient explanation for their ability to terminate all aspects of the migraine attack, and is there evidence that they might work elsewhere in the brain?

Allodynia as a disinhibitory phenomenon. It is well established that dura-sensitive neurons in the trigeminal nucleus are subject to modulation from various levels of the central nervous system. One plausible explanation for sensitization in migraine would be dysfunction of known subcortical trigeminal modulatory nuclei, constituting disinhibitory sensitization rather than sensitization due to abnormal afferent traffic (Goadsby 2003). Most prominent among these inhibitory systems are projections from brainstem structures, such as the periaqueductal gray (PAG), nucleus raphe magnus, and rostroventral medulla, that have a profound antinociceptive effect on these neurons (Behbehani 1995). However, other structures such as the hypothalamus (Benjamin et al. 2004), thalamus (Matharu et al. 2004), and cortical regions also seem to be involved. Recent findings emphasize the role of the ventrolateral division of the PAG (vlPAG) in trigeminal nociception because stimulation of the vlPAG modulates dural nociception and receives input from trigeminovascular afferent fibers (Keay and Bandler 1998; Knight et al. 2002; Bartsch et al. 2004a). We recently described a model of PAG-mediated dural nociception and facilitation of dural nociceptive input after local blockade of P/Q-type voltage-gated calcium channels in the vlPAG (Knight et al. 2002). Missense mutations of these channels seem to be involved in some subforms of migraine (Ferrari et al. 2003). The role of the PAG is also further corroborated by the observation that serotonin 5-HT$_{1B/1D}$ receptor activation to naratriptan injection in the midbrain PAG matter evokes a selective antinociceptive effect of descending pain-modulatory projections on dural nociception (Bartsch et al. 2004a). The involvement of the PAG in migraine finds its correlate in functional imaging studies in patients with spontaneous attacks of migraine without aura, which point to a specific role of the PAG in migraine pathophysiology (Weiller et al. 1995).

Dura-sensitive neurons in the trigeminal nucleus are also subject to a modulation of hypothalamic projections. Recent work has shown that these neurons can be inhibited or facilitated depending on the type of modulation evoked (Bartsch et al. 2004b). These electrophysiological findings may link clinical observations of hypothalamic involvement in primary headache syndromes, such as migraine (Peres et al. 2001) and cluster headache (Goadsby 2002), with the pain phenotypes in these syndromes (Bartsch et al. 2004b). Such findings support the view that the regulation of autonomic and neuroendocrine functions and of nociceptive processing are closely coupled in the hypothalamus.

Taking the experimental, brain-imaging, and clinical evidence together, it seems a more parsimonious argument to suppose that migraine is fundamentally a brain dysmodulatory problem. It is thus entirely plausible that allodynia is due to disinhibition of trigeminal pain processing, and not a result of afferent overactivity as such. Understanding of these basic questions will have great impact on developments such as those in preventive therapy.

MIGRAINE: WHAT NEW TREATMENTS CAN WE EXPECT?

Triptans, serotonin 5-HT$_{1B/1D}$-receptor agonists, served as foot soldiers for the advances in migraine during the latter part of the 20th century. Many migraine sufferers were liberated in a way that they had not anticipated, clinical trial guidelines were refined and revised, and clinical studies became well organized and more uniform. After sumatriptan came zolmitriptan, naratriptan, rizatriptan, almotriptan, eletriptan, and frovatriptan (Goadsby 2000), with donitriptan (John et al. 2000) the latest to have finished preclinical development. Ergotamine, the mainstay of specific acute treatment for most of the 20th century, after its initial description in the 19th century, now has few indications in which it is the treatment of choice (Tfelt-Hansen et al. 2000). It is clear what patients want—rapid, complete, and consistent pain relief—but it has not been established how they make preference decisions amongst available treatments (Cutrer et al. 2004; Dodick et al. 2004; Goadsby et al. 2004). What is established is that most patients do have preferences for individual triptans when asked (Cutrer et al. 2004). I will cover here some of the key clinical issues for new treatments. A more complete account of treatments closer to clinical use is available (Goadsby 2005c), as is an account of more speculative possibilities that as yet only have a good basic science basis (Goadsby 2005a).

NEW TREATMENTS AND UNMET NEEDS

Of the unmet needs, three come readily to mind. First, there is a considerable need for development of preventive medications. On average, two-thirds of patients will have a 50% reduction in headache frequency with most preventives. They can then choose between the potential for sleepiness, exercise intolerance, erectile dysfunction, nightmares, dry mouth, weight gain, tremor, hair loss, or the potential for fetal deformities as possible adverse effects. It is an important statement about the level of disability migraineurs experience that they do make such choices. The recent reporting of positive clinical trials with topiramate (Brandes et al. 2004; Diener et al. 2004; Silberstein et al. 2004) establishes its utility in migraine and, more importantly, has provided good field testing of methods for studies that will now follow. Second, treatments for nonvascular acute attacks are required for those patients who cannot be given triptans and ergot derivatives. A potent specific calcitonin gene-related peptide antagonist was effective in a clinical trial as compared to placebo in acute migraine (Olesen et al. 2004). This study both answers the pressing pathophysiological issue of the primacy of the nerves and vessels and provides the beginning of a crucial advance in therapy. It is useful to observe that the advance was predicted by laboratory work more than a decade ago (Goadsby et al. 1988, 1990). The translation of basic experimental work into clinical practice illustrates the importance of basic neurobiology to advancing clinical practice. It is now clear that vasoconstriction is not necessary for aborting acute migraine. Indeed, a recent demonstration that sildenafil, a phosphodiesterase inhibitor, will induce migraine without changes in cerebral vessel diameter

(Kruuse et al. 2003) provides perhaps the last nail in the coffin of the vascular theory. From a therapeutic viewpoint, the development of non-vasoconstrictor treatments of migraine offers an important development in terms of safety that will be welcomed by clinicians and patients alike.

CONCLUSION

It is no exaggeration to say that the future of headache is bright. A better classification, new understanding of the basic cause in terms of genetics, insights into the pathophysiology from functional brain imaging, detailed analysis of common symptoms such as allodynia, and improved management in terms of novel therapies is very promising. Headache is the most common of human maladies, which is its greatest limitation. Familiarity is a horrible limitation to interrogation of a subject, and so it is with headache. For the pain physician headache is a necessity, for our patients it is a major cause of disability, and for our community it is a major burden of cost. Advances in headache can alleviate both the disability and the burden.

ACKNOWLEDGMENTS

The work of the author has been supported by the Wellcome Trust.

REFERENCES

Ad Hoc Committee on Classification of Headache of the NIH. Classification of headache. *JAMA* 1962; 179:717–718.

Afridi S, Giffin NJ, Kaube H, et al. A PET study in spontaneous migraine. *Arch Neurol* 2005a; 62:1270–1275.

Afridi S, Matharu MS, Lee L, et al. A PET study exploring the laterality of brainstem activation in migraine using glyceryl trinitrate. *Brain* 2005b; 128:932–939.

Amaral DG, Sinnamon HM. The locus coeruleus: neurobiology of a central noradrenergic nucleus. *Prog Neurobiol* 1977; 9:147–196.

Bahra A, Matharu MS, Büchel C, Frackowiak RSJ, Goadsby PJ. Brainstem activation specific to migraine headache. *Lancet* 2001; 357:1016–1017.

Bartsch T, Knight YE, Goadsby PJ. Activation of 5-HT$_{1B/1D}$ receptors in the periaqueductal grey inhibits meningeal nociception. *Ann Neurol* 2004a; 56:371–381.

Bartsch T, Levy MJ, Knight YE, Goadsby PJ. Differential modulation of nociceptive dural input to [hypocretin] Orexin A and B receptor activation in the posterior hypothalamic area. *Pain* 2004b; 109:367–378.

Behbehani MM. Functional characteristics of the midbrain periaqueductal gray. *Prog Neurobiol* 1995; 46:575–605.

Benjamin L, Levy MJ, Lasalandra MP, et al. Hypothalamic activation after stimulation of the superior sagittal sinus in the cat: a Fos study. *Neurobiol Dis* 2004; 16:500–505.

Brandes JL, Saper JR, Diamond M, et al. Topiramate for migraine prevention: a randomized controlled trial. *JAMA* 2004; 291:965–973.

Burstein R, Jakubowski M. Analgesic triptan action in an animal model of intracranial pain: a race against the development of central sensitisation. *Ann Neurol* 2004; 55:27–36.

Burstein R, Yamamura H, Malick A, Strassman AM. Chemical stimulation of the intracranial dura induces enhanced responses to facial stimulation in brain stem trigeminal neurons. *J Neurophysiol* 1998; 79:964–982.

Burstein R, Collins B, Jakubowski M. Defeating migraine pain with triptans: a race against the development of cutaneous allodynia. *Ann Neurol* 2004; 55:19–26.

Carson AJ, Ringbauer B, MacKenzie L, Warlow C, Sharpe M. Neurological disease, emotional disorder, and disability: they are related: a study of 300 consecutive new referrals to a neurology outpatient department. *J Neurol Neurosurg Psychiatry* 2000; 68:202–206.

Cohen AS, Matharu MS, Kalisch R, Friston K, Goadsby PJ. Functional MRI in SUNCT shows differential hypothalamic activation with increasing pain. *Cephalalgia* 2004; 24:1098–1099.

Cohen AS, Matharu MS, Goadsby PJ. Paroxysmal hemicrania in a family. *Cephalalgia* 2006; 26: in press.

Cumberbatch MJ, Hill RG, Hargreaves RJ. Rizatriptan has central antinociceptive effects against durally evoked responses. *Eur J Pharmacol* 1997; 328:37–40.

Cutrer FM, Goadsby PJ, Ferrari MD, et al. Priorities for triptan treatment attributes and the implications for selecting an oral triptan for acute migraine: a study of US primary care physicians (the TRIPSTAR Project). *Clin Ther* 2004; 26:1533–1545.

De Fusco M, Marconi R, Silvestri L, et al. Haploinsufficiency of *ATP1A2* encoding the Na^+/K^+ pump α_2 subunit associated with familial hemiplegic migraine type 2. *Nat Genet* 2003; 33:192–196.

Dichgans M, Freilinger T, Eckstein G, et al. Mutation in the neuronal voltage-gated sodium channel *SCN1A* causes familial hemiplegic migraine. *Lancet* 2005; 366:371–377.

Diener HC, Tfelt-Hansen P, Dahlof C, et al. Topiramate in migraine prophylaxis—results from a placebo-controlled trial with propranolol as an active control. *J Neurol* 2004; 251:943–950.

DiMauro S, Schon EA. Mitochondrial respiratory-chain diseases. *N Engl J Med* 2004; 348:2556–2668.

Dodick DW, Mosek AC, Campbell JK. The hypnic ("alarm clock") headache syndrome. *Cephalalgia* 1998; 18:152–156.

Dodick DW, Brown RD, Britton JW, Huston J. Nonaneurysmal thunderclap headache with diffuse, multifocal, segmental, and reversible vasospasm. *Cephalalgia* 1999; 19:118–123.

Dodick DW, Lipton RB, Ferrari MD, et al. Prioritizing treatment attributes and their impact on selecting an oral triptan: results from the TRIPSTAR project. *Curr Pain Headache Rep* 2004; 8:435–442.

Ducros A, Denier C, Joutel A, et al. The clinical spectrum of familial hemiplegic migraine associated with mutations in a neuronal calcium channel. *N Engl J Med* 2001; 345:17–24.

El Amrani M, Ducros A, Boulan P, et al. Familial cluster headache: a series of 186 index patients. *Headache* 2002; 42:974–977.

Ertel EA, Campbell KP, Harpold MM, et al. Nomenclature of voltage-gated calcium channels. *Neuron* 2000; 25:533–535.

Ferrari MD, Haan J, Palotie A. Genetics of migraine. In: Olesen J, Tfelt-Hansen P, Welch KMA (Ed). *The Headaches*. Philadelphia: Lippincott Williams & Wilkins, 2003.

Gantenbein A, Goadsby PJ. Familial SUNCT. *Cephalalgia* 2005; 25:457–459.

Giffin NJ, Ruggiero L, Lipton RB, et al. Premonitory symptoms in migraine: an electronic diary study. *Neurology* 2003; 60:935–940.

Goadsby PJ. The pharmacology of headache. *Prog Neurobiol* 2000; 62:509–525.

Goadsby PJ. Pathophysiology of cluster headache: a trigeminal autonomic cephalgia. *Lancet Neurol* 2002; 1:37–43.

Goadsby PJ. Migraine pathophysiology: the brainstem governs the cortex. *Cephalalgia* 2003; 23:565–566.

Goadsby PJ. Can we develop neurally-acting drugs for the treatment of migraine? *Nat Rev Drug Discov* 2005a; 4:741–750.

Goadsby PJ. Migraine, allodynia, sensitisation and all of that. *Eur Neurol* 2005b; 53:10–16.

Goadsby PJ. New targets in the acute treatment of headache. *Curr Opin Neurol* 2005c; 18:283–288.

Goadsby PJ. Trigeminal autonomic cephalalgias (TACs): another fancy term or a constructive change to the International Headache Classification? *J Neurol Neurosurg Psychiatry* 2005d; 76:301–305.

Goadsby PJ. Trigeminal autonomic cephalalgias. Pathophysiology and classification. *Rev Neurol (Paris)* 2005e; 161:692–695.

Goadsby PJ, Boes CJ. New daily persistent headache. *J Neurol Neurosurg Psychiatry* 2002; 72: ii6–ii9.

Goadsby PJ, Lipton RB. A review of paroxysmal hemicranias, SUNCT syndrome and other short-lasting headaches with autonomic features, including new cases. *Brain* 1997; 120:193–209.

Goadsby PJ, Edvinsson L, Ekman R. Release of vasoactive peptides in the extracerebral circulation of man and the cat during activation of the trigeminovascular system. *Ann Neurol* 1988; 23:193–196.

Goadsby PJ, Edvinsson L, Ekman R. Vasoactive peptide release in the extracerebral circulation of humans during migraine headache. *Ann Neurol* 1990; 28:183–187.

Goadsby PJ, Zagami AS, Lambert GA. Neural processing of craniovascular pain: a synthesis of the central structures involved in migraine. *Headache* 1991; 31:365–371.

Goadsby PJ, Dodick D, Ferrari M, D., McCrory D, Williams P. TRIPSTAR. Prioritizing triptan treatment attributes in migraine management. *Acta Neurol Scand* 2004; 110:137–143.

Gowers WR. *A Manual of Diseases of the Nervous System.* Philadelphia: P. Blakiston, Son & Co, 1888.

Headache Classification Committee of the International Headache Society. Classification and diagnostic criteria for headache disorders, cranial neuralgias and facial pain. *Cephalalgia* 1988; 8:1–96.

Headache Classification Committee of the International Headache Society. The international classification of headache disorders (second edition). *Cephalalgia* 2004; 24:1–160.

Hoskin KL, Kaube H, Goadsby PJ. Central activation of the trigeminovascular pathway in the cat is inhibited by dihydroergotamine. A c-Fos and electrophysiology study. *Brain* 1996; 119:249–256.

Iversen HK, Olesen J, Tfelt-Hansen P. Intravenous nitroglycerin as an experimental headache model. Basic characteristics. *Pain* 1989; 38:17–24.

Jakubowski M, Levy D, Goor-Aryeh I, et al. Terminating migraine with allodynia and ongoing central sensitization using parenteral administration of COX1/COX2 inhibitors. *Headache* 2005; 45:850–861.

John GW, Perez M, Pawels PJ, et al. Donitriptan, a unique high efficacy 5-HT$_{1B/1D}$ agonist: key features and acute antimigraine potential. *CNS Drug Rev* 2000; 6:278–289.

Jones KW, Ehm MG, Pericak-Vance MA, et al. Migraine with aura susceptibility locus on chromosome 19p13 is distinct from the familial hemiplegic migraine locus. *Genomics* 2001; 78:150–154.

Kaube H, Hoskin KL, Goadsby PJ. Inhibition by sumatriptan of central trigeminal neurones only after blood-brain barrier disruption. *Br J Pharmacol* 1993a; 109:788–792.

Kaube H, Hoskin KL, Goadsby PJ. Intravenous acetylsalicylic acid inhibits central trigeminal neurons in the dorsal horn of the upper cervical spinal cord in the cat. *Headache* 1993b; 33:541–550.

Keay KA, Bandler R. Vascular head pain selectively activates ventrolateral periaqueductal gray in the cat. *Neurosci Lett* 1998; 245:58–60.

Knight YE, Bartsch T, Kaube H, Goadsby PJ. P/Q-type calcium channel blockade in the PAG facilitates trigeminal nociception: a functional genetic link for migraine? *J Neurosci* 2002; 22:1–6.

Kruuse C, Thomsen LL, Birk S, Olesen J. Migraine can be induced by sildenafil without changes in middle cerebral artery diameter. *Brain* 2003; 126:241–247.

Lambert GA, Lowy AJ, Boers P, Angus-Leppan H, Zagami A. The spinal cord processing of input from the superior sagittal sinus: pathway and modulation by ergot alkaloids. *Brain Res* 1992; 597:321–330.

Lance JW, Goadsby PJ. *Mechanism and Management of Headache*. New York: Elsevier, 2005.

Lance JW, McLeod JG. *A Physiological Approach to Clinical Neurology*. Sydney: Butterworths, 1981.

Lauritzen M. Pathophysiology of the migraine aura. The spreading depression theory. *Brain* 1994; 117:199–210.

Leone M, Russell MB, Rigamonti A, et al. Increased familial risk of cluster headache. *Neurology* 2001; 56:1233–1236.

Levy D, Jakubowski M, Burstein R. Disruption of communication between peripheral and central trigeminovascular neurons mediates the antimigraine action of 5HT$_{1B/1D}$ receptor agonists. *Proc Natl Acad Sci USA* 2004; 101:4274–4279.

Manzoni GC, Granella F, Sandrini G, et al. Classification of chronic daily headache by International Headache Society criteria: limits and new proposals. *Cephalalgia* 1995; 15:37–43.

Matharu MS, Boes CJ, Goadsby PJ. Management of trigeminal autonomic cephalalgias and hemicrania continua. *Drugs* 2003; 63:1637–1677.

Matharu MS, Bartsch T, Ward N, et al. Central neuromodulation in chronic migraine patients with suboccipital stimulators: a PET study. *Brain* 2004; 127:220–230.

Matharu MS, Cohen AS, Frackowiak RSJ, Goadsby PJ. Posterior hypothalamic activation in paroxysmal hemicrania using PET. *Ann Neurol* 2006; 54:535–545.

May A, Goadsby PJ. The trigeminovascular system in humans: pathophysiological implications for primary headache syndromes of the neural influences on the cerebral circulation. *J Cereb Blood Flow Metab* 1999; 19:115–127.

May A, Ophoff RA, Terwindt GM, et al. Familial hemiplegic migraine locus on chromosome 19p13 is involved in common forms of migraine with and without aura. *Human Genetics* 1995; 96:604–608.

May A, Bahra A, Büchel C, Frackowiak RSJ, Goadsby PJ. Hypothalamic activation in cluster headache attacks. *Lancet* 1998a; 352:275–278.

May A, Kaube H, Büchel C, et al. Experimental cranial pain elicited by capsaicin: a PET study. *Pain* 1998b; 74:61–66.

May A, Bahra A, Büchel C, Turner R, Goadsby PJ. Functional MRI in spontaneous attacks of SUNCT: short-lasting neuralgiform headache with conjunctival injection and tearing. *Ann Neurol* 1999a; 46:791–793.

May A, Büchel C, Turner R, Frackowiak RSJ, Goadsby PJ. Neurovascular dilatation of intracranial vessels in experimental headache. *Cephalalgia* 1999b; 19:464–465.

May A, Büchel C, Turner R, Goadsby PJ. MR-angiography in facial and other pain: neurovascular mechanisms of trigeminal sensation. *J Cereb Blood Flow Metab* 2001; 21:1171–1176.

Menken M, Munsat TL, Toole JF. The global burden of disease study—implications for neurology. *Arch Neurol* 2000; 57:418–420.

Nyholt DR, Dawkins JL, Brimage PJ, et al. Evidence for an X-linked genetic component in familial typical migraine. *Hum Mol Genet* 1998a; 7:459–463.

Nyholt DR, Lea RA, Goadsby PJ, Brimage PJ, Griffiths LR. Familial typical migraine: linkage to chromosome 19p13 and evidence for genetic heterogeneity. *Neurology* 1998b; 50:1428–1432.

Olesen J, Rasmussen BK. The International Headache Society classification of chronic daily or near daily headaches: a critique of the criticism. *Cephalalgia* 1996; 16:407–411.

Olesen J, Larsen B, Lauritzen M. Focal hyperemia followed by spreading oligemia and impaired activation of rCBF in classic migraine. *Ann Neurol* 1981; 9:344–352.

Olesen J, Diener H-C, Husstedt I-W, et al. Calcitonin gene-related peptide (CGRP) receptor antagonist BIBN4096BS is effective in the treatment of migraine attacks. *N Engl J Med* 2004; 350:1104–1110.

Olesen J, Tfelt-Hansen P, Ramadan N, Goadsby PJ, Welch KMA. *The Headaches.* Philadelphia: Lippincott, Williams & Wilkins, 2005.

Ophoff RA, Terwindt GM, Vergouwe MN, et al. Familial hemiplegic migraine and episodic ataxia type-2 are caused by mutations in the Ca^{2+} channel gene *CACNL1A4. Cell* 1996; 87:543–552.

Peres MF, Sanchez del Rio M, Seabra S, et al. Hypothalamic involvement in chronic migraine. *J Neurol Neurosurg Psychiatry* 2001; 71:747–751.

Pozo-Rosich P, Oshinsky M. Effect of dihydroergotamine (DHE) on central sensitisation of neurons in the trigeminal nucleus caudalis. *Neurology* 2005; 64:A151.

Raieli V, Raimondo D, Gangitano M, et al. The IHS classification criteria for migraine headaches in adolescents need minor modifications. *Headache* 1996; 36:362–366.

Raskin NH. The hypnic headache syndrome. *Headache* 1988; 28:534–536.

Sanin LC, Mathew NT, Bellmeyer LR, Ali S. The International Headache Society (IHS) headache classification as applied to a headache clinic population. *Cephalalgia* 1994; 14:443–436.

Selby G, Lance JW. Observations on 500 cases of migraine and allied vascular headache. *J Neurol Neurosurg Psychiatry* 1960; 23:23–32.

Silberstein SD, Lipton RB, Sliwinski M. Classification of daily and near-daily headaches: a field study of revised IHS criteria. *Neurology* 1996; 47:871–875.

Silberstein SD, Neto W, Schmitt J, Jacobs D. Topiramate in migraine prevention: results of a large controlled trial. *Arch Neurol* 2004; 61:490–495.

Sjaastad O, Spierings EL. Hemicrania continua: another headache absolutely responsive to indomethacin. *Cephalalgia* 1984; 4:65–70.

Storer RJ, Goadsby PJ. Microiontophoretic application of serotonin $(5HT)_{1B/1D}$ agonists inhibits trigeminal cell firing in the cat. *Brain* 1997; 120:2171–2177.

Tfelt-Hansen P, Saxena PR, Dahlof C, et al. Ergotamine in the acute treatment of migraine—a review and European consensus. *Brain* 2000; 123:9–18.

Weiller C, May A, Limmroth V, et al. Brain stem activation in spontaneous human migraine attacks. *Nat Med* 1995; 1:658–660.

Welch KMA, Goadsby PJ. Chronic daily headache: nosology and pathophysiology. *Curr Opin Neurol* 2002; 15:287–295.

Woolf CJ. Evidence for a central component of post-injury pain hypersensitivity. *Nature* 1983; 306:686–688.

Woolf CJ, Salter MW. Neuronal plasticity: increasing the gain in pain. *Science* 2000; 288:1765–1769.

Wolff HG. *Headache and Other Head Pain.* New York: Oxford University Press, 1948.

Correspondence to: Professor Peter J. Goadsby, MD, PhD, Headache Group, Institute of Neurology, The National Hospital for Neurology and Neurosurgery, Queen Square, London WC1N 3BG, United Kingdom. Fax: 44-20-7813-0349; email: peterg@.ion.ucl.ac.uk.

Proceedings of the 11th World Congress on Pain,
edited by Herta Flor, Eija Kalso, and Jonathan O.
Dostrovsky, IASP Press, Seattle, © 2006.

57

Cold Allodynia: From the Molecule to the Clinic

Gunnar Wasner,[a,b] Martin Koltzenburg,[c,d] Ellen Jorum,[e] Ralf Baron,[b] and Troels S. Jensen[f]

[a]Prince of Wales Medical Research Institute, University of New South Wales, Randwick, Sydney, New South Wales, Australia; [b]Division of Neurological Pain Research and Therapy, Department of Neurology, Christian-Albrechts-University, Kiel, Germany; [c]Neural Plasticity Unit, Institute of Child Health, University College London, United Kingdom; [d]National Hospital for Neurology and Neurosurgery, London, United Kingdom; [e]Department of Clinical Neurophysiology, Rikshospitalet University Hospital, Oslo University, Oslo, Norway; [f]Department of Neurology and Danish Pain Research Center, Aarhus University Hospital, Aarhus, Denmark

Neuropathic pains represent a heterogeneous group of pathological conditions resulting from compression of nerves by neoplasms or from traumatic, ischemic, immunological, or endocrinological damage to nervous tissue (Jensen et al. 2001). Despite their heterogeneity in etiology and anatomical location, neuropathic pains share certain characteristics (Jensen et al. 2001; Koltzenburg and Scadding 2001; Jensen and Baron 2003). These characteristics include pain in a neuroanatomical area with partial or complete sensory loss, stimulus-independent ongoing pain, stimulus-dependent evoked types of pain, hypersensitivity, aftersensations, and abnormal summation.

One symptom encountered in neuropathic pain that has attracted particular interest is cold allodynia. Recent findings have enhanced our understanding of the processing of cold under normal conditions and to some extent under pathological conditions. This chapter will highlight biological mechanisms of cold perception, describe human models for cold pain, and discuss clinical aspects of cold allodynia in patients who have been exposed to excessive cold.

PHYSIOLOGICAL BASIS FOR COLD SENSATION

The conscious sensation of innocuous or noxious cold in humans is signaled by thin or unmyelinated sensory fibers. Compression block experiments have suggested that sensitivity to innocuous cold is signaled by Aδ fibers (Torebjörk and Hallin 1973; Mackenzie et al. 1975). Intriguingly, however, recent microneurographic recordings from distal peripheral nerves in humans have found that fibers responding to innocuous cold are conducting in the C-fiber range (Campero et al. 2001). This discrepancy may be explained by the fact that the susceptibility to compression or ischemia correlates with modality and not with axon diameter (Ziegler et al. 1999).

Psychophysical studies have recognized at least three types of cold sensation—cool sensations, painful cold, and freezing pain. Detection of cool sensations is usually sensitive to within 0.5–1.0°C in sensitive areas. The cold pain threshold is usually below 15–20°C but can vary depending on skin area, the rate of cooling, the size of the probe, and the manner in which subjects are instructed (Davis 1998; Harrison and Davis 1999). Some people recognize the burning component of cold pain, whereas others recognize the deep, aching aspects. Pain of freezing is a stinging type of pain that is qualitatively distinct from cool sensations and painful cold (Simone and Kajander 1997). Among the thin myelinated and unmyelinated fibers, three types of responses appear to correlate with these psychophysical responses. First, there are cold-sensitive receptors, which respond vigorously to small reductions of temperature and are often excited by menthol. They show a plateau or even a reduced response to cold temperatures in the noxious range. Second, many mechanosensitive nociceptors respond to cold stimuli in the noxious range. Up to 10% of nociceptive Aδ fibers and up to a third of C fibers in the rat or mouse will respond to noxious cold (Koltzenburg 2004). Units typically discharge vigorously at the onset of a cold stimulus and are rapidly inactivated when the temperature stimulus has passed its nadir. Third, the majority of nociceptive Aδ and C fibers respond to temperatures below freezing, a stimulus that typically evokes a sharp, stinging pain (Simone and Kajander 1996, 1997; Cain et al. 2001).

Consensus is lacking about the cellular and molecular mechanisms that underlie the excitation of different cold-sensitive sensory neurons. Ion channels and cold-sensitive members of the transient receptor potential (TRP) family of ion channels are currently recognized as the principle transducers of thermal stimuli in primary afferents (Clapham 2003; Patapoutian et al. 2003; Tominaga and Caterina 2004), and two are implicated in cold transduction. TRPM8 is expressed in approximately 10% of small-diameter sensory neurons, where it is thought to underlie sensitivity to small decreases in temperature and menthol (McKemy et al. 2002; Peier et al. 2002). Several studies have reported a sensitivity in the range of 8–28°C (Julius and McCleskey 2005). TRPA1 was originally described as a noxious cold-activated channel thought to be activated by temperatures in the range of 12–24°C (Story et al. 2003). However, others failed to find an appreciable cold sensitivity for the cloned rat TRPA1 channel and have therefore questioned its role in thermosensation (Jordt et al. 2004).

Besides TRPM8 and TRPA1, several other potassium and sodium ion channels have been implicated in cold transduction. It has been suggested that depolarization of neurons induced by a cold stimulus is caused by the inhibition of a potassium current (Reid and Flonta 2002; Viana et al. 2002). Furthermore, TREK1, a thermosensitive member of the two-pore-domain potassium channel subfamily, is inhibited by cold (Maingret et al. 2000) and is expressed in a third of cold-sensitive sensory neurons (Nealen et al. 2003). Finally, inward rectifier currents such as I_h and I_{KIR} could also play a role in the modulation of cold sensitivity (Thut et al. 2003). Cold temperatures activate or potentiate the responses of members of the family of degenerin/epithelial sodium channels, Deg/ENaC, which are present in dorsal root ganglia (Askwith et al. 2001).

HUMAN MODELS FOR COLD PAIN

The end of the 19th century, when Thunberg (1896) performed his amazing thermal grill experiment, marked the beginning of a long history of human models for cold pain. Modern imaging techniques (Craig 2002), in combination with quantitative sensory testing in patients suffering from cold allodynia, have contributed to our understanding of the underlying mechanisms and their impact on pathological pain conditions.

THE THERMAL GRILL ILLUSION

In 1896, Thunberg described how concurrent applications of spatially adjacent bands of innocuous warm and cool stimuli to the skin elicited a noxious sensation, described as a "cold burning pain sensation." In reference to the apparatus used in this experiment, which comprised interlaced 40°C warm and 20°C cold bars, this phenomenon is called the thermal-grill illusion. A similar painful sensation, familiar to many of us, can be induced by pouring warm water on cold feet. A psychophysical examination of healthy volunteers demonstrated that this illusion results in the sensation of pain, as well as an increased perception of heat and a decreased perception of cold. Recordings from spinothalamic tract neurons located within lamina I of the dorsal horn of animals have shown that so-called "cool" neurons discharged less during the illusion stimuli than they did with a pure cold stimulus (Craig and Bushnell 1994). On the other hand, the firing rate of nociceptive-specific, "heat-pinch-cold" neurons was the same for pure cold or illusion conditions and hence resulted in a shift in the relative amounts of excitation between the cold-sensitive and nociceptive populations. Based on these data, Craig and Bushnell hypothesized that the burning pain sensation caused by cold-sensitive nociceptors is normally masked centrally by activity in neurons encoding innocuous cold sensations. The thermal grill illusion can therefore be explained physiologically by an unmasking of the cold-evoked activity of polymodal nociceptive lamina I spinothalamic neurons (which are selectively activated by polymodal C nociceptors) due to a reduction in cold-evoked activity of thermosensitive lamina I spinothalamic neurons (which are selectively activated by peripheral cold-specific Aδ fibers) (Craig 2002). The origin of this reduced neuronal activity within the pathways for innocuous cold sensation is not clear. It might be due to spatial summation of the effects of the simultaneous warm stimuli (the warm bars of the thermal grill). However, an interaction between cold- and warm-specific afferents, perhaps via interneurons at the spinal level, cannot be excluded.

Functional imaging has shown that the thermal grill activates the anterior cingulate cortex, which is frequently excited by noxious stimuli, whereas its separate warm and cold components do not (Craig et al. 1996). This finding could reflect an imbalance between the activity of cold-specific and cold-nociceptive cells, resulting in differential excitation of the insular cortex and the medial and lateral aspects of the thalamus.

EFFECTS OF A-FIBER BLOCKADE ON COLD

The central interaction between signals arising from innocuous cold-conducting fibers and cold-activated nociceptive afferents has also been supported by differential nerve block experiments in healthy volunteers. The increased cold perception threshold induced by the selective block of cold-sensitive thermoreceptors, presumably thin myelinated fibers, was paralleled by a decreased cold pain threshold, resulting in the combined symptoms of cold hypoesthesia and cold hyperalgesia (Fruhstorfer 1984; Wahren et al. 1989; Yarnitsky and Ochoa 1990; Wasner et al. 2004). These results support the hypothesis that cold hyperalgesia is due to a change in the central decoding of afferent input related to removal of the inhibition of cold nociceptors normally exerted by concomitant activation of cold-specific A fibers.

TOPICAL MENTHOL APPLICATION

In addition to these central mechanisms, it seems possible that peripheral mechanisms may also have a role in cold hyperalgesia, as is the case for heat hyperalgesia, which is mediated by sensitized nociceptors (Meyer et al. 2005).

Recent investigations have identified a cold- and menthol-sensitive TRP channel (TRPM8) that is activated within the range of 8–28°C. This receptor is expressed in about 10% of all trigeminal and dorsal root ganglion neurons of rats, primarily within small-diameter cells (McKemy et al. 2002). As menthol is a natural ligand of TRPM8, we sought to determine whether menthol can be used to generate cold hyperalgesia in humans by activating and sensitizing nociceptive afferents.

The influence of menthol on pain and cold sensation, on perception evoked by mechanical and thermal stimuli, and on skin perfusion was investigated in volunteers in a double-blind, placebo-controlled, two-way crossover trial (Wasner et al. 2004). We demonstrated that high concentrations of menthol induced ongoing pain and cold sensations as well as punctate and cold hyperalgesia and led to an increase in cutaneous perfusion (at the site of and 3 mm away from the menthol application area) (Figs. 1 and 2). The sensitivity to other mechanosensory and thermal tests (touch, cold, and warm detection thresholds, and heat pain threshold) remained unchanged, and there was no dynamic or static hyperalgesia and no wind-up.

To investigate the underlying mechanisms of menthol-induced cold pain, its effects were tested during an A-fiber conduction blockade. The block itself induced an increase in cold-mediated pain consistent with the removal of the inhibition of C nociceptors, normally exerted by concomitant activation of A fibers. Under these conditions, menthol-induced cold sensation and punctate hyperalgesia were abolished. However, menthol induced spontaneous burning pain, with a trend toward higher ratings than without the block. Furthermore, the hyperalgesia to cold stimuli, which was already present during the A-fiber block, was significantly increased by menthol. These results led to the suggestion that menthol acts to sensitize cold-sensitive peripheral C nociceptors and to activate cold-specific Aδ fibers by mechanisms involving TRPM8. Punctate hyperalgesia has been suggested to be due to central sensitization based on ongoing activity in the sensitized cold-sensitive peripheral C nociceptors, but it might alternatively reflect a direct mechanical sensitization of nociceptors. Whether these cold-sensitive C nociceptors are vasoactive (as suggested by an increase in blood flow) is debatable, because vasoactivity has not been found by others who reproduced these experiments (Namer et al. 2005). In conclusion, topical menthol can be used as a model for cold pain in humans by sensitizing peripheral cold C nociceptors.

ARE HUMAN MODELS FOR COLD PAIN CLINICALLY RELEVANT?

Human models may contribute to our understanding of the cold pain that is found in central and peripheral neuropathic pain conditions, either as ongoing "ice-like" pain or as cold-induced hyperalgesia (Boivie et al. 1989; Craig et al. 1996; Bowsher 1999; Bowsher and Haggett 2005). Cold allodynia is a frequent finding in neuropathic pain of peripheral and central origin. For example, in a study by Andersen et al. (1995), cold allodynia or cold dysesthesia was present in 88% of patients with post-stroke pain, but in only 3% of stroke patients with sensory abnormalities but without pain. The mechanisms of pain in this central condition are not clear, but one possibility is that a lesion of innocuous cold-specific pathways projecting to the lateral thalamus plays a role. Such a lesion may result in unmasking noxious cold-induced activation of the anterior cingulate cortex associated with the burning component of cold pain, consistent

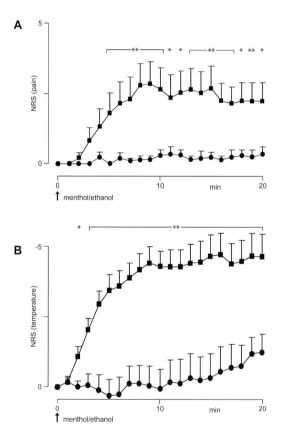

Fig. 1. Group data (10 subjects) showing menthol-induced (black squares) and ethanol-induced (black circles) pain (A) and thermal (B) sensations in a double-blind, two-way cross-over procedure. A gauze pad soaked with menthol dissolved in ethanol placed on the volar forearm for 20 minutes induced a significant sensation of burning pain (A) and coldness (B) in comparison with vehicle (ethanol) applied in exactly the same way. Pain was rated on a numerical rating scale (NRS; A: 0–10; B: minus 10 to plus 10), mean and standard error; * $P < 0.05$, ** $P < 0.01$. Adapted from Wasner et al. (2004), with permission.

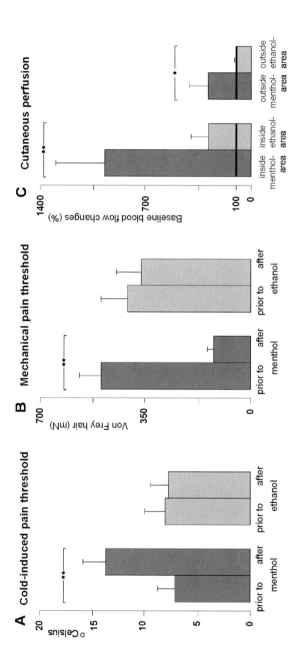

Fig. 2. Effects of menthol (dark columns) and ethanol (light columns) on cold-induced pain thresholds (A), mechanical pain thresholds (B), and on cutaneous perfusion (C) of the volar forearm in 10 subjects. Mean values and standard error prior to and after applying gauze pads soaked with menthol and ethanol, respectively, were compared. Menthol, but not ethanol, induced cold hyperalgesia (A) and punctate hyperalgesia (B) by significantly decreasing the cold pain threshold measured by thermotesting (degrees Celsius) and the mechanical pain threshold tested with von Frey hairs (force measured in milliNewtons). Furthermore, menthol induced a significant cutaneous vasodilatation measured by laser Doppler flowmetry both at the site and outside the area of application compared with ethanol (C). For calculation of relative blood flow changes (%), the baseline blood flow prior to application of the gauze pad was set at 100% (marked by thick lines within the columns). * $P < 0.05$, ** $P < 0.01$. Adapted from Wasner et al. (2004), with permission.

with the essence of the original, prescient conjecture of Head and Holmes (Head and Holmes 1911; Craig et al. 1996).

Paradoxical burning sensations produced by cold stimuli have also been found in patients with peripheral neuropathic pain (Bowsher and Haggett 2005). Given the models above, two underlying mechanisms are possible. On the one hand, a preferential lesion of the peripheral cold-specific $A\delta$-fiber afferents might cause cold pain due to a lack of central inhibition of C nociceptors. In these patients, cold hyperalgesia is combined with cold hypoesthesia due to A-fiber lesions (Ochoa and Yarnitsky 1994). On the other hand, cold pain in peripheral neuropathy might be due to pathological sensitization of cold-specific C nociceptors without lesions of cold-specific A fibers, as suggested by the menthol model. Indeed, the finding of cold hyperalgesia combined with normal cold perception threshold in 9% of 465 patients with different neuropathies suggests that such a mechanism of peripheral sensitization is involved (Verdugo and Ochoa 1992). Studies on neuropathic pain patients have provided evidence that cold hyperalgesia evoked by cold-sensitive nociceptors after central sensitization may be another mechanism (Torebjörk et al. 1995).

Cold allodynia is seen not only in patients with lesions of the peripheral or central nervous system, but also in patients with permanent sequelae after prolonged exposure to cold ambient temperatures (E. Jorum and P.K. Opstad, unpublished manuscript). The differences in the clinical expression of cold hypersensitivity in the two conditions suggest differences in the neurophysiological mechanisms involved. Whereas cold allodynia in neuropathic pain is characterized by a sudden, severe, often irradiating pain at threshold level, which prevents experimenters from attempting suprathreshold stimulation (Jorum et al. 2003), patients with cold injury have a highly pathological cold pain threshold but tolerate suprathreshold stimulation. In neuropathic pain, cold allodynia is most frequently found in addition to other signs of central hyperexcitability, such as mechanical allodynia and hyperalgesia (Jorum et al. 2003), whereas cold allodynia may be the sole finding in patients with injury following prolonged exposure to cold ambient temperatures. Due to normal sensibility mediated by large-diameter $A\beta$ and $A\delta$ fibers, the disinhibition theory may not explain cold allodynia following cold injury. Cold injury is a likely candidate for involving peripheral sensitization of cold-sensitive receptors, whereas central mechanisms most likely will account for cold allodynia in neuropathic pain.

CONCLUDING REMARKS

Cold allodynia and cold hypersensitivity have now been recognized as important symptoms in patients following tissue injury and after lesions of the peripheral or central nervous system. It is unlikely that one single mechanism can explain the clinical picture of these different pathologies. Nevertheless, with the existent knowledge it is now possible to test new and old hypotheses of cold hypersensitivity as they are observed under experimental and pathological conditions.

ACKNOWLEDGMENTS

G. Wasner was supported by the Alexander von Humboldt-Stiftung. R. Baron was supported by the Deutsche Forschungsgemeinschaft (DFG Ba 1921/1-3), the German Ministry of Research and Education within the German Research Network on Neuropathic Pain (BMBF, 01EM05/04), and Pfizer Deutschland (unrestricted educational grant). M. Koltzenburg's work is supported by the Wellcome Trust, the Medical Research Council, and the European Commission.

REFERENCES

Andersen G, Vestergaard K, Ingeman-Nielsen M, Jensen TS. Incidence of central post-stroke pain. *Pain* 1995; 61:187–193.

Askwith C, Benson C, Welsh M, Snyder P. DEG/ENaC ion channels involved in sensory transduction are modulated by cold temperature. *Proc Natl Acad Sci USA* 2001; 98:6459–6463.

Boivie J, Leijon G, Johansson I. Central post-stroke pain—a study of the mechanisms through analyses of the sensory abnormalities. *Pain* 1989; 37:173–185.

Bowsher D. Central pain following spinal and supraspinal lesions. *Spinal Cord* 1999; 37:235–238.

Bowsher D, Haggett C. Paradoxical burning sensation produced by cold stimulation in patients with neuropathic pain. *Pain* 2005; 117:230.

Cain DM, Khasabov SG, Simone DA. Response properties of mechanoreceptors and nociceptors in mouse glabrous skin: an in vivo study. *J Neurophysiol* 2001; 85:1561–1574.

Campero M, Serra J, Bostock H, Ochoa JL. Slowly conducting afferents activated by innocuous low temperature in human skin. *J Physiol* 2001; 535:855–865.

Clapham DE. TRP channels as cellular sensors. *Nature* 2003; 426:517–524.

Craig AD. How do you feel? Interoception: the sense of the physiological condition of the body. *Nat Rev Neurosci* 2002; 3:655–666.

Craig AD, Bushnell MC. The thermal grill illusion: unmasking the burn of cold pain. *Science* 1994; 265:252–255.

Craig AD, Reiman EM, Evans A, Bushnell MC. Functional imaging of an illusion of pain. *Nature* 1996; 384:258–260.

Davis KD. Cold-induced pain and prickle in the glabrous and hairy skin. *Pain* 1998; 75:47–57.

Fruhstorfer H. Thermal sensibility changes during ischemic nerve block. *Pain* 1984; 20:355–361.

Harrison JL, Davis KD. Cold-evoked pain varies with skin type and cooling rate: a psychophysical study in humans. *Pain* 1999; 83:123–135.

Head H, Holmes G. Sensory disturbances from central lesions. *Brain* 1911; 34:102–254.

Jensen TS, Baron R. Translation of symptoms and signs into mechanisms in neuropathic pain. *Pain* 2003; 102:1–8.

Jensen TS, Gottrup H, Bach FW, Sindrup SH. The clinical picture of neuropathic pain. *Eur J Pharmacol* 2001; 429:1–11.

Jordt SE, Bautista DM, Chuang HH, et al. Mustard oils and cannabinoids excite sensory nerve fibres through the TRP channel ANKTM1. *Nature* 2004; 427:260–265.

Jorum E, Warncke T, Stubhaug A. Cold allodynia and hyperalgesia in neuropathic pain: the effect of *N*-methyl-D-aspartate (NMDA) receptor antagonist ketamine: a double-blind, cross-over comparison with alfentanil and placebo. *Pain* 2003; 101:229–235.

Julius D, McCleskey EW. Cellular and molecular properties of primary afferent neurons. In: McMahon SB, Koltzenburg M (Eds). *Wall and Melzack's Textbook of Pain*. Philadelphia: Elsevier, 2005, pp 35–48.

Koltzenburg M. Thermal sensitivity of sensory neurons. In: Villanueva L, Dickenson AH, Ollat H (Eds). *The Pain System in Normal and Pathological States: A Primer for Clinicians,* Progress in Pain Research and Management, Vol. 31. Seattle: IASP Press, 2004.

Koltzenburg M, Scadding J. Neuropathic pain. *Curr Opin Neurol* 2001; 14:641–647.

Mackenzie RA, Burke D, Skuse NF, Lethlean AK. Fibre function and perception during cutaneous nerve block. *J Neurol Neurosurg Psychiatr* 1975; 38:865–873.

Maingret F, Lauritzen I, Patel A, et al. TREK-1 is a heat-activated background K+ channel. *EMBO J* 2000; 19:2483–2491.

McKemy DD, Neuhausser WM, Julius D. Identification of a cold receptor reveals a general role for TRP channels in thermosensation. *Nature* 2002; 416:52–58.

Meyer RA, Ringkamp M, Campbell JN, Raja SN. Peripheral mechanisms of cutaneous nociception. In: McMahon SB, Koltzenburg M (Eds). *Wall and Melzack's Textbook of Pain,* 5th ed. Philadelphia: Elsevier, 2005, pp 3–34.

Namer B, Seifert F, Handwerker HO, Maihofner C. TRPA1 and TRPM8 activation in humans: effects of cinnamaldehyde and menthol. *Neuroreport* 2005; 16:955–959.

Nealen ML, Gold MS, Thut PD, Caterina MJ. TRPM8 mRNA is expressed in a subset of cold-responsive trigeminal neurons from rat. *J Neurophysiol* 2003; 90:515–520.

Ochoa JL, Yarnitsky D. The triple cold syndrome. Cold hyperalgesia, cold hypoaesthesia and cold skin in peripheral nerve disease. *Brain* 1994; 117:185–197.

Patapoutian A, Peier AM, Story GM, Viswanath V. Thermo-TRP channels and beyond: mechanisms of temperature sensation. *Nat Rev Neurosci* 2003; 4:529–539.

Peier AM, Moqrich A, Hergarden AC, et al. A TRP channel that senses cold stimuli and menthol. *Cell* 2002; 108:705–715.

Reid G, Flonta ML. Ion channels activated by cold and menthol in cultured rat dorsal root ganglion neurones. *Neurosci Lett* 2002; 324:164–168.

Simone DA, Kajander KC. Excitation of rat cutaneous nociceptors by noxious cold. *Neurosci Lett* 1996; 213:53–56.

Simone DA, Kajander KC. Responses of cutaneous A-fiber nociceptors to noxious cold. *J Neurophysiol* 1997; 77:2049–2060.

Story GM, Peier AM, Reeve AJ, et al. ANKTM1, a TRP-like channel expressed in nociceptive neurons, is activated by cold temperatures. *Cell* 2003; 112:819–829.

Thunberg T. Förnimmelserne vid till samma ställe lokaliserad, samtidigt pågående köld-och värmeretning. *Uppsala Läkfören Förh* 1896; 2:489–495.

Thut PD, Wrigley D, Gold MS. Cold transduction in rat trigeminal ganglia neurons in vitro. *Neuroscience* 2003; 119:1071–1083.

Tominaga M, Caterina MJ. Thermosensation and pain. *J Neurobiol* 2004; 61:3–12.

Torebjörk HE, Hallin RG. Perceptual changes accompanying controlled preferential blocking of A and C fibre responses in intact human skin nerves. *Exp Brain Res* 1973; 16:321–332.

Torebjörk E, Wahren L, Wallin G, Hallin R, Koltzenburg M. Noradrenaline-evoked pain in neuralgia. *Pain* 1995; 63:11–20.

Verdugo R, Ochoa JL. Quantitative somatosensory thermotest. A key method for functional evaluation of small calibre afferent channels. *Brain* 1992; 115:893–913.

Viana F, de la PE, Belmonte C. Specificity of cold thermotransduction is determined by differential ionic channel expression. *Nat Neurosci* 2002; 5:254–260.

Wahren LK, Torebjörk E, Jorum E. Central suppression of cold-induced C fibre pain by myelinated fibre input. *Pain* 1989; 38:313–319.

Wasner G, Schattschneider J, Binder A, Baron R. Topical menthol—a human model for cold pain by activation and sensitization of C nociceptors. *Brain* 2004; 127:1159–1171.

Yarnitsky D, Ochoa JL. Release of cold-induced burning pain by block of cold-specific afferent input. *Brain* 1990; 113:893–902.

Ziegler EA, Magerl W, Meyer RA, Treede RD. Secondary hyperalgesia to punctate mechanical stimuli. Central sensitization to A-fibre nociceptor input. *Brain* 1999; 122:2245–2257.

Correspondence to: Priv.-Doz. Dr. med. Gunnar Wasner, Prince of Wales Medical Research Institute, University of New South Wales, Barker Street, Randwick, Sydney, NSW 2031, Australia. Fax: 61-2-93991034; email: g.wasner@unsw.edu.au.

Proceedings of the 11th World Congress on Pain,
edited by Herta Flor, Eija Kalso, and Jonathan O.
Dostrovsky, IASP Press, Seattle, © 2006.

58

Postherpetic Neuralgia: A Disease with Many Faces

Gunnar Wasner,[a,b] Susan M. Fleetwood-Walker,[c]
Emer M. Garry,[c] Catherine Abbadie,[d] Ralf Baron,[b]
Robert W. Johnson[e]

*[a]Prince of Wales Medical Research Institute, University of New South Wales,
Randwick, Sydney, New South Wales, Australia; [b]Division of Neurological
Pain Research and Therapy, Department of Neurology, Christian-Albrechts
University, Kiel, Germany; [c]Centre for Neuroscience Research, Division
of Veterinary Biomedical Sciences, University of Edinburgh, Edinburgh, United
Kingdom; [d]Department of Pharmacology, Merck Research Laboratories, Rahway,
New Jersey, USA; [e]Pain Management Clinic, Bristol Royal Infirmary, Bristol,
United Kingdom*

Postherpetic neuralgia (PHN) is a neuropathic pain syndrome associated with the reactivation of varicella zoster virus, which resides in latent form in sensory trigeminal and dorsal root ganglia following primary infection as varicella. The severe chronic pain may persist for month to years, becoming a major reason for reduced quality of life and decreased ability to participate in daily activities, mostly affecting the elderly and immune-compromised individuals.

Clinically, PHN is typically characterized by a constant, spontaneous burning pain in combination with several forms of allodynia and hyperalgesia and intermittent lancinating pain. Dynamic mechanical allodynia, perceived as a sharp radiating pain evoked by very light touching of the skin, is often the most unpleasant aspect of the patient's pain (Fields et al. 1998).

The disorder is often taken as a paradigm for neuropathic pain in research and treatment studies. However, therapy is often unsatisfactory. This chapter focuses on recent epidemiological, animal, and patient data that may improve our understanding of the underlying pathophysiology of PHN and lead to better treatment options.

EPIDEMIOLOGY

VARICELLA ZOSTER VIRUS INFECTION

The varicella zoster virus (VZV), like other herpes viruses, is capable of causing primary disease (Seward 2000), followed by latency and reactivation, resulting in a secondary condition. With VZV, the primary disease is varicella (chickenpox); latency is usually prolonged, and reactivation results in herpes zoster (HZ, also known as shingles). During the period of latency, the virus is asymptomatic. Primary infection produces long-term immunity to varicella. Protection from reactivation depends upon intact cell-mediated immunity, which gradually declines with age (immune senescence), in certain diseases (some malignancies, HIV/AIDS), and as a result of immunosuppressive therapy (therapy after organ transplantation, chemotherapy, and steroids). Varicella produces an enduring humoral response and a less prolonged cell-mediated response. It is believed, with good evidence, that immune mechanisms are boosted by two natural phenomena: first, from regular contact of seropositive (at-risk) adults with children who have varicella (exogenous boosting) (Thomas et al. 2002), and second, from silent reactivations of latent virus (endogenous boosting) (Arvin 2005) (Fig. 1). In addition, vaccination with a live attenuated OKA vaccine, named after the child with varicella in Japan from which it was isolated by Takahashi, affords protection against varicella when given to children or seronegative adults and, in a more potent preparation, against herpes zoster if administered to adults aged 60 or above (Oxman et al. 2005).

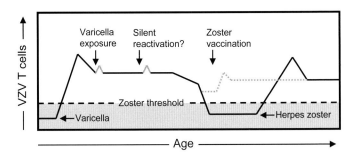

Fig. 1. Lifetime changes in cell-mediated immunity to varicella zoster virus (VZV). Varicella is the primary infection caused by VZV, and its resolution is associated with the induction of VZV-specific memory T cells (black line). Memory immunity to VZV may be boosted periodically by exposure to varicella or by silent reactivation from latency (gray peaks). VZV-specific memory T cells decline with age. The decline below a threshold (dashed black line) correlates with an increased risk of zoster. The occurrence of zoster, in turn, is associated with an increase in VZV-specific T cells. The administration of zoster vaccine to older persons may prevent VZV-specific T cells from dropping below the threshold for zoster occurrence (dashed gray line). Adapted from Arvin (2005), with permission.

INCIDENCE OF HERPES ZOSTER AND ROLE OF VACCINATION

Data for incidence of HZ arise from a number of sources, and all show a clear increase with age. Despite the correlation with age, HZ is not rare in younger persons. The median age for HZ is approximately 64 years. Published data for all ages include those of Hope-Simpson (1965), De Moragas and Kierland (1957), and Helgason et al. (2000) and, for a population aged 60 years and above, from the Shingles Prevention Study (Oxman et al. 2005).

It is probable that the incidence of HZ will change over coming decades as a result of increasing longevity of the population, changes in therapy for malignant and autoimmune disease, increasing use of organ transplantation, and childhood vaccination against varicella. It is also probable that adult vaccination against HZ will follow the recently published Shingles Prevention Study (Oxman et al. 2005).

In the developed world, and perhaps elsewhere, significant increases in the elderly population are predicted. In the United Kingdom, 2001 census data showed the population aged 65 years and over to be approximately 9 million (16%); the projected figure for 2025 is 13 million. Data from the Scientific Registry of Transplant Recipients draft analysis in the United States has shown a year-by-year increase in solid organ transplants from 12,300 in 1988 to 24,200 in 2003; all these patients receive immunosuppressant drugs. Use of the OKA vaccine in children to protect against varicella was introduced in the United States in 1995, and other countries that have adopted the strategy include Japan, South Korea, Germany, Australia, and Israel. Surveillance of sentinel sites in the United States to date has not shown an effect on HZ, but mathematical modeling based on valid assumptions indicates that a significant effect could occur (Edmunds and Brisson 2002). As vaccination reduces the number of children with varicella, it will also severely reduce exogenous boosting as a means of enhancing cell-mediated immunity and delaying the reactivation of latent virus. Seropositive adults without contact with children with varicella will be more likely to develop HZ than those exposed to varicella on a regular basis. Edmunds and Brisson (2002) have proposed that the incidence of HZ might rise significantly from about 3.4 to 4.2 per 1,000 person-years, peaking between 10 and 20 years after adoption of childhood vaccination and only returning to baseline after 30 to 40 years. Subsequently, there should be a significant decline in incidence, as the adult population carrying latent virus declines. Adult vaccination with a modified OKA-based vaccine has been shown in the Shingles Prevention Study of nearly 39,000 adults aged 60 years and above to reduce the incidence of HZ by 51.3% and that of PHN by 66.5% compared with placebo (Oxman et al. 2005).

EPIDEMIOLOGY OF PHN

Epidemiology of PHN is difficult to quantify with confidence because of the widely varying definitions of PHN that have been used in surveys and publications. The advent of studies of antiviral drugs has driven the development of valid definitions and has provided large databases from which reliable information may be derived. It is now accepted that the term "zoster-associated pain" may be used to cover a continuum of pain from start of prodrome to its resolution and that "postherpetic neuralgia" should be reserved for cases of significant pain or painful abnormal sensations persisting beyond approximately 4 months after HZ rash appearance. In particular, work by Dworkin and Portenoy (1994) as well as that of Arani and colleagues (2001) provides credence to the proposed terminology. Whether only pain that scores 3 or greater on a 0–10 scale should be included (Lydick et al. 1995) remains undecided. An option is to present data according to both definitions (Scott et al. 2006) (Fig. 2).

What is certain is that the prevalence of PHN increases with age and that more severe acute pain and rash, as well as prodromal pain, are predictors for

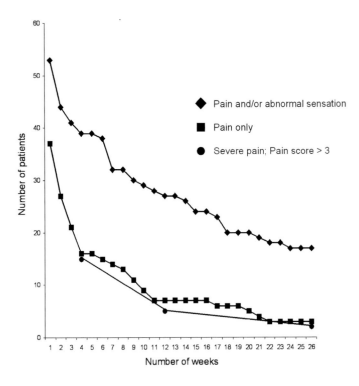

Fig. 2. Cohort incidence of postherpetic neuralgia utilizing three different criteria for pain assessment. Adapted from Scott et al. (2006), with permission.

its development (Wood et al. 1994; Dworkin et al. 2001; Nagasako et al. 2002; Jung et al. 2004).

ANIMAL STUDIES

A RODENT MODEL OF CHRONIC PAIN INDUCED BY VARICELLA ZOSTER VIRUS

The striking PHN symptoms of hyperalgesia and allodynia can be produced for a period of at least 3 months in animal models of latent VZV infection by injection of virus into the rat footpad (Fig. 3) (Sadzot-Delvaux et al. 1990; Fleetwood-Walker et al. 1999; Dalziel et al. 2004; Garry et al. 2005).

In these models, there is no development of skin lesions and generally little development of behavioral sensitization on the contralateral (uninjured) side (Fleetwood-Walker et al. 1999; Dalziel et al. 2004; Garry et al. 2005). The pain behaviors exhibited are specific to infection with the varicella virus and are thought to be independent of virus replication (Dalziel et al. 2004). Viral infection in the sensory dorsal root ganglia (DRG) is confirmed by the presence of the immediate early (IE) protein VZV IE62 (Kinchington et al. 1992; Sato et al. 2003; Garry et al. 2005). The development of the sensitized pain response in this model is dependent on the viral titer injected and correlates with the levels of the viral protein IE62 in the DRG (Garry et al. 2005). When xenografts of human DRG in immunodeficient mice were infected with VZV, varicella zoster virions were found widely throughout neurons and myelinated axons (Zerboni

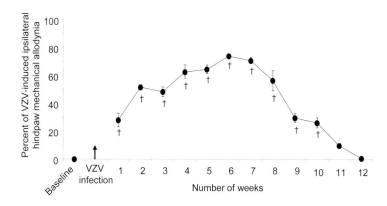

Fig. 3. Mechanical allodynia produced by injection of VZV into the rat footpad. Allodynia is expressed as a percentage of baseline pre-infection responses. There is a significant induction of allodynia in this model lasting for 10 weeks. Symbols (†) represents a significant difference between post-infection and pre-infection baseline responses ($P < 0.05$; Kruskal-Wallis ANOVA followed by a Dunn's test).

et al. 2005). Immunofluorescent confocal analysis of VZV-infected DRG shows that VZV IE62 is expressed in >80% of myelinated and unmyelinated cells (Garry et al. 2005). Expression is largely limited to the ipsilateral side, with <21% of cells showing expression in the contralateral DRG. Under these conditions, the VZV IE62 protein appeared to be localized in the cytoplasm with no apparent nuclear staining, characteristic of latent infection (Lungu et al. 1998).

While the role of these viral proteins in the generation of a chronic pain state is unknown, the association of VZV IE62 expression with particular subtypes of nociceptive afferents suggests an influence on cellular mechanisms within these afferents. Phenotypic changes in the neuropeptide content of DRG neurons play a role in the nervous system plasticity that leads to development of neuropathic pain states following nerve injury. There is an increased expression of neuropeptide Y, the neuropeptide galanin, and activating transcription factor-3 (ATF-3) in DRG ipsilateral to VZV infection (Garry et al. 2005), indicating damage to large-diameter DRG neurons (neuropeptide Y and galanin) and axonal damage (ATF-3) (Hökfelt et al. 1994; Villar et al. 1989; Tsujino et al. 2000).

UNDERLYING MECHANISMS THAT CONTRIBUTE TO VZV-INDUCED PAIN IN RODENTS

Voltage-gated sodium channels. Peripheral nerve injury can cause an increase in the excitability of both injured and adjacent uninjured afferents, which contributes to chronic pain states. Changes in the expression of voltage-gated sodium channel subunits following nerve damage may play an important role in this hyperexcitability (Waxman et al. 1999; Baker and Wood 2001). Expression of the tetrodotoxin-sensitive $Na_V1.3$ sodium channel is markedly increased in infected DRG (Garry et al. 2005), paralleling the upregulation that was seen following peripheral nerve damage (Cummins et al. 2000; Kim et al. 2001). The related tetrodotoxin-resistant channel $Na_V1.8$ is also upregulated following VZV infection (Garry et al. 2005), matching a report of the effectiveness of $Na_V1.8$ knockdown in reducing nerve-injury-induced pain behaviors (Porreca et al. 1999). These changes in expression may lead to altered sodium current characteristics, spontaneous ectopic discharge, and reduced neuronal activation thresholds in primary afferents (Novakovic et al. 1998; Cummins et al. 2000; Gold et al. 2003; Roza et al. 2003) that could contribute to VZV-induced hyperalgesia and allodynia. In agreement with these findings, the sodium-channel-blocking agents mexiletine and lamotrigine are effective in alleviating VZV-induced behavioral sensitization (Garry et al. 2005).

Voltage-gated calcium channels. A further phenotypic alteration seen following VZV infection in rodent is an upregulation of the $\alpha_2\delta_1$ subunit of voltage-gated calcium channels in the DRG (Garry et al. 2005), matching reports of increases following nerve injury in both the DRG and spinal cord (Newton et al. 2001; Luo et al. 2002; Bayer et al. 2004). This finding is of particular interest, because $\alpha_2\delta_1$ has been proposed as one of the targets of gabapentin, which is effective in the treatment of PHN (Rowbotham et al. 1998; Beydoun 1999; Mao and Chen 2000). Animal experiments have demonstrated that gabapentin can suppress ectopic discharges of injured primary afferents and reverse injury-induced allodynia (Hunter et al. 1997; Abdi et al. 1998; Pan et al. 1999; Erichsen and Blackburn-Munro 2002; Laughlin et al. 2002; Kanai et al. 2004). This drug is now known to reduce VZV-induced behavioral reflex sensitization (Garry et al. 2005).

NMDA receptors. N-methyl-D-aspartate (NMDA) receptors have a well-established role in central sensitization in the spinal cord (Davies and Lodge 1987; Dickenson and Sullivan 1987), and their antagonists are effective in treating some kinds of neuropathic pain in patients (Nelson et al. 1997). Interestingly, local spinal application of an antagonist to the glutamatergic NMDA receptor also attenuates VZV-induced pain behaviors (Garry et al. 2005). However, trials in PHN patients with some oral NMDA-receptor antagonists have not shown any benefit (Sang et al. 2002).

Opioid receptors. Unlike treatment studies in PHN in humans showing efficacy of opioids (Watson and Babul 1998; Boureau et al. 2003), VZV infection in laboratory rodents is unresponsive to opioid-mediated analgesia, as shown by the lack of effect of the selective μ-opioid receptor agonist DAMGO on virus-induced behavioral reflex sensitization (Garry et al. 2005).

In summary, a rodent model of chronic pain induced by VZV infection has shown similarities to models of chronic pain from peripheral nerve injury, although more investigation will reveal whether there are physiological changes specific to this model. Rodent models of VZV-induced pain states and underlying molecular changes in afferents have revealed a clearly neuropathic-like profile of changes. These findings will help to guide strategies for the development of novel analgesics for clinical VZV-induced pain states including PHN.

HUMAN RESEARCH

PATHOPHYSIOLOGICAL MECHANISMS OF PAIN GENERATION IN PHN PATIENTS

Based on results from animal studies as described above, we hypothesize that distinct pathophysiological mechanisms lead to specific sensory symptoms and signs in patients. If this is the case, a thorough analysis of sensory symptoms and signs may reveal the most active underlying mechanisms in a particular patient. This analysis could provide a basis for a mechanism-based treatment approach that should increase therapeutic efficacy. The key method by which to create a detailed sensory profile of the affected painful area is quantitative sensory testing (QST), which comprises various psychophysiological methods that are used, for example, to investigate the function of small-fiber afferents including nociceptive pathways. Interestingly, two major subtypes of distinct sensory symptom constellations can be identified in PHN, which may be caused by different pathophysiological mechanisms.

Type I. Peripheral and central sensitization of nociceptive neurons. Increased excitability of primary afferent neurons after peripheral nerve injury is associated with increased expression of certain voltage-gated sodium channels, which leads to a lowering of the action potential threshold.

As a consequence of peripheral nociceptor hyperactivity, the excitability of the central nociceptive neurons within the dorsal horn also increases, a process known as central sensitization (Tal and Bennett 1994). Once central sensitization is established, normally innocuous tactile stimuli become capable of activating spinal cord pain-signaling neurons via Aβ low-threshold mechanoreceptors (Tal and Bennett 1994). By this mechanism, light touching of the skin induces mechanical allodynia.

Several clinical observations support the concept of sensitized nociceptors and central sensitization in PHN patients. When patients with PHN who suffered from ongoing pain and severe dynamic mechanical allodynia were tested with QST, about 30% did not show any loss of sensory function in the affected area, indicating that in these particular patients, loss of neurons is minimal or absent (Wasner et al. 2005). Accordingly, thermotesting, a key method in QST, revealed that heat pain thresholds in their region of greatest pain are decreased (Rowbotham et al. 1996; Pappagallo et al. 2000), a well-known phenomenon of peripheral nociceptor sensitization (Jensen and Baron 2003).

Type II. Predominant degeneration of nociceptive neurons. About 70% of PHN patients who also suffer from ongoing pain and severe dynamic mechanical allodynia show considerable signs of neuronal degeneration and loss of function within the affected tissues. Immunohistochemical investigations and punch biopsies of the affected dermatome showed degeneration of small-fiber afferents in the skin (Rowbotham et al. 1996; Oaklander 2001). Furthermore, functional studies investigating C-fiber axon reflexes demonstrated a significant loss of cutaneous C-fiber afferents in skin regions with intense dynamic allodynia (Baron and Saguer 1993, 1995). Accordingly, quantitative thermal sensory testing showed greatly increased heat pain thresholds in the affected dermatome of some patients with chronic PHN (Nurmikko and Bowsher 1990). Thus, a subset of PHN patients have pain and *loss* of cutaneous C-nociceptor function in a region that is coextensive with allodynic skin. Mechanisms underlying allodynia in these patients are still unclear. They might be related to hyperexcitability of second-order nociceptive neurons at the spinal level due to loss of inhibitory GABAergic interneurons, which occurs after peripheral nerve lesion (Scholz et al. 2005).

MECHANISM-BASED TREATMENT APPROACH IN POSTHERPETIC NEURALGIA

Based on the two different types of PHN patients described above, the first prospective mechanism-based treatment approach was performed using topical lidocaine (Wasner et al. 2005). The group studied included 18 patients who suffered from spontaneous burning pain and mechanical allodynia but differed concerning their cutaneous nociceptor function, as shown by QST. Six patients had evidence for sensitized nociceptors in the affected dermatome. The other 12 patients demonstrated severe partial nerve injury associated with functional deafferentation, including damage to nociceptive C-fiber afferents of the affected skin area. Topical lidocaine (5% patch) was chosen for treatment, because it has been proven to be effective in PHN (Meier et al. 2003). Additionally, it is generally assumed that its pain-relieving effect is caused by acting on sensitized cutaneous nociceptors that have expressed voltage-gated sodium channels within the superficial layers of the skin (Argoff 2000). Therefore, it was hypothesized that patients with sensitized nociceptors would respond well to lidocaine. Surprisingly, topical lidocaine was more effective in patients with predominant degeneration of nociceptive neurons, and did not provide significant relief in patients with sensitized nociceptors (Fig. 4). Although the heterogeneous distribution of the patients in the two groups ($n = 6$ vs. 12) weakens the statistical analyses, the striking finding that patients with nociceptor-deprived skin responded significantly to dermal lidocaine therapy cannot be ignored.

DISTINCT SENSORY PROFILES IN PHN PATIENTS: CLINICAL RELEVANCE?

As attractive as the PHN subtype-classification based on nociceptor function and evoked pain types might be, data from the study described above demonstrate that the ideal hypothesis of translating one symptom into one mechanism needs to be modified.

It is suggested that several underlying pain mechanisms probably have not yet been identified. For example, an explanation for the lidocaine effect in nociceptor-deprived skin might be that other intact afferents that have survived the virus infection are targeted by lidocaine after expression of sodium channels during the acute inflammatory disease process. Future studies are needed

Nociceptor Sensitization   Nociceptor Degeneration

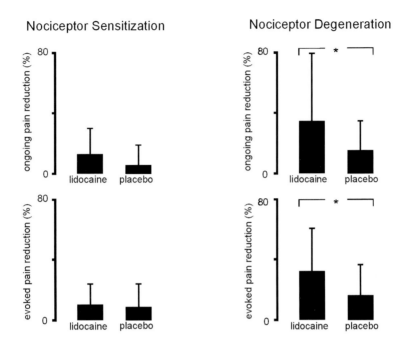

Fig. 4. Percentage reduction of ongoing pain and mechanical allodynia after lidocaine and placebo treatment in postherpetic neuralgia patients with sensitized nociceptor function versus impaired nociceptor function. Data are mean and SD; * $P < 0.05$. Adapted from Wasner et al. (2005), with permission.

to further evaluate the advantages and limitations of such mechanism-based treatment approaches to establish an optimal therapy with drugs that address the specific mechanisms in each patient.

TREATMENT

PREVENTION OF PHN

Recent results from the Shingles Prevention Study show that vaccination of adults is effective at preventing PHN (Oxman et al. 2005). If vaccination of adults is adopted, and if it shows similar long-term effects, a dramatic reduction of PHN is possible in decades to come. In the case of acute herpes zoster, early antiherpetic therapy, in particular with modern antiviral drugs (Wassilew 2005), significantly reduced the development of PHN. An indicative pilot study by Bowsher (1997) demonstrated that starting treatment with amitriptyline at the onset of shingles had a positive effect on PHN at this stage. Furthermore, gabapentin showed promising results in animal experiments (Kuraishi et al.

2004). However, large, prospectively designed studies are needed to estimate the effect on PHN of neuropathic pain treatment for shingles.

TREATMENT OF POSTHERPETIC NEURALGIA

We have not reached a point at which a mechanism-based treatment approach can be recommended, but a broad evidence base for treatment of PHN has been constructed from clinical trials of analgesics that have examined PHN as a single disease entity (Sindrup and Jensen 1999; Dworkin et al. 2003a; Finnerup et al. 2005; Hempenstall et al. 2005).

Tricyclic antidepressants. Tricyclic antidepressants (e.g., amitriptyline, desipramine, and nortriptyline) are effective in the treatment of postherpetic pain (Sindrup et al. 2005). These compounds are inhibitors of the reuptake of monoaminergic transmitters. They are believed to potentiate the effects of biogenic amines in pain modulation by the central nervous system, in particular, pain-inhibiting pathways projecting from the brainstem to the spinal cord. In addition, tricyclics block voltage-dependent sodium channels and α-adrenergic receptors.

Anticonvulsants. Placebo-controlled trials show that gabapentin is effective for PHN (Rowbotham et al. 1998). The drug acts on the $\alpha_2\delta$ subunit of presynaptic calcium channels on primary nociceptive endings. Gabapentin has a low potential for adverse interactions with other drugs, and no negative impact on cardiac function.

Pregabalin, the successor drug of gabapentin, was shown to be efficacious in PHN in recent controlled studies (Dworkin et al. 2003b). One major advantage over gabapentin is its superior bioavailability, which makes it easier to use without the need for long titration periods. Both gabapentin and pregabalin were noted to considerably improve sleep, overall mood, and other measures of quality of life in neuropathic pain patients (Rowbotham et al. 1998; Sabatowski et al. 2004).

Opioid analgesics. Double-blind, placebo-controlled studies have demonstrated that acute infusions of morphine or fentanyl give significant pain relief to patients with PHN (Rowbotham et al. 1991). Furthermore, recent controlled trials have demonstrated sustained efficacy for several weeks of oral oxycodone (Watson and Babul 1998) and tramadol (Boureau et al. 2003) in patients with PHN. Additionally, in a non-placebo-controlled parallel group study comparing two doses of levorphanol, significant dose-dependent pain relief was found in PHN patients who entered the study (Rowbotham et al. 2003). In one study, investigators analyzed the effect of oral morphine in a group of PHN patients, comparing the effect of tricyclic antidepressants in the same cohort. Both drugs were similarly effective. However, there was no correlation in the response rate between the two drugs, indicating that different mechanisms are active in these PHN patients (Raja et al. 2002). We recommend using long-acting opioid analgesics (e.g., a sustained-release morphine preparation) when alternative approaches to treatment have failed.

Topical medications. Topical capsaicin reduces pain in PHN (Watson et al. 1993). Capsaicin is an agonist of the vanilloid receptor, which is present on the sensitive terminals of primary nociceptive afferents. On initial application it has an excitatory action and produces burning pain. However, with repeated or prolonged application it inactivates the receptive terminals of nociceptors. Therefore, this approach is reasonable for those patients whose pain is maintained by anatomically intact sensitized nociceptors.

Topical lidocaine patches (5%) can also bring significant pain relief in PHN (Galer et al. 1999; Meier et al. 2003). Lidocaine patch therapy is a safe and well-tolerated supplemental modality for PHN pain relief.

Intrathecally administered drugs. Intrathecal administration of lidocaine and methyl prednisolone combined appears to be associated with remarkable benefit in PHN patients (Kotani et al. 2000). However, the therapy has potentially dangerous short- and long-term side effects, and the trial has not yet been replicated. Therefore, further high-quality controlled trials of this therapy are required before definite recommendations can be made (Hempenstall et al. 2005).

TREATMENT GUIDELINES

Adult vaccination seems to be effective for prevention of shingles and PHN (Fig. 5). In acute herpes zoster, early antiviral therapy is recommended, and pain treatment with amitriptyline or gabapentin should be attempted (Fig. 5). The medical management of PHN consists of three main classes of oral medication—tricyclic antidepressants, anticonvulsants (calcium channel blockers), and opioids—and two categories of topical medications (lidocaine is preferred to capsaicin, because of fewer side effects) (Fig. 5). Since more than one mechanism of pain is at work in most patients, a combination of two or more analgesic agents to cover multiple types of mechanisms will generally produce greater pain relief and fewer side effects. Therefore, early combinations of two or three compounds from different classes may be more appropriate for some patients than a stepwise strategy with successive monotherapies. This approach is indicated in the circles in Fig. 5. Indeed, in a recent controlled four-period crossover trial, gabapentin and morphine combined achieved better analgesia at lower doses of each drug than either as a single agent (Gilron et al. 2005). Therefore, this combination might be preferred (small square connecting both classes of medication in Fig. 5).

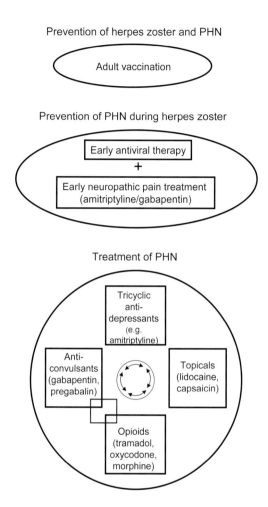

Fig. 5. Prevention and treatment guidelines for postherpetic neuralgia (PHN). The empty box connecting anticonvulsants and opioids indicates a combination of these therapies.

If this treatment strategy fails, further drugs should be considered that have been effective in animal models, in smaller studies, or in other neuropathic pain conditions, for example NMDA-receptor antagonists, anticonvulsants other than calcium channel blockers, such as lamotrigine or carbamazepine, and the selective serotonin and norepinephrine reuptake inhibitors venlafaxine and duloxetine. In particular cases, intrathecal administration of lidocaine and methyl prednisolone combined, or invasive stimulation techniques such as epidural spinal cord stimulation, may be indicated. Transcutaneous electrical nerve stimulation may be effective in some cases and has minimal side effects.

Beyond these pharmacological treatment approaches, the importance of the biopsychosocial model of chronic pain should be considered by additional management of psychological and social aspects (Haythornthwaite and Benrud-Larson 2000; Hempenstall et al. 2005).

ACKNOWLEDGMENTS

This work was supported by the Alexander von Humboldt-Stiftung, the Deutsche Forschungsgemeinschaft (DFG Ba 1921/1-3), the German Ministry of Research and Education within the German Research Network on Neuropathic Pain (BMBF, 01EM05/04), Pfizer Deutschland (unrestricted educational grant), Merck & Co. Inc., and The Wellcome Trust.

REFERENCES

Abdi S, Lee DH, Chung JM. The anti-allodynic effects of amitriptyline, gabapentin, and lidocaine in a rat model of neuropathic pain. *Anesth Analg* 1998; 87:1360–1366.

Arani RB, Soong SJ, Weiss HL, et al. Phase specific analysis of herpes zoster associated pain data: a new statistical approach. *Stat Med* 2001; 20:2429–2439.

Argoff CE. New analgesics for neuropathic pain: the lidocaine patch. *Clin J Pain* 2000; 16(Suppl 2):S62–66.

Arvin A. Aging, immunity, and the varicella-zoster virus. *N Engl J Med* 2005; 352:2266–2267.

Baker MD, Wood JN. Involvement of Na⁺ channels in pain pathways. *Trends Pharmacol Sci* 2001; 22:27–31.

Baron R, Saguer M. Postherpetic neuralgia. Are C-nociceptors involved in signalling and maintenance of tactile allodynia? *Brain* 1993; 116(Pt 6):1477–1496.

Baron R, Saguer M. Mechanical allodynia in postherpetic neuralgia: evidence for central mechanisms depending on nociceptive C-fiber degeneration. *Neurology* 1995; 45(Suppl 8): S63–65.

Bayer K, Ahmadi S, Zeilhofer HU. Gabapentin may inhibit synaptic transmission in the mouse spinal cord dorsal horn through a preferential block of P/Q-type Ca^{2+} channels. *Neuropharmacology* 2004; 46:743–749.

Beydoun A. Postherpetic neuralgia: role of gabapentin and other treatment modalities. *Epilepsia* 1999; 40 (Suppl 6):S51–56; discussion S73–154.

Boureau F, Legallicier P, Kabir-Ahmadi M. Tramadol in post-herpetic neuralgia: a randomized, double-blind, placebo-controlled trial. *Pain* 2003; 104:323–331.

Bowsher D. The effects of pre-emptive treatment of postherpetic neuralgia with amitriptyline: a randomized, double-blind, placebo-controlled trial. *J Pain Symptom Manage* 1997; 13:327–331.

Cummins TR, Dib-Hajj SD, Black JA, Waxman SG. Sodium channels and the molecular pathophysiology of pain. *Prog Brain Res* 2000; 129:3–19.

Dalziel RG, Bingham S, Sutton D, et al. Allodynia in rats infected with varicella zoster virus—a small animal model for post-herpetic neuralgia. *Brain Res Brain Res Rev* 2004; 46:234–242.

Davies SN, Lodge D. Evidence for involvement of *N*-methylaspartate receptors in 'wind-up' of class 2 neurones in the dorsal horn of the rat. *Brain Res* 1987; 424:402–406.

De Moragas JM, Kierland RR. The outcome of patients with herpes zoster. *AMA Arch Derm* 1957; 75:193–196.

Dickenson AH, Sullivan AF. Evidence for a role of the NMDA receptor in the frequency dependent potentiation of deep rat dorsal horn nociceptive neurones following C fibre stimulation. *Neuropharmacology* 1987; 26:1235–1238.

Dworkin RH, Portenoy RK. Proposed classification of herpes zoster pain. *Lancet* 1994; 343:1648.

Dworkin RH, Nagasako EM, Johnson RW, Griffin DR. Acute pain in herpes zoster: the famciclovir database project. *Pain* 2001; 94:113–119.

Dworkin RH, Backonja M, Rowbotham MC, et al. Advances in neuropathic pain: diagnosis, mechanisms, and treatment recommendations. *Arch Neurol* 2003a; 60:1524–1534.

Dworkin RH, Corbin AE, Young JP II, et al. Pregabalin for the treatment of postherpetic neuralgia: a randomized, placebo-controlled trial. *Neurology* 2003b; 60:1274–1283.

Edmunds WJ, Brisson M. The effect of vaccination on the epidemiology of varicella zoster virus. *J Infect* 2002; 44:211–219.

Erichsen HK, Blackburn-Munro G. Pharmacological characterisation of the spared nerve injury model of neuropathic pain. *Pain* 2002; 98:151–161.

Fields HL, Rowbotham M, Baron R. Postherpetic neuralgia: irritable nociceptors and deafferentation. *Neurobiol Dis* 1998; 5:209–227.

Finnerup NB, Otto M, McQuay HJ, Jensen TS, Sindrup SH. Algorithm for neuropathic pain treatment: an evidence based proposal. *Pain* 2005; 118:289–305.

Fleetwood-Walker SM, Quinn JP, Wallace C, et al. Behavioural changes in the rat following infection with varicella-zoster virus. *J Gen Virol* 1999; 80(Pt 9):2433–2436.

Galer BS, Rowbotham MC, Perander J, Friedman E. Topical lidocaine patch relieves postherpetic neuralgia more effectively than a vehicle topical patch: results of an enriched enrollment study. *Pain* 1999; 80:533–538.

Garry EM, Delaney A, Anderson HA, et al. Varicella zoster virus induces neuropathic changes in rat dorsal root ganglia and behavioral reflex sensitisation that is attenuated by gabapentin or sodium channel blocking drugs. *Pain* 2005; 118:97–111.

Gilron I, Bailey JM, Tu D, et al. Morphine, gabapentin, or their combination for neuropathic pain. *N Engl J Med* 2005; 352:1324–1334.

Gold MS, Weinreich D, Kim CS, et al. Redistribution of $Na_V1.8$ in uninjured axons enables neuropathic pain. *J Neurosci* 2003; 23:158–166.

Haythornthwaite JA, Benrud-Larson LM. Psychological aspects of neuropathic pain. *Clin J Pain* 2000; 16(2 Suppl):S101–105.

Helgason S, Petursson G, Gudmundsson S, Sigurdsson JA. Prevalence of postherpetic neuralgia after a first episode of herpes zoster: prospective study with long term follow up. *BMJ* 2000; 321:794–796.

Hempenstall K, Nurmikko TJ, Johnson RW, A'Hern RP, Rice AS. Analgesic therapy in postherpetic neuralgia: a quantitative systematic review. *PLoS Med* 2005; 2:e164.

Hökfelt T, Zhang X, Wiesenfeld-Hallin Z. Messenger plasticity in primary sensory neurons following axotomy and its functional implications. *Trends Neurosci* 1994;17:22–30.

Hope-Simpson RE. The nature of herpes zoster: a long-term study and a new hypothesis. *Proc R Soc Med* 1965; 58:9–20.

Hunter JC, Gogas KR, Hedley LR, et al. The effect of novel anti-epileptic drugs in rat experimental models of acute and chronic pain. *Eur J Pharmacol* 1997; 324:153–160.

Jensen TS, Baron R. Translation of symptoms and signs into mechanisms in neuropathic pain. *Pain* 2003; 102:1–8.

Jung BF, Johnson RW, Griffin DR, Dworkin RH. Risk factors for postherpetic neuralgia in patients with herpes zoster. *Neurology* 2004; 62:1545–1551.

Kanai A, Sarantopoulos C, McCallum JB, Hogan Q. Painful neuropathy alters the effect of gabapentin on sensory neuron excitability in rats. *Acta Anaesthesiol Scand* 2004; 48:507–512.

Kim CH, Oh Y, Chung JM, Chung K. The changes in expression of three subtypes of TTX sensitive sodium channels in sensory neurons after spinal nerve ligation. *Brain Res Mol Brain Res* 2001; 95:153–161.

Kinchington PR, Hougland JK, Arvin AM, Ruyechan WT, Hay J. The varicella-zoster virus immediate-early protein IE62 is a major component of virus particles. *J Virol* 1992; 66:359–366.

Kotani N, Kushikata T, Hashimoto H, et al. Intrathecal methylprednisolone for intractable postherpetic neuralgia. *N Engl J Med* 2000; 343:1514–1519.

Kuraishi Y, Takasaki I, Nojima H, Shiraki K, Takahata H. Effects of the suppression of acute herpetic pain by gabapentin and amitriptyline on the incidence of delayed postherpetic pain in mice. *Life Sci* 2004; 74:2619–2626.

Laughlin TM, Tram KV, Wilcox GL, Birnbaum AK. Comparison of antiepileptic drugs tiagabine, lamotrigine, and gabapentin in mouse models of acute, prolonged, and chronic nociception. *J Pharmacol Exp Ther* 2002; 302:1168–1175.

Lungu O, Panagiotidis CA, Annunziato PW, Gershon AA, Silverstein SJ. Aberrant intracellular localization of Varicella-Zoster virus regulatory proteins during latency. *Proc Natl Acad Sci USA* 1998; 95:7080–7085.

Luo ZD, Calcutt NA, Higuera ES, et al. Injury type-specific calcium channel alpha 2 delta-1 subunit up-regulation in rat neuropathic pain models correlates with antiallodynic effects of gabapentin. *J Pharmacol Exp Ther* 2002; 303:1199–1205.

Lydick E, Epstein RS, Himmelberger D, White CJ. Herpes zoster and quality of life: a self-limited disease with severe impact. *Neurology* 1995; 45(Suppl 8):S52–53.

Mao J, Chen LL. Gabapentin in pain management. *Anesth Analg* 2000; 91:680–687.

Meier T, Wasner G, Faust M, et al. Efficacy of lidocaine patch 5% in the treatment of focal peripheral neuropathic pain syndromes: a randomized, double-blind, placebo-controlled study. *Pain* 2003; 106:151–158.

Nagasako EM, Johnson RW, Griffin DR, Dworkin RH. Rash severity in herpes zoster: correlates and relationship to postherpetic neuralgia. *J Am Acad Dermatol* 2002; 46:834–839.

Nelson KA, Park KM, Robinovitz E, Tsigos C, Max MB. High-dose oral dextromethorphan versus placebo in painful diabetic neuropathy and postherpetic neuralgia. *Neurology* 1997; 48:1212–1218.

Newton RA, Bingham S, Case PC, Sanger GJ, Lawson SN. Dorsal root ganglion neurons show increased expression of the calcium channel alpha2delta-1 subunit following partial sciatic nerve injury. *Brain Res Mol Brain Res* 2001; 95:1–8.

Novakovic SD, Tzoumaka E, McGivern JG, et al. Distribution of the tetrodotoxin-resistant sodium channel PN3 in rat sensory neurons in normal and neuropathic conditions. *J Neurosci* 1998; 18:2174–2187.

Nurmikko T, Bowsher D. Somatosensory findings in postherpetic neuralgia. *J Neurol Neurosurg Psychiatry* 1990; 53:135–141.

Oaklander AL. The density of remaining nerve endings in human skin with and without postherpetic neuralgia after shingles. *Pain* 2001; 92:139–145.

Oxman MN, Levin MJ, Johnson GR, et al. A vaccine to prevent herpes zoster and postherpetic neuralgia in older adults. *N Engl J Med* 2005; 352:2271–2284.

Pan HL, Eisenach JC, Chen SR. Gabapentin suppresses ectopic nerve discharges and reverses allodynia in neuropathic rats. *J Pharmacol Exp Ther* 1999; 288:1026–1030.

Pappagallo M, Oaklander AL, Quatrano-Piacentini AL, Clark MR, Raja SN. Heterogenous patterns of sensory dysfunction in postherpetic neuralgia suggest multiple pathophysiologic mechanisms. *Anesthesiology* 2000; 92:691–698.

Porreca F, Lai J, Bian D, et al. A comparison of the potential role of the tetrodotoxin-insensitive sodium channels, PN3/SNS and NaN/SNS2, in rat models of chronic pain. *Proc Natl Acad Sci USA* 1999; 96:7640–7644.

Raja SN, Haythornthwaite JA, Pappagallo M, et al. Opioids versus antidepressants in postherpetic neuralgia: a randomized, placebo-controlled trial. *Neurology* 2002; 59:1015–1021.

Rowbotham MC, Reisner-Keller LA, Fields HL. Both intravenous lidocaine and morphine reduce the pain of postherpetic neuralgia. *Neurology* 1991; 41:1024–1028.

Rowbotham MC, Yosipovitch G, Connolly MK, et al. Cutaneous innervation density in the allodynic form of postherpetic neuralgia. *Neurobiol Dis* 1996; 3:205–214.

Rowbotham M, Harden N, Stacey B, Bernstein P, Magnus-Miller L. Gabapentin for the treatment of postherpetic neuralgia: a randomized controlled trial. *JAMA* 1998; 280:1837–1842.

Rowbotham MC, Twilling L, Davies PS, et al. Oral opioid therapy for chronic peripheral and central neuropathic pain. *N Engl J Med* 2003; 348:1223–1232.

Roza C, Laird JM, Souslova V, Wood JN, Cervero F. The tetrodotoxin-resistant Na+ channel Nav1.8 is essential for the expression of spontaneous activity in damaged sensory axons of mice. *J Physiol* 2003; 550(Pt 3):921–926.

Sabatowski R, Galvez R, Cherry DA, et al. Pregabalin reduces pain and improves sleep and mood disturbances in patients with post-herpetic neuralgia: results of a randomised, placebo-controlled clinical trial. *Pain* 2004; 109:26–35.

Sadzot-Delvaux C, Merville-Louis MP, Delree P, et al. An in vivo model of varicella-zoster virus latent infection of dorsal root ganglia. *J Neurosci Res* 1990; 26:83–89.

Sang CN, Booher S, Gilron I, Parada S, Max MB. Dextromethorphan and memantine in painful diabetic neuropathy and postherpetic neuralgia: efficacy and dose-response trials. *Anesthesiology* 2002; 96:1053–1061.

Sato B, Ito H, Hinchliffe S, et al. Mutational analysis of open reading frames 62 and 71, encoding the varicella-zoster virus immediate-early transactivating protein, IE62, and effects on replication in vitro and in skin xenografts in the SCID-hu mouse in vivo. *J Virol* 2003; 77:5607–5620.

Scholz J, Broom DC, Youn DH, et al. Blocking caspase activity prevents transsynaptic neuronal apoptosis and the loss of inhibition in lamina II of the dorsal horn after peripheral nerve injury. *J Neurosci* 2005; 25:7317–7323.

Scott FT, Johnson RW, Leedham-Green M, et al. The burden of herpes zoster: a prospective population based study. *Vaccine* 2006; 24:1308–1314.

Seward J. *Epidemiology of varicella*. In: Arvin AM, Gershon AA (Eds). *Varicella-Zoster Virus: Virology and Clinical Management*. Cambridge: Cambridge University Press, 2000, pp 187–205.

Sindrup SH, Jensen TS. Efficacy of pharmacological treatments of neuropathic pain: an update and effect related to mechanism of drug action. *Pain* 1999; 83:389–400.

Sindrup SH, Otto M, Finnerup NB, Jensen TS. Antidepressants in the treatment of neuropathic pain. *Basic Clin Pharmacol Toxicol* 2005; 96:399–409.

Tal M, Bennett GJ. Extra-territorial pain in rats with a peripheral mononeuropathy: mechano-hyperalgesia and mechano-allodynia in the territory of an uninjured nerve. *Pain* 1994; 57:375–382.

Thomas SL, Wheeler JG, Hall AJ. Contacts with varicella or with children and protection against herpes zoster in adults: a case-control study. *Lancet* 2002; 360:678–682.

Tsujino H, Kondo E, Fukuoka T, et al. Activating transcription factor 3 (ATF3) induction by axotomy in sensory and motoneurons: a novel neuronal marker of nerve injury. *Mol Cell Neurosci* 2000; 15:170–182.

Villar MJ, Cortes R, Theodorsson E, et al. Neuropeptide expression in rat dorsal root ganglion cells and spinal cord after peripheral nerve injury with special reference to galanin. *Neuroscience* 1989; 33:587–604.

Wasner G, Kleinert A, Binder A, Schattschneider J, Baron R. Postherpetic neuralgia: topical lidocaine is effective in nociceptor-deprived skin. *J Neurol* 2005; 252:677–686.

Wassilew S. Brivudin compared with famciclovir in the treatment of herpes zoster: effects in acute disease and chronic pain in immunocompetent patients. A randomized, double-blind, multinational study. *J Eur Acad Dermatol Venereol* 2005; 19:47–55.

Watson CP, Babul N. Efficacy of oxycodone in neuropathic pain: a randomized trial in postherpetic neuralgia. *Neurology* 1998; 50:1837–1841.

Watson CP, Tyler KL, Bickers DR, et al. A randomized vehicle-controlled trial of topical capsaicin in the treatment of postherpetic neuralgia. *Clin Ther* 1993; 15:510–526.

Waxman SG, Dib-Hajj S, Cummins TR, Black JA. Sodium channels and pain. *Proc Natl Acad Sci USA* 1999; 96:7635–7639.

Wood MJ, Johnson RW, McKendrick MW, et al. A randomized trial of acyclovir for 7 days or 21 days with and without prednisolone for treatment of acute herpes zoster. *N Engl J Med* 1994; 330:896–900.

Zerboni L, Ku CC, Jones CD, Zehnder JL, Arvin AM. Varicella-zoster virus infection of human dorsal root ganglia in vivo. *Proc Natl Acad Sci USA* 2005; 102:6490–6495.

Correspondence to: Priv.-Doz. Dr. med. Gunnar Wasner, Prince of Wales Medical Research Institute, University of New South Wales, Barker St, Randwick, Sydney, NSW 2031, Australia. Tel: 61-2-93991039; email: g.wasner@neurologie.uni-kiel. de.

Proceedings of the 11th World Congress on Pain,
edited by Herta Flor, Eija Kalso, and Jonathan O.
Dostrovsky, IASP Press, Seattle, © 2006.

59

Urogenital Pain:
Taking Management Forward

Andrew Baranowski,[a] Beverly Collett,[b]
Toby Newton-John,[c] and Ursula Wesselmann[d]

*[a]The Pain Management Centre, The National Hospital for Neurology and
Neurosurgery, University College London Hospitals, NHS Foundation Trust,
London, United Kingdom; [b]Pain Management Service, University Hospitals
of Leicester, Leicester, United Kingdom; [c]Innervate Pain Management, Hunter
Specialist Medical Centre, Broadmeadow, New South Wales, Australia;
[d]Department of Neurology, Johns Hopkins University School of Medicine,
Baltimore, Maryland, USA*

Chronic pelvic pain in men and women can be a complex clinical problem.
Patients initially visit their primary care doctor, a urologist, a gynecologist, or
a gastroenterologist for investigation with the full expectation that a cause will
be found for their pain and that treatment will be given and a cure obtained.
While the outcome is good in many patients, in an unfortunate few an etiology cannot be identified, nor does treatment result in a cure. This situation is
frustrating for both the doctor and the patient. The patient may seek multiple
medical opinions, undergoing numerous negative investigations and often many
invasive treatments.

Management of chronic pelvic pain requires sensitive and empathetic clinical care. Doctors who specialize in pain management appreciate that a biopsychosocial approach needs to be taken. However, patients may resent what they
perceive as intrusive questioning into their social and sexual functioning.

This chapter aims to illustrate the points made above by describing the case
of a patient with pelvic pain, in which a multidisciplinary approach was necessary. We discuss current animal and clinical research and explore the potential
impact of recent findings on clinical management.

BACKGROUND

Several guidelines have been published based on evidence-based medicine for the management of various chronic pelvic pains (Fall et al. 2004; Hanno et al. 2005). These guidelines often neglect the role of pain medicine, including medical and cognitive-behavioral therapies. First among the reasons for this omission is the poor understanding of the mechanisms involved, along with a failure to accept that urogenital disorders are often complex, involving multiple systems. Second, the classification system reflects the confusion over mechanisms and tends to be very end-organ based (focusing primarily on pathology within the peripheral organ and not taking into account pathologies within other systems and more centrally within the nervous system). Third, the resulting lack of evidence-based information on the role of pain medicine to guide decisions means that more research is necessary. Finally, many doctors who are treating an "end-organ condition" fail to see the importance of treating a pain syndrome, and this situation will not change until the first three issues are resolved.

This chapter describes the case of a 45-year-old man with penile pain and allodynia secondary to a sarcoid pudendal neuralgia. This case illustrates the multiple investigations, both physical and psychological, that may be performed and introduces multiple pain medicine interventions that can be considered as well as an approach to cognitive-behavioral pain management. This case demonstrates that appropriately chosen patients may benefit from a combined physical and psychological approach.

THE ROLE OF MEDICAL INVESTIGATIONS

Magnetic resonance imaging (MRI) scans may have a limited role in the evaluation of chronic pelvic pain (Cody and Ascher 2000). They should be considered to rule out significant pathology, such as spinal pathology (Holley et al. 1999). MR neurography has been suggested as useful for the evaluation of peripheral nerve injuries, but whether it will be helpful for pudendal neuralgia still has to be established. Superficial, minimally invasive pelvic floor electromyography (EMG) may have a role in both the diagnosis and treatment of patients with chronic pelvic pain. There is strong evidence that EMG is helpful in women (Glazer 2000) and some evidence for this in men, for instance in those with non-infective, non-inflammatory prostatitis (type IIIb according to the National Institutes of Health classification [Krieger et al. 1999]) (Cornel et al. 2005). Nerve conduction studies may have a limited role in the assessment of patients with chronic pelvic pain, and they are unlikely to be abnormal in the absence of some clinical signs. The role of EMG of the bulbocavernosus muscle needs to be further investigated as there is some suggestion that early pathology of the pudendal nerve may be detected in this muscle.

THE ROLE OF MEDICAL TREATMENTS

Pelvic floor exercises are recognized as important in the management of painful pelvic floor dysfunction. Core muscle exercises and stretches can be discussed with patients and endorsed. The role of the physiotherapist, both for assessment and intervention, may be important. Internal trigger point release may also be considered. As with most chronic pains, a role for nerve blocks probably exists. Specific nerve injuries, such as pudendal neuralgia, may be both investigated and treated with nerve blocks (Roberts et al. 2005). In certain cases, surgery may be indicated.

In patients with suspected visceral hyperalgesia or neuropathic pain, neuromodulating drugs should be considered. It has been suggested that interventional neuromodulation techniques such as stimulation of the sacral root (S3) and spinal cord stimulation may be of help for the management of chronic pelvic pain. Neuromodulation (primarily S3 root stimulation) has been used with success to treat incontinence in unstable painful bladders (Jonas and Grunewald 2002). Only limited data are available to support interventional neuromodulation for chronic pelvic pain, and further clinical research is required (Peters and Konstandt 2004).

PSYCHOLOGICAL INTERVENTIONS

The most common format in contemporary pain clinic practice is for pain treatments to run in a serial fashion. In other words, attempts are made during the initial treatment phase to relieve pain, but if these are not successful then efforts are redirected toward teaching coping strategies for the ongoing pain problem. The rationale for the serial treatment approach is that a patient who is being offered the chance of pain relief through medical treatment is less likely to invest the necessary time and effort to learn the self-management techniques espoused by pain psychologists. Only when all reasonable efforts to obtain a resolution of the pain have been exhausted does management move onto increasing function in the context of pain. Although this approach has not been empirically verified, there is certainly plenty of anecdotal evidence to indicate that many patients will only give "lip service" to the idea of pain self-management while efforts are being made to obtain a cure or the elimination of their symptoms.

However, this rule is not fixed by any means, and it might be argued that the serial approach to pain treatment inadvertently reinforces the Cartesian dualistic model by separating out physical and psychosocial interventions. Furthermore, patients can feel that a referral for pain self-management training represents a failure on the part of the physician (or themselves), or they may see it as an expression of the physician's hopelessness about their treatment progress. The case study presented is an example of pain treatment in parallel, with the intervention by pain doctor and pain psychologist occurring simultaneously. The psychological input consisted of one assessment session and eight treatment sessions taking place over an 8-month period. The psychological assessment followed standard cognitive-behavioral procedure in drawing on the clinical interview, self-report questionnaire data (see Table I), and self-monitoring data (Newton-John 2002).

CASE REPORT: THE PSYCHOLOGICAL PERSPECTIVE

The patient was a 45-year-old man with a 9-month history of chronic intractable penile pain. Assessment revealed high levels of pain-related disability; the patient was virtually housebound, spending most of the day lying flat because moving around provoked extreme allodynia. Coping strategies for pain were predominantly passive: for example, the patient placed wads of protective cotton wool in his underwear if he needed to dress to go out, and the psychometric profile revealed low confidence for managing pain. Although not frankly depressed, he had impaired mood and a high frequency of alarmist thoughts when in pain.

Table I
The outcome of a psychological pain management approach combined with
medical management in a patient with chronic intractable penile pain

Measures	Pretreatment	Post-Treatment	3-Year Follow-up
Pain intensity (0–100 numeric rating scale)	55	10	15
Pain Disability Index (0–70)	54	25	4
Pain Self-Efficacy Questionnaire (0–60)	12	47	52*
Coping Strategies Questionnaire			
Catastrophizing (0–30)	20	2	3
Coping Self-Statement (0–30)	7	24	13
Beck Depression Inventory (0–63)	18	6	6

* Questions included "I can cope with my pain without medication."

As is often the case with persistent pain problems, the assessment also revealed significant disturbance within the man's primary relationship (Schwartz and Edhe 2000). The onset of the pain had coincided with a casual sexual experience that occurred outside the relationship, the first time this had happened. Although the patient was experiencing considerable guilt about this event (and held a belief that his pain was somehow a punishment for his infidelity), he also had several reasons for dissatisfaction with the relationship that were affecting the degree of support he was receiving.

The psychological intervention consisted of two integrated but distinct elements: pain management and relationship therapy (Turk and Meichenbaum 1994). Pain management began with education concerning the influence of the affective state on pain perception and continued with an outline of the principles of activity pacing. These sessions increased the patient's understanding of the impact of mood on pain experience, underlining the importance of addressing catastrophic thoughts and heightened fears of pain. Pacing was applied to "up time" during the day, particularly in relation to time spent engaging in work activities (the patient was self-employed and worked from home). Pain management then moved onto the systematic desensitization of the allodynic areas, through regular timed periods of manual pressure as well as a gradual decrease in the use of padding in the underwear. The patient was encouraged to consider time constraints rather than pain level when determining his activities. This strategy allowed the patient to resume going swimming, which was one of his favorite activities.

Cognitive therapy was introduced, with an emphasis on the appraisal of pain when at its most severe (Sullivan et al. 2001). The patient readily grasped the concept of "catastrophizing" and was able to appreciate the interplay between his extreme beliefs about the pain, the distress that resulted from these beliefs, and the negative enhancement of his pain experience. Successfully generating alternative, less extreme interpretations of pain was critical to a more proactive response to periods of increased discomfort.

While this skills-based intervention was proceeding, time was set aside during each therapy session for a broader discussion of the patient's primary relationship, including its history and the patient's expectations of its future. Efforts were made to normalize the patient's sexual urges and to reframe the belief that the pain was retribution for the infidelity that had occurred. As discussion of these issues progressed, it was apparent that there had been some significant rifts within the relationship for some time, but both parties had chosen to avoid confronting them. In an environment of impartiality, the patient was given the opportunity to explore his beliefs about the relationship and how it might be improved or even ended.

Table I shows the outcome of the intervention. It does not solely reflect the psychological component because medical investigations and treatments were also being carried out during this time. The results were positive and proved to be durable over the next 3 years. It should be noted, however, that while the patient's total score for confidence to manage pain on the Pain Self-Efficacy Questionnaire (Asghari and Nicholas 2001) at the 3-year follow-up was relatively high, the individual item concerning confidence to manage pain without pain medication was very low (reported as 1/6). This result suggests that the patient relies on continuing use of pain medications in order to retain his high level of functioning.

DISCUSSION OF PSYCHOLOGY

It can only be speculated as to why a parallel treatment model was successful in this case, but the following set of factors may serve as a guide for other pain psychologists and physicians considering working in this way.

PATIENT FACTORS

The patient had high expectations of success and was prepared to make efforts in order to obtain a positive outcome. He understood that learning to manage pain was not invalidated by efforts to seek relief from pain (through medical investigations or treatments); both were equally important endeavors rather than being mutually exclusive approaches. The patient had the capacity to discuss potentially embarrassing or distressing information in an open and honest way.

CLINICIAN FACTORS

Efforts were made to communicate regularly using letters, phone calls, and meetings so that each member of the treatment team was aware of the progress of the other. The patient occasionally commented that the "team work" that he perceived taking place boosted his confidence in the approach being taken. When flare-ups of pain did occur, the response was not one of exasperation or apprehension. Alternatively, these episodes were viewed in an empathic light, but were interpreted as sources of new and potentially important information from which the patient could learn more about the modulators of his pain condition.

At no stage was the mistake made of inferring that because of the time contingency between the patient's casual sexual encounter and the onset of pain, the patient's pain was psychogenic in origin. Previous psychiatrists had made much of this assumption, and the patient had come to distrust this unidimensional view. He experienced this view as a patient-blaming, critical stance that closed off further consideration of the biological causes of pain. An integrated, biopsychosocial perspective allowed the patient to openly discuss all factors that might be relevant to his condition, both physical and psychological.

UROGENITAL PAIN AND TRANSLATIONAL RESEARCH ASPECTS

UROGENITAL PAIN: A CHRONIC PAIN SYNDROME

The recognition of chronic urogenital pain as a "chronic visceral pain syndrome" is fairly new in the clinical subspecialties of urology and gynecology (Wesselmann et al. 1997; Wesselmann 2001; Abrams et al. 2002; ACOG Committee on Practice Bulletins—Gynecology 2004; Fall et al. 2004). Although chronic nonmalignant pain syndromes of the urogenital tract have been well described in the literature in the last 100 years (Wesselmann et al. 1997), their etiology is poorly understood. Pain in these areas of the body is usually very embarrassing for both male and female patients, who may be afraid to discuss their symptoms with family members, friends, and health care providers. The controversy that surrounds these pain syndromes ranges from questioning their existence to dismissing them as purely psychosomatic. This view is counterbalanced by an extensive literature attesting to their organic basis. Patients with these pain syndromes often suffer for many years, have seen numerous physicians in numerous subspecialties, and have undergone numerous diagnostic tests, which have all been negative. The difficulties in diagnosing chronic urogenital pain by identifying a testable abnormality are due to the fact that even now we still lack the tools to objectively measure sensory abnormalities that result in painful sensations. A similar diagnostic dilemma is observed when patients with chronic headache are evaluated. The diagnostic work-up is typically negative (imaging studies show no pathology and the spinal fluid is normal), and the diagnosis of chronic headache is made based on exclusion of brain lesions and infections. However, chronic headaches are usually considered to be "legitimate diseases," whereas chronic urogenital pain is only recently gaining consideration as a "real" pain syndrome.

NEUROANATOMY

A basic understanding of the neuroanatomy of the pelvic floor is a prerequisite for gaining insight into some of the neurophysiological mechanisms responsible for the clinical presentation of patients with chronic urogenital pain. The urogenital tract is a highly specialized area of the body, responsible for carrying out a host of basic biological functions including micturition, copulation, and reproduction (for review see Burnett and Wesselmann 1999). The innervation of the genitourinary area involves both components of the autonomic nervous system, the sympathetic and parasympathetic divisions, as well as the somatic nervous systems (Figs. 1 and 2). In a broad neuroanatomical view, dual projections from the thoracolumbar and sacral segments of the spinal cord carry out this innervation, converging mostly into peripheral neuronal plexuses from which nerve fibers ramify throughout the pelvic floor. The inferior hypogastric plexus is the major neuronal coordinating center that supplies visceral structures of the pelvis and the pelvic floor. Nociception and pain arising from within the pelvis and pelvic floor involve diverse neuronal mechanisms. In general, sensations from the pelvic viscera are conveyed within the sacral afferent parasympathetic system, with a far lesser afferent supply from thoracolumbar sympathetic origins. Receptive fields in the perineum are understood to be generated primarily by sensory-motor discharges associated with pudendal nerve afferents. While the interactions of sensory afferents are quite complex, likely mechanisms by which these pathways exert effects on autonomic efferent function include mediatory effects on spinal cord reflexes and modulatory effects on efferent release in peripheral autonomic ganglia and in peripheral organs. These neural structures in the periphery comprise the first of numerous relays of sensory neurons, which transmit painful sensations from the abdominal/pelvic cavity to the brain. Traditionally it was thought that ascending pathways for visceral and other types of pain were mainly the spinothalamic and spinoreticular tracts. However, three previously undescribed pathways that carry visceral nociceptive information have been discovered: the dorsal column pathway, the spino(trigemino)-parabrachio-amygdaloid pathway, and the spino-hypothalamic pathway (Cervero and Laird 1999; Willis and Westlund 2001; Gebhart 2004). In addition, descending facilitatory influences may contribute to the development of maintenance of hyperalgesia, thus contributing to the development of chronic urogenital pain.

VISCERO-VISCERAL AND VISCERO-SOMATIC INTERACTIONS

There are two components of visceral pain, which were first described more than 100 years ago: "true visceral pain" (deep visceral pain arising from inside the body) and "referred visceral pain" (pain that is referred to segmentally related somatic structures, such as skin and muscles, and also to other visceral structures). Secondary hyperalgesia usually develops at the referred site. A number of explanations have been offered for the existence of referred pain (for review see Giamberardino and Vecchiet 1994). When examining and treating a patient with chronic urogenital pain it is important for the clinician to consider

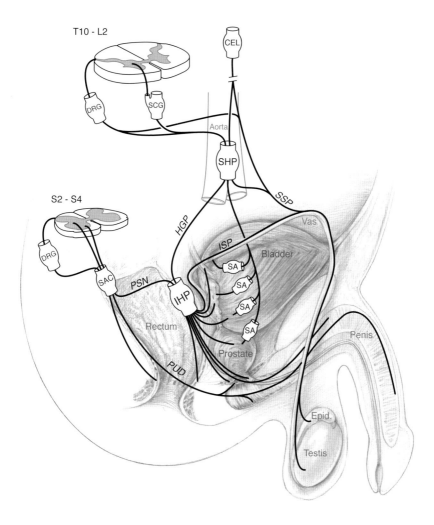

Fig. 1. Schematic drawing showing the innervation of the pelvic floor in males. Although this diagram attempts to show the innervation in humans, much of the anatomical information is derived from animal data. CEL = celiac plexus, DRG = dorsal root ganglion, HGP = hypogastric plexus, IHP = inferior hypogastric plexus, ISP = inferior spermatic plexus, PSN = pelvic splanchnic nerve, PUD = pudendal nerve, Epid. = epididymis, SA = short adrenergic projections, SAC = sacral plexus, SCG = sympathetic chain ganglion, SHP = superior hypogastric plexus, SSP = superior spermatic plexus. (From Wesselmann et al. 1997, with permission.)

both aspects of the pain syndrome (local and referred pain), including the pain deep in the pelvic cavity and pain referred to somatic structures (i.e., the lower back and legs) and other visceral organs. The mechanisms of referred viscerovisceral pain might explain the substantial overlap observed in epidemiological

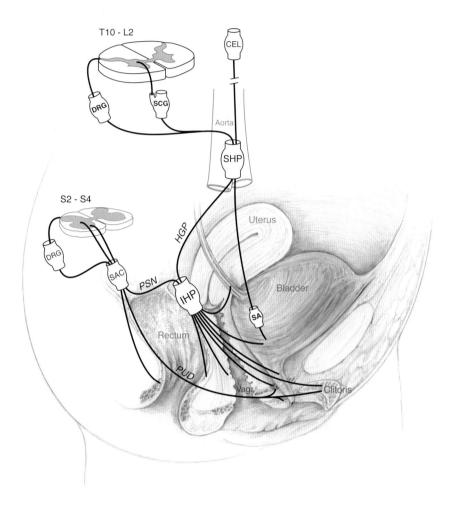

Fig. 2. Schematic drawing showing the innervation of the pelvic floor in females. Although this diagram attempts to show the innervation in humans, much of the anatomical information is derived from animal data. Abbreviations as in Fig. 1; Vag. = vagina. (From Wesselmann et al. 1997, with permission.)

studies between different urogenital pain syndromes (i.e., interstitial cystitis and vulvodynia; interstitial cystitis and prostatodynia) and between urogenital floor pain and pelvic pain (i.e., vulvodynia and pain with endometriosis). Referred viscero-somatic mechanisms can explain the clinical observation that patients with urogenital pain often complain about pain radiating to the upper legs and to the back. Considering the concept of referred visceral pain will allow the therapist to look at the global picture of visceral dysfunction, rather than chasing after one aspect of the urogenital pain syndrome out of context. In addition, many patients with urogenital pain report chronic pain outside the referred areas, including headache and generalized joint and muscle pain. This clinical impression has been confirmed by epidemiological studies (Alagiri et al. 1997; Erickson et al. 2001). These observations suggest that generalized alterations in pain-modulatory mechanisms may occur in patients with chronic urogenital pain.

FROM BENCH TO BEDSIDE: WHAT CAN WE LEARN FROM BASIC SCIENCE STUDIES FOR CLINICAL CARE?

Wesselmann et al. (1998) and Wesselmann and Lai (1997) have developed an animal model of inflammatory pelvic pain in the rat. This model has allowed us to gain insights into some of the mechanisms of referred pain. Inflammation of the uterus in rats pretreated with Evans blue dye resulted in dye extravasation in the skin over the abdomen, groin, lower back, thighs, perineal area, and proximal tail, thus providing the first evidence for some of the trophic changes observed in the area of referred visceral pain in an animal model of pelvic pain (Wesselmann and Lai 1997). The neuronal pathways mediating the observed dye extravasation in the skin after uterine inflammation may include dichotomizing afferent fibers or afferent-afferent interactions via a spinal cord pathway or a sympathetic reflex. These pathways were activated within minutes of pelvic inflammation, indicating that the pathways for referred pain are already in place. This indication is further confirmed by the anecdotal clinical observation that patients with acute pelvic pain (such as labor pain) experience referred pain to somatic structures (the urogenital area and the back) in distribution similar to that of patients with chronic urogenital or pelvic pain.

We have further used this animal model to study interventions aimed at alleviating chronic pelvic and urogenital pain. Using reduction in spontaneous pain behavior as an outcome measure, we have shown that opioids were effective in this model of pelvic pain (Czakanski and Wesselmann 2002). Based on the clinical observation that patients with chronic pelvic and urogenital pain often have significant pain relief with a combination of pharmacological and psychological treatment approaches, we explored whether environmental enrichment alters spontaneous pain behavior in this model of visceral pain. Our results suggest that environmental enrichment significantly reduces visceral pain behavior (Czakanski and Wesselmann 2005). Future studies will allow to explore the underlying mechanisms of environmental enrichment in this rat model of visceral pain and might provide further insights into the mechanisms of psychological modulations (such as reduction of stressors in the environment or relaxation techniques) of clinical visceral pain.

CONCLUSIONS

In summary, clinical observations and studies in animal models of visceral pain indicate that a spectrum of different insults might lead to chronic urogenital pain syndromes. Different underlying pathogenic mechanisms may require different pain treatment strategies for patients with chronic urogenital pain syndromes, and multiple pathogenic pain mechanisms may coexist in the same patient, requiring several different pain treatment strategies.

It is essential that all factors should be taken into account when managing patients with chronic urogenital pain syndromes. The clinical history, together with an examination and appropriate investigation, should not only encompass the physical factors but also put these into a psychosocial context, both to gain an understanding of the pain and to improve its management.

ACKNOWLEDGMENTS

Ursula Wesselmann is supported by NIH grants DK57315 (NIDDK), DK066641 (NIDDK), and HD39699 (NICHD, Office of Research for Women's Health).

REFERENCES

Abrams P, Cardozo L, Fall M, et al. The standardisation of terminology of lower urinary tract function: report from the Standardisation Sub-committee of the International Continence Society. *Neurourol Urodyn* 2002; 21:167–178.

ACOG Committee on Practice Bulletins—Gynecology. ACOG Practice Bulletin No. 51. Chronic pelvic pain. *Obstet Gynecol* 2004; 103:589–605.

Alagiri M, Chottiner S, Ratner V, et al. Interstitial cystitis: unexplained associations with other chronic disease and pain syndromes. *Urology* 1997; 49:52–57.

Asghari A, Nicholas MK. Pain self-efficacy beliefs and pain behaviour: a prospective study. *Pain* 2001; 94: 85–100.

Burnett AL, Wesselmann U. Neurobiology of the pelvis and perineum: principles for a practical approach. *J Pelvic Surgery* 1999; 5:224–232.

Cervero F, Laird JMA. Visceral pain. *Lancet* 1999; 353:2145–2148.

Cody RF, Ascher SM. Diagnostic value of radiological tests in chronic pelvic pain. *Best Pract Res Clin Obstet Gynaecol* 2000; 14:433–466.

Cornel EB, van Haarst EP, Schaarsberg RW, Geels J. The effect of biofeedback physical therapy in men with Chronic Pelvic Pain Syndrome Type III. *Eur Urology* 2005; 47:607–611.

Czakanski PP, Wesselmann U. Modulation of uterine pain by kappa-opioids. *Abstracts: 10th World Congress on Pain*. Seattle: IASP Press, 2002, p 288.

Czakanski PP, Wesselmann U. Environmental enrichment modulates pain behavior in an animal model of pelvic pain. *Abstracts: 11th World Congress on Pain*, Seattle: IASP Press, 2005, p 48.

Erickson DR, Morgan KC, Ordille S, et al. Nonbladder related symptoms in patients with interstitial cystitis. *J Urol* 2001; 166:557–561.

Fall M, Baranowski AP, Fowler CJ, et al. EAU guidelines on chronic pelvic pain. *Eur Urol* 2004; 46:681–689.

Gebhart GF. Descending modulation of pain. *Neurosci Biobehav Rev* 2004; 27:729–737.

Giamberardino MA, Vecchiet L. Experimental studies on pelvic pain. *Pain Rev* 1994; 1:102–115.

Glazer HI. Long term follow-up of dysesthetic vulvodynia patients after completion of successful treatment by surface electromyography assisted pelvic floor muscle rehabilitation. *J Reprod Med* 2000; 45:798–801.

Hanno P, Baranowski A, Fall M, et al. Painful ladder syndrome (including interstitial cystitis). In: Abrams P, Cardozo L, Khoury S, Wein A (Eds). *Management,* Incontinence, Vol. 2. Health Publications, 2005, pp 1455–1520.

Holley RL, Richter HE, Wang L. Neurologic disease presenting as chronic pelvic pain. *South Med J* 1999; 92:1105–1107.

Jonas U, Grunewald V (Eds). *New Perspectives in Sacral Nerve Stimulation for Control of Lower Urinary Tract Dysfunction.* Martin Dunitz, 2002.

Krieger JN, Nyberg L, Nickel JC. NIH Consensus definition and classification of prostatitis. *JAMA* 1999; 282:236–237.

Newton-John TRO. Psychological effects of chronic pain and their assessment in adults. In: Jensen T, Wilson PR, Rice ASC (Eds). *Chronic Pain,* Clinical Pain Management. Vol. 3. London: Arnold Press, 2002, pp 101–111.

Peters KM, Konstandt D. Sacral neuromodulation decreases narcotic requirements in refractory interstitial cystitis. *BJU Int* 2004; 93:777–779.

Roberts R, Labat JJ, Bensignor M, et al. Decompression and transposition of the pudendal nerve in pudendal neuralgia: a randomized controlled trial and long-term evaluation. *Eur Urol* 2005; 47:403–408.

Schwartz L, Edhe DM. Couples and chronic pain. In: Schmaling KB, Goldman Sher T (Eds). *The Psychology of Couples and Illness*. Washington, DC: American Psychological Association, 2000.

Sullivan MJL, Thorn B, Haythornthwaite JA, et al. Theoretical perspectives on the relation between catastrophizing and pain. *Clin J Pain* 2001; 17:52–64.

Turk DC, Meichenbaum D. A cognitive-behavioural approach to pain management. In: Wall PD, Melzack RM (Eds). *Textbook of Pain,* 3rd ed. Edinburgh: Churchill Livingstone, 1994, pp 1337–1348.

Wesselmann U. Interstitial cystitis: a chronic visceral pain syndrome. *Urology* 2001; 57:32–39.

Wesselmann U, Lai J. Mechanisms of referred visceral pain: uterine inflammation in the adult virgin rat results in neurogenic plasma extravasation in the skin. *Pain* 1997; 73:309–317.

Wesselmann U, Burnett AL, Heinberg LJ. The urogenital and rectal pain syndromes. *Pain* 1997; 73:269–294.

Wesselmann U, Czakanski PP, Affaitati G, et al. Uterine inflammation as a noxious visceral stimulus: behavioral characterization in the rat. *Neurosci Lett* 1998; 246:73–76.

Willis WD, Westlund KN. The role of the dorsal column pathway in visceral nociception. *Curr Pain Headache Rep* 2001; 5:20–26.

Correspondence to: Andrew Baranowski, MB BS, MD, FRCA, The Pain Management Centre, University College London Hospitals, NHS Foundation Trust, The National Hospital for Neurology and Neurosurgery, Queen Square, London WC1N 3BG, United Kingdom. Fax: 44-207-419-1714; email: andrew.baranowski@uclh.org.

Proceedings of the 11th World Congress on Pain,
edited by Herta Flor, Eija Kalso, and Jonathan O.
Dostrovsky, IASP Press, Seattle, © 2006.

60

Central Pain in Multiple Sclerosis: Clinical Characteristics and Sensory Abnormalities

Anders Österberg[a,b] and Jörgen Boivie[a]

*[a]Division of Neurology, Department of Neurosience and Locomotion,
Faculty of Health Science, University of Linköping, Linköping, Sweden;
[b]Department of Geriatrics, Motala Hospital, Motala, Sweden*

In older clinical descriptions of multiple sclerosis (MS), pain is hardly mentioned at all, with the exception of pain from optic neuritis, trigeminal neuralgia, painful tonic seizures, and possibly pain related to spasticity, reflecting the notion that pain rarely occurs in patients with this disorder. However, studies from the last 20 years have shown that pain is common in MS patients, with a prevalence of 50–85% (for references see Österberg et al. 2005). These recent studies recognized several pain conditions, but did not attempt a thorough differentiation between central neuropathic pain, peripheral neuropathic pain, and nociceptive pain. One or more of these types of pain may occur in a given patient.

This chapter describes a study designed to identify the various pain conditions in a large, unselected population of MS patients, with special emphasis on central pain, defined as pain caused by a lesion or dysfunction in the brain or spinal cord (Merskey and Bogduk 1994). Another aim was to identify the features of central pain in MS, such as its location, quality, intensity, and temporal pattern and the coexistence of other symptoms and signs.

In the best-studied central pain condition so far—central post-stroke pain (CPSP)—the pain is always accompanied by abnormal temperature and pain sensitivity. This finding forms the basis for the hypothesis that central pain develops only in patients who have lesions affecting the spinothalamocortical pathways (Boivie et al. 1989; Andersen et al. 1995; Vestergaard et al. 1995; Bowsher et al. 1998; Boivie 1999). We decided to test whether this hypothesis applies to central pain in MS. This chapter reports the results from the analysis of 364 patients, including the incidence of pain, the characteristics of central pain, and sensory abnormalities in patients with central pain.

PATIENTS AND METHODS

All patients with a diagnosis of definite MS in the patient register at our neurology department (429 patients) formed the basis for the study (66% women, 34% men). Patients were sent a questionnaire with 24 questions asking about pain and sensory symptoms experienced at the time they received the questionnaire and previously during the course of the disease; 371 patients replied, of whom 7 were excluded because of dementia, confusion, or psychiatric illness, thus replies from 364 patients were used in our analysis. Patients were asked to report all forms of pain, to describe the character, location, onset, and duration of the pain, and to indicate the location and quality of the pain on a pain map. All patients who reported pain were interviewed by telephone, and those with suspected central pain or with an unclear pain history were asked to come in for an examination and extended interview at the outpatient clinic.

The diagnosis of central pain was partly based on exclusion, and partly on specific criteria (Boivie 1999). Patients with back pain were not included due to difficulties in determining whether their pain was neuropathic or non-neuropathic. Clinical examination of patients suspected of having central pain included a detailed pain history including pain location, quality, time of onset, present and past time profile, intensity, and influence of physical activity. Patients also received a neurological examination, blood tests, and magnetic resonance imaging of the brain and spinal cord. Electroneurography of the median, peroneal, and sural nerves and quantitative sensory testing (QST) were performed, and pain intensity was assessed using a 0–100 visual analogue scale.

Examination of sensitivity was done using conventional clinical and quantitative methods. The clinical examination included tests for touch sensitivity by stroking with cotton wool and with a light pinprick and tests for cold sensitivity by applying the round surface of a tuning fork at room temperature. Tests were also performed for dermalaxia, in which the examiner wrote a number from 2 to 9 with his index finger on the dorsum of the patient's foot or hand and asked the patient to say which number he had written, and for kinesthesia.

In the quantitative sensory tests (QST), perception thresholds for vibration, touch, warmth, cold, cold pain, and heat pain were examined using the method of limits (Boivie et al. 1989). The tests were performed on standardized regions of the body, including the hands and feet, as well as one or more parts of the painful region. Threshold for vibration (cut-off limit 200 μm) was measured using a vibrometer (for references see Boivie et al. 1989). The threshold for touch was measured by von Frey filaments (10 mg–300 g, cut-off limit 300 g).

The quantitative assessment of sensitivity for temperature utilized a thermotesting apparatus (for references see Boivie et al. 1989). From a baseline
corresponding to the patient's skin temperature, the temperature was increased
or decreased at a rate of 1°C/second (with cut-off limits of 50.0° and 0°C). The
examination was made using the method of limits, using alternating warming
and cooling stimuli. In addition to the perception thresholds recorded, the difference between the thresholds for perception of warmth and cold was used as
a measure of sensitivity to innocuous temperature (Fruhstorfer et al. 1976). In
patients with severe loss of sensitivity, failure to respond to cut-off limits resulted in the cut-off limit being recorded as the threshold value. The thresholds
we recorded were compared with published material on thresholds for vibration,
warmth, and cold in healthy volunteers (for references see Boivie et al. 1989).

Perception thresholds normally are higher on the feet than on the hands. It
is not possible to pool the measurements from the hands and feet in an analysis
of possible differences between painful and nonpainful regions, due to the large
standard deviations. Thus a scale was required to grade the abnormalities of
the thresholds on the extremities. The following index values were used: 0 =
up to 50% of the normal threshold (NT); 1 = 50% to 200% of NT; 2 = >200%
to 500% of NT; 3 = >500% of NT, but not total loss; 4 = total loss. Statistical
tests used were Fisher's exact test and Student's t-test.

RESULTS

Valid replies were received from 364 patients (67% women, 33% men), i.e.,
86% of all patients. Two hundred and nine patients (58%) reported pain (other
than headache) during the course of their disease. The prevalence of various
pain conditions is presented in Table I.

Seventy-six patients had nociceptive pain, generally low back pain (58%)
or neck and shoulder pain (22%). The pain was ongoing in the majority (88%),
was constant, and had one pain quality (55%), and this quality was usually
aching (57%). Eight patients had peripheral neuropathic pain. Four of these
had nerve root pain, two had meralgia paresthetica, one had polyneuropathy
pain, and one had painful carpal tunnel syndrome. Only three patients had pain
directly related to uncontrolled muscle contraction (i.e., spasticity).

One hundred patients (27.5% of the 364 patients) currently had central pain,
and 86 patients (23.5%) had nontrigeminal central pain while 10 patients had
trigeminal neuralgia and 4 patients had both trigeminal and nontrigeminal pain.
The location, quality, temporal aspect, duration, and intensity of nontrigeminal
central pain in these patients are shown in Table II; examples of pain drawings
appear in Fig. 1. Eighteen patients (4.9%) had trigeminal neuralgia, and four
of these patients also had nontrigeminal central pain.

Table I
Demographic data of the pain population (364 patients), including number (and
percentage) of patients with various pain conditions, gender, age (in years), and
duration of pain and disease (in years)

Pain Condition	No. of Patients (% of All)	Percent Female/ Male	Mean Age (Range)	Mean Disease Duration (Range)	Mean Pain Duration (Range)
Central pain (excluding TN)	86 (23.6)	70/30	51 (25–79)	19 (2–43)	12 (<1–40)
Trigeminal neuralgia	18 (4.9)	72/28	60 (28–79)	30 (7–54)	11 (2–34)
Probable nontrigeminal CP	15 (4.1)	87/13	54 (32–77)	22 (7–46)	13 (3–46)
Peripheral neuropathic pain	8 (2.2)	87/13	57 (41–81)	21 (6–50)	12 (2–16)
Nociceptive pain	76 (20.9)	70/30	56 (24–88)	25 (<1–57)	–
Spasticity pain	3 (0.8)	33/66	57 (52–62)	22 (12–30)	14 (5–29)
Pain of uncertain origin	3 (0.8)	33/66	64 (55–78)	29 (23–34)	–

Abbreviations: CP = central pain; TN = trigeminal neuralgia.

Almost all patients (98% of those with nontrigeminal pain) had ongoing pain, mostly daily and constant, at the time of examination. Some patients had pain-free periods lasting from minutes to hours. The intensity of the pain was almost always constant, but it could vary for shorter or longer periods. One-fifth of the patients had an increase in pain during the afternoon or evening, or at night (resulting in insomnia or disturbed sleep). In other patients the pain was of greatest intensity in the morning. In 36% of the patients, physical activity such as walking increased the pain. Central pain was the first symptom of MS in five patients and preceded other symptoms by months to years. In 14% of all the MS patients with central pain, the pain began the same year as other MS symptoms. Among the other patients, the onset of pain commonly occurred within the first 5–10 years of their disease. As with other MS symptoms, central pain can be the only symptom or one of several symptoms in a relapse, as reported by three of our patients, and as previously reported by Clifford and Trotter (1984).

The most common neurological sign in patients with nontrigeminal central pain was sensory disturbance (97%), whereas paresis was found in 60% and ataxia in 38%. Sixty-two MS patients with nontrigeminal central pain and 16 MS patients with sensory symptoms but without pain (designated as controls) were examined with QST. All central pain patients except two had abnormal sensitivity for one or more of the modalities tested. Details of the results from the quantitative and clinical sensory examinations are presented in Table III.

Table II
Characteristics of pain in 86 MS patients with nontrigeminal central pain; figures are
given as percentages of patients

Location			Duration	
Uni (U)- versus bilateral (B)	U	B	<10 years	56
Upper extremity	16	15	10–20 years	27
Arm (hand excluded)	8	6	21–30 years	10
Hand (arm included)	8	5	>30 years	7
Hand (arm excluded)	0	5		
Trunk	13	20	*Temporal Aspects*	
Lower extremity	15	72	Onset before other symptoms	7
Leg (foot excluded)	7	26	Onset the same year as other symptoms	16
Foot (leg included)	8	38	Onset 1–5 years after other symptoms	35
Foot (leg excluded)	0	8	Onset 6–10 years after other symptoms	16
			Onset >10 years after other symptoms	26
Pain Qualities			Ongoing pain at examination	98
Superficial	22		Constant pain	62
Deep	27		Daily pain with pain-free periods	26
Superficial and deep	51			
			Intensity	
Aching	40		Constant intensity	42
Burning	40		Episodic increase	19
Pricking	24		Increased with time	7
Stabbing	15		Increased by physical activity	36
Smarting	13			
Squeezing	13		Highest intensity in the morning	4
Cutting	12		Highest intensity in the afternoon	3
Others	19		Highest intensity in the evening	12
			Highest intensity at night	4
One pain quality	18			
Two pain qualities	43		Pain intensity VAS (mean)	
Three pain qualities	22		Minimal: 20 (5–83)	
Four or more pain qualities	17		Maximal: 74 (10–100)	

Significant differences ($P < 0.05$–0.001) in sensitivity were found in the feet between regions with central pain and regions without pain for the difference in threshold between innocuous warmth and cold ("difference limen" in Table III) and for warmth, cold, and cold pain. In the comparisons based on the index values, which enabled a comparison between the lower and upper extremities, there were significant differences ($P < 0.001$) between regions with central pain and regions without central pain for the difference in threshold between innocuous warmth and cold ("difference limen"), and for heat pain and cold pain combined. To summarize, all patients except two (97%) had abnormal sensitivity to temperature and/or pain in the painful region, compared to 81% in the symptomatic region in the control group ($P < 0.05$).

Central pain patients (27%) and controls (44%) commonly experienced various kinds of nonpainful dysesthesias when stimulated with painful heat or cold. They usually reported pricking sensations or some other kind of unpleasant

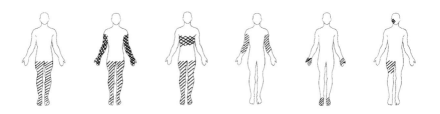

Fig. 1. Pain drawings showing examples of the location of nontrigeminal central pain in six patients with multiple sclerosis.

sensation. Pinprick was abnormally perceived in the painful region by 63% of the central pain patients and by 81% of the control patients (n.s). Eleven percent of the central pain patients reported dysesthesia or hyperalgesia to pinprick, compared to 25% of the controls (n.s).

QST for touch showed an increased threshold in 57% of the central pain patients vs. 69% of the controls (n.s), and the threshold was often more abnormal in the controls. In the clinical test, tactile hypoesthesia was seen in 66% of central pain patients vs. 87% of controls (n.s.), including 5% vs. 13% (n.s.), respectively, with allodynia.

DISCUSSION

The results from this study of 364 MS patients confirm and expand on previous knowledge, showing that central pain is common in MS. The finding of an overall prevalence for pain of 58% (other than headache) is of the same magnitude as in other studies published over the last 20 years (54–86%; for references see Österberg et al. 2005).

In this study the prevalence of definite central pain was 27.5%, including 4.9% with trigeminal neuralgia. There is reason to suspect that the figure for nontrigeminal central pain is higher, because we did not include patients with probable, but not definite, central pain, or patients with back pain, and it is possible that some of this pain was in fact central pain.

Half of the patients with central pain experienced their pain both superficially in the skin and in deeper parts of the body, and more than 80% experienced two or more pain qualities, a similar finding to that of Leijon et al. (1989) for CPSP. The most common qualities in both disease entities were burning and aching.

Central pain can be a presenting symptom in MS, as was found in 20% of our sample with central pain. Although there was a long interval between the clinical onset of MS and the onset of central pain (ranging from 7 years before

Table III
Perception thresholds in patients with nontrigeminal central pain (CP) and in controls

	Central Pain				Non-Central Pain					Controls with Sensory Symptoms				
	Mean	Median	SD	No.	Mean	Median	SD	No.	P	Mean	Median	SD	No.	P
Feet														
Warmth (°C)	43.3	43.5	5.7	96	38.7	36.9	4.3	96	<0.001	40.9	40.0	4.6	27	<0.05
Cold (°C)	15.5	20.5	13.5	96	21.2	26.4	11.8	96	<0.05	23.5	26.3	8.3	27	<0.01
Difference limen (°C)	27.7	23.5	17.0	96	17.5	11.6	14.7	96	<0.01	17.5	13.5	11.3	27	<0.01
Heat pain (°C)	46.9	47.9	3.4	96	46.1	47.2	3.3	96	0.3	47.3	48.1	2.3	27	0.6
Cold pain (°C)	6.3	0.0	9.0	96	12.5	14.0	9.3	96	<0.01	7.6	7.7	8.0	27	0.5
Touch (mg)	26230	2200	78091	96	1889	1100	1817	96	0.1	5446	2200	6887	25	0.2
Vibration (µg)	67.8	22.5	80.3	94	11.6	5.0	19.7	94	<0.001	61.2	30.0	64.5	27	0.7
Hands														
Warmth (°C)	33.7	33.0	2.7	31	33.4	33.2	2.2	93	0.5	31.9	31.6	2.2	15	<0.05
Cold (°C)	28.4	29.3	6.0	31	29.4	30.3	3.9	93	0.3	28.7	28.4	1.4	15	0.9
Difference limen (°C)	5.3	3.5	7.6	31	4.0	2.5	4.9	93	0.3	3.2	2.7	2.1	15	0.3
Heat pain (°C)	41.5	41.2	4.1	31	41.7	41.5	4.1	93	0.8	42.1	42.6	2.8	15	0.6
Cold pain (°C)	13.0	13.9	6.4	31	14.9	14.0	7.3	93	0.2	12.8	13.4	6.8	15	0.9
Touch (mg)	1547	730	3940	31	904	200	2175	31	0.3	1074	2200	21942	13	<0.05
Vibration (µg)	6.4	0.6	12.7	30	2.7	0.4	7.8	30	0.06	23.3	2.3	51.5	15	0.09
Extremities														
Difference limen (°C)	2.5	3.0	1.2	127	1.7	2.0	1.1	127	<0.001	2	2.0	0.8	42	<0.05 / <0.00
Heat pain/cold pain (°C)	1.1	1.0	1.0	127	0.4	0.0	0.8	127	<0.001	0.5	0.0	0.7	42	1
Touch (mg)	1.3	1.0	1.3	127	0.5	0.0	0.9	127	<0.001	1.4	2.0	1.3	38	0.7
Vibration (µg)	2.0	3.0	1.5	127	0.8	0.0	1.2	127	<0.001	2.4	3.0	1.4	42	0.1

Note: In the CP patients, the thresholds are listed for regions with CP and regions without CP. *P* values show the results of statistical tests of differences between these regions, and between the thresholds in the regions with CP and the thresholds in the controls (two-sample *t*-test). Difference limen is the difference in sensitivity to non-noxious cold vs. warmth.

to 25 years after other symptoms), in most patients central pain started within 5 years of the onset of the disease (57%).

Most central pain conditions appear to be truly chronic, frequently lasting the rest of the patient's life (Boivie 1999), and this also seems to be the case for MS patients with central pain. Long-term follow-up of patients with CPSP has shown that only in a small minority of patients does the pain gradually subside (Leijon and Boivie 1996). In only 12 of the MS patients in this study did the central pain disappear, and most of these had trigeminal neuralgia.

Central pain in MS was usually experienced daily, as reported by 88% of the patients, of whom only 30% had pain-free periods lasting minutes to hours. The intensity of the pain varied somewhat, but 44% of the patients experienced constant intensity, and for many, this situation had gone on for years.

In the most studied central pain condition, CPSP, the contralateral non-painful site has been used as a reference for sensitivity disturbances (Boivie et al. 1989; Andersen et al. 1995; Vestergaard et al. 1995). This strategy was not possible in the present study because many MS patients have bilateral pain, and thus the other side could not be used as a control.

The results from this study show that almost all MS patients with central pain have severe sensory abnormalities in the painful regions, dominated by disturbances in sensibility to temperature and pain. All but two patients with nontrigeminal central pain (97%) had abnormal thresholds for innocuous and/or noxious temperatures, compared to 81% in the control group ($P < 0.05$), whereas there was a tendency toward the opposite regarding sensitivity to touch, which was decreased in 66% vs. 87% (n.s.) and joint movement (32% vs. 62%; $P < 0.04$).

In comparisons of painful and nonpainful regions, both the absolute threshold values and the indexed values were significantly ($P < 0.05$–0.001) abnormal in the central pain regions for warmth, cold, difference between innocuous warmth and cold, cold pain, and heat pain/cold pain combined, but only in the lower extremities. There were also similar significant ($P < 0.05$–0.001) differences between central pain regions and regions with sensory symptoms in the controls for warmth, cold, the difference between innocuous warmth and cold, and heat pain/cold pain combined, in the lower extremities.

The results of this study concerning sensitivity to temperature in central pain regions are similar to those from corresponding investigations on patients with central pain due to other diseases, such as stroke (Boivie et al. 1989; Vestergaard et al. 1995) and spinal cord injury (Finnerup et al. 2003; Finnerup and Jensen 2004).

In a recently published study of the sensory abnormalities and pain in MS, Svendsen et al. (2005) found that all patients with central pain had signs of "spinothalamic dysfunctions" at the maximal pain site as examined with clinical methods. They also found that these patients had cold or mechanical allodynia and temporal summation more often than patients with musculoskeletal pain. In the 50 patients with mixed pains (musculoskeletal, central pain, and other types of pain), QST revealed that only the threshold for pressure pain was different from that among the patients without pain. Svendsen et al. also reported that in patients with central pain, the "detection or pain thresholds for temperature, tactile stimulation, vibration or pressure" were not different from those of patients with musculoskeletal pain. However, this sentence refers to examination "at the maximal pain site," which means that the values were obtained in different body regions including areas on the torso. Thus, the normal threshold values at the examined sites varied over a large range, which means that there is a large risk that one cannot show a significant difference unless large groups of patients are examined. It is therefore our conclusion that their results do not contradict our own, nor do they contradict our conclusion that the profile of sensory abnormalities in MS patients with nontrigeminal central pain supports the hypothesis that central pain only develops in patients who have lesions affecting the spinothalamocortical pathways.

SUMMARY

Central pain in MS is severe and causes the patient a great deal of suffering. At least 27.5% of MS patients have central pain, including trigeminal neuralgia (4.9%). Central pain, which may be the very first clinical manifestation of MS, tends to start early in the course of the disease and may be the only symptom of a relapse. Central pain in MS is mostly constant and long-lasting. Nontrigeminal central pain in MS may have any quality, but aching, burning, and pricking are the most common. Nontrigeminal central pain in MS is predominantly located in the lower extremities (87%). Nontrigeminal central pain can be extensive or restricted to a small area of the body; in MS this condition is accompanied by sensory abnormalities, dominated by decreased sensitivity to temperature and pain. MS patients with nontrigeminal central pain, like patients with CPSP, have sensory abnormalities indicating lesions affecting the spinothalamocortical pathways (temperature and pain sensitivity); these lesions affect the medial lemniscal pathways (touch, position sense, and vibration) to a lesser degree. These results support the hypothesis that among patients with MS, only those who have lesions affecting the spinothalamocortical pathways run the risk of developing central pain.

ACKNOWLEDGMENTS

The study was supported by grants from the County Council of Östergötland, the Swedish Medical Research Council (MFR), the Bank of Sweden Tercentenary Foundation, and the Swedish Association of Neurologically Disabled.

REFERENCES

Andersen G, Vestergaard K, Ingeman-Nielsen M, Jensen TS. Incidence of central post-stroke pain. *Pain* 1995; 61:187–193.

Boivie J. Central pain. In: Wall PD, Melzack R (Eds). *Textbook of Pain,* 4th ed. New York: Churchill Livingstone, 1999, pp 879–914.

Boivie J, Leijon G, Johansson I. Central post-stroke pain: a study of the mechanisms through analyses of the sensory abnormalities. *Pain* 1989; 37:173–185.

Bowsher D, Leijon G, Thuomas K-Å. Central poststroke pain: correlation of MRI with clinical pain characteristics and sensory abnormalities. *Neurology* 1998; 51:1352–1358.

Clifford DB, Trotter JL. Pain in multiple sclerosis. *Arch Neurol* 1984; 41:1270–1272.

Finnerup NB, Jensen TS. Spinal cord injury pain-mechanisms and treatment. *Eur J Neurol* 2004; 11:73–82.

Finnerup NB, Johannesen IL, Fuglsang-Frederiksen A, Bach FW, Jensen TS. Sensory function in spinal cord injury patients with and without central pain. *Brain* 2003; 126(Pt 1):57–70.

Fruhstorfer H, Lindblom U, Schmidt WC. Method for quantitative estimation of thermal thresholds in patients. *J Neurol Neurosurg Psychiatry* 1976; 39:1071–1075.

Leijon G, Boivie J. Central post-stroke pain (CPSP)—a long term follow up. In: *Abstracts: 8th World Congress on Pain.* Seattle: IASP Press, 1996, p 380.

Leijon G, Boivie J, Johansson I. Central post-stroke pain-neurological symptoms and pain characteristics. *Pain* 1989; 36(1):13–25.

Merskey H, Bogduk N. *Classification of Chronic Pain: Descriptions of Chronic Pain Syndromes and Definitions of Pain Terms,* 2nd ed. Seattle: IASP Press, 1994.

Osterberg A, Boivie J, Thuomas KA. Central pain in multiple sclerosis: prevalence and clinical characteristics. *Eur J Pain* 2005; 9:531–542.

Svendsen KB, Jensen TS, Hansen HJ, Bach FW. Sensory function and quality of life in patients with multiple sclerosis and pain. *Pain* 2005; 114:473–481.

Vestergaard K, Nielsen J, Andersen G, et al. Sensory abnormalities in consecutive, unselected patients with central post-stroke pain. *Pain* 1995; 61:177–186.

Correspondence to: Anders P. Osterberg, MD, Verkstadsvagen 16 A, Motala 591 37, Sweden. Email: anders.osterberg@lio.se.

Proceedings of the 11th World Congress on Pain,
edited by Herta Flor, Eija Kalso, and Jonathan O.
Dostrovsky, IASP Press, Seattle, © 2006.

61

Pathological Coupling between Afferent Nociceptive C Fibers and Sympathetic Nerve Fibers in a Patient with Sympathetically Maintained Pain

Ellen Jørum,[a] Kristin Ørstavik,[a] Roland Schmidt,[b]
Barbara Namer,[c] Richard W. Carr,[c] Gunnvald
Kvarstein,[d] Marita Hilliges,[e] Hermann Handwerker,[c]
Erik Torebjörk,[b] and Martin Schmelz[f]

*[a]Laboratory of Clinical Neurophysiology, Department of Neurology,
Rikshospitalet University Hospital, Oslo, Norway; [b]Department of Clinical
Neurophysiology, University Hospital, Uppsala, Sweden; [c]Department
of Physiology and Experimental Pathophysiology, University of Erlangen,
Nürnberg, Germany; [d]Department of Anesthesiology, Rikshospitalet University
Hospital, Oslo, Norway; [e]Department of Basic Oral Sciences, Karolinska
Institute, Huddinge, Sweden; [f]Department of Anesthesiology and Operative
Intensive Care, University of Heidelberg, Mannheim, Germany*

Sympathetically maintained pain (SMP) is present in many neuropathic pain disorders, but it is first and foremost associated with complex regional pain syndrome (CRPS). Despite the many questions related to the effect of sympathetic blockade (Verdugo and Ochoa 1994; Verdugo et al. 1994), the fact that some patients obtain pain relief indicates that the sympathetic nervous system is involved in the generation of pain. This assertion is supported by the fact that application of norepinephrine to the painful area of skin may exacerbate the pain (Wallin et al. 1976; Torebjörk et al. 1995; Ali et al. 2000). Sympathetic arousal may increase the pain in patients with CRPS (Drummond and Finch 2004), but the question still remains as to how sympathetic activity may affect the activity of afferent nociceptive neurons.

There is no evidence for increased sympathetic outflow in patients with CRPS (Wallin et al. 1976; Casale and Elam 1992). Studies have found no increase in the venous concentration of norepinephrine in the affected limb (Drummond et al. 1991) and no increase in reflex vasoconstrictor response in the sympathetic extremity (Christensen and Henriksen 1983; Rosen et al. 1988). Therefore, α-adrenergic receptor supersensitivity to catecholamines has been postulated as a likely mechanism for both the hyperalgesia and the autonomic disturbances associated with SMP (Raja 1995). Another hypothesis postulates a coupling of afferent and efferent axons via ephaptic interaction (McMahon 1991; Jänig et al. 1996). Specific sympathetic-sensory contacts suggesting functional interaction between sympathetic and sensory neurons have been observed both in vitro (Belenky and Devor 1997) and in vivo (Chen et al. 1996).

Previous microneurographic recordings in healthy volunteers have failed to show any coupling between activity in efferent sympathetic nerve fibers and activity in cutaneous afferents, including both unmyelinated C fibers (Elam et al. 1999) and myelinated A fibers (Elam and Macefield 2004). In this chapter we present data from single C-fiber recordings in a patient with SMP that show nociceptors being activated by endogenous catecholamine release and exogenous application of norepinephrine.

METHODS

Prior to the microneurography experiments, the patient was examined clinically with a special emphasis on the assessment of pain, including evaluation of areas of allodynia to light brush as well as to punctate hyperalgesia. Electromyography and neurography were also included. Measurement of thermal thresholds (heat detection, cold detection, and heat-pain detection thresholds) was performed on the dorsum of both feet with a Somedic thermotest. The method of microneurography employed in this study has been described in detail elsewhere (Schmidt et al. 1995).

THE "MARKING METHOD"

During iterative intracutaneous electrical stimulation at a constant frequency of 0.25 Hz for several minutes, the C-fiber responses stabilized at latencies characteristic for each unit. Even a single additional spike induced in a C fiber by a conditioning stimulus produces an increased delay of the subsequent electrically induced spike by about 1 ms (Schmelz et al. 1995). This "marking" technique is very useful to identify which C fiber in a multi-unit recording responds to a particular stimulus (Torebjörk and Hallin 1974b; Schmidt et al. 1995). In this study we used the "marking" technique to determine whether

C-fiber units were spontaneously active and to determine the responsiveness of afferent C nociceptors to mechanical and heat stimuli and the responsiveness of efferent sympathetic C-fiber units to reflex sympathetic activation.

ACTIVITY-DEPENDENT SLOWING

Activity-dependent slowing of conduction velocity is a well-known characteristic of unmyelinated nerve fibers. Thought to be due to prolonged changes in membrane potential that occur after impulse conduction (Torebjörk and Hallin 1974a), it can be used to differentiate functional subtypes of C fibers (Raymond et al. 1990; Thalhammer et al. 1994; Serra et al. 1999; Weidner et al. 1999, 2000; Bostock et al. 2003). It is much more pronounced for mechanoinsensitive C nociceptors than for mechanoresponsive ones in human skin, particularly at low stimulation frequencies (Weidner et al. 1999). This feature has been used to reliably separate these unit classes in healthy subjects.

In our study, after a rest period of at least 2 minutes, intracutaneous electrical stimuli were applied in a train consisting of 20 pulses at 0.125 Hz, immediately followed by a second train of 20 pulses at 0.25 Hz and a third train of 30 pulses at 0.5 Hz. The accumulated increase in conduction latency during the entire stimulation protocol was measured in milliseconds ("total slowing").

SYMPATHETIC PROVOCATION

Sympathetic units were identified by their responses to arousing stimuli, such as an unexpected loud noise, mental stress, or deep inhalation, which are known to elicit sympathetic reflexes in human skin nerves (Hallin and Torebjörk 1970; Hagbarth et al. 1972). The efficacy of these stimuli was controlled by recording the background activity of sympathetic burst discharges.

CHEMICAL STIMULATION

Ten microliters of norepinephrine (0.05% [0.3 mM] in saline) was injected intracutaneously in the innervation territory of identified C fibers. To test for afferent responses, low pH solution (phosphate buffer, pH 6) containing prostaglandin E_2 (10^{-6} M) was also injected in another part of the innervation territory. For both injections, the insertion of the cannula and the injection of the stimulating agent were separated by about 30 seconds to allow us to differentiate between the response to the mechanical stimulus of cannula insertion and a response to norepinephrine or low pH.

CLASSIFICATION OF C FIBERS

Signals from the recording electrodes were amplified and recorded on line by a personal computer using an interface card and SPIKE2 software. According to the receptive and reflex properties assessed as described above, C fibers were classified into three main classes: efferent sympathetic fibers, afferent mechanoresponsive fibers, and afferent mechanoinsensitive fibers (also called "sleeping nociceptors").

RESULTS

THE PATIENT

The patient was a 41-year-old male who developed a compartment syndrome in both legs following a 5-hour abdominal surgical operation in October 2002. The initial deep aching pain diminished over a period of 3 weeks, but a new burning, aching pain appeared that was located in both legs over a skin region from 12–15 cm above the ankle to the dorsum of the feet and the toes, within the innervation territory of the peroneal nerve. The pain varied spontaneously in intensity, but sometimes it would reach 10/10 on a visual analogue scale. After the initial phase there were no signs of edema, no trophic changes of the skin, and no skin discoloration. However, the patient did exhibit signs of autonomic dysfunction, evidenced by profuse sweating in both feet.

Electromyographic recordings confirmed minor damage to the deep peroneal nerve, with signs of reinnervation in muscles innervated by that nerve. Measurement of thermal thresholds revealed reduced sensibility to both heat and cold on the dorsum of both feet (heat detection threshold of 47.8° in the left and 45.8°C in the right foot), and the patient was unable to detect cold stimuli on either foot. Areas of allodynia to light brush and hyperalgesia to punctate stimuli are shown in Fig. 1. The patient responded to sympathetic blockade by 30 mg guanethidine diluted in 100 mg lidocaine.

MICRONEUROGRAPHY

In two sessions, a total of 19 C fibers (conduction velocity 0.82 ± 0.26 m/s; mean $\pm$ standard deviation) were recorded from the left and right peroneal nerve. According to their responses to mechanical and sympathetic provocations, eight units were classified as polymodal nociceptors, six as mechanoinsensitive nociceptors, and none as sympathetic efferent fibers. The response pattern of five fibers did not allow us to classify them definitively. The total slowing of conduction velocity in the electrical stimulation protocol was significantly less pronounced in mechanosensitive fibers (10.9 ± 3 ms) as compared to

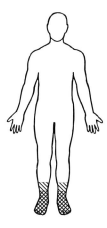

Fig. 1. Areas of allodynia to brush and punctate hyperalgesia. Areas of punctate hyperalgesia (hatched) and mechanical allodynia (cross-hatched) in both legs of the patient are depicted.

mechanoinsensitive nociceptors (34.6 ± 9.4 ms). The most pronounced separation was found at the lowest stimulation frequency of 0.125 Hz, which provoked a slowing of 0.5 ± 1.1 ms in mechanosensitive nociceptors, but 7.1 ± 2.0 ms in mechanoinsensitive fibers. No overlap between the two classes of nociceptors was found in their slowing behavior.

ACTIVATION OF AFFERENT FIBERS BY ENDOGENOUS CATECHOLAMINES

Two additional C fibers displaying the typical slowing behavior of mechanoinsensitive units were spontaneously active during the electrical protocol (Fig. 2). While the activity in one of these units was irregular, the other was activated only when the stimulation frequency was changed. Changes in stimulation frequency led to a pronounced increase of the number of sympathetic bursts. The patient was forewarned of changes in stimulation frequency, and this expectation may have increased the arousal response. The activation of the fiber was not directly correlated with the sympathetic burst, but had a delay of more than 4 seconds. In addition, the extent of the "marking" appeared to be related to the magnitude of the sympathetic burst. The unit was also activated by arousal stimuli.

ACTIVATION OF AFFERENT FIBERS BY EXOGENOUS CATECHOLAMINES

Intracutaneous injection of norepinephrine caused a burning pain sensation that lasted for about 2 minutes with a maximum pain rating of 3 on a numerical

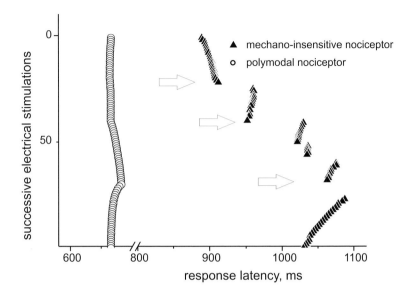

Fig. 2. Activation of afferent mechanoinsensitive C fibers by sympathetic arousal. Responses of two C fibers to repetitive electrical stimulation in their innervation territory on the foot dorsum. Action potentials of the units are symbolized by circles (polymodal nociceptor) and by triangles, respectively, for the mechanoinsensitive unit. Abrupt shifts in response latency ("marking") indicate spontaneous activity in the units. When stimulation frequency was switched (arrows), activation of the mechanoinsensitive unit occurred, combined with sympathetic arousal reactions.

scale (0 = "no pain"; 10 = "maximum pain"). The skin at the injection site was blanched within a circular area about 5 mm in diameter. The injection caused a massive response of the two spontaneously active units. However, it was difficult to determine whether the mechanosensitive nociceptor was also activated. The insertion of the needle produced an instantaneous response in the mechanosensitive unit, whereas the two spontaneously active fibers were activated following a delay of about 8 seconds, suggesting a chemical response rather than activation by the mechanical stimulus.

RESPONSE TO MECHANICAL STIMULATION

Mechanical stimulation with a von Frey filament (750 mN) readily activated the mechanosensitive nociceptor. One of the spontaneously active fibers did not respond at all to the stimulation, whereas the spontaneously active unit that had an initially longer conduction latency was activated by repetitive poking with the stiff filament (Fig. 3).

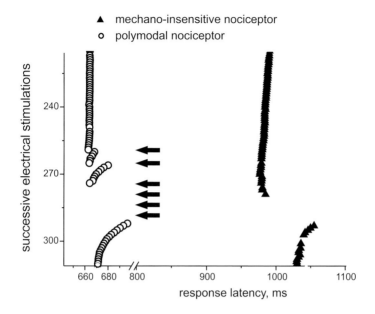

Fig. 3. Responses of two C fibers to repetitive electrical stimulation in their innervation territory on the foot dorsum. Action potentials of the units are symbolized by circles (polymodal nociceptor) and by triangles, respectively, for the mechanoinsensitive unit. Abrupt shifts in response latency ("marking") indicate activity in the units. Mechanical stimulation with a 750-mN von Frey filament (arrows) readily activates the early polymodal unit. The second fiber initially is not activated by these mechanical stimuli, but upon repetitive poking it also shows some activity, as indicated by the shift in response latency.

ACTIVATION BY LOW pH SOLUTION

Intracutaneous injection of a phosphate buffer solution at pH 6 containing prostaglandin E_2 caused a burning pain sensation that lasted about 30 seconds with a maximum pain rating of 5 on a numeric scale (0 = "no pain"; 10 = "maximum pain"). The injection caused a massive response in the two spontaneously active units, but it was difficult to determine whether the mechanosensitive nociceptor was activated. The heat threshold of the unit that initially had a longer conduction latency fell from 44°C to 39°C after the injection.

DISCUSSION

Sympathetically maintained pain is a common feature of neuropathic pain states such as CRPS. Activity of sympathetic efferents could affect the nociceptors either by direct coupling via ephaptic interaction (McMahon 1991; Jänig et al. 1996) or by chemical interaction of released catecholamines in the vicinity of sensitized nociceptors ("soft coupling"). While interruption of the sympathetic chain would interfere with both mechanisms, depletion of catecholamines would be expected to suppress soft coupling while leaving ephaptic coupling intact. Thus, from the reduction in persistent pain following catecholamine depletion (Raja et al. 1991), one might indirectly conclude that the coupling between sympathetic efferents and nociceptors in the periphery is dominated by catecholamine release rather than by ephaptic interactions.

There is ample evidence for norepinephrine-induced pain in patients with SMP (Wallin et al. 1976; Torebjork et al. 1995; Ali et al. 2000; Mailis-Gagnon and Bennett 2004), indicating that α_1 adrenergic receptors play a major role in mediating SMP. However, some evidence suggests that α_2 adrenergic receptors may be involved (Davis et al. 1991). Sensitization of nociceptors to catecholamines has been shown in single-fiber recordings during inflammation (Sato et al. 1993) and following partial nerve injury (Sato and Perl 1991; O'Halloran and Perl 1997; Lee et al. 1999; Moon et al. 1999) in animal models. In humans, catecholamines induce acute heat hyperalgesia, but not mechanical hyperalgesia, when injected intracutaneously in healthy volunteers (Fuchs et al. 2001). Moreover, in healthy skin, catecholamines do not generate an axon reflex erythema (Zahn et al. 2004). Release of endogenous catecholamines does not affect the firing behavior of either cutaneous C nociceptors (Elam et al. 1999) or Aβ mechanoreceptors (Elam and Macefield 2004), as has been shown with single-fiber recordings in humans. Thus, under normal conditions, activation of catecholamine receptors on nociceptors will not generate excitation or mechanical sensitization in humans.

Human data on neuronal changes under conditions of sympathetically maintained pain are sparse. Histological examination reveals no gross structural changes in skin innervation (Drummond et al. 1996), and functional changes have been difficult to measure. Microneurographic recordings of mass activity in the sympathetic nervous system did not provide any evidence for increased sympathetic activity (Casale and Elam 1992). Our current results are based on the recent refinement of microneurographic techniques, including the discovery of specific patterns of activity-dependent slowing in different C-fiber classes in humans (Serra et al. 1999; Weidner et al. 1999, 2000; Bostock et al. 2003; Serra et al. 2004). Activity-dependent slowing can be used as an independent criterion for classification of nociceptor classes, and it is of particular importance under pathophysiological conditions (Orstavik et al. 2003). Although the number of mechanoinsensitive units being activated by endogenous and exogenous catecholamines is small, the present results are of principal importance showing for the first time in human a pathological coupling between the sympathetic nervous system and afferent nociceptive C fibers.

CONCLUSION

In patients with SMP, C fibers, identified as nociceptors by their response to heat and sensitization, by their extensive activity-dependent slowing of conduction velocity, and by their long-lasting response to low pH solution, become activated following sympathetic bursts. The delay between the sympathetic bursts and the activity, however, lasted for several seconds. This delay clearly speaks against a direct axonal coupling between the sympathetic efferent fibers and the nociceptors. More probably, it reflects the time needed for the release of norepinephrine from sympathetic efferents and for its diffusion and binding to catecholamine receptors on the nociceptors. This interpretation is supported by the observation of long-lasting activation in two units in response to exogenous norepinephrine.

ACKNOWLEDGMENTS

This work was supported by the Norwegian Research Council through a PhD fellowship to Dr. K. Ørstavik, by the Swedish Research Council K2005-04x-15300-01A, and by the Deutsche Forschungsgemeinschaft (Clinical Research Unit 107).

REFERENCES

Ali Z, Raja SN, Wesselmann U, et al. Intradermal injection of norepinephrine evokes pain in patients with sympathetically maintained pain. *Pain* 2000; 88:161–168.

Belenky M, Devor M. Association of postganglionic sympathetic neurons with primary afferents in sympathetic-sensory co-cultures. *J Neurocytol* 1997; 26:715–731.

Bostock H, Campero M, Serra J, Ochoa J. Velocity recovery cycles of C fibres innervating human skin. *J Physiol* 2003; 553:649–663.

Casale R, Elam M. Normal sympathetic nerve activity in a reflex sympathetic dystrophy with marked skin vasoconstriction. *J Auton Nerv Syst* 1992; 41:215–219.

Chen Y, Michaelis M, Jänig W, Devor M. Adrenoreceptor subtype mediating sympathetic-sensory coupling in injured sensory neurons. *J Neurophysiol* 1996; 76:3721–3730.

Christensen K, Henriksen O. The reflex sympathetic dystrophy syndrome. An experimental study of sympathetic reflex control of subcutaneous blood flow in the hand. *Scand J Rheumatol* 1983; 12:263–267.

Davis KD, Treede RD, Raja SN, Meyer RA, Campbell JN. Topical application of clonidine relieves hyperalgesia in patients with sympathetically maintained pain. *Pain* 1991; 47:309–317.

Drummond PD, Finch PM. Persistence of pain induced by startle and forehead cooling after sympathetic blockade in patients with complex regional pain syndrome. *J Neurol Neurosurg Psychiatry* 2004; 75:98–102.

Drummond PD, Finch PM, Smythe GA. Reflex sympathetic dystrophy: the significance of differing plasma catecholamine concentrations in affected and unaffected limbs. *Brain* 1991; 114:2025–2036.

Drummond PD, Finch PM, Gibbins I. Innervation of hyperalgesic skin in patients with complex regional pain syndrome. *Clin J Pain* 1996; 12:222–231.

Elam M, Macefield VG. Does sympathetic nerve discharge affect the firing of myelinated cutaneous afferents in humans? *Auton Neurosci* 2004; 111:116–126.

Elam M, Olausson B, Skarphedinsson JO, Wallin BG. Does sympathetic nerve discharge affect the firing of polymodal C-fibre afferents in humans? *Brain* 1999; 122:2237–2244.

Fuchs PN, Meyer RA, Raja SN. Heat, but not mechanical hyperalgesia, following adrenergic injections in normal human skin. *Pain* 2001; 90:15–23.

Hagbarth KE, Hallin RG, Hongell A, Torebjörk HE, Wallin BG. General characteristics of sympathetic activity in human skin nerves. *Acta Physiol Scand* 1972; 84:164–176.

Hallin RG, Torebjörk HE. Afferent and efferent C units recorded from human skin nerves in situ. A preliminary report. *Acta Soc Med Ups* 1970; 75:277–281.

Jänig W, Levine JD, Michaelis M. Interactions of sympathetic and primary afferent neurons following nerve injury and tissue trauma. *Prog Brain Res* 1996; 113:161–184.

Lee DH, Liu X, Kim HT, Chung K, Chung JM. Receptor subtype mediating the adrenergic sensitivity of pain behavior and ectopic discharges in neuropathic Lewis rats. *J Neurophysiol* 1999; 81:2226–2233.

Mailis-Gagnon A, Bennett GJ. Abnormal contralateral pain responses from an intradermal injection of phenylephrine in a subset of patients with complex regional pain syndrome (CRPS). *Pain* 2004; 111:378–384.

McMahon SB. Mechanisms of sympathetic pain. *Br Med Bull* 1991; 47:584–600.

Moon DE, Lee DH, Han HC, et al. Adrenergic sensitivity of the sensory receptors modulating mechanical allodynia in a rat neuropathic pain model. *Pain* 1999; 80:589–595.

O'Halloran KD, Perl ER. Effects of partial nerve injury on the responses of C-fiber polymodal nociceptors to adrenergic agonists. *Brain Res* 1997; 759:233–240.

Orstavik K, Weidner C, Schmidt R, et al. Pathological C-fibres in patients with a chronic painful condition. *Brain* 2003; 126:567–578.

Raja SN. Role of the sympathetic nervous system in acute pain and inflammation. *Ann Med* 1995; 27:241–246.

Raja SN, Treede RD, Davis KD, Campbell JN. Systemic alpha adrenergic blockade with phentolamine a diagnostic test for sympathetically maintained pain. *Anesthesiology* 1991; 74:691–698.

Raymond SA, Thalhammer JG, Popitz BF, Strichartz GR. Changes in axonal impulse conduction correlate with sensory modality in primary afferent fibers in the rat. *Brain Res* 1990; 526:318–321.

Rosen L, Ostergren J, Fagrell B, Stranden E. Skin microvascular circulation in the sympathetic dystrophies evaluated by videophotometric capillaroscopy and laser Doppler fluxmetry. *Eur J Clin Invest* 1988; 18:305–308.

Sato J, Perl ER. Adrenergic excitation of cutaneous pain receptors induced by peripheral nerve injury. *Science* 1991; 251:1608–1610.

Sato J, Suzuki S, Iseki T, Kumazawa T. Adrenergic excitation of cutaneous nociceptors in chronically inflamed rats. *Neurosci Lett* 1993; 164:225–228.

Schmelz M, Forster C, Schmidt R, et al. Delayed responses to electrical stimuli reflect C-fiber responsiveness in human microneurography. *Exp Brain Res* 1995; 104:331–336.

Schmidt R, Schmelz M, Forster C, et al. Novel classes of responsive and unresponsive C nociceptors in human skin. *J Neurosci* 1995; 15:333–341.

Serra J, Campero M, Ochoa J, Bostock H. Activity-dependent slowing of conduction differentiates functional subtypes of C fibres innervating human skin. *J Physiol* 1999; 515:799–811.

Serra J, Campero M, Bostock H, Ochoa J. Two types of C nociceptors in human skin and their behaviour in areas of capsaicin-induced secondary hyperalgesia. *J Neurophysiol* 2004; 91:2770–2781.

Thalhammer JG, Raymond SA, Popitz Bergez FA, Strichartz GR. Modality-dependent modulation of conduction by impulse activity in functionally characterized single cutaneous afferents in the rat. *Somatosens Mot Res* 1994; 11:243–257.

Torebjörk HE, Hallin RG. Identification of afferent C units in intact human skin nerves. *Brain Res* 1974a; 67:387–403.

Torebjörk HE, Hallin RG. Responses in human A and C fibres to repeated electrical intradermal stimulation. *J Neurol Neurosurg Psychiatry* 1974b; 37:653–664.

Torebjörk HE, Wahren L, Wallin G, Hallin R, Koltzenburg M. Noradrenaline-evoked pain in neuralgia. *Pain* 1995; 63:11–20.

Verdugo RJ, Ochoa JL. 'Sympathetically maintained pain.' I. Phentolamine block questions the concept. *Neurology* 1994; 44:1003–1010.

Verdugo RJ, Campero M, Ochoa JL. Phentolamine sympathetic block in painful polyneuropathies. II. Further questioning of the concept of 'sympathetically maintained pain'. *Neurology* 1994; 44:1010–1014.

Wallin BG, Torebjörk HE, Hallin RG. Preliminary observations on the pathophysiology of hyperalgesia in the causalgic pain syndrome. In: Zotterman Y (Ed). *Sensory Functions of the Skin*. New York: Pergamon Press, 1976, pp 489–499.

Weidner C, Schmelz M, Schmidt R, et al. Functional attributes discriminating mechano-insensitive and mechano-responsive C nociceptors in human skin. *J Neurosci* 1999; 19:10184–10190.

Weidner C, Schmidt R, Schmelz M, et al. Time course of post-excitatory effects separates afferent human C fibre classes. *J Physiol* 2000; 527:185–191.

Zahn S, Leis S, Schick C, Schmelz M, Birklein F. No alpha-adrenoreceptor-induced C-fiber activation in healthy human skin. *J Appl Physiol* 2004; 96:1380–1384.

Correspondence to: Ellen Jørum, MD, PhD, Laboratory of Clinical Neurophysiology, Rikshospitalet, Sognsvannsveien 20, 0027 Oslo, Norway. Email: ellen.jorum@rikshospitalet.no.

Part VIII

Pain Assessment and Outcome Measurement

Proceedings of the 11th World Congress on Pain,
edited by Herta Flor, Eija Kalso, and Jonathan O.
Dostrovsky, IASP Press, Seattle, © 2006.

62

Challenges of Pain Measurement in Vulnerable Populations

Bonnie J. Stevens

*The University of Toronto Centre for the Study of Pain,
Toronto, Ontario, Canada*

Current definitions of pain suggest that self-report is the gold standard for pain assessment for those capable of communication, with behavioral and physiological indicators being acceptable proxies if the individual is incapable of self-report (Merskey and Bogduk 1994; IASP Task Force on Taxonomy 2006). Although this stance provides validity for incorporating these pain indicators into pain measurement, it is not ideal, because indicators such as those obtained through behavioral observation are subject to factors associated with the observer, the individual being observed, and the environment in which the behavior is occurring. Observer factors include knowledge, attitudes and beliefs concerning pain in a particular population, and availability of resources such as sufficient time to assess the patient and access to interventions. Individual characteristics such as age, severity of illness, or level of neurological or cognitive development also require consideration, as do environmental factors including the physical setting or the organizational climate in which pain is experienced. Individuals who are incapable of self-report—whether due to developmental immaturity or deterioration or due to neurological, cognitive, physiological, or pharmacological impairment—are thus more vulnerable to pain than those who can engage in verbal report and therefore are more at risk for the consequences of unrelieved pain. This chapter explores the concept of vulnerability and defines populations that are vulnerable in terms of pain assessment. A critical review of pain measures for these populations will provide the background for addressing existing pain measurement challenges and determining future directions.

VULNERABILITY AND VULNERABLE POPULATIONS

Vulnerability implies a weakness that renders a system open to an external stressor that could be injurious or undesirable. Vulnerable, from the Latin *vulnerare*, means to wound or to be easily wounded or injured. "At risk," from the epidemiological literature, refers to those persons who experience a biological event that can impair their health. The factors associated with risk can be fixed and unalterable such as gender or age, or they may be acquired, such as exposure to a toxin, disease, or injury. Vulnerability to such risk can be defined as a varying state of weakness or strength that can modify risk responses (Leffers et al. 2004).

Flaskerud and Winslow (1998) have conceptualized vulnerability as the interplay among resource availability, relative risk, and health status. "Resource availability" refers to the availability of socioeconomic and environmental resources; "relative risk" is the ratio of risk of poor outcome in groups exposed to risk factors and not receiving resources compared to that of groups who do receive such resources; and "health status" is measured by disease prevalence and by morbidity and mortality rates. This conceptualization may also serve as a framework for considering how pain assessment (as a health care resource) might modify the vulnerability (as a result of exposure to noxious stimuli) of populations such as infants, children with neurological or cognitive impairments, and the elderly with dementia, and thus might affect their health outcomes. The complexity of the health care environment and the potential for altered physical and behavioral responses or adverse neurological sequelae must be considered along with exposure to pain and the inherent vulnerability of the specific population.

Vulnerability varies greatly with context. In the human context, we could consider those populations who cannot engage in self-report for a variety of reasons as vulnerable and at risk. Specifically, they are vulnerable because they must rely on others to assess their pain, advocate for effective pain management interventions, safely implement those interventions, and appropriately evaluate their effectiveness. Pain assessment involves complex measurement processes. However, as assessment is the cornerstone for effective advocacy and pain management, it is the crucial first step to ensuring the highest quality of care for these individuals and thus warrants careful scrutiny. When this rationale is used to conceptualize vulnerability, pain in infants, the elderly, and those individuals with neurological or cognitive impairments will be addressed in terms of the adequacy of pain assessment measures. As infant pain assessment has progressed substantially in the past 15 years and many lessons have been learned, it will serve as a template for addressing pain measurement issues in other vulnerable populations.

PAIN IN INFANTS

CAPACITY FOR PAIN

The notion of capacity for pain in the human neonate is in constant flux due to the ever-decreasing age of viability, such that we now need to consider the capacity for pain in those born at very low birth weight/gestational age (<1500 g; 29–32 weeks; VLBW/GA) or even at extremely low birth weight/gestational age (<1000 g; ≤28 weeks; ELBW/GA) (Bakewell-Sachs and Blackburn 2001). What we have learned concerning capacity for pain in the extra-uterine environment is now being applied to the fetal environment, where the issue of conscious awareness and the ability to experience pain prior to birth is currently under scrutiny (Mellor et al. 2005).

There has been substantial focus on the development of nociceptive pathways at the peripheral and spinal level, the balancing of inhibitory and excitatory synaptic transmission in developing pain pathways, and the short- and long-term effects of early tissue damage on the developing nervous system (Fitzgerald 2005). Pain responses in VLBW, and especially ELBW, preterm infants are thought to be largely subcortical, with functional maturation of higher brain centers being required to produce a pain experience (Fitzgerald 2005).

In VLBW and ELBW neonates, cells in the dorsal horn are more excitable than in more mature infants. Inhibition is weak and immature and therefore "may not modulate excitatory inputs with precision" (Fitzgerald 2005, p. 14). Cutaneous receptive fields of dorsal horn cells are enlarged (Torsney and Fitzgerald 2002) and are subject to prolonged hypersensitivity following early skin injury, with a greater number of third-order dorsal horn neurons being activated by a given stimulus. The result is reduced spatial discrimination and increased input to and reduced thresholds of tertiary cells such as motor neurons and thalamic neurons. Expanded receptive fields can contribute to enhanced sensitivity and lower behavioral thresholds such that previously ineffective or subthreshold input at the motor neuron or thalamic level may now be capable of evoking reflex behavior or activating nociceptive neurons to noxious mechanical stimulation such as heel lance. The most immature infants have the lowest thresholds and display widespread reflex responses at the spinal level, thus reflecting the lack of balance between excitatory and inhibitory synaptic transmission in the immature nervous system (Fitzgerald 2005).

INFANT PAIN RESPONSES

Spinal responses such as cutaneous reflex responses have consistently been shown to decrease with age (Saito 1979) and with repeated stimulation (Andrews and Fitzgerald 1994, 1999; Andrews et al. 2002), making them less useful indicators of pain over time. However, Fitzgerald (2005) has indicated that cortical responses increase with age; thus, these responses are important to consider as future pain indicators. The most important caveat with very premature infants is that noxious information is processed by a spinal cord and cortex within a system in constant change and development.

Behavioral responses including facial actions and expression, body movements, and crying currently represent the mainstays of acute pain assessment in neonates and young infants. Early infant behavioral assessment research by Grunau and Craig (1987), through the development of the Neonatal Facial Coding Scale, clearly articulated 10 individual neonatal facial actions associated with pain in healthy preterm infants. The majority of validated infant pain measures now comprise multidimensional behavioral indicators or a composite of behavioral and physiological indicators. Only a few researchers have examined the validity of these indicators of pain in ELBW infants. Grunau and colleagues have suggested that in ELBW neonates, flexing and extending of the extremities, finger splaying, fisting, and mouthing are movements consistent with pain, while startles, twitches, jitters, and tremors are not associated with pain (Grunau et al. 2000; Holsti et al. 2004). The context in which noxious stimulation occurs, such as gestational age, experience with painful procedures in the neonatal intensive care unit, and severity of illness, should be carefully considered because it will provide additional clues to account for exaggerated or diminished responses demonstrated by the most vulnerable infants.

EXISTING INFANT PAIN MEASURES

More than three dozen multidimensional behavioral and composite infant pain measures have been published (Duhn and Medves 2004). However, only a few measures take context into account or have well-established psychometric properties (i.e., reliability and validity) and clinimetric properties (i.e., feasibility and clinical utility; Stevens and Gibbins 2002) (see Table I). Many other infant pain measures are reconstitutions of existing indicators, and frequently they have limited psychometric properties, thus adding little to exploring new ways of assessing pain in vulnerable infants. A few recently developed measures with additional or novel configurations of indicators have demonstrated some initial or limited psychometric properties (e.g., Hudson-Barr et al. 2002; Puchalski and Hummel 2002; Guinsburg et al. 2003; Suominen et al. 2004) and hold promise in furthering measurement approaches in infants.

PHYSIOLOGICAL INDICATORS AND BIOMARKERS

There are now novel insights into the use of physiological indicators and biomarkers in the measurement of pain in vulnerable infants (Oberlander et al. 1999, 2000; Grunau et al. 2001a,b). Physiological responses to a painful event should be accepted as evidence of pain reactivity, not simply as a "surrogate measure" of pain in infants (Anand and Craig 1996). Whether the response is specific to pain or stress continues to be debated, although hospitalized neonates are likely to be exposed repeatedly to both. Crucial information is gleaned about the infant's capacity to mount and regulate a response following a painful event. In this sense, "pain biomarkers" can be regarded as measuring reactivity rather than as a direct measure of "infant pain."

"Biomarkers of pain" can be defined as a response or physiological process that reflects one or more systems that respond to a painful event (see reviews by Goldman and Koren 2002; Oberlander and Saul 2002). Within the context of pain, reactivity occurs at multiple levels of a highly diverse physiological system that includes central and peripheral neurons, neurotransmitters, genes, inflammatory mediators, "wound hormones" such as cortisol, β-endorphins, and growth hormone. Pain biomarkers can be characterized by cellular, molecular, and physiological pain processes and by generalized stress responses.

Biomarkers can be utilized as outcome measures (e.g., to quantify the effect of an analgesic intervention), as predictors of health and development, and as probes of the integrity of the central nervous system. Ideally, the biomarker should be a meaningful biological signal that reflects some component of the stress or pain system. Measures of the autonomic nervous system function are well suited biomarkers. Specific measures of autonomic function can be derived from heart rate, and those variations that are linked to respiratory patterns (vagal tone), thus making it one of the most commonly used autonomic biomarkers. Salivary cortisol has also been widely used as a biomarker of acute stress/pain responses of the hypothalamic- pituitary-adrenal system (Walker et al. 2000). Understanding the cumulative impact of stress in the neonatal intensive care unit may be advanced by using a more definitive biological marker such as hair cortisol (Yamada et al. 2003).

While biomarkers may be appealing as they are readily and inexpensively obtained, their use as measurable and identifiable indicators is frequently challenging. As with behavioral indicators, consideration of the context in which they are measured needs to be taken. For example, neurological compromise from birth asphyxia and intraventricular hemorrhage reduces heart rate variability (HRV) (Prietsch et al. 1994). The administration of opioid analgesics, conceptual age, and postnatal maturation may also influence biomarker response to a painful stimulus. Typically, mean heart rate among term born infants increases

Table I
Validated multidimensional behavioral and composite infant pain measures

Measure	Age Level	Scale Type/Indicators	Psychometric and Clinimetric Properties
Neonatal Facial Coding System (Grunau and Craig 1987)	Preterm infants >25 weeks GA to term infants	Multidimensional behavioral scale: Brow bulge, eye squeeze, nasolabial furrow, open lips, horizontal and vertical mouth stretch, lips pursed, taut tongue, chin quiver, tongue protrusion	Interrater reliability, $r = 0.88$ Intrarater reliability, $r = 0.88$ Content validity Face validity Construct validity Convergent validity Feasibility
Douleur Aigue du Nouveau-né (DAN; Carbajal et al. 1997, 2005)	25 weeks GA: full-term newborns	Multidimensional behavioral scale: facial expression, limb movement, vocalizations/attempts at vocalizations	Internal consistency, $r = 0.88$ Interrater reliability, $r = 0.91$ Content validity Convergent and divergent validity across pain management conditions and pain conditions, $P = 0.004–0.0001$
Echelle Douleur Inconfort Nouveau-Né (EDIN; Debillon et al 2001)	26–36 weeks GA	Multidimensional behavioral scale: Facial expression, movement, sleep, consolability	Interrater reliability, $r = 0.59–0.74$ Intrarater reliability Content validity Construct validity, $P < 0.0001$
Liverpool Infant Distress Scale (LIDS; Horgan and Choonara 1996; Horgan et al. 2002)	Neonates	Multidimensional behavioral scale: Facial expression, sleep pattern, cry quantity, cry quality, spontaneous movement, spontaneous excitability, flexion of fingers and toes, tone	Internal consistency, $r = 0.84–0.94$ Interrater reliability, $r = 0.74–0.88$ Intrarater reliability, $r = 0.81–0.96$ Content validity Discriminant validity, $P = 0.004–0.0000$

Instrument	Population	Components	Psychometric Properties
Pain Assessment Tool (PAT, Hodgkinson et al. 1994; Spence et al. 2005)	27 weeks to full-term neonates	Composite scale: Posture/tone, sleep pattern, expression, color, crying, respirations, heart rate, oxygen saturation, blood pressure, nurse perception	Interrater reliability, $r = 0.85$ Content validity Convergent validity, $r = 0.38$ Concurrent validity, $r = 0.76$
Crying, Requires increased oxygen, Increased vital signs, Expression, Sleeplessness (CRIES, Krechel and Bildner 1995)	Neonates 32–60 weeks	Composite scale: Crying, requires increased oxygen, increased vital signs, expression, sleeplessness	Inter-rater reliability, $r = 0.72$ Content validity Concurrent validity, $r = 0.49$–0.73 Discriminant validity, $P < 0.0001$ Concurrent validity for first 24 hours (ICC = 0.34–0.65; McNair et al. 2004)
Premature Infant Pain Profile (PIPP, Stevens et al. 1996; Ballantyne et al. 1999; McNair et al. 2003; Schiller et al. 2003)	Term and preterm neonates	Composite scale: Gestational age, behavioral state, heart rate, oxygen saturation, brow bulge, eye squeeze, nasolabial furrow	Inter-rater reliability (ICC = 0.93–0.96) Intra-rater reliability (ICC = 0.94–0.98) Internal consistency ($\alpha = 0.59$–0.76) Content validity Construct validity in preterm neonates, $P = 0.0001$–0.02; in term neonates, $P < 0.02$ Construct validity in clinical setting, $P < 0.0001$. Concurrent validity with crying Feasibility Clinical utility

Abbreviations: GA = gestational age; ICC = intraclass correlation coefficient.

to a maximum in the first 2 months of life and then decreases through infancy (Doussard-Roosevelt et al. 1997). In contrast, HRV undergoes opposite changes, and after the first 2 months of life it is generally positively correlated with age (Massin and von Bernuth 1997). In preterm infants, HRV increases with age but remains lower at term compared with term-born infants, suggesting continued maturational delay (Porges 1992). Maximum heart rate response to a heel lance in infants born at 28 weeks GA, but studied at 4 weeks of extra-uterine life, was higher when compared with infants born at 32 weeks GA (Johnston and Stevens 1996). Craig et al. (1993), in preterm infants from 25–27 weeks to term, also reported increasing heart rate responses to heel lance with increasing gestational age. In contrast, Johnston et al. (1996) reported no differences in maximum heart rate to painful events among infants born at 28 weeks GA studied at 2-week intervals over the succeeding 8 weeks of life.

While multiple biomarkers are readily available for use in studies of neonatal pain reactivity, no single biomarker characterizes all aspects of neonatal pain, and there is little research to suggest how well the available biomarkers correlate with clinical pain scales. The pain system has complex interrelationships with other reactivity systems, and it remains impossible to make any conclusion based on only one system. Contexts vary and may influence a marker to "behave" differently under different contextual and illness conditions. Questions about how to quantify the acute response and regulation of that response and how to use biomarkers modeled as outcome measures or developmental probes must be addressed by investigators studying pain and developmental outcomes of vulnerable neonates.

LESSONS LEARNED FROM MEASUREMENT OF PAIN IN INFANTS

We have gained much from human and animal research to further our understanding of the developmental neurobiology, behavior, and physiology of infant pain responses. This understanding provides a strong basis for developing infant pain measures, yet this trajectory has been challenging. Lessons learned could strengthen assessment of pain in infants as well as in other vulnerable populations. Most notably, there has been an overproliferation of invalidated or poorly validated pain measures in infants. Recommendations to further validate or adapt existing measures often go unheeded, and new measures are developed, even though several valid and reliable measures exist. The most valid measures are those that have received considerable attention to establishing psychometric and clinimetric properties. However, within the validation process, content and face validity, inter-rater reliability, and feasibility are frequently overemphasized, with internal consistency, construct validity, and clinical utility often being discounted. The most neglected property is clinical utility. Clinically useful infant pain measures provide the user with the information to plan, implement, and evaluate pain interventions and services. Clinical utility ensures that the needs of a particular infant, in a particular circumstance and setting, are met. Clinical utility differs from feasibility, where the reliability and validity of the measure are considered in light of whether the care provider can apply the measure effectively and efficiently at the bedside. Validity ensures that the score on the measure is truly measuring the construct pain, while reliability is the extent to which the true score is represented in the measured score. Feasibility involves evaluating the length of time for measure completion, the simplicity of scoring and interpretation, cost, format, and training time (Stevens and Gibbins 2002). Schiller (1999) evaluated the clinical utility of the Premature Infant Pain Profile (PIPP; Stevens et al. 1996) and the CRIES (an acronym for Crying, Requires increased oxygen, Increased vital signs, Expression, Sleeplessness; Krechel and Bildner 1995) with regard to time, cost, instructions, acceptability, and format. Both measures were rated as clinically useful, although the CRIES rated higher on completion time and cost while the PIPP rated higher on acceptability.

Although many validated infant pain measures are multidimensional, they comprise a limited cadre of behavioral and physiological indicators with little imaginative exploration for novel markers or indices of infant pain. As our understanding of the neurobiology of pain increases, new clues to indicators reflecting both spinal and cortical responses may be possible. Furthermore, very few measures consider the context of the pain experience. Factors associated with the infant (e.g., conceptual or gestational age, maturational status, risk of impairment, and severity of illness), the observer (e.g., attitudes and beliefs toward pain), and the environment (e.g., time and measures available to measure pain) influence individual pain indicators, measures, and approaches (Stevens et al. 2003; Breau et al. 2004).

Behavioral and physiological indicators within the multidimensional milieu are either uncorrelated or weakly correlated ($r = 0.3$) across situations and studies (Stevens et al. 1994). This dissociation in responsive systems suggests that physiological systems may be only loosely coupled to behavioral responsive systems (Barr 1998) and impedes both our judgment about pain intensity and our decision making about the effectiveness of interventions. An overall understanding of different behavioral and physiological indicators leads many to assert that the assessment of infant pain should be multidimensional or composite, because no unitary measure captures all the phenomena of infant pain. Conversely, the question of whether combining physiological, behavioral, and other types of indicators is the ideal approach across clinical and research settings needs attention. Ensuring assessment across both physiological and behavioral assessment modalities will help overcome discrepancies between these two approaches and help decipher the presence of distress and the need for deeper investigation of pain. The limitation is that the understanding of unique changes in individual pain indicators is often lost in the processes of summation and averaging of indicator scores.

Finally, there is no consensus on which scale, indicator, or approach should be used to assess pain across ages and stages of infant development, various types of pain, and differing pain situations. The emphasis has been on the development of measures to assess acute or prolonged (e.g., postoperative) pain. Consensus on an assessment approach and measure may allow movement beyond assessment of acute pain toward effective management for infants who suffer prolonged, persistent, or chronic pain.

PAIN IN COGNITIVELY OR NEUROLOGICALLY IMPAIRED INFANTS AND CHILDREN

In comparison to the amount of emphasis given to the measurement of pain in healthy term and preterm infants, relatively little attention has been paid to measuring pain in infants and children with cognitive or neurological impairments. Risk for neurological impairment in infants is the result of a multiplicity of factors including congenital syndrome/chromosomal abnormalities, birth trauma, extreme preterm birth, and acquired illnesses with central nervous system involvement. The frequency of painful procedures also appears to vary due to risk for neurological impairment. In a study of 194 infants, Stevens et al. (2003) compared the number of procedures conducted for infants at high, moderate, and low risk for neurological impairment. Although there was no overall difference in the number or type of procedures performed over the first 7 days of admission to the neonatal intensive care unit, infants at high risk for neurological impairment did receive significantly more painful procedures than those at moderate or low risk on their first day of life. Infants at high risk also received two to three times fewer bolus opioids than infants at moderate or low risk over the first 2 days of admission, and the difference was not related to duration of ventilation. There was a significant relationship between the number of procedures performed and analgesic use and sedation for the low and moderate risk groups, but no relation in infants at highest risk.

Two studies have addressed pain responses in infants with neurological impairment. In a comparative cohort study of pain reactivity in VLBW infants with and without parenchymal brain injury (PBI), no differences in facial action or measures of cardiac autonomic reactivity were identified following an acute painful event. The only significant difference between groups was that infants with PBI exhibited more tongue protrusion following the heel lance (Oberlander et al. 2002). Although most of the infants with PBI went on to develop cerebral palsy, pain responses appeared to remain intact in the neonatal period. Contrasting results come from a prospective observational study of behavioral and physiological responses to a heel lance of 149 neonates (GA >25–40 weeks) at high risk (cohort A, $n = 54$), moderate risk (cohort B, $n = 45$), and low risk (cohort C, $n = 50$) for neurological impairment. Although all infants responded to the most painful phase of the heel lance with the greatest change from baseline, infants at the moderate and highest risk for neurological impairment exhibited the least change in facial expression and some physiological indicators (B.J. Stevens et al., unpublished manuscript). Infants with the highest severity of illness demonstrated the highest-pitched cries. These results demonstrate that infants at all risk levels for neurological impairment are capable of demonstrating behavioral and physiological responses to painful procedures, although these responses vary in magnitude based on risk status and severity of illness. Differences in these two studies warrant further research in this area, prior to the validation of indicators for pain measurement.

Inherent difficulties in measuring pain in children with cognitive or neurological impairment are compounded because the behavior of these children when they are not in pain, such as thrashing their limbs, may resemble pain behavior. Frequently these children cannot provide self report, so proxy reports by parents or other methods must be used. Biological measures may not be as easily obtained; for example, these children may not tolerate measurement of heart rate and blood pressure; moreover, they may have unusual ranges of baseline physiological activity and may have complex known comorbid conditions (e.g., spasticity and muscle contractures) or unknown ones (e.g., gastroesophageal reflux and central and peripheral neuropathies). Autonomic reactivity as signaled by changes in heart rate and sweating may also be different and thus will confound the clinician's discernment of the cause of pain. Caregivers and parents may presume that these children are less sensitive or insensitive to pain when compared with children without cognitive and neurological impairment. All of these factors make assessment of pain difficult for the clinician and family care provider.

Self-injury has also been reported as a maladaptive behavior that coincides with persistent or repeated pain in infants and older children. McCann et al. (2004) examined rates of self-injury in infants who had sustained brachial plexus birth injury and found that 6.8% of the 133 infants who underwent surgery to correct the injury displayed self-injurious behavior, compared to only 1.4% of the 147 infants who did not undergo surgery. Of the total of 11 children who injured themselves, self-injury most often began 8 months after surgery and was frequently directed at the affected limb. In a retrospective chart review of 25 children with severe cognitive impairments who displayed self-injury, Bosch et al. (1997) determined that seven children had undiagnosed medical conditions that would be expected to cause pain. Treatment resulted in decreased self-injury for six of the children. Self-injury has also been reported as an indicator of pain by caregivers of children with severe cognitive impairments (McGrath et al. 1998) and is included in some pain assessment tools for children with impairments.

Assessment in children with neurological and cognitive impairments is just as challenging as it is with infants. However, the reasons for this difficulty may differ. The best validated measures for children with cognitive impairment include the San Salvadore Scale (Collignon and Giusiano 2001), the Non-Communicating Children's Pain Checklist (McGrath et al. 1998; Breau et al. 2000, 2002), the Pediatric Pain Profile (Hunt et al. 2004), and the Pain Indicator for Communicatively Impaired Children (Stallard et al. 2002). It is important not to repeat the over-proliferation of scales that have been developed in infants. Instead, a more fruitful approach will be to focus on establishing better construct validity, feasibility, and clinical utility for existing measures and fostering investigation of new indicators that are superior either alone or in combination with existing indicators.

PAIN IN THE ELDERLY

Similar to other vulnerable populations, the elderly often have pain that is inadequately assessed and undertreated (Gagliese 2001). This situation is even more dire in the cognitively impaired elderly or those with dementia. Dementia is associated with the progressive decline of cognitive function, including deterioration of emotional control, social behavior, and motivation (World Health Organization 1990), and widespread neurodegeneration. The prevalence of dementia increases with age, with an incidence of approximately 1% at 65 years old and 25% at 85 years old (Jorm et al. 1993), with speculation that the number of persons affected will increase dramatically as the current population ages. This speculation emphasizes the urgency for the development of valid and reliable pain assessment measures in the elderly.

The question as to whether inadequate assessment is the cause of poor pain management in this vulnerable age group also needs to be considered. Research indicates that postoperative and chronic pain receives less attention in the elderly compared to younger adults. Older postoperative patients as compared to younger patients are asked about pain less often, are given less frequent analgesia, and receive a lower percentage of their prescribed dosage (de Rond et al. 2000). Researchers report that 47–80% of elderly people who report pain do not receive any treatment (Woo et al. 1994). Bernabei et al. (1998) also have determined that the frailest elderly (those more than 85 years old) with cancer are more likely either to receive no analgesia or to be given non-opioid analgesics or weak opioids than those who are either 65–74 or 75–84 years of age. These frail elderly also are administered significantly less opioids as compared with their less elderly counterparts. Generally, predictors of poor analgesic administration include those who are more than 85 years old, male, and of non-white ethnicity and those with increased cognitive impairment (Won et al. 1999).

Just as with vulnerable populations of infants and children, assessing pain in the elderly poses significant challenges, and particularly in those with dementia. Clinicians must consider recall interval and memory impairment, the validity and reliability of pain questions, understanding of the task, decline in vision and hearing, and dysphasias. Verbal descriptor scales (VDS; e.g., no pain, mild, moderate, severe pain), numerical rating scales (NRS; e.g., 0–10), facial scales, and visual analogue scales (VAS) have all been evaluated for use with the elderly. Gagliese et al. (2005) recently compared the face validity of the NRS, VDS, McGill Pain Questionnaire, and VAS (vertical and horizontal) across younger and older surgical patients. In terms of ease, accuracy, and preference of use, the NRS was consistently rated the highest in all three domains across age groups, while the VAS (both vertical and horizontal) was rated the lowest. Also, the error rate was highest and increased with age on the horizontal VAS ($P \leq 0.05$).

The question of whether the experience of pain is different in individuals with dementia must also be considered. The particular challenge is to differentiate pain measurement issues in relation to either cognitive or verbal problems and to consider their interactions. Also, can the elderly with dementia complete pain scales in a valid and reliable way? In a study of 217 institutionalized, verbal, demented elderly, which compared the use of five pain scales, only 32% of subjects could complete all five scales, and 17% were unable to complete any of them; the highest failure rate was with the VAS (56%) (Ferrell et al. 1995).

Self-report of pain is associated with high failure rates and has been generally devoid of adequate demonstration of reliability, validity, and sensitivity in existing scales such that nonverbal elderly with dementia are almost completely excluded from pain assessment. Additionally, those with dementia display fewer facial expressions and more facial action units than those elderly who are cognitively intact (Hadjistavropoulos et al. 2000). Other studies of patients with dementia who have a history of "painful" disorders also have indicated that most had no pain behaviors, but reported changes from normal behavior; interindividual differences were considerable (Marzinski 1991).

Fuchs-Lacelle and Hadjistavropoulos (2004) developed the Pain Assessment Checklist for Seniors with Limited Ability to Communicate, which included activity/body movement, facial expressions, vocal behaviors, aggressive behaviors, social/personality/mood indicators, eating/sleeping changes, and physiological indicators. These authors reported high inter-rater reliability (0.97), internal consistency (0.86), and good levels of sensitivity and specificity. This measure is one example of a composite measure where the authors have included multiple types of behavioral, physiological, and contextual indicators and worked to establish the psychometric properties. However, many other measures are being developed with much less attention to both psychometric and clinimetric properties, especially clinical utility. Justina et al. (2005) recently reviewed 12 observational measures that were developed to assess pain in the elderly. The authors considered these measures in terms of construct clarity, sample representativeness, reliability and validity, sensitivity, and clinical usefulness. Of the 12, there were 9 with moderate clinical utility, but collectively they exhibited limitations either in terms of structures of the measures or in the rigor of the psychometric validation studies. It is hoped that the development of further measures for this vulnerable group will benefit from the lessons learned from other groups such as infants.

CONCLUSION

Pain must be assessed adequately to be effectively managed. Assessment is one aspect of pain that requires further efforts to expand our understanding. There can be little movement on ameliorating pain's effects until we can measure it reliably and validly and utilize these assessments in the clinical world. Pain assessment in vulnerable populations presents particular challenges. In order to address these challenges, we must pay close attention to underlying pain mechanisms. Assessment must also move beyond acute pain and pain intensity in those who are most vulnerable, taking into consideration a multitude of unexplored contextual factors.

We must prevent further proliferation of measures with common indicators. Rather, we need to focus on establishing stronger psychometric properties in those measures that are the most valid and reliable. Feasibility, which is generally overemphasized, must give way to determining clinical utility, which is generally under-addressed. We also need to consider why some individuals are devoid of pain responses and seek reasonable explanations. Inconsistency in proxy reporting among lay and professional care providers must be addressed, as well as attitudes and beliefs of health care providers that may prevent optimal pain assessment.

In summary, vulnerable populations including infants, children with neurological and cognitive impairments, and the elderly have not received adequate attention in terms of pain measurement. Contrary to conventional practice, these individuals are equally deserving of the attention of those who develop and validate pain measures. Therefore, our attention must be refocused in their direction so that they may receive equal opportunity for the most optimal pain management available.

ACKNOWLEDGMENTS

Dr. Stevens is the Signy Hildur Eaton Chair in Paediatric Nursing Research at the Hospital for Sick Children and Professor, Faculties of Nursing and Medicine, University of Toronto. Her current research is supported primarily through the Canadian Institutes of Health Research.

REFERENCES

Anand KJS, Craig KD. New perspectives on the definition of pain. *Pain* 1996; 67:3–6.

Andrews K, Fitzgerald M. The cutaneous withdrawal reflex in human neonates: sensitization, receptive fields and the effects of contra lateral stimulation. *Pain* 1994; 56:95–102.

Andrews K, Fitzgerald M. Cutaneous flexion reflex in human neonates: a quantitative study of threshold and stimulus response characteristics after single and repeated stimuli. *Dev Med Child Neurol* 1999; 41:696–703.

Andrews K, Desai D, Dhillon H, et al. Abdominal sensitivity in the first year of life: comparison of infants with and without prenatally diagnosed unilateral hydronephrosis. *Pain* 2002; 100:35–46.

Ballantyne M, Stevens B, McAllister M, et al. Validation of the premature infant pain profile in the clinical setting. *Clin J Pain* 1999; 15:297–303.

Barr RG. Reflections on measuring pain in infants: dissociation in responsive systems and "honest signalling." *Arch Dis Child Fetal Neonatal Ed* 1998; 79:152–156.

Bakewell-Sachs S, Blackburn S. *Discharge and Follow-up of the High-Risk Preterm Infant*. White Plains: March of Dimes Education Services, 2001, p 20.

Bernabei, Gambassi G, Lapane K, et al. Management of pain in elderly patients with cancer. SAGE (Systematic Assessment of Geriatric Drug Use via Epidemiology) study group. *JAMA* 1998; 279:1877–1882.

Bosch J, Van Dyke DC, Smith SM, Poulton S. Role of medical conditions in the exacerbation of self-injurious behavior: an exploratory study. *Ment Retard* 1997; 35:124–130.

Breau LM, McGrath PJ, Camfield C, Rosmus C, Finley GA. Preliminary validation of an observation pain checklist for cognitively-impaired, non-communicating persons. *Dev Med Child Neurol* 2000; 42:609–616.

Breau LM, Finley AG, McGrath PJ, Camfield C. Validation of the Non-Communicating Children's Pain Checklist-Postoperative version. *Anesthesiology* 2002; 96:528–535.

Breau L, McGrath PJ, Stevens B, et al. Healthcare professionals' perceptions of pain in infants at risk for neurologic impairment. *BMC Pediatr* 2004; 4:23.

Carbajal R, Paupe A, Hoenn E, et al. DAN: une echelle comportementale d'evaluation de la douleur aigue du nouveau-né. [APN: evaluation behavioral scale of acute pain in newborn infants.] *Arch Pediatr* 1997; 4:623–628.

Carbajal R, Lenclen R, Jugie M, et al. Morphine does not provide adequate analgesia for acute procedural pain among preterm neonates. *Pediatrics* 2005; 115:1494–1500.

Collignon P, Giusiano B. Validation of a pain evaluation scale for patients with severe cerebral palsy. *Eur J Pain* 2001; 5:433–442.

Craig KD, Whitfield MF, Grunau RVE, Linton J, Hadjistavropoulos HD. Pain in the preterm neonate: behavioural and physiological indices. *Pain* 1993; 52:287–299.

Debillon T, Zupan V, Ravault N, Magny J-F, Dehan M. Development and initial validation of the EDIN scale, a new tool for assessing prolonged pain in preterm infants. *Arch Dis Child* 2001; 85:F36–F40.

de Rond ME, de Witt R, van Dam FS, Muller MJ. A pain monitoring program for nurses: effects on administration of analgesics. *Pain* 2000; 89: 25–38.

Doussard-Roosevelt JA, Porges SW, Scanlon JW, et al. Vagal regulation of heart rate in the prediction of developmental outcome for very low birth weight preterm infants. *Child Dev* 1997; 68:173–186.

Duhn L, Medves J. A systematic integrative review of infant pain assessment tools. *Adv Neonatal Care* 2004; 4:126–140.

Ferrell BA, Ferrell BA, Rivers L. Pain in cognitively impaired nursing home residents. *J Pain Symptom Manage* 1995; 591–598.

Fitzgerald M. The development of nociceptive circuits. *Nat Rev Neurosci* 2005; 6:507–520.

Flaskerud JH, Winslow BJ. Conceptualizing vulnerable populations health related research. *Nurs Res* 1998; 47:69–78.

Fuchs-Lacelle S, Hadjistavropoulos T. Development and preliminary validation of the pain assessment checklist for seniors with limited ability to communicate (PACSLAC). *Pain Manag Nurs* 2004; 5:37–49.

Gagliese L. Assessment of pain in the elderly. In: Turk DC, Melzack R (Eds). *Handbook of Pain Assessment*. New York: Guilford Press, 2001, pp 119–133.

Gagliese L, Weizblit N, Ellis W, Chan VW. The measurement of postoperative pain: a comparison of intensity scales in younger and older surgical patients. *Pain* 2005;117:412–420.

Goldman R, Koren G. Biologic markers of pain in vulnerable infant. *Clin Perinatol* 2002; 29:415–425.

Grunau RVE, Craig KD. Pain expressions in neonates: facial action and cry. *Pain* 1987; 28:395–410.

Grunau RVE, Holsti L, Whitfield MF, et al. Are twitches, startles, and body movements pain indicators in extremely low birth weight infants? *Clin J Pain* 2000; 16:37–45.

Grunau RVE, Oberlander TF, Whitfield MF, et al. Demographic and therapeutic determinants of pain reactivity in very low birth weight neonates at 32 weeks' postconceptional age. *Pediatrics* 2001a; 107:105–112.

Grunau RVE, Oberlander TF, Whitfield MF, et al. Pain reactivity in former extremely low birth weight infants at corrected age 8 months compared with term born controls. *Infant Behavior Develop* 2001b; 24:41–55.

Guinsburg R, de Almeida MF, Peres C, Shinzato A, Kopelman B. Reliability of two behavioural tools to assess pain in preterm neonates. *Sao Paulo Med J* 2003; 121(2):72–76.

Hadjistavropoulos T, LaChapelle DL, MacLeod FK, Snider B, Craig KD. Measuring movement-exacerbated pain in cognitively impaired frail elders. *Clin J Pain* 2000; 16:54–63.

Hodgkinson K, Bear M, Thorn J, Van Blaricum S. Measuring pain in neonates: evaluating an instrument and developing a common language. *Aust J Adv Nurs* 1994; 12:17–22.

Holsti L, Grunau R, Oberlander T, Whitfield M. Specific newborn individualized developmental care and assessment program movements are associated with acute pain in preterm infants in the neonatal intensive care unit. *Pediatrics* 2004; 114:65–72.

Horgan M, Choonara I. Measuring pain in neonates: an objective score. *Pediatr Nurs* 1996; 8:24–27.

Horgan M, Glenn S, Choonara I. Further development of the Liverpool Infant Distress Scale. *J Child Health Care* 2002; 6:96–106.

Hudson-Barr D, Capper-Michel B, Lambert S, et al. Validation of the Pain Assessment in Neonates (PAIN) scale with the Neonatal Infant Pain Scale (NIPS). *Neonatal Netw* 2002; 21:15–21.

Hunt A, Goldman A, Seers K, et al. Clinical validation of the paediatric pain profile. *Dev Med Child Neurol* 2004; 46:9–18.

IASP Task Force on Taxonomy. *IASP Pain Terminology.* Available at: www.iasp-pain.org/terms-p.html. Accessed February 9, 2006.

Johnston CC, Stevens B. Experience in a neonatal intensive care unit affects pain response. *Pediatrics* 1996; 98(5):925–930.

Johnston CC, Stevens B, Yang F, et al. Developmental changes in response to heelstick in preterm infants: a prospective cohort study. *Dev Med Child Neurol* 1996; 38:438–445.

Jorm AF, Henderson S, Scott R, et al. The disabled elderly living in the community: care received from family and formal services. *Med J Aust* 1993; 158(6):383–385, 388.

Justina LY, Jose CS, Briggs M. A critical appraisal of 12 observational pain tools for use with cognitively impaired elderly people. In: *Abstracts: 11th World Congress on Pain.* Seattle: IASP Press, 2005, p 84.

Krechel S, Bildner J. CRIES: a new neonatal postoperative pain measurement score: initial testing of validity and reliability. *Paediatr Anaesth* 1995; 5:53–61.

Lawrence J, Alcock D, McGrath P, et al. The development of a tool to assess neonatal pain. *Neonatal Netw* 1993; 12:59–66.

Leffers J, Martins D, McGrath, et al. Development of a theoretical construct for risk and vulnerability from six empirical studies. *Res Theory Nurs Pract* 2004; 18:15–34.

Marzinski LR. The tragedy of dementia: clinically assessing pain in the confused, nonverbal elderly. *J Gerontol Nurs* 1991; 17:25–28.

Massin M, von Bernuth G. Normal ranges of heart rate variability during infancy and childhood. *Pediatr Cardiol* 1997; 18:297–302.

McCann ME, Waters P, Goumnerova LC, Berde C. Self-mutilation in young children following brachial plexus birth injury. *Pain* 2004; 110:123–129.

McGrath PJ, Rosmus C, Camfield C, Campbell MA, Hennigar AW. Behaviours caregivers use to determine pain in non-verbal, cognitively impaired individuals. *Dev Med Child Neurol* 1998; 40:340–343.

McNair C, Ballantyne M, Dionne K, Stephens D, Stevens B. Postoperative pain assessment in the neonatal intensive care unit. *Arch Dis Child Fetal Neonatal Ed* 2004; 89:537–541.

Mellor DJ, Diesch TJ, Gunn AJ, Bennet L, et al. The importance of "awareness" for understanding fetal pain. *Brain Res Rev* 2005; 1–16.

Merskey H, Bogduk N (Eds). *Classification of Chronic Pain: Descriptions of Chronic Pain Syndromes and Definitions of Pain Terms,* 2nd ed. Seattle: IASP Press, 1994, pp 209–214.

Oberlander TF, Saul JP. Methodological considerations for the use of heart rate variability as a measure of pain reactivity in vulnerable infants. *Clin Perinatol* 2002; 29:427–443.

Oberlander TF, Grunau RE, Pitfield S, et al. The developmental character of cardiac autonomic responses to an acute noxious event in 4- and 8-month-old healthy infants. *Pediatr Res* 1999; 45:519–525.

Oberlander TF, Grunau RVE, Whitfield MF, et al. Biobehavioral pain responses in former extremely low birth weight infants at four months' corrected age. *Pediatrics* 2000; 105:e6.

Oberlander TF, Grunau RVE, Fitzgerald C, et al. Does parenchymal brain injury affect biobehavioral pain responses in very low birth weight infants at 32 weeks' postconceptional age? *Pediatrics* 2002; 110(3):570–576.

Porges SW. Vagal tone: a physiologic marker of stress vulnerability. *Pediatrics* 1992; 90:498–504.

Prietsch V, Knoepke U, Obladen M. Continuous monitoring of heart rate variability in preterm infants. *Early Hum Dev* 1994; 37:117–131.

Puchalski M, Hummel P. The reality of neonatal pain. *Adv Neonatal Care* 2002; 2:233–244.

Saito K. Development of spinal reflexes in the rat fetus studied *in vitro. J Physiol* 1979; 294:581–594.

Schiller CJ. Clinical utility of two neonatal pain assessment measures. Master's thesis. Toronto: Faculty of Nursing, University of Toronto, 1999.

Spence K, Gillies D, Harrison D, Johnston L, Nagy S. A reliable pain assessment tool for clinical assessment in the neonatal intensive care unit. *J Obstet Gynecol Neonatal Nurs* 2005; 34:80–86.

Stallard P, Williams L, Velleman R. et al. The development and evaluation of the pain indicator for communicatively impaired children (PICIC). *Pain* 2002; 145–149.

Stevens B, Gibbins S. Clinical utility and clinical significance in the assessment and management of pain in vulnerable infants. *Clin Perinatol* 2002; 29:459–468.

Stevens BJ, Johnston CC, Horton L. Factors that influence the behavioural pain responses of premature infants. *Pain* 1994; 59:101–109.

Stevens B, Johnston C, Petryshen P, Taddio A. Premature Infant Pain Profile: development and initial validation. *Clin J Pain* 1996; 12:13–22.

Stevens B, McGrath PJ, Gibbins S, et al. Procedural pain in newborns at risk for neurologic impairment. *Pain* 2003; 105:27–35.

Suominen P, Caffin C, Linton S, et al. The cardiac analgesic assessment scale (CAAS): a pain assessment tool for intubated and ventilated children after cardiac surgery. *Paediatr Anaesth* 2004; 14:336–343.

Torsney C, Fitzgerald M. Age-dependent effects of peripheral inflammation on the electrophysiological properties of neonatal rat dorsal term neurons. *J Neurophysiol* 2002; 87(3):1311–1317.

Walker C, Anand KJS, Plotsky PM. Development of the hypothalamic-pituitary-adrenal axis and the stress response. In: McEwen B, Goodman H (Eds). *Coping with the Environment: Neural and Endocrine Mechanisms.* Oxford: Oxford University Press, 2000, pp 237–270.

Won A, Lapane K, Gambassi G, et al. Correlates and management of nonmalignant pain in the nursing home. SAGE Study Group. Systematic assessment of geriatric drug use via epidemiology. *J Am Geriatr Soc* 1999; 47:936–942.

Woo J, Ho SC, Lau J, et al. Musculoskeletal complaints and associated consequences in elderly Chinese aged 70 and over. *J Rheumatol* 1994; 21:1927–1931.

Yamada J, Stevens B, de Silva N, Klein J, Koren G. Hair cortisol as a biologic marker of chronic stress in neonates: a pilot study. *Pain Res Manag* 2003; Suppl 8:59B.

Correspondence to: Bonnie J. Stevens, RN, PhD, Hospital for Sick Children, 555 University, Room 4734B, Toronto, ON, Canada M5G 1X8. Fax: 416-813-8273; email: b.stevens@utoronto.ca.

Proceedings of the 11th World Congress on Pain,
edited by Herta Flor, Eija Kalso, and Jonathan O.
Dostrovsky, IASP Press, Seattle, © 2006.

63

Clinicians' Cognitions and Clinical Style in Relation to Patient Outcome

Donna Kalauokalani,[a] Jenny Keating,[b] Peter Kent,[b,c] and Tamar Pincus[d]

[a]*Division of Pain Medicine, Department of Anesthesiology and Pain Medicine, University of California, Davis Medical Center, Sacramento, California, USA;* [b]*Physiotherapy, School of Primary Health, Faculty of Medicine, Nursing and Health Sciences, Monash University, Victoria, Australia;* [c]*Monash University Department of Clinical Epidemiology and Preventive Medicine, Cabrini Hospital, Victoria, Australia;* [d]*Department of Psychology, Royal Holloway, University of London, United Kingdom*

The focus of research on risk factors for the development of chronic pain syndromes has concentrated on patient characteristics (psychological and social), but these explain only a small proportion of the variance. It is possible that clinicians' behavior, advice, and even treatment methods indirectly contribute to maintaining the problem by creating, maintaining, and reinforcing an illness paradigm. The opposite is also possible: clinicians' beliefs and motivations may encourage patients to recover in the absence of any active treatment. Either way, there is a remarkable lack of research into the interaction between clinicians' beliefs and decision-making procedures and patients' outcome. This chapter describes three original studies, each investigating a different angle of the interaction between beliefs, behaviors, and outcomes. Different methodologies used to assess this rich and complex subject are presented, including mixed methods and survey methodologies. New specific measurements are presented that can help researchers to reliably assess clinicians' cognitions about low back pain.

CLINICIANS' COGNITIONS ABOUT BACK PAIN: THE ATTITUDES TO BACK PAIN SCALE

Little is known about practitioners' beliefs and attitudes regarding the treatment of low back pain or to what extent these beliefs influence clinical decisions, intervention strategies, and patient-centered outcomes. We chose a two-stage study so that we could combine rich and novel data from interviews with a reduced data set from a new survey. Stage I was a qualitative approach with two aims: first, to investigate to what extent clinicians treating individuals with low back pain continue to offer long-term treatment even when they fail to see any improvement; and second, to study the beliefs that allow chiropractors, osteopaths, and physiotherapists to continue to treat patients whose low back pain does not appears to be improving. Stage II was a quantitative approach designed to develop, test, and explore the underlying dimensions of a new questionnaire, the Attitudes to Back Pain Scale, in a specific group of clinicians: practitioners who specialize in musculoskeletal therapy.

METHODS AND RESULTS

In Stage I of the study (Pincus et al. 2006a), we mailed a questionnaire survey to 200 chiropractors, 200 osteopaths, and 200 physiotherapists. Responses were received from 354/600 (59%) clinicians, equally distributed among the three types of professionals. Clinicians who reported treating at least one patient more than eight times over 3 months with little improvement were invited to be interviewed ($N = 42$). Methodological techniques ranged from grounded theory analysis to sorting of categories by both the research team and the subjects themselves.

The findings suggest that the practitioners' self-image and their view of their role as health educator rather than problem solver were the main reasons behind this practice. In addition, the clinicians' understanding of psychosocial risk and of the circumstances that encourage disclosure from patients can result in extended treatment in the absence of objective signs of recovery, in contrast to current guidelines. These cognitions will affect whether clinicians choose to implement guidelines, whether they engage with their patients' psychological problems, and how they make decisions about appropriate referral.

In Stage II of the study, we constructed a new questionnaire from the transcripts of the interviews. Where possible, we used verbatim quotes in the construction of our items. The draft questionnaire (52 items) sought to assess practitioners' attitudes concerning role and self-image as well as their beliefs about treatment goals and about the prognosis of low back pain. The questionnaire was sent to a random selection of 300 practitioners from each professional group, and 546 (61%) responded. Split-sample analyses were performed using exploratory and confirmatory factor analysis. The questionnaire has been demonstrated to have good reliability (> 0.95) and validity (Pincus et al. 2006b). The Attitudes to Back Pain Scale: Musculoskeletal Practitioners contains two sections, personal interaction and treatment orientation. The personal interaction section consists of four factors: (1) *Limitations on Sessions,* with items about practitioners' policy on limiting the length of treatment; (2) *Psychological,* with items measuring practitioners' willingness to engage with psychological issues with their patients; (3) *Connection to Healthcare System,* with items measuring practitioners' perception of the health care system and provision of available services; and (4) *Confidence and Concern,* with items measuring practitioners' confidence in themselves and concern about the quality of treatment received by others. The treatment orientation section consists of two factors: (1) *Re-activation,* with items concerning return to work, resumption of daily activity, and increasing mobility; and (2) *Biomedical,* with items concerning advice to restrict activities and to be vigilant, and concerning the belief that there is an underlying structural cause of back pain.

DISCUSSION

Clearly, such self-report tools are only a measure of explicit attitudes, which may not reflect behavior and decision-making, let alone have an impact on clinical practice. While future research should address the relationship between explicit and implicit attitudes, behavior, and outcome, we have already demonstrated that the Attitudes to Back Pain Scale can be used to compare subtle differences between chiropractors, osteopaths, and physiotherapists (Pincus et al. 2006b). In addition, it is the first tool of its kind to address the health care network within which clinicians operate and to show how clinicians' sense of connection to this network can affect their attitudes.

THE EFFECTS OF DIAGNOSTIC UNCERTAINTY ON CLINICIANS' APPROACH TO TREATMENT OF LOW BACK PAIN

Most low back pain (LBP) remains a diagnostic enigma, with approximately 80% of primary care LBP presentations being most accurately labeled as "nonspecific LBP." As a result, clinicians routinely deal with diagnostic uncertainty in designing interventions for LBP. It appears that clinicians either tailor treatment to address individual patient characteristics or prescribe a "one size fits all" intervention. Manual therapy clinicians (chiropractors, osteopaths, and physiotherapists) are trained to think that subgroups exist within the nonspecific LBP population. We sought to identify the extent to which these beliefs are widely held in primary care (Kent and Keating 2004). We also sought to identify the subgroups that clinicians believe are recognizable within that heterogeneity (Kent and Keating 2005). We describe how clinicians currently assess nonspecific LBP and how these assessment practices influence clinicians' capacity to identify subgroups.

METHODS

We conducted a survey of 1,093 Australian primary contact clinicians from six professional disciplines (physiotherapists, manipulative physiotherapists, chiropractors, osteopaths, general medical practitioners, and musculoskeletal medicine practitioners). Clinicians were randomly selected from their disciplines. Descriptive statistics, chi-square tests, and cluster analysis were used to analyze clinician responses.

RESULTS AND DISCUSSION

Completed questionnaires were returned by 651 (60%) of the clinicians. Of the primary-contact clinicians who responded, 93% did not think nonspecific LBP is one condition. Seventy-four percent thought it currently possible to recognize nonspecific LBP subgroups. Ninety-three percent treated nonspecific LBP differently based on patterns of signs and symptoms. The proportion of clinicians who held these views was highest for physiotherapists and manipulative physiotherapists and smallest for general medical practitioners and musculoskeletal medicine practitioners. Most primary care clinicians thought that nonspecific LBP is heterogeneous and treated patients differently based on that heterogeneity (Table I).

Table I
Primary care clinicians' attitudes and self-reported behaviors with regard to assessment of nonspecific low back pain (NSLBP)

	Percentage (95% CI)
A) Attitudes about NSLBP	
Percentage who think NSLBP is a number of conditions (subgroups)	93 (91–95)
Percentage who treat NSLBP differently based on patterns of signs and symptoms	93 (91–95)
Percentage who think it currently possible to recognize NSLBP subgroups	74 (71–77)
Percentage of clinician-nominated NSLBP subgroups that have labels that imply putative pathoanatomy	88
Percentage consensus regarding the three most frequent symptoms and signs that identify commonly nominated NSLBP subgroups	<9
B) Behaviors in the Assessment of Recent-Onset NSLBP	
Percentage who at any time assess symptoms and signs from the health domain of:	
Physical impairment	100
Pain	99 (98–100)
Activity limitation	42 (35–49)
Psychosocial functioning	25 (19–31)

There was little consensus among participating clinicians regarding the signs and symptoms that identify subgroups of nonspecific LBP. Most clinicians give labels to nonspecific LBP subgroups that imply putative pathoanatomy; however, the evidence that these labels are valid is scant and controversial. Clinicians commonly assessed symptoms and signs from the health domains of physical impairment and pain. Clinicians believe that information from these assessment domains can identify nonspecific LBP subgroups. The assessment of symptoms and signs from the domains of activity limitation and psychosocial function was uncommon, although there is evidence that this information can be prognostically important and useful for outcome assessment. It may be that the identification of clinically important nonspecific LBP subgroups will require the assessment of symptoms and signs across a broader range of health domains than are currently routinely assessed.

CONCLUSIONS

Although assigning nonspecific LBP patients to subgroups has not been validated, it is common in primary care settings and influences case management. If subgroups exist within the LBP population, there are implications for research into the effects of treatment. A lack of consensus among participating clinicians regarding subgroups of nonspecific LBP and a lack of evidence for the validity of such subgrouping are a compelling argument for further research into this clinical practice.

TREATMENT EXPECTATIONS: WHAT THE PATIENT BRINGS TO THE CLINICAL ENCOUNTER

Aside from clinician cognitions and diagnostic uncertainties, the patient also brings significant perspectives to the clinical encounter. In primary care settings, patient expectations regarding treatment benefit can have profound effects on treatment outcomes, depending on which treatment is prescribed (Kalauokalani et al. 2001). Patients with chronic pain presenting to a specialized pain clinic undoubtedly have predetermined expectations to benefit from any of a number of potential treatments typically offered at such clinics. The potential effects such expectations may have on clinical outcome notwithstanding, the assessment of these patient expectations may also be useful in guiding the patient-provider interaction and influencing decision-making.

METHODS

We surveyed a consecutive cohort of patients presenting for an initial consultation visit at a specialty pain clinic. We elicited expectations for benefiting from specific types of therapies typically offered at a pain clinic (opioid medication, intervention procedures, non-opioid medications, psychological counseling, active physical therapies, and passive physical therapies). For each of the six modalities, patients were asked to rate their expectations on a 0 to 10 scale anchored by 0 (not helpful at all) and 10 (extremely helpful). Examples of each modality were given parenthetically as part of the question, for example: "How helpful do you believe *active physical therapies* (such as *stretching, strengthening,* and *conditioning exercises*) will be for your current pain problem?"

The survey also elicited expectations for symptomatic improvement at 1 and 6 months using a 7-point Likert scale. For example: "One month from now, do you expect your current pain problem to be: (1) completely gone; (2) much better; (3) a little better; (4) moderately better; (5) about the same; (6) a little worse; (7) much worse." For both the modality-specific and the global prognostic questions, patients had the option of responding with "don't know."

RESULTS AND DISCUSSION

Findings were consistent with the notion that patients have pre-existing expectations regarding specific types of treatments before they are seen by the physician and that these can be assessed using a simple questionnaire format. Interestingly, patients generally had, on initial presentation, high expectations for symptomatic improvement despite having persistent and severe pain symptoms. Moreover, patients had stronger expectations to benefit from interventional procedures and opioid medications than from non-opioid medications or physical or psychological therapies (Fig. 1).

Even before interaction with a physician, patients demonstrate discernible prognostic and treatment expectations. Low expectations to benefit from important elements of multidisciplinary pain management such as non-opioid medications, rehabilitative physical therapies, and psychological therapies may adversely affect patient compliance and outcomes. Exploring how processes of care may reshape or influence patient expectations can have implications for compliance as well as for developing educational interventions. Further research is needed to understand how patient expectations are formulated and how the assessment of these expectations can facilitate clinical interactions and optimize outcomes.

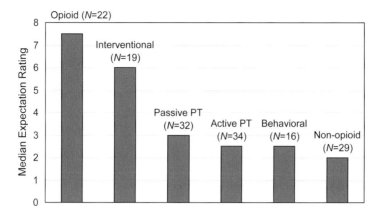

Fig. 1. Patient expectation ratings for specific therapies. PT = physical therapy. Data from D. Kalauokalani et al. (unpublished manuscript).

SUMMARY

Clinicians and patients each bring important elements to the clinical encounter. The perspectives of each party can influence their interaction, determining the degree of engagement and choices made, which can then influence clinical outcomes. The stage for optimal healing appears to be set well before actual treatments are rendered. Further exploration into characterizing elements of the clinical encounter that lend themselves to modification through education and training may lead to improved quality and value of care.

ACKNOWLEDGMENTS

Supported in part by the Faculty of Health Sciences (La Trobe University), Joint Coal Board Health and Safety Trust (Australia), Musculoskeletal Physiotherapy Association (Victoria), Washington University Pain Center, and the Washington University School of Medicine Summer Research Fellowship Program (USA).

REFERENCES

Kalauokalani D, Cherkin DC, Sherman KJ, Koepsell TD, Deyo RA. Lessons from a trial of acupuncture and massage for low back pain: patient expectations and treatment effects. *Spine* 2001; 26:1418–1424.

Kent PM, Keating JL. Do primary-care clinicians think that non-specific low back pain is one condition? *Spine* 2004; 29:1022–1031.

Kent PM, Keating JL. Classification in non-specific low back pain—what methods do primary care clinicians currently use? *Spine* 2005; 30:1433–1440.

Pincus T, Vogel S, Breen A, Foster N, Underwood M. Persistent back pain: why do physical therapy clinicians continue treatment? A mixed methods study of chiropractors, osteopaths and physiotherapists. *Eur J Pain* 2006a; 10:67–76.

Pincus T, Vogel S, Santos R, et al. The Attitudes to Back Pain Scale in musculoskeletal practitioners (ABS-mp); the development and testing of a new questionnaire. *Clin J Pain* 2006b; in press.

Correspondence to: Donna Kalauokalani, MD, MPH, UC Davis Division of Pain Medicine, 4860 Y Street, Suite 3020, Sacramento, CA 95817, USA. Fax: 916-734-6827; email: dkalauokalani@ucdavis.edu.

Proceedings of the 11th World Congress on Pain,
edited by Herta Flor, Eija Kalso, and Jonathan O.
Dostrovsky, IASP Press, Seattle, © 2006.

64

Classification, Diagnosis, and Outcome Measures in Patients with Orofacial Pain

Joanna M. Zakrzewska,[a] Alain Woda,[b] Christian S. Stohler,[c] and E. Russell Vickers[d]

[a]Clinical and Diagnostic Oral Sciences, Dental Institute, Barts and the London Queen Mary's School of Medicine and Dentistry, London, United Kingdom; [b]Dental Faculty, Clermont-Ferrand, France; [c]Baltimore College of Dental Surgery, University of Maryland, Baltimore, Maryland, USA; [d]Pain Management Research Institute, University of Sydney, Royal North Shore Hospital, St Leonards, New South Wales, Australia

In order to conduct multicenter epidemiological and clinical studies on chronic orofacial pain, it is important to first establish consensus on classification, diagnostic criteria, and outcome measures. This chapter brings together new perspectives to challenge our current thinking and provide insights into future developments in orofacial pain. This chapter presents details of a study that provides us with an evidence-based classification that can be a framework for the development of diagnostic criteria (Woda et al. 2005). While acknowledging the impact of the Research Diagnostic Criteria for Temporomandibular Disorders (Dworkin and LeResche 1992), we suggest the need for a new version that takes into account our increased understanding of the multifactorial nature of these conditions. Outcome measures used in trials need to be valid, reliable, and reproducible; biological markers used alongside more traditional outcome measures may improve our ability to show positive outcomes after treatment.

CLASSIFICATION OF OROFACIAL PAIN

The different forms of idiopathic orofacial pain (stomatodynia, atypical odontalgia, atypical facial pain, and facial arthromyalgia) are sometimes considered as separate entities and sometimes grouped together. Since there is no current consensus (Zakrzewska 2004), we used a new approach to help to place these different painful syndromes in the general classification of chronic facial pain. This approach was based on multivariate analysis to reveal the patterns of clustering of a wide range of items related to various clinical dimensions in a consecutive series of patients with oral or facial pain conditions (Mongini 2000). Our working hypothesis was that syndromes such as atypical facial pain, atypical odontalgia (toothache), stomatodynia (burning pain in the mouth), and disorders of the temporomandibular joint and masticatory muscles display some common clinical characteristics and thus may correspond to a single disease expressed in different tissues—the bones, teeth, oral mucosa, muscles, and joints (Feinmann 1996; Harris 1996; Woda and Pionchon 1999, 2000). Based on this hypothesis, it should be possible to propose a classification of these syndromes according to the presence of similar signs and/or symptoms, which may reflect similar pathophysiological mechanisms, rather than according to topography, organs, or tissues. This proposal would be in line with the mechanism-based classification of chronic pain (Woolf et al. 1998).

Woda and colleagues (2005) conducted a prospective multicenter study in Clermont-Ferrand, Paris, Saint-Etienne, and Sainte Foy, Quebec. We recruited consecutive patients attending specialized facial pain clinics presenting with any kind of chronic facial pain that had lasted for more than 4 months without any identified cause. Each patient was seen by two experts, who provided a 111-item self-administered questionnaire that was constructed to cover all symptoms that could possibly be relevant to reach the various diagnoses expected to be found according to the inclusion criteria. We listed the needed signs and symptoms from the existing diagnostic criteria described in the classification systems based on expert opinion (Dworkin and LeResche 1992; Merskey and Bogduk 1994; Okeson 1996; International Headache Society 2004) and in other relevant reviews (Truelove et al. 1992; Clark et al. 1993; Woda and Pionchon 1999). A standardized 68-item examination form was then completed. At the end of the first visit, the examiners put forward a proposed diagnosis for their patients using the systems described above, which included atypical facial pain, atypical odontalgia, stomatodynia, facial arthromyalgia, migraine, post-traumatic neuralgia, trigeminal neuralgia, cluster headache, tension-type headache, and other pain. Three meetings were held for piloting (i.e., to ensure that the forms were designed in a way that yielded consistent data) and calibration (i.e., to ensure everyone collected the data in the same way and came to the same diagnosis).

Statistical processing included four steps. Step 1 involved preselection of signs and symptoms by univariate analyses to select the significant signs or symptoms among the 179 items (111 questions contained in the self-administered questionnaire plus 68 items from the investigators' examination form). Signs and symptoms were retained only if they permitted the discrimination of at least one orofacial pain entity, as diagnosed by the examiners, with significance determined at $P < 0.001$. In step 2, composite signs and symptoms were formed by using a multiple correspondence analysis (homogeneity analysis by alternating least squares; De Leeuw et al. 1980). In step 3, clustering of the patients' conditions was determined following multidimensional analyses and an ascendant hierarchical classification. In step 4, the clusters were labeled by searching the signs and symptoms characterizing the subjects of each cluster. The labeling of each cluster was also facilitated by unblinding the initial clinical diagnoses.

A total of 245 patients (81.2% women) participated in the study. The mean age of the sample was 53.9 years, with a standard deviation of 18.05 years. Preselection by univariate analyses and formation of composite items led to the formation of two lists of signs and symptoms. The detailed composition of these combined signs and symptoms is reported in Table I.

List 1 ($n = 29$) differed from List 2 ($n = 49$) in that it comprised only the signs and symptoms related to the general characteristics of pain. This list excluded signs or symptoms referring to a topographical site, organ, or tissue so as to obtain a classification based on nontopographic signs or symptoms. We also had initially included four psychological signs or symptoms (anxiety, depression, and somatization with or without pain) taken from the Symptom Checklist-90 Revised (Derogatis 1983), but we excluded them after another multiple correspondence analysis showed that they were tightly clustered, but in an area of the multidimensional space completely separate from the areas of all the other data, and consequently remote from the main information.

Identification of a homogeneous group of subjects by multidimensional analysis (step 3) and labeling of the resulting clusters (step 4) led to different conclusions depending on the list used. With List 1 (not including the items related to anatomy), seven clusters were identified. The seven clusters were organized in two first-order dendrites, which appeared to represent two well-differentiated groups of clusters as indicated by their individualization very early in the dendritic tree. One dendrite included the two types of neuralgia, and the other one also rapidly split into two groups. One sub-dendrite later split toward the migraine and tension-type headache clusters, and the other gave three clusters, of which two were labeled as idiopathic orofacial pain because they did not discriminate between the different idiopathic conditions and the other was labeled as stomatodynia. The stomatodynia cluster, though clearly individualized, appeared to be linked to the other idiopathic conditions, and although it separated very late from its neighboring idiopathic groups, it was very homogeneous. Clinical cases diagnosed as stomatodynia amounted to 77% of the cluster labeled stomatodynia, and 79% of the diagnoses of stomatodynia in the whole sample were gathered in this cluster.

Table I
Signs and symptoms used as variables in the multidimensional analyses

Signs and Symptoms	List†
Pain duration within the day (from seconds to continuous)	1–2
Pain duration within 3 months (<7 days, <3 months, daily)	1–2
Pain at night or during the day	1–2
Burning pain	1–2
Throbbing pain	1–2
Paroxysmal pain	1–2
Constrictive pain (pressure)	1–2
Effectiveness of analgesics	1–2
Neurological signs revealed by clinical examination	1–2
Laterality of the pain (unilateral, bilateral, alternatively)	1–2
Pain that follows a nerve path	1–2
Superficial or deep pain	1–2
Possible link with a traumatic event	1–2
Similar pain in other family members	1–2
Female without sex hormones	1–2
Associated back pain	1–2
Associated diurnal bruxism	1–2
Pain elicited or triggered by noise, light, or odor*	1–2
Pain elicited or triggered by eating, speaking, or yawning*	1–2
Pain elicited or triggered by light touch	1–2
Pain elicited or triggered by menstruation	1–2
Pain increased by noise, light, odor, effort, or activity*	1–2
Pain increased by menstruation	1–2
Pain increased by yawning	1–2
Pain increased by certain foods	1–2
Nausea or vomiting accompanying the pain	1–2
Claude Bernard Homer syndrome	1–2
Indigestion, diarrhea	1–2
Flooding nose, tearing*	1–2
Pain felt in one upper quadrant of the face	2
Pain felt in one lower quadrant of the face	2
Pain felt bilaterally in the periorbital area	2
Pain felt unilaterally in the lateral part of the face	2
Pain felt in the nape	2
Pain felt in the mouth	2
Pain felt in the teeth	2
Pain felt in the bone	2
Pain felt in the mucosae	2
Pain felt in the temporomandibular joint (TMJ)	2
Pain felt in the masticatory muscles	2
Pain felt in the tongue	2
Pain felt in the skull	2
Pain felt in the eyes	2
Saliva abnormality	2
Xerostomia	2
Crackling, cracking, or clicking*	2
Pain or stiffness during muscle contraction*	2
TMJ pain at rest, active opening, against resistance*	2
Pain induced by muscle palpation	2

† Each sign or symptom was entered in List 1 (signs and symptoms related to the general characteristics of pain) and/or List 2 (also including signs and symptoms referring to a topographical site, organ, or tissue). Composite variables, marked with an asterisk (*), were formed with several single variables from the results of multidimensional analysis.

Adding the topographic signs and symptoms (List 2) strongly modified the dendritic tree and the clusters. The two neuralgias were no longer closely linked, migraine and tension-type headache were mixed, and the different idiopathic conditions tended to be more individualized. Dendrites leading to stomatodynia and arthromyalgia clusters became individualized early in the tree. Most atypical facial pain and atypical odontalgia were concentrated in two different clusters, which separated very late in the dendritic tree. These two clusters could therefore be labeled by a single term and so reduced to one cluster.

Using the variables forming List 1, we tested the reliability of the obtained classification in 10 subsamples, each including 75% of the total sample selected at random. The same statistical procedure was performed, and similar clustering was found. The validity of these present results was tested in the 107 patients who suffered from the five most well-known orofacial pain conditions (migraines, tension-type headaches, cluster headaches, classical trigeminal neuralgia, and post-traumatic trigeminal neuralgia). The reliability of the clinical diagnoses was also checked and was found to be satisfactory. These results suggested a classification of the chronic orofacial pain conditions, shown in Fig. 1, which includes proposals for the naming of the different clusters.

The strength of this approach is that it does not rely on any a priori decision and therefore can be regarded as aiming to achieve an evidence-based classification of idiopathic orofacial pain. Most previous studies of this type were based on a different approach. Usually, the different groups of patients are defined on the basis of a priori clinical criteria proposed on an authority-based consensus (Merskey and Bogduk 1994; Okeson 1996; Bierma-Zeinstra et al. 2001; International Headache Society 2004). It must also be emphasized that List 1 did not allow a clear separation between the different forms of idiopathic conditions, indicating that their individualization relies mainly on topographical criteria. It was only after the addition of items related to anatomy that entities such as arthromyalgia, atypical facial pain, and atypical odontalgia were identified. These idiopathic pain syndromes thus may involve similar pathophysiological mechanisms and may correspond to a single disease expressed in different tissues (Woolf et al. 1998).

In conclusion, these data provide grounds for an evidence-based classification of idiopathic facial pain entities and indicate that the current subclassification of these syndromes relies primarily on the topography of the symptoms.

TEMPOROMANDIBULAR JOINT DISEASES AND DISORDERS: CLASSIFICATION TO BE REVISITED

In the early 1990s, the University of Washington Pain Research Group, under the leadership of Dworkin and LeResche, spearheaded the development

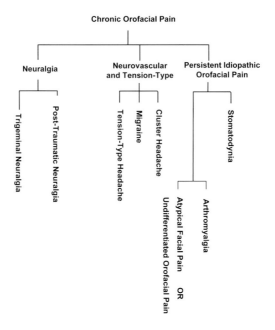

Fig. 1. Proposed classification for orofacial pain after multidimensional analyses. The term "arthromyalgia" is intended to exclude the temporomandibular joint and masticatory muscle disorders with well-identified causes or mechanisms. Undifferentiated orofacial pain includes the former atypical facial pain and atypical odontalgia. Persistent idiopathic orofacial pain includes stomatodynia, arthromyalgia, and undifferentiated orofacial pain. Because arthromyalgia and undifferentiated orofacial pain can be separated only by topographic signs and symptoms, they are located lower in the classification tree.

of a classification system for temporomandibular joint diseases and disorders (TMJD), referred to as the Research Diagnostic Criteria for Temporomandibular Disorders (RDC/TMJD) (Dworkin and LeResche 1992). The impact of this diagnostic construct on our understanding of these conditions has been greater than that of any other work in the field of TMJD. During the intervening years, the RDC/TMJD has fostered new understanding of what these conditions are and what they are not. Prior to their formulation, the TMJD were poorly defined with respect to identifying features, and no single case definition was universally applied.

The construct proposed in 1991–1992 was based on the best available data at that time, comprising rigorously acquired community-based epidemiological data sets, and was better than anything seen before in the TMJD literature in terms of the quality of the scientific methodology employed. It allowed the designation of a threshold upon which a subject became a case based on the presence of operationally defined, observable symptoms and signs. Notably, the case-identifying thresholds were adjusted so that they best matched the historical perceptions of the clinical communities with respect to the prevalence of cases in the general population (Dworkin et al. 1990).

Prior to publication of these criteria, little had been published in any systematic way about patients observed in tertiary care environments, including academic health care centers, the ultimate migration point for those cases refractory to otherwise successful therapeutic interventions. However, most clinicians had experienced frustration with the occasional case that appeared to be nonresponsive to interventions offered in the primary care environment. The huge range of case complexities did not escape scholarly explanation and was conceptualized by an appealing intellectual construct (Dworkin 1991). Fifteen years later, Dworkin's intellectual construct continues to attract those interested in trying to understand the underlying neurobiological mechanisms that distinguish the range of cases encountered in community-based settings and in the primary and tertiary care environments.

While Dworkin's intellectual construct offers an appealing explanatory model to rationalize the case complexity encountered in clinical practice, the question arises as to whether the RDC/TMJD construct itself—optimized for sensitivity at the threshold level of disease to be a satisfactory field research tool to be used in a community setting—is sufficiently sensitive to describe the full range of the case phenomenology in a valid and useful manner. References made to validity in this context are not to be confused with the validity of measurement of disease attributes, such as intra-examiner and inter-examiner reliabilities. Instead, the term—in the present context—should be understood as construct validity to express the fidelity by which the current understanding of the disease phenomenon is truthfully represented in the assigned diagnosis. The question arises: "Is the state of the patient's disease truthfully and comprehensively captured in the assigned case description?" On the other hand, when assigned a diagnostic label, the patient may wonder: "Does my care provider understand the full extent of my problem, or are further qualifying data required that must contain information of greater significance to me as a patient than was implied in the assigned diagnosis?" Specifically, is there reason to believe that the RDC/TMJD classification scheme captures the most severely affected patients in such a way that meaningful data are generated in support of scientific endeavors focusing on those patients who need help the most? Because TMJD cases, taken from different environments (e.g., the community setting or primary or tertiary care), can be forced into the RDC/TMJD framework, does it mean that their pathogenesis is sufficiently similar to warrant the pooling of cases for which personally critical disease factors are not even included?

Dworkin suggested, and few would disagree, that chronic pain associated with TMJD should be viewed as the worst possible outcome (Dworkin 1991). Unlike any other classification system, the RDC/TMJD incorporate this thinking in the Axis II data, making this portion of the diagnostic matrix the strongest piece of the system (Von Korff et al. 1992). In fact, it has become clear over the past 15 years that—although they lack disease specificity—case attributes related to psychosocial status and pain-related disability are the best predictors of current and future states of patients with TMJD. On the other hand, the core of the RDC/TMJD, Axis I, includes anatomical specificity with little or no evidence that the differentiation into its subsets (e.g., muscle, disk, joint) has any notable utility with respect to the prediction of the clinical course or treatment response. Furthermore, factors such as gender or sex constitute better predictors of a bad outcome than the anatomical RDC/TMJD classifiers that we so carefully guard.

Patients who are not being helped to any satisfactory degree usually have not embraced the concepts of psychosocial function and pain-related disability included in Axis II. Furthermore, patients increasingly express dissatisfaction about the fact that—mostly for those in the tertiary care environment—the medical problem is bigger than just a matter of muscle, disk, or joint. In fact, pain is often widespread, and only in a small portion of cases is it limited to the face. Comorbid conditions that are not listed in the RDC/TMJD are more likely than not to represent a key health issue for those seeking continued care (Turp et al. 1998a,b). Overall, this issue raises concern among patients—again, mostly among those in the tertiary care environment—that our records paint an insufficiently comprehensive picture of the patient's disease state.

It has now become necessary to consider ways of improving the construct validity of the RDC/TMJD diagnostic system. We may need to classify the various disease manifestations into categories that have etiologic and pathogenetic significance instead of adhering to anatomical classifiers of little or no significance for the patient's present and future states. It is probably time to incorporate what we have learned from applying the RDC/TMJD for more than a decade with respect to the extent to which comorbid conditions affect tertiary care cases. It may be necessary to capture comorbid conditions beyond Axis II criteria so that patients perceive our descriptions to be a truthful reflection of the totality of their disease state. We believe that the time for a revision is right and suggest that the incorporation of some of these concepts may improve the value of our favored diagnostic system, especially in the tertiary care sector.

CONCLUSIONS

Given the prevalence of orofacial pain both in the community and in secondary and tertiary centers, there is a need to accurately diagnose and then provide appropriate treatment for patients with this type of pain. The studies described in this chapter have shown that many of the orofacial conditions share common signs and symptoms and suggest that the nomenclature we have used is no longer appropriate. It is time to drop the term "atypical facial pain" and to rationalize the RDC/TMJD classification in the light of our increasing knowledge that orofacial pain is multifactorial and often widespread. Newer, more robust diagnostic criteria now need to be proposed and validated, and we need more objective measures both to diagnose and assess the outcomes of our treatments.

REFERENCES

Bierma-Zeinstra SMA, Bohnen AM, Bernsen RMD, et al. Hip problems in older adults: classification by cluster analysis. *J Clin Epidemiol* 2001; 54:1139–1145.

Clark GT, Delcanho RE, Goulet JP. The utility and validity of current diagnostic procedures for defining temporomandibular disorder patients. *Adv Dent Res* 1993; 7:97–112.

De Leeuw J, Van Rijckevorsel K. Homals and princals. Some generalizations of principal component analysis. In: Diday E (Eds). *Data Analysis and Informatics.* Amsterdam: Elsevier, 1980.

Derogatis LR. *SCL-90R: Administration, Scoring, and Procedures Manual-II.* Towson, MD: Clinical Psychometric Research, 1983.

Dworkin SF. Illness behavior and dysfunction: review of concepts and application to chronic pain. *Can J Physiol Pharmacol* 1991; 69:662–671.

Dworkin SF, LeResche L. Research diagnostic criteria for temporomandibular disorders: review, criteria, examinations and specifications, critique. *J Craniomandib Pract* 1992; 6:301–55.

Dworkin SF, Huggins KH, LeResche L, et al. Epidemiology of signs and symptoms in temporomandibular disorders: clinical signs in cases and controls, *J Am Dent Assoc* 1990; 120:273–281.

Feinmann C. Idiopathic orofacial pain: a multidisciplinary problem: the contribution of psychiatry and medicine to diagnosis and management. In: Campbell JN (Ed). *Pain 1996—An Updated Review.* Seattle: IASP Press, 1996, pp 397–402.

Harris M. The surgical management of idiopathic facial pain produces intractable iatrogenic pain? *Br J Oral Maxillofac Surg* 1996; 34:1–3.

International Headache Society (Headache Classification Committee). The international classification of headache disorders. *Cephalgia* 2004; 24:1–136.

Merskey H, Bogduk N. *Classification of Chronic Pain: Description of Chronic Pain Syndromes and Definitions of Pain Terms,* 2nd ed. Seattle: IASP Press, 1994.

Mongini F, Ciccone G, Ibertis F, Negro C. Personality characteristics and accompanying symptoms in temporomandibular joint dysfunction, headache, and facial pain. *J Orofac Pain* 2000; 14:52–58.

Okeson JP. *Orofacial Pain: Guidelines for Assessment, Classification, and Management.* Chicago: Quintessence, 1996.

Truelove EL, Sommers EE, LeResche L, Dworkin SF, Von Korff M. Clinical diagnostic criteria for TMD, new classification permits multiple diagnoses. *J Am Dent Assoc* 1992; 123:47–54.

Turp JC, Kowalski CJ, O'Leary TJ, Stohler CS. Pain maps from facial pain patients indicate a broad pain geography. *J Dent Res* 1998a; 77:1465–1472.

Turp JC, Kowalski CJ, Stohler CS. Treatment-seeking patterns of facial pain patients: many possibilities, limited satisfaction. *J Orofac Pain* 1998b; 12:61–66.

Von Korff MR, Dworkin SF, Fricton JR, Ohrbach R. Research diagnostic criteria. B. Axis II: Pain-related disability and psychological status. *J Craniomandib Disord Facial Oral Pain* 1992; 6:330–334.

Woda A, Pionchon P. A unified concept of idiopathic orofacial pain: clinical features. *J Orofac Pain* 1999; 13:172–184.

Woda A, Pionchon P. A unified concept of idiopathic orofacial pain: pathophysiologic features. *J Orofac Pain* 2000; 14:196–212.

Woda A, Tubert-Jeannin S, Bouhassira D, et al. Towards a new taxonomy of idiopathic orofacial pain. *Pain* 2005; 116:396–406.

Woolf CJ, Bennett GJ, Doherty M, et al. Towards a mechanism-based classification of pain. *Pain* 1998; 77:227–229.

Zakrzewska JM. Classification issues related to neuropathic trigeminal pain. *J Orofac Pain* 2004; 18:325–331.

Correspondence to: Professor Joanna M. Zakrzewska, MD, Clinical and Diagnostic Oral Sciences, Dental Institute, Barts and the London Queen Mary's School of Medicine and Dentistry, Turner Street, London E1 2AD, United Kingdom. Fax: 44-20-7377-7627; email: j.m.zakrzewska@qmul.ac.uk.

Proceedings of the 11th World Congress on Pain, edited by Herta Flor, Eija Kalso, and Jonathan O. Dostrovsky, IASP Press, Seattle, © 2006.

65

Clinical Decision-Making in Multidisciplinary Clinics

Stephen Loftus[a] and Joy Higgs[b]

[a]Pain Management Research Institute, University of Sydney, Royal North Shore Hospital, St Leonards, New South Wales, Australia; [b]Faculty of Health Sciences, University of Sydney, Lidcombe, New South Wales, Australia

Clinical decisions frequently are made by individual health care professionals alone. However, multidisciplinary pain clinics require the collaboration of different health care professions. Clinical meetings require individuals to articulate and justify their decision-making for each other as they negotiate and formulate the patients' problems and decide on management. We investigated the ways in which this interprofessional experience affects the clinical decision-making of the health care professionals involved in a multidisciplinary setting in order to come to a deeper understanding of clinical reasoning. This project, which sought to explore clinical reasoning from the philosophical perspective of hermeneutic phenomenology, was informed by insights from the work of Vygotsky (1978) and Wittgenstein (1958).

Phenomenology has evolved into many different forms since its introduction by Husserl (1973), having been modified by philosophers such as Heidegger (1996) and Gadamer (1989). Briefly, phenomenology seeks to understand phenomena by exploring the ways in which human beings experience them. Hermeneutic inquiry refers to the theory and practice of interpretation, and hermeneutic phenomenology combines the two strategies by seeking to explore people's interpretations of their experience.

A STUDY OF CLINICAL REASONING

We conducted our research in a multidisciplinary pain center. Twelve participants from the center were interviewed by the first author, who also attended the multidisciplinary team clinical meetings as a non-participating observer.

Participants included doctors, dentists, nurses, physiotherapists, and clinical psychologists. Interviews were recorded and transcribed, at which point participants were made anonymous (through the use of pseudonyms and the removal of identifying descriptors) in accordance with ethical principles. The transcripts were used for data analysis, along with the field notes from the observations of the meetings. Interview questions focused on topics such as patient assessment, communication with colleagues, aspects of practice that clinicians changed because they were working in the center and in a multidisciplinary team, procedures that they thought new staff needed to learn, and formative experiences that had occurred during their time in the center. Participants were encouraged to provide concrete examples of the experiences they described.

Data analysis followed typical practice for hermeneutic phenomenology. First, there was "immersion in the data," which involves close reading of all transcripts several times to attain a deep familiarity with the text. Second, themes or meaning units relevant to the research questions were identified. Third, these themes were brought together and used to develop a rich description of the phenomenon. Selected key findings are summarized below.

HOW LANGUAGE AFFECTS CLINICAL REASONING

It was apparent that a number of aspects of language permeated and informed the participants' understanding and use of clinical reasoning when dealing with chronic pain patients. The first was the notion of categories.

CATEGORIES

Health care professionals working at the multidisciplinary center needed to categorize patients' problems according to the biopsychosocial model (Engel 1977), which is frequently represented by the "onion skin" diagram (e.g., Loeser 2005). Practitioners in the pain center formulated a patient's problems according to this model, attempting to describe and understand what was happening at each layer of the "onion" rather than coming up with one definitive pathological diagnosis. The biopsychosocial model recognizes that in chronic cases, in addition to the original pathology, numerous problems have time to develop that must also be confronted. Simply focusing on pain to the exclusion of the other problems leads to frustration for both patients and practitioners. The practitioners in the center recognized pain not as an isolated entity, but as one category among other problems that they needed to assess and manage. The notion of categories led into the next major finding, which was the use of the underlying metaphors of health care.

METAPHOR

Lakoff and Johnson (1980) argued that thought and language are fundamentally metaphorical. Metaphor is not simply an embellishment of language exploited by writers and poets. It can be argued that language and thought are intensely and inherently metaphorical and that metaphor use goes largely unnoticed because it is so completely natural to us (Ortony 1993). Recent years have seen growing recognition of the extent to which metaphor underlies scientific and medical practice and shapes the ways in which both health professionals and their patients conceptualize their health problems and the possible solutions (e.g., Draaisma 2001; Reisfield and Wilson 2004). The health professionals in the pain center had to change the metaphors they used when working with chronic patients in the multidisciplinary environment. A key metaphor underlying the biomedical model is "the body is a machine." This is also the underlying metaphor with which patients in Western societies tend to conceptualize their bodily problems. In acute care, this metaphor could be appropriate. The implication of this metaphor is that we can always, in principle at least, repair a broken machine. However, the metaphor frequently falls down in the chronic situation in which repeated attempts at repair have failed, resulting in frustration and disappointment for both patients and health professionals. Often such patients are "discarded" by the system as "failed" patients (Alder 2003). The ways in which pain center staff described their work indicated that different metaphors were at work that were more in keeping with caring for chronic patients. For example, one metaphor that suggested itself repeatedly is "life is a journey." Rather than trying to cure patients, the staff provided interventions, from dorsal column stimulators to cognitive-behavioral therapy, that can help patients adjust their lives so that they can continue to live a relatively normal life despite pain. Such metaphors, in turn, provide the basis for different narratives.

NARRATIVE

The patients in the center have to cope with lives that have been drastically altered by pain. Pain has forced them to live out a different narrative from the one they lived before the pain came along. Patients seemed to be living out a narrative of increasing deterioration and distress. Much of the activity of the pain center can be seen as providing patients with an opportunity to develop a new narrative, a new sense of identity. Instead of seeing themselves as semipermanent invalids, dependent on the health professions and their families, the patients were encouraged to set achievable goals that would enable them to live relatively normal lives in which pain might be a factor, but one that was no longer dominant or overwhelming. The staff were careful not to impose new narratives, but let the patients work these out for themselves, using a problem-solving approach and what they sometimes described as "Socratic questioning," meaning that they would engage the patients in an ongoing dialogue in which the old narrative of being an invalid was gently, but persistently, questioned and the way opened for patients to reinterpret their own lives into a more able-bodied narrative. The various interventions of the clinic can be seen as providing the patients with the various "cognitive tools" they need to live out the new narrative and to give them a new lease on life.

COGNITIVE TOOLS

Cognitive tools, as described by Vygotsky (1978) also featured in the findings, not only for patients, but also for the staff. The staff learned to use a variety of cognitive tools from mnemonic devices, such as being aware of red and yellow flags during assessment, to formal questionnaires that were administered to patients. One extremely important cognitive tool used by all health professionals in their clinical meetings was the summary each wrote about every patient. (Each new patient is assessed individually by a doctor or dentist, a physiotherapist, and a clinical psychologist or psychiatrist during the course of one morning.) These summaries played a formal and important role in the clinical meetings that would immediately follow the assessments.

RITUAL/RHETORIC

The clinical meetings provided the setting for the practitioners to meet to compare findings and decide on treatment options. The meetings always adhered to a set pattern, with the doctor (or dentist) presenting a summary first, followed by the physiotherapist and then the psychologist. This pattern was formal enough to be regarded as a medical ritual, as described by Atkinson (1995). The formality and the way in which summaries were presented lent the proceedings a distinctive rhetorical force. Presenting an adequate summary was a crucial aspect of the clinical meetings, and new practitioners had to learn rapidly how to construct and present their summaries for these meetings. Summaries had to present only salient points about patients, rather than all the assessment findings. The summaries were, in essence, compressed narratives about the patients, as practitioners consciously tried to adopt a holistic view of the patient and the ways in which available management options could fit into the patients' lives.

The physiotherapists and psychologists also had to acquire the skill of dynamically adjusting their summaries as they listened to their predecessors describe the same patient they had seen. The purpose of this dynamic adjustment was to avoid needless repetition, to raise issues that others had not addressed, and to add emphasis and more detail to issues that were considered of key importance for the case being discussed.

Of particular interest was the way in which differing metaphors of health care were combined in what can be best described as a dialectical synthesis. Although all practitioners subscribed to the biopsychosocial model, this approach manifested itself in distinctive ways. The doctors tended to assess patients from a clinico-pathological approach, looking for organic features that could be treated (i.e., following the "body is a machine" metaphor). This approach was in contrast to that of the psychologists and physiotherapists, who tended to assess patients from a more functional viewpoint, looking for ways to improve a patient's lifestyle regardless of any organic diagnosis (following the "life is a journey" metaphor). The doctors were well aware that they could be accused of adhering to a biomedical model, but felt that they had to provide a balance to the functional approach of the other team members. The two models or metaphors do not have to be seen as contradictory. A dialectical perspective would see them as complementary, and together they can constitute a rigorous and catalytic application of the biopsychosocial approach. Similar findings have also been found in the management of atherosclerosis (Mol 2002).

CONCLUSION

It can be argued that qualitative aspects of clinical decision-making in relation to pain management have been under-researched compared to the wealth

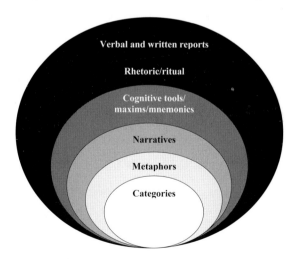

Fig. 1. Verbal and written reports are the audible and visual results of clinical reasoning. The skill of clinical reasoning in a multidisciplinary setting depends on the complex interaction of many aspects of specialized language use.

of effort poured into fields such as neurobiology. If we accept pain as a phenomenon that is subjectively experienced and appreciated, then the subjectivity of both patients and practitioners needs to be better understood. The recent interest in pain and narrative (Carr et al. 2005) is a welcome development in this direction.

Our research into clinical decision-making falls within this interpretive tradition. We propose a model of collective, interdisciplinary clinical reasoning that is focused in process around a community of practice using the primary tool of a shared language and is similar in structure to the onion skin metaphor of pain (Fig. 1). Clinical reasoning, like pain, is a multidimensional phenomenon in which the various aspects, such as narrative and metaphor, are intimately related. In order to serve our patients better and enable them to optimize the quality of their lives, we need to come to a deeper understanding of the ways in which we make decisions about our patients and with them.

REFERENCES

Alder S. *Beyond the Restitution Narrative*. Thesis. The University of Western Sydney, 2003.

Atkinson P. *Medical Talk and Medical Work: The Liturgy of the Clinic*. London: Sage Publications, 1995.

Carr DB, Loeser JD, Morris DB (Eds). *Narrative, Pain, and Suffering,* Progress in Pain Research and Management, Vol. 34. Seattle: IASP Press, 2005.

Draaisma D. The tracks of thought. *Nature* 2001; 414:153.

Engel GL. The need for a new medical model: a challenge for biomedicine. *Science* 1977; 196:129–136.

Gadamer H-G. *Truth and Method,* 2nd revised ed. New York: Continuum, 1989.

Heidegger M. *Being and Time: A Translation of Sein und Zeit* (Stambaugh J, Trans). Albany, NY: State University of New York Press, 1996.

Husserl E. *Cartesian Meditations: An Introduction to Phenomenology* (Cairns D, Trans). The Hague: Nijhoff, 1973.

Lakoff G, Johnson M. *Metaphors We Live By*. Chicago: University of Chicago Press, 1980.

Loeser JD. Pain, suffering, and the brain: a narrative of meanings. In: Carr DB, Loeser JD, Morris DB (Eds). *Narrative, Pain and Suffering,* Progress in Pain Research and Management, Vol. 34. Seattle: IASP Press, 2005, pp 17–27.

Mol A. *The Body Multiple: Ontology in Medical Practice*. Durham, NC: Duke University Press, 2002.

Ortony A (Ed). *Metaphor and Thought,* 2nd ed. Cambridge: Cambridge University Press, 1993.

Reisfield GM, Wilson GR. Use of metaphor in the discourse on cancer. *J Clin Oncol* 2004; 22(19):4024–4027.

Vygotsky LS. *Mind in Society: The Development of the Higher Psychological Processes*. Cambridge, MA: MIT Press, 1978.

Wittgenstein L. *Philosophical Investigations,* 3rd ed (Anscombe GEM, Trans). Upper Saddle River, NJ: Prentice Hall, 1958.

Correspondence to: Stephen Loftus, MSc, Pain Management Research Institute, Royal North Shore Hospital, St Leonards, Sydney, NSW 2065, Australia. Email: sloftus@nsccahs.health.nsw.gov.au.

Proceedings of the 11th World Congress on Pain,
edited by Herta Flor, Eija Kalso, and Jonathan O.
Dostrovsky, IASP Press, Seattle, © 2006.

66

A Prospective Approach to Defining Chronic Pain

Michael Von Korff and Diana L. Miglioretti

Center for Health Studies, Group Health Cooperative, Seattle, Washington, USA

This chapter provides an overview of a prospective approach to defining chronic pain in probabilistic terms, recognizing that predicting the future course of pain is inherently uncertain. Valid, reproducible operational criteria for classifying chronic pain are needed for epidemiological and clinical research, and for clinical practice (Andersson 1999). Prevalence estimates of chronic pain conditions often vary widely due to lack of reproducible operational criteria. In clinical research, it is often unclear how chronic pain status is defined and evaluated, making it difficult to understand whether patient populations are comparable across studies. In clinical practice, existing definitions of chronic pain have been difficult to apply. Cedraschi et al. (1998) observed that "difficulties in defining and classifying ... pain may lead to communication problems among health professionals as well as between patients and health professionals."

Chronic pain has been defined as: "pain which persists past the normal time of healing. ... With nonmalignant pain, three months is the most convenient point of division between acute and chronic pain, but for research purposes six months will often be preferred" (Merskey and Bogduk 1994). Although this definition seems simple, it can be difficult to apply. The term "chronic" is as much a prognostic statement as a description of pain history, but chronic pain classifications have rarely been evaluated in terms of predictive validity.

Three approaches to classifying chronic pain can be contrasted: pain history, concurrent, and prognostic. Classifications based on *pain history* focus on pain persistence, for example, episode duration (Merskey and Bogduk 1994) or number of days with pain in a defined time period (Olesen et al. 2003). *Concurrent* classifications employ multiple measures of pain intensity, interference with activities, and psychosocial variables to identify patients with significant pain dysfunction (Turk and Rudy 1988). A *prognostic* classification extends the concurrent approach by using measures of current pain status and prognostic variables to predict future pain severity. This chapter summarizes work on a prospective approach to classifying chronic back pain.

METHODS

The details of the data and methods employed here are reported in depth elsewhere (Von Korff and Miglioretti 2005). This chapter provides an overview of concepts and empirical results that led us to propose defining chronic back pain in terms of outcome probabilities.

Definitions. Using a prognostic approach, chronic pain is defined as clinically significant pain likely to be present one or more years in the future. Specifically, *possible chronic back pain* is defined by a 50% or greater probability of future clinically significant back pain. *Probable chronic back pain* is defined by an 80% or greater probability of future clinically significant back pain.

Setting and sample. Patients at Group Health Cooperative aged 18 to 75 years making back pain visits in primary care during 1989–1990 were identified through appointment logs.

Data collection. Three to six weeks after the back pain visit resulting in study enrollment, eligible patients were contacted and asked to participate in a 20–30-minute telephone interview after providing informed consent. Follow-up interviews were carried out by telephone 1, 2, and 5 years later.

Pain severity. Pain severity was assessed using multiple measures of pain intensity, interference with activities, and role disability using measures described in other reports (Von Korff and Miglioretti 2005).

Prognostic variables. Three prognostic variables were employed: the Symptom Checklist (SCL)-90 depression scale (Derogatis 1983), the number of days with back pain in the past 6 months (Von Korff et al. 1992), and the number of other pain sites (including headache, abdominal pain, chest pain, and facial pain).

Statistical methods. Latent transition regression analysis (LTRA) was used to identify a set of ordered categories constituting latent pain severity classes. The LTRA methods developed for this research are described in a prior report (Miglioretti 2003). The classes identified by LTRA were: (1) no pain; (2) mild pain; (3) moderate pain and limitation; and (4) severe, limiting pain. LTRA was used to assess the course of pain severity over time by modeling transitions among these pain severity classes.

Consistent with prior research, we observed that only persons with severe, limiting back pain at one observation point were at high risk (50% or greater) of having such pain a year or more later. For that reason, we initially focused on the probability that a person with severe, limiting back pain would continue to have severe pain at a subsequent observation point (at least 1 year later). These analyses helped elucidate the population dynamics of chronic back pain, and suggested classifying chronic pain in terms of outcome probabilities.

Drawing on the LTRA results, a risk-based approach to classification of chronic back pain was developed. A risk score was estimated from pain severity and prognostic variables that predicted future clinically significant back pain. For these analyses we defined clinically significant back pain at follow-up by Chronic Pain Grades 2, 3 or 4 (Von Korff et al. 1992). We chose this criterion for clinically significant back pain because these grades identify persons with intense back pain accompanied by mild to severe dysfunction, whereas persons with Grade 1 back pain have low levels of pain and dysfunction.

A smoothed probability plot was fit to the baseline risk score. Using this plot, we identified the baseline risk score levels at which 50% and 80% of patients were found to have clinically significant back pain at 1 year follow-up. We then assessed whether these risk score thresholds achieved comparable levels of prediction when applied to year 1 and year 2 data in predicting Grade 2–4 back pain at subsequent follow-ups.

RESULTS

Prevalence of severe, limiting pain. The prevalence (percentage) of each of the four pain severity classes (no pain; mild pain; moderate pain and limitation; and severe, limiting pain) was estimated by the LTRA model at baseline and at years 1, 2, and 5. At baseline, 30% of study patients were estimated to have severe, limiting pain, while the prevalence of such pain declined to 15% at the 1-year follow-up, 14% at the 2-year follow-up, and 12% at the 5-year follow-up. The prevalence of moderate pain and limitation was 52% at baseline, and was reduced to 39% at 1 year, 34% at 2 years, and 30% at 5 years. Relatively few patients were completely free of back pain at long-term follow-up, reaching a maximum of 23% at 5 years. The high prevalence of mild to moderate back pain, typically recurrent, suggests the difficulty in defining chronic back pain by duration alone.

Back pain outcomes over time. LTRA analyses revealed that the most common pattern was to remain in the same pain severity class from one observation point to the next. For example, from baseline to year 1, 67% of patients with mild pain continued to have mild pain, 50% of the moderate pain patients continued to have moderate pain, and 43% of those with severe pain continued to have severe pain 1 year later. The second most likely outcome was to improve by one pain severity class.

The transition probabilities from severe, limiting pain at one observation point to severe, limiting pain at the next are of particular interest in understanding chronicity. The probability that severe pain would be present at the following observation were: 43% from baseline to year 1, 69% from year 1 to year 2, and 57% from year 2 to year 5. Thus, the presence of severe, limiting pain identified patients with high probabilities of future severe pain, consistent with the proposed definition of chronic pain. In contrast, the probabilities of transitioning to severe, limiting pain at follow-up among persons with moderate pain or mild pain were substantially lower. Among persons with moderate pain initially, the percent with severe, limiting pain at the following observation were 5% from baseline to year 1, 9% from year 1 to year 2, and 10% from year 2 to year 5. The probability of developing severe, limiting pain among persons with mild back pain was less than 3% at all follow-up interviews. These observations indicated the utility of pain severity measures in predicting risks of future clinically significant back pain.

Prognostic variables.   When we examined the effect of prognostic variables among persons with mild or moderate back pain, we found that even high levels of pain persistence, diffuse pain, or depressive symptoms did not predict risks of future severe pain approaching 50%. Persons with mild or moderate pain, although back pain often continued, were at low risk of future severe back pain, *even when unfavorable prognostic indicators were present.*

By considering prognostic variables other than pain severity among patients with severe, limiting pain, we sought to differentiate persons with lower versus higher risk of enduring, clinically significant pain. Fig. 1 shows the probabilities of having severe, limiting pain at year 1 among persons with severe, limiting pain at baseline for varying levels of each of the three prognostic variables (depicted from each variable's minimum to maximum value). Similar results were observed for the prediction of severe, limiting back pain by these prognostic variables from year 1 to year 2 and from year 2 to year 5.

From baseline to year 1, high levels of depressive symptoms raised the risk of future severe back pain above the 50% threshold and toward the 80% level. Conversely, persons with low levels of depressive symptoms were at much lower risk. From baseline to year 1, the presence of pain at multiple body sites increased the risk of future severe back pain above the 50% level, as did increasing numbers of days with back pain.

Prediction of future severe back pain by risk score.   To develop a practical means to identify patients with possible or probable chronic back pain, we created an empirical risk score drawing on items and scales used in the LTRA models. This risk score included ratings of pain intensity and interference with activities, days of activity limitation, depressive symptoms, number of days with back pain, and number of other pains (see Von Korff and Miglioretti 2005 for details).

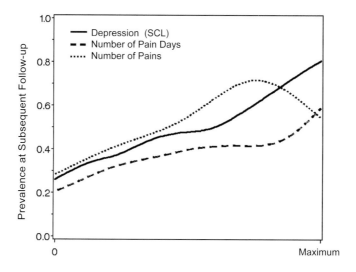

Fig. 1. Percentage with severe, limiting back pain at year 1 among persons with severe, limiting back pain at baseline by level of three prognostic variables: depression scores on the Symptom Checklist-90 (SCL), number of back pain days in the last 6 months, and number of other pain problems.

The ability of the baseline risk score to predict Chronic Pain Grades 2–4 was assessed by a smoothed probability plot (Fig. 2). Using this plot, a threshold risk score for probable chronic back pain was set at the value corresponding to an 80% probability of future clinically significant back pain (Chronic Pain Grades 2–4). The threshold risk score for possible chronic back pain corresponded to a 50% probability of future clinically significant back pain. As indicated in Fig. 2, low and intermediate risk levels were differentiated by a 20% probability of future clinically significant back pain.

At baseline, 6.1% of patients were classified as having probable chronic back pain, and an additional 20.3% were classified as having possible chronic back pain. Using the same risk score cut-off points for possible and probable chronic pain but using pain status measures assessed at subsequent observations, 4.4% were scored as having probable chronic back pain at year 1, and an additional 12.5% were scored as having possible chronic back pain at year 1. At year 2, 3.4% of study patients surpassed the risk score threshold for probable chronic pain, and an additional 10.5% fell in the risk score range for possible chronic pain.

As might be expected, these risk score groups were found to strongly predict future clinically significant back pain from baseline to 1 year, with 58.7% of possible and 82.1% of probable chronic back pain patients having back pain

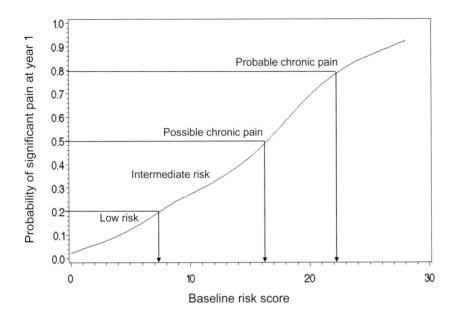

Fig. 2. Probability of clinically significant back pain (Chronic Pain Grades 2–4) at year 1 predicted from baseline risk score.

at Chronic Pain Grades 2–4 one year later (Table I). Baseline risk score group also strongly predicted the percentage with clinically significant back pain (Chronic Pain Grades 2–4) at year 2 and year 5. As shown in Table I, about half of the patients classified as having possible chronic back pain at baseline were found to have clinically significant back pain at years 2 and 5, while about 70% of the probable chronic back pain patients had clinically significant back pain at years 2 and 5.

Replicating the baseline results, risk score groups assessed at year 1 (using the cut-off points established at baseline) also strongly predicted the presence of clinically significant back pain at years 2 and year 5 (Table I). Among persons with probable chronic back pain at year 1, 90.9% and 76.5% had clinically significant back pain at years 2 and 5, respectively. Well over half of the patients with possible chronic back pain at year 1 had clinically significant back pain at years 2 and 5. Among persons with a risk score at or above the threshold for probable chronic pain at year 2, 74% had clinically significant back pain 3 years later, while 68% of those with possible chronic pain at year 2 had clinically significant back pain at year 5. The differences in the percentage at Chronic Pain Grades 2–4 between the four chronic pain risk groups in Table I were highly statistically significant at all time points ($P < 0.0001$), as assessed by Chi-square tests.

Table I
Probability of clinically significant pain in primary care back pain patients at 1,
2, and 5 years by risk level determined at baseline and at year 1

	Percentage with Chronic Pain		
	1 Year	2 Years	5 Years
Baseline Risk Score Group			
Low risk (0–7) (30.6%, *n* = 339)	10.9	8.0	11.7
Intermediate risk (8–15) (43.0%, *n* = 476)	32.1	27.6	24.6
Possible chronic pain (16–21) (20.3%, *n* = 225)	58.7	51.7	46.4
Probable chronic pain (22+) (6.1%, *n* = 67)	82.1	71.7	68.2
Year 1 Risk Score Group			
Low risk (0–7) (54.4%, *n* = 550)		10.9	13.1
Intermediate risk (8–15) (28.8%, *n* = 291)		40.6	33.8
Possible chronic pain (12.5%, *n* = 126)		62.7	58.8
Probable chronic pain (4.4%, *n* = 44)		90.9	76.5

DISCUSSION

PREDICTING PAIN OUTCOMES

Consistent with prior research (Turk and Rudy 1988; Von Korff et al 1992), multiple measures of pain intensity, interference with activities, and role disability could be used to assess pain severity. These results support a multi-variable approach to assessing chronic pain.

Back pain outcomes are highly variable (Von Korff et al. 1993; Cedraschi et al. 1999; McGorry et al. 2000). A prognostic approach discards the notion that "chronic" means unlikely to change. There was not a clear demarcation distinguishing persons with possible or probable chronic back pain from those with less severe back pain. This finding suggests that a classification of chronic back pain should be viewed as a prognostic guide whose future implications are uncertain and mutable. The potential for change, indeed the likelihood of change, is an important and often neglected feature of chronic pain. For these reasons, the terms *possible* and *probable* chronic back pain appropriately emphasize the inherent uncertainty of long-term back pain outcomes. The focus shifts from the potentially stigmatizing question of whether a person is a "chronic pain patient" to the *likelihood* that clinically significant back pain will continue and, by extension, to steps that might be taken to reduce future risks of significant pain and dysfunction.

FUTURE RESEARCH

Prognostic variables that might improve prediction of future pain status in future research include other psychological measures (e.g., catastrophizing and fear-avoidance beliefs), clinical assessments specific to back pain, and genetic or psychophysiological variables that may be found to predict back pain outcomes in future research. The common denominator of a prospective approach is the ability to predict clinically significant pain at a distal time point, rather than the content or nature of the specific measures employed. It would be useful to use logistic regression methods to optimize prediction of future pain status.

CONCLUSIONS

In conclusion, our results support a prognostic approach to defining chronic back pain. There appeared to be a continuum of chronic back pain, rather than a distinct class of chronic back pain patients. Because back pain outcomes were highly variable across individuals and over time, chronic back pain should be viewed as an uncertain prognostic statement, rather than a static trait identifying patients unlikely to improve. The term "chronic pain" has come to carry negative connotations for patients and clinicians alike. By shifting the focus from pain history to prognosis, and by defining chronicity in probabilistic terms, the assessment of chronic pain may be less stigmatizing for patients and more focused on steps that can be taken to reduce risks of an unfavorable outcome.

ACKNOWLEDGMENTS

This research was supported by NIH grant P01 DE08773. Kathleen Saunders' contributions to this research are gratefully acknowledged. This chapter includes material published in extended form elsewhere (Von Korff and Miglioretti 2005) and is presented here with permission of the International Association for the Study of Pain.

REFERENCES

Andersson GB. Epidemiological features of low back pain. *Lancet* 1999; 14:581–585.
Cedraschi C, Nordin M, Nachemson AL, Vischer TL. Health care providers should use a common language in relation to low back pain patients. *Bailleres Clin Rheumatol* 1998; 12:1–8.
Cedraschi C, Robert J, Goerg D, et al. Is chronic non-specific low back pain chronic? Definitions of a problem and problems of a definition. *Br J Gen Pract* 1999; 49:358–362.
Derogatis LR. *SCL-90-R: Administration, Scoring and Procedures Manual-II for the Revised Version*. Towson, MD: Clinical Psychometric Research, 1983.

McGorry RW, Webster BS, Snook SH, Hsiang SM. The relation between pain intensity, disability, and the episodic nature of chronic and recurrent low back pain. *Spine* 2000; 25:834–841.

Merskey H, Bogduk N. *Classification of Chronic Pain: Descriptions of Chronic Pain Syndromes and Definitions of Pain Terms.* Seattle: IASP Press, 1994.

Miglioretti DL. Latent transition regression for mixed outcomes. *Biometrics* 2003; 59:710–720.

Olesen J, Goadsby P, Steiner T. The International Classification of Headache Disorders, 2nd edition (ICHD-II): revision of criteria for 8.2 Medication-overuse headache. *Lancet Neurol* 2003; 2:720.

Turk DC, Rudy TE. Toward an empirically derived taxonomy of chronic pain patients: integration of psychological assessment data. *J Consult Clin Psychol* 1988; 56:233–238.

Von Korff M, Miglioretti DL. A prognostic approach to defining chronic pain. *Pain* 2005; 117:304–313.

Von Korff M, Ormel J, Keefe F, Dworkin SF. Grading the severity of chronic pain. *Pain* 1992; 50:133–149.

Von Korff M, Deyo RA, Cherkin D, Barlow W. Back pain in primary care: outcomes at one year. *Spine* 1993; 18:855–862.

Correspondence to: Michael Von Korff, ScD, Center for Health Studies, Group Health Cooperative, 1730 Minor Avenue, Suite 1600, Seattle, WA, 98101, USA. Fax: 206-287-2871; email: vonkorff.m@ghc.org.

Part IX

Psychological Interventions, Occupational Therapy, and Physical Approaches

Proceedings of the 11th World Congress on Pain,
edited by Herta Flor, Eija Kalso, and Jonathan O.
Dostrovsky, IASP Press, Seattle, © 2006.

67

Developing Multidisciplinary Cognitive-Behavioral Pain Management Programs in Asia

Michael K. Nicholas, Mary Cardosa, and P.P. Chen

*Pain Management and Research Institute, University of Sydney at Royal North
Shore Hospital, Sydney, Australia; Department of Anesthesiology, Selayang
Hospital, Kuala Lumpur, Malaysia; Department of Anesthesiology
and Operating Services, Alice Ho Miu Ling Nethersole Hospital and North
District Hospital, Hong Kong*

Systematic reviews and meta-analyses have provided strong evidence of the effectiveness of cognitive-behavioral interventions for enhancing pain self-management in a wide range of chronic pain populations (Morley et al. 1999; Guzmán et al. 2001). These interventions aim to equip chronic pain patients with the necessary skills to improve their social, occupational, and psychological functioning and decrease their reliance on passive modalities, such as taking unnecessary medication and undergoing repeated procedures (Nicholas 2003). The vast majority of this work has been conducted in Western countries, especially in Europe and North America. In Asia, self-management techniques for chronic pain have not been adopted as rapidly as other advances in Western medicine. Furthermore, cultural and language differences in the different populations raise questions about the acceptability and suitability of these techniques for many Asian patients. No outcomes have been reported previously on the application of this approach in Asian countries. Nevertheless, epidemiological findings indicate that persisting pain conditions are a problem in those countries. Pain clinics have been established in a number of Asian countries, and there is growing recognition of the need for improved pain management services in Asia.

This chapter describes the pioneering work at two Asian pain clinics that are attempting to establish multidisciplinary pain management programs. Accounts of these clinics not only provide a valuable source of information on the challenging processes involved in establishing a new health care venture, but in common with much of the history of pain medicine, they illustrate how dependent the development of new services is on individuals who are prepared to go beyond the normal expectations of traditional professional roles and to grapple with health systems that can be as challenging as many persisting pain conditions.

THE MENANG PROGRAM IN MALAYSIA

SOCIAL AND HEALTH SYSTEM CONTEXTS

Malaysia has a multiethnic, multicultural population of 24 million, with 65% Bumiputeras (Malays and indigenous peoples), 26% Chinese, and 8% Indians. The dominant religion is Islam (60%), but there are significant numbers of Buddhists (19%), Christians (9%), and Hindus (6%) (Department of Statistics Malaysia 2005). The Ministry of Health is the main provider of health care in Malaysia, with an annual health care expenditure of 3.8% of the gross domestic product (World Health Organization 2005). Priority areas for the Ministry of Health are primary community health, infectious diseases, cancer, and heart disease. Recent years have seen an additional emphasis on computerization of hospitals and on the provision of subspecialty services in tertiary hospitals using the latest diagnostic and therapeutic techniques. As a result, Malaysians have high expectations of technical medical solutions from modern hospitals using state-of-the-art techniques and equipment.

CHRONIC PAIN AND PAIN MEDICINE IN MALAYSIA

Pain medicine is a relatively new specialty in Malaysia for which funding has only been available since 1997. The first of Malaysia's eight current multidisciplinary pain clinics was established in 2000. No studies have focused on the prevalence of chronic pain in Malaysia, but we can assume that it affects around 15–20% of the population (e.g., Elliott et al. 1999; Moore and Brödsgaard 1999; Blyth et al. 2001). For the estimated 3–4 million Malaysians with chronic pain, access to pain specialists is limited; most pain patients are treated by general practitioners and other specialists.

INJURY COMPENSATION SCHEMES

Most workers are covered by the Social Security Organisation, a statutory body that receives compulsory monthly contributions from workers and employers. There is little recognition of the disability that may result from chronic pain, which merits an additional 3–5% given on top of a baseline disability assessment that is usually limited to loss of limb or of mobility of joints.

THE MENANG PAIN MANAGEMENT PROGRAM

The Multidisciplinary Pain Clinic at Hospital Selayang, a Ministry of Health Hospital in Kuala Lumpur, opened in June 2000. A pain management program based on cognitive-behavioral therapy principles was an early priority because there were no such programs in the country, let alone the region. The first MENANG program, conducted in 2002, was modeled on the ADAPT pain management program of the Pain Management and Research Centre at the Royal North Shore Hospital in Sydney, Australia (Nicholas et al. 2000). "Menang" means "win" in the official Malaysian language (Bahasa Malaysia) and is derived from "program menangani kesakitan," which literally means "program to manage pain."

INITIAL PLANNING AND IMPLEMENTATION

In late 2001, a team of four Malaysians (an anesthetist, a psychiatrist, a nurse, and a physiotherapist) received funds from the Ministry of Health to spend 3 weeks at the Royal North Shore Hospital in Sydney, where they observed the ADAPT program, participated in discussions with the experienced staff there, and developed an implementation plan for the MENANG program. Further discussions were held in Malaysia that settled issues such as the schedule (2 weeks instead of ADAPT's 3 weeks, mainly because of the staff's other duties and time constraints), the role of each team member, and criteria for selection of patients. Support was sought from other staff and hospital authorities, and funding and space were assigned.

The first MENANG program involved the Malaysian staff and two experienced Australian pain clinic staff—a clinical psychologist (Michael Nicholas) and a physiotherapist (Lois Tonkin). A training workshop for staff (and other health workers) was conducted prior to the program, and supervision was provided by Dr. Nicholas and Ms. Tonkin over the 2 weeks.

Since the initial program, two MENANG programs a year have been conducted. Clinical psychologists (three from Australia and one from the United Kingdom) experienced in running pain management programs have been invited to assist in each of the subsequent four programs. Over this time, further work has concentrated on expanding the team, sharing the knowledge and skills with other staff (physiotherapists, psychiatrists, clinical psychologists, anesthetists, and nurses) from other hospitals, educating health care administrators and other doctors about the principles of pain management programs, and integrating MENANG into the pain clinic.

DESCRIPTION OF THE MENANG PROGRAM

The program is conducted in English and Bahasa Malaysia, with translation into Tamil and Mandarin when necessary. It runs daily from 8:30 a.m. to 4:30 p.m. for 2 weeks (10 days), with approximately 10 patients per group. Sessions include education about pain and reformulation of the pain (as chronic but not sinister); training in skills including relaxation, goal setting, and identifying and challenging unhelpful cognitions (beliefs and thought processes); problem-solving and pain management strategies (e.g., activity pacing and daily planning); and an exercise component that encourages patients to perform activities on a graded basis, to limit avoidance behaviors, and to regain confidence in functioning despite pain. Patients also discontinue their pain medications in a gradual, guided fashion. Patient selection is based on persisting high levels of disability and distress and on a clinical opinion that no further medical or surgical treatments are appropriate. Participants attend as either inpatients or outpatients, depending on the distance of their home from the hospital (see Table I for a description of patient characteristics). The team running the program includes a clinical psychologist, a psychiatrist, physiotherapists, physicians, and nurses. The team meets regularly during the program to discuss each patient's progress. Follow-up review sessions are conducted at 1, 3, 6, and 12 months.

Table I
Demographic details of patients in the Malaysian program

Variable	
Number of patients	47
Mean age in years (SD); range	44 (10.6); 17–68
Gender	F: 26 (55.3%)
Ethnic Group	
Malay, n (%)	10 (21.3%)
Chinese, n (%)	10 (21.3%)
Indian, n (%)	27 (57.4%)
Pain Types	
Neuropathic, n (%)	15 (31.9%)
Musculoskeletal, n (%)	22 (46.8%)
Mixed, neuropathic/musculoskeletal, n (%)	2 (4.3%)
Visceral, n (%)	8 (17.0%)
Mean duration of pain in months (SD); range	84.7 (79.9); 8–360
Language	
English-speaking *(n)*	34 (73.3%)
Bahasa Malaysia speaking *(n)*	45 (95.7%)

OUTCOMES

No major differences have been found in pain-related disability and distress, reactions to pain, or beliefs about pain among Malaysian patients compared to those reported in Western countries, and the methods used in Western programs have been equally applicable in Malaysia (e.g., Nicholas et al. 1992; Williams et al. 1999). The results achieved to date (see Table II) show that median scores on self-report questionnaires and activity measures improved at the end of the 2-week program and that these changes were maintained at the 1-month follow-up. Data from the 12-month follow-up are currently being collected, but indications are that most improvements have been maintained. Disability and catastrophizing scores were reduced, and level of function was

Table II
Medians and quartile (25th to 75th percentile) ranges of outcome measures across different time frames with the Malaysian program ($n = 47$ participants)

Measure (Range of Scores)*	Pretreatment	Post-treatment	At 1 Month	At 1 Year
N (range on different measures)	47 (45–47)	47 (46–47)	46 (42–46)	20 (18–20)
Usual pain, NRS (0–10)	6.0 (5.0–7.0)	5.0 (4.0–6.0)[a]	5.0 (4.0–6.5)[b]	5.0 (3.3–6.0)
Disability, R&M (0–24)	14 (10–18)	6 (3–15)[a]	4 (2–12)[b,c]	6.5 (3.0–13.3)[e]
Depression, DASS (0–42)	12.5 (6.8–21.5)	5.0 (1.0–13.9)[a]	3.0 (0–12.0)[b]	3.0 (0–15.0)
Self-efficacy, PSEQ (0–60)	33 (24–43)	49 (35–55)[a]	45 (34.5–52)[b]	43.5 (30–58.3)[f]
Catastrophizing (0–5)	2.8 (2.1–3.6)	1.4 (0.4–2.2)[a]	1.2 (0.3–2.1)[b]	1.6 (0.6–2.8)[g]
20-m walk (seconds)	20 (17.5–28.5)	16 (14.4–23)[a]	16 (14–24.8)[b]	NA
Stairs climbed in 2 minutes	60 (36–84)	69 (48–96)[a]	84 (50–108)[b,d]	NA

Note: Data were analyzed with nonparametric, Wilcoxon matched-pairs signed-rank tests. [a]Change from pre- to post-treatment, $P < 0.001$; [b]change from pretreatment to 1 month, $P < 0.001$; [c]change from post-treatment to 1 month, $P < 0.001$; [d]change from post-treatment to 1 month, $P < 0.02$; [e]change from pretreatment to 1 year, $P < 0.002$; [f]change from pretreatment to 1 year, $P < 0.02$; [g]change from pretreatment to 1 year, $P < 0.01$.

* Pain: 0–10 numerical rating scale of usual pain in last week; R&M: Modified Roland and Morris scale (24 = maximum disability) (Asghari and Nicholas 2001); DASS: Depression Anxiety and Stress Scale (depression subscale, 42 = maximum depression) (Taylor et al. 2005); PSEQ: Pain Self-Efficacy Questionnaire (60 = maximum confidence in being active despite pain) (Nicholas et al. 1992); Catastrophizing: Pain Response Self-Statements Scale (5 = maximum catastrophizing) (Flor et al. 1993); NA: not available.

improved. Mood and confidence to manage despite the pain also improved, and median pain scores were reduced despite the use of less medication for pain, although this outcome was not one of the goals of the program (see Table III). Return-to-work outcomes were also very promising (see Table IV), although there were many obstacles such as the unavailability of graded return-to-work schemes and prejudice among employers against those with chronic pain. In addition, use of health care services for pain (visits to pain clinics, emergency departments, and other doctors) has been noticeably reduced and even discontinued by many patients since their participation in the program.

CHALLENGES

Establishing the Malaysian program posed many challenges. Patients are from multiethnic, multicultural backgrounds with varying levels of literacy. Sessions were conducted in both Bahasa Malaysia and English, but some patients could understand neither language, requiring translation into Tamil or Mandarin. This process is time consuming, but on the positive side, translation has meant the repetition and reinforcement of messages conveyed. The different religious and cultural beliefs, while adding to the complexity of the group, have turned out to be a positive factor because patients have shared the helpful teachings and principles from their own religion or cultural group with others. The staff, also a multiethnic and multicultural group, has also learned from the patients, who have provided examples or stories that have helped staff to address difficult concepts with subsequent groups.

Another challenge has been the possible scepticism regarding this new "treatment" and its place vis-a-vis the more established modalities of treatment for pain as well as the variety of traditional remedies available in Malaysia such as herbal remedies, massage, and acupuncture. One advantage in favor of the team was that they had already established relationships of trust with the patients before the program started. This trust encouraged the patients to try out the "new" treatment. Continuing to show concern for the patient as a person,

Table III
Medication use in the Malaysian program

No. Drug Types Used Regularly	Pre-admission ($n = 47$)	Post-treatment ($n = 47$)	At 1-month Follow-up ($n = 47$)
0	14 (29.8%)	42 (89.4%)	31 (66%)
1	12 (25.5%)	4 (8.5%)	11 (23.4%)
2	11 (23.4%)	1 (2.1%)	5 (10.6%)
3	3 (6.3%)	0	0
Taking an opioid	19 (40.4%)	1 (2.1%)	10 (21.3%)

Note: Opioids includes weak opioids, e.g., tramadol, dihydrocodeine.

Table IV
Work status for the Malaysian program

Work Status	Pre-admission ($n = 47$)	At 6–12-month Follow-up ($n = 46$)
Not working*	16 (34.0%)	10 (21.3%)
Working full-time	16 (34.0%)	20 (42.6%)
Working part-time	5 (10.6%)	4 (8.5%)
Retired	5 (10.6%)	7 (14.9%)
Domestic duties	4 (8.5%)	4 (8.5%)
Student	1 (2.1%)	1 (2.1%)

* Includes those who are unemployed and those who are on long-term sick leave due to pain.

while maintaining a consistent message as a team, was important in ensuring adherence to the program and good outcomes.

Staffing has posed a special challenge because each of the team members had a host of other responsibilities, and running a pain management program was not included in their official duties. During this initial period the program has depended on the dedication of individuals willing to make many personal sacrifices. This exceptional effort is not sustainable, and the management team is exploring ways of "mainstreaming" this modality of treatment and lobbying administrators to recognize pain management programs as an important and worthwhile treatment for chronic pain patients. Issues of long-term funding and training also must be addressed if the program is to continue and even expand to cater for the growing population in need of pain management programs.

Yet another challenge is educating others in the health services and in the community generally. Physicians and other health care professionals need to understand the principles of the program, especially that its goal is not pain relief, but rather improvement in function and mood. Friends and family of patients need to know that chronic pain can be seen as a disease in its own right and that self-management is critical, allowing patients with chronic pain to return to normal lives. Patients can be encouraged to communicate with others about their pain and about how they are managing. Publicity in the local press regarding the concepts of self-management of chronic pain has been an important aspect of educating the community.

Perhaps the biggest challenge is in the area of return to work. Currently, there is no incentive for employers to retain an injured person at work, rehabilitation facilities are limited, and there are no graded return-to-work or retraining schemes. Employers must understand that persons with chronic pain can continue to work and that they need to be able to incorporate pain management strategies such as pacing, stretching, and relaxation into their work.

THE COPE PROGRAM IN HONG KONG

SOCIAL AND HEALTH CARE CONTEXTS

Hong Kong is a Special Administrative Region of China that is governed under the "one country, two systems" policy by which the Chinese government guarantees full autonomy in local governance except on sovereign matters. A capitalist environment continues to flourish in Hong Kong, where the British common law system still prevails. Public health care in Hong Kong is provided by the Hospital Authority, which manages all public hospitals and general outpatient clinics, and by the Department of Health, which manages public health issues such as health promotion and prevention and control of infectious diseases. Both organizations are government funded. There is little private practice in the public system. Health care expenditure in 2003–2004 was U.S.$4.4 billion, representing 5.8% of the gross domestic product (Census and Statistics Department 2005). Public health care is generously subsidized, with local residents having to pay a small nominal fee for hospital services. Fees are waived for those on social welfare benefit. At present there is no structured family physician system in Hong Kong. General practitioners and specialists in private practices compete for patients, and "doctor-shopping" is common. Private health care is financed mainly by individuals, and only about 20% of the population subscribe to health insurance schemes.

CHRONIC PAIN STATUS

The prevalence of persistent pain in Hong Kong is estimated at 10.8% (Ng et al. 2002). The quality of life and mood of patients with persistent pain are severely impaired when compared to the normal population (Lee at al. 2005; Wong et al. 2005) and are similar to Western population findings (Becker et al. 1997). A significant proportion of local Chinese patients with chronic pain also show impaired self-efficacy and pain catastrophizing (Yap et al. 2004; Lim et al. 2005; Wong et al. 2005).

The Employee's Compensation Ordinance protects the welfare of employees who sustain a work-related injury in Hong Kong (Labour Department 2005). Employers are responsible for this liability. Injured workers are entitled to 80% of their normal salary during their sick leave for up to 2 years (after which a court order is required for further extension). During this time it is illegal for the employer to dismiss an injured employee. An employee compensation assessment may be held during this time, but appeals can be lodged by either party, which may further delay the final result. The prolonged legal process often delays and interferes with rehabilitation. A recent survey found that about 35% of the patients attending a regional pain center had a work-related injury and that over 80% of these patients were involved in compensation claims and litigation (Chen et al. 2004).

PAIN MEDICINE IN HONG KONG

While acute pain services have advanced rapidly since the early 1990s (Kwan 1996), the development of chronic pain services has been slow. Currently, six public hospitals have pain clinics. Many pain patients are managed by specialists from different disciplines in their respective clinics. Most of the funding for pain management in public hospitals comes from the budgets for existing clinical services such as anesthesiology. The current public health priority on infectious diseases such as avian flu, and the focus on medical technology make it difficult to obtain funding for pain management. Public interest and awareness regarding chronic pain are also limited.

THE COPE PAIN MANAGEMENT PROGRAM

In 2001, in the face of increasing demands on the health care system due to often complex chronic pain patients the Hospital Authority allocated funding for a half-time dedicated clinical psychologist to work at four pain management centers in Hong Kong for a 3-year trial period. Previously, pain patients often waited 6–12 months to attend the clinical psychology outpatient clinic. With a clinical psychologist attached to the pain management team, other relevant specialists, including physiotherapists, occupational therapists, medical social workers, pain nurses, a dietician, and the hospital chaplain were invited to contribute to a new multidisciplinary pain management program at the Alice Ho Miu Ling Nethersole hospital, a district hospital. At that time, none of the staff involved in the program had any formal training in conducting a pain management program. Staffing depended on the goodwill of participating disciplines to allocate dedicated staff from their existing teams to the program on a part-time basis. Dedicated staff members also sacrificed significant personal time to plan the first program that was conducted in 2002. The program was based on information from the literature and from Web sites, on the experience gained from another local program, and on the knowledge and experience from the disciplines of participating specialists.

FIRST PROGRAM

The Comprehensive Outpatient Pain Engagement (COPE) program was designed as a 6-week program, held two days a week. Patients were referred to the program from the hospital's pain clinic as well as from other pain clinics. Strict selection criteria were employed, and eight Chinese patients were recruited into the first program, which was conducted in Cantonese.

Different team members had their own views about the role of their discipline in the program. Consequently, the first program included several novel sessions such as fit-ball and Tai Chi exercises, spiritual aspects, and nutrition education. There was little integration among the different staff, who attended their allocated sessions and then left. Monitoring of patients' progress was limited and there was no graduated exercise and activity regimen. Nonetheless, all patients completed the first program and appeared generally satisfied. Most had improved in terms of social interactions, but their (physical) functional improvement was limited, and they remained dependent on passive (symptom-focused) therapies.

Team members were concerned about the conduct of the program, and they were disappointed with the results. As a result funding for specific training for the team was obtained later in 2002 and was used to send a six-member team to the ADAPT program at the Royal North Shore Hospital in Sydney. During this visit, the team observed a 3-week program and learned about the principles and conduct of an integrated pain management program. They became familiar with the course content and learned the importance of regular reviews of progress by individual patients and opportunities to discuss this feedback with the patients. They recognized the importance of all team members being familiar with the principles of a pain management program. These lessons were instrumental in a number of changes being made to the COPE program.

Further training in cognitive-behavioral pain management was also obtained with funding from the Hong Kong Hospital Authority Commissioned Training scheme for a week of workshops and discussions with Dr. Nicholas in early 2004, as well as a week of training from the senior nurse on the ADAPT program (Lee Beeston) in late 2004.

OUTCOMES

The results of 27 patients from four groups who have completed the program are now available. The mean age of the patients was 43 years (SD = 6 years), and the median duration of their pain was 46 months. A general trend of improvement was found in measures of quality of life and physical functions, including sitting and standing tolerance (Chen et al. 2005). Dependence on regular use of pain-related medication was substantially reduced, with 37% and 42.3% of the patients not on regular medication at 6 months and 12 months, respectively, compared to 22.2% in this category at baseline. Return-to-work outcomes are shown in Table V. Although the results are limited by the small sample size, they suggest that the multidisciplinary pain management program is useful in improving patients' health-related quality of life and physical function.

Table V
Work status for Hong Kong program ($n = 27$)

Work Status	At Baseline	At 6 Months	At 12 Months
Have a full-time job	7.4%	14.8%	22.2%
Are looking for employment	3.7%	14.8%	11.1%
Are not working in any capacity	70.4%	33.4%	33.4%

CHALLENGES

Considerable challenges arose during the establishment of the pain management program. A major obstacle was finding adequate resources (funding and staff). As the program is funded through the hospital, it is clearly essential that hospital administrators should be aware of the program and its potential benefits. This challenge was addressed by involving senior administrators in aspects of the program, such as officiating at the farewell session at the end of each program. This opportunity allows them to see how the program has helped the patients, it gives them a sense of ownership of the program, and links the program to the hospital's overall services. However, further thought still needs to be given to seeking other sources of funding in addition to the hospital's contribution. These could include donations from charitable or business organizations, the health industry, and research grants. It is also hoped that establishing local epidemiological data and research on pain and pain management will highlight the size and costs of pain problems in the community and promote interest and support for this work. Increasing the awareness of pain patients, the community, and health care workers generally about pain and the pain management program are other avenues to be explored in seeking support for these programs. Ongoing efforts include public lectures and exhibitions, educational material and media publications, and education for health care workers.

Another concern identified by the program staff is that many of the patients appeared poorly motivated to attend the program. It is unlikely that the issue was financial because the hospital fee is usually not a concern, although public transport costs can be onerous for some. A more likely source of low motivation is that many patients had not accepted the chronicity of their pain and continued to search for a cure. This tendency is reinforced by easy access to culturally accepted, low-cost traditional Chinese medicine alternatives, especially in nearby mainland China. A recent survey of a local pain center found that 50% of patients were receiving traditional Chinese medicine in addition to their prescribed care (Chen et al. 2004). Like many pain patients in other countries, by the time they are referred to a pain clinic many patients have developed a well-entrenched "sick role" lifestyle, and they may find it difficult to embrace a self-management approach to their pain. Patients with unresolved compensation and litigation issues may also be cautious about making changes that could place their financial security at risk.

It is also possible that cultural perceptions of receiving psychological management could create reluctance to actively participate in such a program in case of the insinuation that they had a form of "mental illness." This embarrassment and resulting avoidance could be related to the reputed "face-saving" mentality or pride of the Chinese culture. At a more practical level, the staff also found that many of the patients were slow to acquire new concepts such as thought challenging and goal setting. In part, this reluctance may be related to the low socioeconomic and educational backgrounds of many patients. Another difficulty the patients may have had could be related to the Cantonese language used in the program. Many of the English concepts and terms do not have a Cantonese equivalent, and the explanations offered by the staff may not have been adequate in some areas. It was also notable that compared to the Australian pain patients observed in Sydney, the Hong Kong patients appeared to be more guarded and slow to open up and become interactive within the group. This finding may be attributed to the cultural tendency to avoid disclosure of shameful experiences.

Despite these difficulties, a substantial proportion of the patients treated in the COPE program have responded well, and the task now is to develop better ways of addressing the problems identified and to obtain more broad-based financial and institutional support for the program.

CONCLUSION

Our experience shows that despite the challenges posed by their multiethnicity, Malaysian and Hong Kong pain patients can benefit from a structured pain management program applying the same methods and principles used successfully in Western countries. Critical factors for success include planning, lobbying administrators and colleagues, being creative in utilizing available resources, being positive but realistic, and learning about the local systems (e.g., compensation schemes). Working in a team, keeping the team together, and gaining the trust of patients and other team members are also important principles. Last but not least, sharing patients' stories with other patients, medical practitioners, health administrators, other health care workers, and the public seems crucial in contributing to the sustainability of such programs.

While there are some cultural and language barriers to the acceptance of a self-management approach to persisting pain, these problems are surmountable, especially with well-trained and dedicated pain clinic staff. What is required, as always, is more reliable funding and institutional support for these programs. In addition, both programs illustrate the importance of access to suitable training and expert guidance that should be available in situ. Thus, major challenges remain to be overcome to meet the goal of further development and consolidation of pain management programs in Asia. In the longer run, this work cannot rely upon the extraordinary efforts of a dedicated few.

ACKNOWLEDGMENTS

Malaysia: We would like to acknowledge a number of people and organizations whose support and contributions have been essential to the development and operation of the MENANG pain management program. In particular, we would like to thank the members of the MENANG team: Dr. Zubaidah Jamil, Clinical Psychologist, University Putra Malaysia; Dr. Ramli Mohd Ali, Psychiatrist, Hospital Selayang; Dr. Siti Nor Aizah, Psychiatrist, Hospital Kuala Lumpur; Khuzaimah Abdul Aziz, Physiotherapist, Hospital Kuala Lumpur; Chan Chooi Leng and Chan Sook Ching, physiotherapists from the Physiotherapy College, Kuala Lumpur; Dr. Nor Ridah Muhammad Yassin and Norhayati Shariff, program coordinators; and Marzimi Morad, clinic nurse. We would also like to thank the Directors, Hospital Selayang; the Ministry of Health, Malaysia; Pfizer Malaysia; Lois Tonkin, Professor Michael Cousins, and clinical psychologists Dr. Robin Murray, Caroline Perry, and Dr. Toby Newton-John at the Pain Management and Research Centre, Royal North Shore Hospital in Sydney; and clinical psychologist Dr. Amanda Williams from University College London.

Hong Kong: We would like to acknowledge the enormous contribution of current and past COPE team members from Alice Ho Miu Ling Nethersole Hospital, including Dr. M.C. Chu (Anesthesiologist); Ms. Marlene Ma and Ms. Josephine Chen (Nurses), Mr. Tony Wong (Clinical Psychologist), Mr. Leo Cheung (Physiotherapist); Mr. Ewert Tse, Mr. Adrian Leung, and Ms. Hellen Yung (Occupational Therapists); Ms. Emily Cheng and Ms. Jamie Wan (Social Workers); Ms. Sally Leung (Dietitian); and Ms. Jenny Poon, Ms. Helen Lei, and Mr. William Lam (Chaplains). We would also like to acknowledge the Hospital Executive Committee, our former Hospital Chief Executive Dr. Raymond Chen, Dr. Nancy Tung (Hospital Chief Executive), Ms. Elsa Tsang (retired General Manager, Nursing), Mr. Calvin Leung (General Manager, Administrative Services), Professor Tony Gin (Chairman, Department of Anesthesia and Intensive Care), Mr. Anthony Lau (Physiotherapy Department), Ms. Frances Louie (Occupational Therapy Department), and Mr. Victor Tam (Social Work Department). Lastly but not least, we are immensely thankful for the continuing advice and training from the ADAPT team at the Royal North Shore Hospital, Sydney.

REFERENCES

Asghari A, Nicholas MK. Pain self-efficacy beliefs and pain behaviour: a prospective study. *Pain* 2001; 94:85–100.

Becker N, Thomsen AB, Olsen AK, et al. Pain epidemiology and health related quality of life in chronic non-malignant pain patients referred to a Danish multi-disciplinary pain center. *Pain* 1997; 73:393–400.

Blyth FM, March LM, Brnabic AJM, et al. Chronic pain in Australia: a prevalence study. *Pain* 2001; 891(2,3):127–134.

Census and Statistics Department. Hong Kong Special Administrative Region of the People's Republic of China. Available at: www.info.gov.hk. Accessed 2005.

Chen PP, Chen J, Gin T, et al. Out-patient chronic pain service in Hong Kong: prospective study. *Hong Kong Med J* 2004; 10:150–155.

Chen PP, Ma M, Wong T, et al. Six-month results of a multidisciplinary pain management program in Chinese patients with chronic pain. *Abstracts: 11th World Congress on Pain.* Seattle: IASP Press, 2005, p 264.

Department of Statistics Malaysia. Available at: www.statistics.gov.my. Accessed 2005.

Elliott AM, Smith BH, Penny KJ, Smith WC, Chambers WA. The epidemiology of chronic pain in the community. *Lancet* 1999; 354:1248–1252.

Flor H, Behle DJ, Birbaumer N. Assessment of pain related cognitions in chronic pain patients. *Behav Res Ther* 1993; 31:63–73.

Guzmán J, Esmail R, Karjalainen K, et al. Multidisciplinary rehabilitation for chronic low back pain: systematic review. *BMJ* 2001; 322:1511–1516.

Kwan A. Acute pain management in Hong Kong. *Hong Kong Med J* 1996; 2:381–384.

Labour Department. Liability of employer. In: *A Concise Guide to the Employees' Compensation Ordinance.* Hong Kong: Government of Hong Kong Special Administrative Region, 2005, p. 4.

Lee S, Chen PP, Lee A, et al. A prospective evaluation of health related quality of life in Chinese patients with chronic non-cancer pain. *Hong Kong Med J* 2005; 11:174–180.

Lim HS, Chen PP, Wong CM, et al. Validation of the Chinese (Hong Kong) version of the Pain Self-efficacy Questionnaire (PSEQ-HK). *Abstracts: 11th World Congress on Pain.* Seattle: IASP Press, 2005, p 343.

Moore R, Brödsgaard I. Cross-cultural investigations of pain. In: Crombie IK, Crofts PR, Linton SJ, Von Korff M (Eds). *Epidemiology of Pain.* Seattle: IASP Press, 1999, pp 53–80.

Morley S, Eccleston C, Williams A. Systematic review and meta-analysis of randomised controlled trials of cognitive behaviour therapy and behaviour therapy for chronic pain in adults, excluding headache. *Pain* 1999; 80:1–13.

Ng JKF, Tsui SL, Chan WS. Prevalence of common chronic pain in Hong Kong adults. *Clin J Pain* 2002; 18:275–281.

Nicholas MK. Cognitive behavioural therapy for chronic pain patients. *Medicine Today Suppl* 2003; August:12–17.

Nicholas MK, Wilson PH, Goyen J. Comparison of cognitive-behavioural group treatment and an alternative, non-psychological treatment for chronic low back pain patients. *Pain* 1992; 48:339–347.

Nicholas MK, Molloy AM, Tonkin L, Beeston L. *Manage Your Pain.* Sydney: ABC Books, 2000.

Taylor R, Lovibond PF, Nicholas MK, et al. The utility of somatic items in the assessment of depression in chronic pain patients: a comparison of the Zung Self-rating Depression Scale (SDS) and the Depression Anxiety Stress Scales (DASS) in chronic pain, clinical and community samples. *Clin J Pain* 2005; 21:91–100.

Williams AC de C, Nicholas MK, Richardson PH, Pither CE, Fernandes J. Generalizing from a controlled trial: the effects of patient preference versus randomization on the outcome of inpatient versus outpatient chronic pain management. *Pain* 1999; 83:57–65.

Wong S, Hung CT, Chen PP, et al. Profile of Chinese chronic pain patients attending multidisciplinary pain clinics in Hong Kong. *Abstracts: 11th World Congress on Pain.* Seattle: IASP Press, 2005, p 473.

World Health Organization. *World Health Report 2005.* Available at: www.who.int/whr/2005/annex/indicators_country_g-o.pdf.

Yap JC, Chen PP, Lau JTF, et al. Validation of the Chinese pain catastrophizing scale (HK_PCS) in chronic pain patients. *Qual Life Res* 2004; 13:1529.

Correspondence to: Prof. Michael K. Nicholas, PhD, Pain Management and Research Centre, University of Sydney at Royal North Shore Hospital, St Leonards, NSW 2065, Australia. Email: miken@med.usyd.edu.au.

Proceedings of the 11th World Congress on Pain,
edited by Herta Flor, Eija Kalso, and Jonathan O.
Dostrovsky, IASP Press, Seattle, © 2006.

68

Behavioral Therapies for the Management of Cancer Pain: A Systematic Review

Amy P. Abernethy, [a,b] Francis J. Keefe, [c] Douglas C. McCrory, [b,d] Cindy D. Scipio, [e] and David B. Matchar [b,d]

[a]*Department of Medicine, Division of Medical Oncology,* [b]*Duke Center for Clinical Health Policy Research,* [c]*Department of Psychiatry and Behavioral Sciences,* [d]*Department of Medicine, Division of General Internal Medicine, Duke University Medical Center, and* [e]*Department of Psychology, Social and Health Sciences, Duke University, Durham, North Carolina, USA*

The literature strongly supports an association between cancer pain and psychological factors such as distress, pain catastrophizing, self-efficacy, social functioning, and coping (Wilkie and Keefe 1991; Jacobsen and Butler 1996; Lin 1998; Zaza and Baine 2002; Bishop and Warr 2003). Given the importance of psychological factors in the ways in which pain is experienced, interpreted, and coped with, it follows that behavioral therapies should be effective adjuvant interventions for cancer pain.

Established behavioral therapies for cancer pain fall into three categories: (1) comprehensive cognitive-behavioral therapy (CBT), (2) hypnosis and imagery-based CBT, and (3) psychoeducational interventions. Comprehensive CBT comprises varied packages of adaptive strategies taught to a patient to maximize coping. Strategies may include providing patients with a rationale that emphasizes pain as a complex experience influenced by thoughts, feelings, and behavior; systematic training in one or more cognitive or behavioral strategies for controlling pain, such as progressive relaxation training, imagery, goal setting, and activity pacing, typically provided over a series of sessions; and home practice (Redd et al. 2001; Keefe et al. 2005). In hypnosis-based CBT, a trained therapist helps the patient achieve a relaxed state and then actively provides specific hypnotic suggestions designed to enhance pain control and relaxation (Syrjala and Roth-Roemer 2002). In imagery-based CBT, patients are taught how to intentionally focus their attention on specific mental images so as to divert attention away from pain (Syrjala and Roth-Roemer 2002). Psychoeducational interventions combine patient education with behavioral techniques such as skills training, personal interactions between the educator and the learner, and repeat visits to reinforce key messages and skills (Keefe et al. 2005).

Most cancer pain management guidelines focus on pharmacological and procedural interventions, and there is uncertainty about the role of behavioral therapies as adjuvant interventions. In conjunction with the Centers for Medicare and Medicaid Services (CMS), the Agency for Healthcare Research and Quality (AHRQ) commissioned a systematic review and meta-analysis to determine the demonstrated efficacy of behavioral therapies for cancer pain on patients' physical health status. This chapter provides an outline of this study, which will be published in detail elsewhere (A. Abernethy et al., unpublished manuscript).

METHODS

Definitions. Cancer-related pain was defined as pain caused by neoplastic disease or its treatment, including cancer-related procedures such as diagnostic procedures, chemotherapy, radiotherapy, and surgery (Jacox et al. 1994). Behavioral therapies or interventions were initially defined broadly to capture all relevant interventions that met the criteria of the 2004 Medicare current procedural terminology manual (American Medical Association 2003). This definition was refined after an initial review of abstracts. To determine whether an intervention should be included or excluded in this review, we defined behavioral interventions as meeting at least two of three criteria: (1) they included more than one session, (2) they involved cognitive or behavioral skills training, and (3) they were interactive. Studies meeting two out of the three criteria were included if they demonstrated the impact of the behavioral intervention on pain or pain-related outcomes.

Search strategy. MeSH terms *neoplasms* and *pain* were exploded and combined. Cancer pain articles were combined with a behavioral therapy concept using the exploded MeSH terms "*behavioral disciplines and activities*"/ or *cognitive therapy*/ as well as a patient education concept using the MeSH term *patient education*/. Both strategies were combined with a standard search for randomized controlled trials (Dickersin et al. 1994). Strategies were executed in MEDLINE, CINAHL, and PsychINFO and were limited to articles published from 1966 through May 2004 pertaining to human adults and published in the English language. Reference lists of identified studies and relevant systematic reviews were hand-checked. Additional articles were identified through ongoing searches and discussions with field experts.

Literature screening. Abstracts and full-text versions of articles were screened against six exclusion criteria: (1) the study did not address cancer-related pain, (2) the subjects were not adults, (3) the study was not a randomized controlled trial, (4) no pain or pain-related medical outcomes were reported, (5) no behavioral intervention was included, and (6) "other" reasons (e.g., the article was an editorial or review article, or no post-intervention pain data were included). All abstracts were reviewed by two internists, an oncologist, and a psychologist. Any abstract selected by one or more reviewers was included for full-text review. Selected full-text articles were reviewed by an oncologist and psychologist to identify included articles that met all eligibility criteria. Differences in judgments were resolved by discussion.

Data abstraction and analysis. Basic study parameters were abstracted into evidence tables summarizing eligibility criteria, design, subjects, interventions, treatment duration, outcomes, and quality (available at http://clinpol. mc.duke.edu). Pain intensity ratings, measured on 0–10 and 0–7 scales, were normalized to a 0–100 scale.

Effect on pain intensity was reported as the proportion of studies that indicated a statistically positive effect on pain control. Given that statistically significant results would only be expected in 5% of studies by chance alone, this criterion provided a general-purpose, albeit crude, assessment of the efficacy of a treatment in a pool of diverse studies. Meta-analyses were conducted for those studies in which pain intensity means and variances could be estimated from published reports. Relationships between categorical variables were tested using Fisher's exact test. Relationships between continuous variables were described using the Student t test and analysis of variance (ANOVA) as appropriate. Statistical analyses were conducted using the computer programs SPSS for Windows version 11.5 and Comprehensive Meta Analysis. Two-sided P values are reported, and statistical significance was assumed if $P < 0.05$.

RESULTS

Article review. Of 631 citations reviewed, 490 abstracts were excluded and 141 (22%) full-text articles were reviewed. One hundred sixteen of the full-text articles were excluded. The final set of 25 abstracted articles represents data from 21 different studies; 4 papers were different pain-related reports from previously presented study datasets. All identified studies focused on one or more of the following CBT intervention protocols: comprehensive CBT ($n = 7$, 33%, Table I), imagery and hypnosis-based CBT ($n = 8$, 38%, Table II), and (3) education-focused interventions with brief CBT ($n = 9$, 42%, Table III). Three studies compared comprehensive CBT and imagery and hypnosis-based CBT interventions and were considered in both categories.

Table I
Comprehensive cognitive-behavioral therapy (CBT) studies and components of the CBT packages.

Study	N	Coping Skills Training	Information Provision	Cognitive Restructuring	Self-Efficacy Training	Progressive Muscle Relaxation	Guided Imagery	Physical Training	Group Interactions	Outcome*
Arathuzik 1994	24	X	X	X		X	X			Neg
Berglund et al. 1994a,b	199	X	X					X	X	Pos
Dalton et al. 2004	121	X	X	X	X		X			Pos
Gaston-Johansson et al. 2000	110	X	X	X		X	X			Neg
Jacobsen et al. 2002	411	X	X			X	X			Neg
Syrjala et al. 1992	45	X	X	X	X	X				Neg
Syrjala et al. 1995	94	X	X	X	X	X	X			Pos

* Outcome is designated as positive (Pos) if the comprehensive CBT intervention arm was effective for pain or negative (Neg) if it was ineffective.

Participant characteristics. The 21 studies represented 2,296 adult participants with an average age of 54 years; 68% were female, and 82% were Caucasian. Nineteen studies involved adults with current cancer, one study involved cancer survivors, and one involved people undergoing a cancer-related diagnostic procedure. Baseline mean pain intensity was 41.6 (standard deviation [SD] = 14, median = 42.1, range = 19–72), representing moderate pain intensity.

Intervention characteristics. Features of the interventions are presented in Tables I–III. The median number of contacts per study was 3.0 (mean = 6.9 contacts, SD = 11, range = 1–52). The median total duration of intervention contact per study was 82 minutes, with a range of 10–520 minutes; mean contact time for an individual intervention session was 34 minutes (SD = 27).

Disciplines of treatment providers included nurses ($n = 12$, 57%), psychologists with doctorates ($n = 4$, 19%), a psychiatrist ($n = 1$, 5%), a social worker ($n = 1$, 5%), and a graduate student ($n = 1$, 5%). Two imagery and hypnosis-based CBT studies did not comment on the provider discipline. Across all studies, training for the providers in the intervention was rarely described.

Four studies representing five intervention arms occurred at times of expected acute transient high levels of pain, namely during bone marrow transplant ($n = 3$ intervention arms), hyperthermia therapy ($n = 1$), and breast biopsy ($n = 1$); the studies were of comprehensive CBT ($n = 1$), imagery and hypnosis-based CBT interventions ($n = 3$), or both ($n = 1$). All other studies occurred at more general times in the course of the cancer illness.

Treatment efficacy. Fig. 1 presents a global assessment of efficacy, where a score of >50% indicates that the intervention generally improves pain outcomes.

Table II
Imagery and hypnosis-based CBT studies and components of the interventions

Study	N	Infor-mation Provision	Progressive Muscle Relaxation	Guided Imagery	Hypnosis	Outcome
Arathuzik 1994	24	X	X	X		Neg
Graffam and Johnson 1987	30	X	X	X		Neg
Montgomery et al. 2002	20	?	?		X	Pos
Reeves et al. 1983	28	?	?		X	Pos
Sloman et al. 1994	67	X	X	X		Pos
Spiegel and Bloom 1983	58	X	X		X	Pos
Syrjala et al. 1992	45	?	?		X	Pos
Syrjala et al. 1995	94	X	X	X		Pos

Table III
Studies of education-focused interventions plus brief CBT
and components of the interventions

Study	N	Information Provision	>1 Session	CBT Skills Training	Interactive	Outcome
Dalton 1987	30	X	X	X	X	Neg
de Wit et al. 1997, 2001a,b,c	313	X	X	X	X	Pos
Ferrell et al. 1993	40	X	X	X	X	Pos
Given et al. 2002	113	X	X	?	X	Neg
Lai et al. 2004	30	X	X	X	X	Pos
Miaskowski et al. 2004	212	X	X	X	X	Pos
Oliver et al. 2001	78	X		X	X	Pos
Rimer et al. 1987	230	X		X	X	Neg
Ward et al. 2000	43	X	X	?	X	Neg

Overall, CBT interventions were effective (65% were positive), although the success rate differed by intervention category (see Fig. 1, with supplementary information in Tables I–III).

Of the 21 studies, 7 (33%) provided sufficient data to calculate effect sizes post-treatment, corresponding to 10 active interventions. The results confirmed the findings of the proportion-based analyses. Behavioral therapies were globally effective for the control of cancer pain, with a mean effect size of 0.232 (95% confidence interval [CI] = 0.072–0.392, $P = 0.004$). On a 0–100 pain intensity scale, an effect size of this magnitude (0.20–0.30) implies a 7–9-point difference between groups. The test for homogeneity had a $P = 0.45$ for the overall effect size analysis, indicating that studies in this group are sufficiently similar to combine in a meta-analysis. The Forest plot for the meta-analysis will be presented in the journal publication of this study (A. Abernethy et al., unpublished manuscript).

Effect sizes were also calculated for each subgroup. The results were consistent with the general efficacy estimates presented in Fig. 1. Imagery and hypnosis-based CBT ($n = 3$ studies) was effective for controlling cancer pain, with a mean effect size of 0.419 (95% CI = 0.059–0.779, $P = 0.023$). Education-focused interventions with brief CBT ($n = 4$ studies) were borderline effective, with a mean effect size of 0.207 (95% CI = –0.017–0.431, $P = 0.070$).

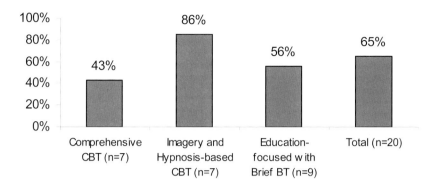

Fig. 1. Percentage of positive studies, by study category. A study was defined as positive when the cognitive-behavioral therapy (CBT) and behavioral therapy (BT) intervention groups showed significant improvements in pain intensity in comparison to the control groups that did not receive such therapy. The one study without a non-intervention control group was not included in this analysis (Graffam and Johnson 1987).

Comprehensive CBT ($n = 3$) was not effective, with a mean effect size of 0.148 (95% CI = –0.151–0.446, $P = 0.330$).

The findings in the three studies that evaluated comprehensive CBT interventions versus imagery and hypnosis-based CBT interventions supported the general conclusions of this review. No other outcomes were presented consistently enough across studies to allow comparisons.

The relationship between positive or negative study outcome and various study characteristics was investigated. Potential predictors included timing of intervention, treatment intensity, and provider discipline. None of these factors showed any association with study outcome, although the numbers were small.

DISCUSSION

Cognitive-behavioral therapies were effective at reducing pain intensity when used as an adjuvant to the overall cancer pain management plan, with a mean effect size of 0.232 (CI = 0.072–0.392; $P = 0.004$), translating to a 7–9-point reduction in pain intensity on a 0–100-point pain intensity rating scale.

When evaluating pharmacological interventions, most pain clinicians would consider a 10-point reduction in pain intensity as clinically meaningful. The nonpharmacological interventions included in this review are presumed to be safer, and therefore even smaller differences between groups may represent clinically meaningful evidence for beneficial effects. Another interpretation is that all of the effect sizes had wide confidence intervals due to the limited number of available studies, wide between-study variation (although the test for heterogeneity was negative), and small numbers of patients in individual studies. These wide confidence intervals mean that the true effect size could fall into the range that is not clinically meaningful.

Interventions did not need to be intensive to have an impact, and differences among the intervention categories were striking. This body of evidence most clearly supports the role of imagery and hypnosis-based CBT in cancer pain management, especially in settings of expected acute and transient moderate to severe pain. The role of education-focused interventions with brief CBT was less clear, and comprehensive CBT strategies were not clearly effective when evaluated on their own. An extensive consideration of potential factors influencing these findings and other limitations of this study is available in the full AHRQ report available at http://clinpol.mc.duke.edu.

In summary, the literature generally supported the claim that CBT, and particularly imagery and hypnosis-based therapies, are effective in reducing cancer pain. Psychological interventions are advantageous because they can improve pain control without drug-related side effects. Further, these interventions can be combined with most other cancer pain interventions, can foster an increased sense of self-efficacy among patients, and are easily administered. Increased evidence of their role and effectiveness is needed; the evidence that does exist also needs to be adequately disseminated. Sorting out a variety of critical issues such as likely responders and timing of interventions will require significant expansion and improvement of this body of empirical evidence.

ACKNOWLEDGMENTS

Research support was provided by the U.S. Agency for Healthcare Research and Quality, the Doris Duke Charitable Foundation (New York), and the U.S. National Cancer Institute.

REFERENCES

American Medical Association. *Current Procedural Terminology (CPT): 2004 Professional Edition*. Chicago: American Medical Association, 2003.

Arathuzik D. Effects of cognitive-behavioral strategies on pain in cancer patients. *Cancer Nurs* 1994; 17:207–214.

Berglund G, Bolund C, Gustafsson UL, Sjoden PO. One-year follow-up of the 'Starting Again' group rehabilitation program for cancer patients. *Eur J Cancer* 1994a; 30A:1744–1751.

Berglund G, Bolund C, Gustavsson UL, Sjoden PO. A randomized study of a rehabilitation program for cancer patients: the 'starting again' group. *Psychooncology* 1994b; 3:109–120.

Bishop SR, Warr D. Coping, catastrophizing and chronic pain in breast cancer. *J Behav Med* 2003; 26:265–281.

Dalton JA. Education for pain management: a pilot study. *Patient Educ Couns* 1987; 9:155–165.

Dalton JA, Keefe FJ, Carlson J, Youngblood R. Tailoring cognitive-behavioral treatment for cancer pain. *Pain Manag Nurs* 2004; 5:3–18.

de Wit R, van Dam F. From hospital to home care: a randomized controlled trial of a Pain Education Programme for cancer patients with chronic pain. *J Adv Nurs* 2001; 36:742–754.

de Wit R, van Dam F, Zandbelt L, et al. A pain education program for chronic cancer pain patients: follow-up results from a randomized controlled trial. *Pain* 1997; 73:55–69.

de Wit R, van Dam F, Loonstra S, et al. Improving the quality of pain treatment by a tailored pain education program for cancer patients in chronic pain. *Eur J Pain* 2001a; 5:241–256.

de Wit R, van Dam F, Loonstra S, et al. The Amsterdam Pain Management Index compared to eight frequently used outcome measures to evaluate the adequacy of pain treatment in cancer patients with chronic pain. *Pain* 2001b; 91:339–349.

de Wit R, van Dam F, Litjens MJ, et al. Assessment of pain cognitions in cancer patients with chronic pain. *J Pain Symptom Manage* 2001c; 22:911–924.

Dickersin K, Scherer R, Lefevre C. Identifying relevant studies for systematic reviews. *BMJ* 1994; 309:1286–1291.

Ferrell BR, Rhiner M, Ferrell BL. Development and implementation of a pain education program. *Cancer* 1993; 72:3426–3432.

Gaston-Johansson F, Fall-Dickson JM, Nanda J, et al. The effectiveness of the comprehensive coping strategy program on clinical outcomes in breast cancer autologous bone marrow transplantation. *Cancer Nurs* 2000; 23:277–285.

Given B, Given CW, McCorkle R, et al. Pain and fatigue management: results of a nursing randomized clinical trial. *Oncol Nurs Forum* 2002; 29:949–956.

Graffam S, Johnson A. A comparison of two relaxation strategies for the relief of pain and its distress. *J Pain Symptom Manage* 1987; 2:229–231.

Jacobsen PB, Butler RW. Relation of cognitive coping and catastrophizing to acute pain and analgesic use following breast cancer surgery. *J Behav Med* 1996; 19:17–29.

Jacobsen PB, Meade CD, Stein KD, et al. Efficacy and costs of two forms of stress management training for cancer patients undergoing chemotherapy. *J Clin Oncol* 2002; 20:2851–2862.

Jacox A, Carr DB, Payne R, et al. *Management of Cancer Pain,* Clinical Practice Guideline No. 9. Rockville, MD: Agency for Health Care Policy and Research, Public Health Service, U.S. Department of Health and Human Services, 1994.

Keefe FJ, Abernethy AP, Campbell L. Psychological approaches to understanding and treating disease-related pain. *Annu Rev Psychol* 2005; 56:601–630.

Lai YH, Guo SL, Keefe FJ, et al. Effects of brief pain education on hospitalized cancer patients with moderate to severe pain. *Support Care Cancer* 2004; 12(9):645–652.

Lin CC. Comparison of the effects of perceived self-efficacy on coping with chronic cancer pain and coping with chronic low back pain. *Clin J Pain* 1998; 14:303–310.

Miaskowski C, Dodd M, West C, et al. Randomized clinical trial of the effectiveness of a self-care intervention to improve cancer pain management. *J Clin Oncol* 2004; 22:1713–1720.

Montgomery GH, Weltz CR, Seltz M, Bovbjerg DH. Brief presurgery hypnosis reduces distress and pain in excisional breast biopsy patients. *Int J Clin Exp Hypn* 2002; 50:17–32.

Oliver JW, Kravitz RL, Kaplan SH, Meyers FJ. Individualized patient education and coaching to improve pain control among cancer outpatients. *J Clin Oncol* 2001; 19:2206–2212.

Redd WH, Montgomery GH, DuHamel KN. Behavioral intervention for cancer treatment side effects. *J Natl Cancer Inst* 2001; 93:810–823.

Reeves JL, Redd WH, Managawa RY, Storm CK. Hypnosis in the control of pain during hyperthermia treatment of cancer. *Advances in Pain Research.* Philadelphia: Raven Press, 1983, pp 857–861.

Rimer B, Levy MH, Keintz MK, et al. Enhancing cancer pain control regimens through patient education. *Patient Educ Couns* 1987; 10:267–277.

Sloman R, Brown P, Aldana E, Chee E. The use of relaxation for the promotion of comfort and pain relief in persons with advanced cancer. *Contemp Nurse* 1994; 3:6–12.

Spiegel D, Bloom JR. Group therapy and hypnosis reduce metastatic breast carcinoma pain. *Psychosom Med* 1983; 45:333–339.

Syrjala K, Roth-Roemer S. Nonpharmacologic management of pain. In: Berger AM, Portenoy RK, Weissman DE (Eds). *Principles and Practice of Palliative Care and Supportive Oncology.* Philadelphia: Lippincott Williams & Wilkins, 2002, p 1176.

Syrjala KL, Cummings C, Donaldson GW. Hypnosis or cognitive behavioral training for the reduction of pain and nausea during cancer treatment: a controlled clinical trial. *Pain* 1992; 48:137–146.

Syrjala KL, Donaldson GW, Davis MW, Kippes ME, Carr JE. Relaxation and imagery and cognitive-behavioral training reduce pain during cancer treatment: a controlled clinical trial. *Pain* 1995; 63:189–198.

Ward S, Donovan HS, Owen B, Grosen E, Serlin R. An individualized intervention to overcome patient-related barriers to pain management in women with gynecologic cancers. *Res Nurs Health* 2000; 23:393–405.

Wilkie DJ, Keefe FJ. Coping strategies of patients with lung cancer-related pain. *Clin J Pain* 1991; 7:292–299.

Zaza C, Baine N. Cancer pain and psychosocial factors: a critical review of the literature. *J Pain Symptom Manage* 2002; 24:526–542.

Correspondence to: Amy P. Abernethy, MD, Duke University Medical Center, Box 3436, Durham, NC 27710, USA. Fax: 919-684-5325; email: amy.abernethy@ duke.edu.

Proceedings of the 11th World Congress on Pain,
edited by Herta Flor, Eija Kalso, and Jonathan O.
Dostrovsky, IASP Press, Seattle, © 2006.

69

Moving with Pain

Maureen J. Simmonds,[a] Liesbet Goubert,[b]
G. Lorimer Moseley,[c] and Jeanine A. Verbunt[d]

*[a]School of Physical and Occupational Therapy and Faculty of Medicine,
McGill University, Centre for Interdisciplinary Rehabilitation Research, and
McGill Centre for Research on Pain, Montreal, Quebec, Canada; [b]Department
of Experimental Clinical and Health Psychology, Ghent University, Ghent,
Belgium; [c]Centre for fMRI of the Brain, and Department of Physiology, Anatomy
and Genetics, University of Oxford, Oxford, United Kingdom; [d]Rehabilitation
Foundation Limburg, Hoensbroek, The Netherlands*

For many years, motor dysfunction in individuals with pain was generally
understood to be a simple consequence of an aversive sensory input. Not surprisingly, research has shown that the link between pain and motor dysfunction
is complex and involves physiological, psychological, and social domains. In
fact, current concepts suggest that motor dysfunction associated with pain constitutes one dimension of a disorder rather than a consequence of that disorder.
This chapter discusses this subtle but important distinction by summarizing
a selection of studies that explore the relationships between pain, mind, and
movement and attempt to utilize these relationships in treatment. We discuss
three key issues, each with clear clinical implications: (1) the relevance of
dysfunction of movement variability and velocity associated with pain, (2) the
concept that both pain and motor output reflect a perceived threat to body tissue, and (3) the concept of fear of pain and injury or re-injury. The final section
focuses on a common result of each of the above—a reduction in activity—and
challenges commonly held clinical beliefs and assumptions about disability,
physical deconditioning, and disuse in individuals with pain.

PAIN AND MOVEMENT: COMPLEX MULTIDIMENSIONAL CONSTRUCTS

Perception and action are fundamentally linked, as are pain and movement. Myriad sensory, emotional, cognitive, and social factors contribute not only to an individual's anticipated and experienced pain, but also to how that individual might move. It is no surprise, then, that there is great variability in the way people move, both within and between individuals, just as there is great variability in the way people hurt. Two aspects of movement that are particularly relevant are variability and velocity.

MOVEMENT VARIABILITY

The variability in movement patterns makes it difficult to identify "normal" movement and to determine what was normal for a particular individual prior to having pain. For example, Fig. 1 presents kinematic data (movement patterns)

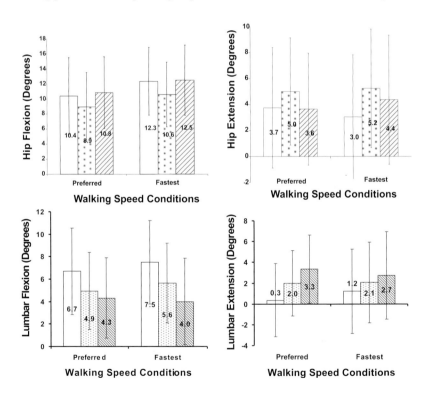

Fig. 1. Illustrates the large magnitude of variability in movement at the hip and lumbar spine during walking in an age and gender matched control group ($n = 20$; white bars), in individuals with back pain only ($n = 20$; shaded bars), and in individuals with referred leg pain ($n = 20$; hatched bars).

that illustrate inter-individual variability in movement strategies during walking. These data support the assertion that everybody walks differently—an assertion that holds true across tasks and across different patient groups, i.e., *everybody moves, but everybody moves differently.* Within-subject variability is evident even at the level of postural adjustments during simple limb movements (Moseley and Hodges 2005). Such variability, inherent in motor systems, may undermine conclusions drawn from studies that involve specific activities or motor tasks, particularly if they implicate "abnormal" strategies as a cause, or consequence, of pain. Fig. 2 further illustrates the limitations of examining the recruitment order of specific muscles. Although a distinct pattern of electromyographic (EMG) activity (relative "on" and "off" times for individual muscle groups) occurs in control subjects, patients with pain demonstrate a general increase in EMG activity throughout the performance of the specific physical task. The identification of recruitment timing (i.e., when specific muscles are active and inactive; "on" and "off" periods) and of the order of timing is open to interpretation. These data emphasize the need for teasing out fundamental principles of movement and movement differences between patients and matched control groups and validating these principles in longitudinal studies.

Taken together, the dynamic, variable, and integrated pain and movement systems make for a difficult research problem because multiple factors need to be controlled, or at least considered. The complexity is compounded by the fact that many individuals with pain and movement problems frequently have other symptoms such as fear, fatigue, and depression. Such symptom clusters, in addition to the specific impairment or disorder, can influence the magnitude of perceived pain as well as its threat value. Thus, there is a bidirectional higher-order complexity: movement changes reflect and affect not only pain, but other aspects of the individual's experience.

VELOCITY

In addition to movement variability, another fundamental and robust movement finding in disorders and disease states is reduced movement velocity. Slowing of movement occurs regardless of the specific disease or disorder; it is also a phenomenon of aging (Simmonds et al. 1998, 2005; Simmonds 2002). We have shown that in age- and gender-matched groups, healthy individuals outperform those with disease symptoms (e.g., pain and fatigue) by a factor of four (Simmonds 2002; Simmonds et al. 2005). This movement slowing appears to be generalized across activities and across self-selected movement speed conditions, e.g., slow, preferred, or fastest speed (Simmonds and Rebelo 2003a,b). Slow movement is relatively inefficient and requires more energy (Lee et al. 2002a). Why those with disease move more slowly is not fully understood.

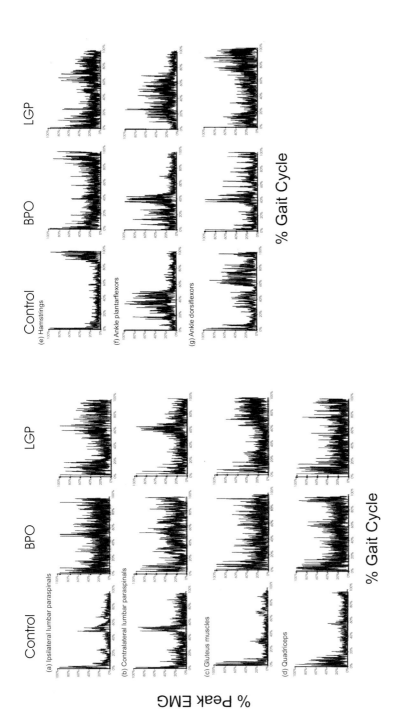

Fig. 2. Rectified and normalized electromyographic (EMG) activity during one gait cycle in a typical individual with back pain only (BPO), back pain and referred leg pain (LGP), and a control subject. The control subject shows a distinct pattern of relative "on" and "off" times for each muscle during the gait cycle. The patients demonstrate a generalized increase and no decrease in EMG activity in all muscles throughout the gait cycle.

Clearly the impairment itself offers a partial explanation. For example, individuals with pain are not able to generate (or sometimes tolerate) relatively large muscle forces (Lee et al. 2002b). Thus, in walking at their "preferred" speed, individuals with back pain generate less "push-off" force than a pain-free cohort, which contributes to slower walking speeds. Interestingly, when challenged to walk faster, individuals with back pain can achieve walking speeds close to those of healthy controls. However, those with a greater level of impairment (i.e., referred leg pain) do not have the same reserve capacity, and although these individuals can speed up, they are unable to walk as fast as those with back pain only. It is noteworthy that—at least in our experience—individuals with referred leg pain not only have a higher level of pain and impairment than individuals with back pain only, but they also score higher on a fear avoidance questionnaire. However, fear avoidance is not a significant predictor of walking performance (i.e., walking speed); rather, pain distribution alone is the strongest predictor of walking performance (Lee and Simmonds 2002).

It would appear that *individuals with pain can move faster but do not*. Perhaps the acute response to reduce movement velocity simply persists because of ongoing impairment or because there is no challenge to move faster (see Fig. 3). The former is intuitive. Our preliminary work however, also supports the latter by suggesting that anticipated pain prevents patients from increasing their movement speed. We have found that individuals with pain systematically overestimate the magnitude of pain intensity and pain unpleasantness that they will experience with faster movements and systematically underestimate the magnitude of pain associated with slow movements (MJ. Simmonds, unpublished data). It is certainly possible that these erroneous expectations contribute to the persistence of slower movements. However, we have found that pain reduction by topical heat wrap (worn as the subject performs the task) can increase preferred speed of movement (Simmonds and Rebelo 2003b). Our ongoing work involves testing speed-targeted interventions across different subject groups. Preliminary results are promising and suggest that a simple modified Wingate protocol (simply incorporating into a walking program a 30-second sprint walk, i.e., "walk as fast as possible") not only increases walking efficiency (e.g., by about 20% in a healthy elderly group (M.J. Simmonds, unpublished data), but also increases performance speed across other physical tasks e.g., repeated sit-to-stand.

Why some patients *anticipate* pain at faster movement and others do not is not clear. We have emphasized the interrelationships between pain, mind, and movement and contend that these interrelationships offer possible explanations. One explanation involves the proposal that for some individuals, both pain and motor control reflect the brain's perception of threat to body tissue.

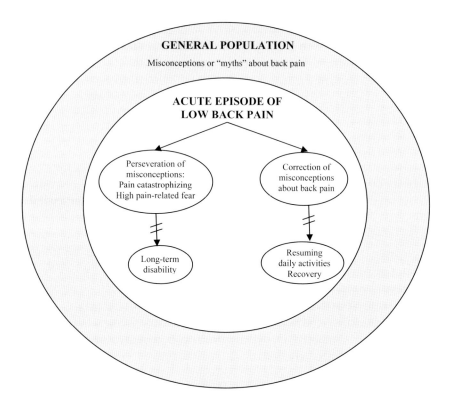

Fig. 3. Model showing the crucial role of correction of misconceptions about back pain in recovery from an acute episode of low back pain.

A THREAT RESPONSE MODEL OF PAIN AND MOTOR CONTROL

Several groups have investigated the *control* of movement in people with pain. As noted earlier, it has been established that people with recurrent back pain adopt a strategy that reduces velocity and range of excursion of spinal segments (Simmonds et al. 1998; Hodges and Moseley 2003). Asymptomatic volunteers given experimentally induced pain demonstrate a similar postural response (Hodges et al. 2003). Moreover, when asymptomatic persons just expect their back to hurt, they also adopt a similar response (Moseley et al. 2004a), which normally returns to normal when the experimentally induced expectation is extinguished. These studies are important because the postural command associated with the perceived threat to the back is probably problematic if it is maintained long-term, since it limits movement and is associated with increased spinal loads (Van Dieen et al. 2003). Such changes in postural control may not always resolve. Preliminary data suggest that when the threat value of back pain is higher than usual, it is associated with non-resolution of changes (Moseley and Hodges 2005), whereas a cognitive intervention to reduce the threat value of back pain can help to normalize postural changes (Moseley 2005a,b).

Implementation of a motor control training approach within the framework of graded exposure to threat can result in large reductions in pain and disability in patients with complex regional pain syndrome (Moseley 2005a,b) and in those with chronic and disabling spinal pain (Moseley 2002, 2003). Another strategy is to attempt to reduce the threat value of pain by explaining, in detail, the biology of pain. Explaining to patients how the nervous system produces pain and changes with persistent pain reduces the threat value of pain (Moseley 2004a,b), which is not surprising, because it emphasizes the sensitivity of the nervous system rather than tissue pathology. When combined with motor control and conventional physiotherapy approaches, explaining pain biology reduces pain and disability (Moseley 2002). Such strategies provide a platform on which better treatments can be developed and tested and corroborate mounting evidence that effective treatments tend to incorporate strategies from across cognitive, behavioral, biomechanical and rehabilitation domains. Moreover, although specific treatment strategies may target specific domains, they have an effect across domains. *This important insight suggests that we can utilize the links between pain, mind, and movement to effect change across all three domains.*

FEAR OF PAIN AND (RE-)INJURY AND GRADED EXPOSURE TO MOVEMENT

Another approach to embracing links between pain, mind, and movement is to focus on fear of pain and (re-)injury. For some individuals with pain, fear that physical movements may cause pain or (re-)injury can lead to severe debilitation and disability. Two opposing behavioral responses to pain have been postulated: confrontation and avoidance. Confrontation, i.e., gradual resumption of daily activities despite pain, is considered adaptive and should lead to reduction of fear and recovery. In contrast, avoidance is considered maladaptive and may initiate a vicious circle of fear, avoidance, and functional disability (Vlaeyen and Linton 2000).

A largely unexplored issue is how catastrophic thinking about pain and pain-related fear could be corrected. There are few opportunities to correct these cognitions because the strategy is effective—avoidance prevents the activity. Philips (1987) suggested that graded exposure should be undertaken to produce disconfirmations between expectations of pain and actual pain experiences. In graded exposure, patients are exposed to physical activities that they fear.

Usually, their worst expectations do not come true (e.g., that they will re-injure themselves, or that a certain movement will hurt a lot).

That graded exposure decreases fear is established, but it is not known whether the effect is generalizable to other activities. We investigated this possibility in 39 patients with chronic low back pain (LBP) (Goubert et al. 2002), and found that high-catastrophizing patients overpredicted pain associated with an activity but readily corrected this overprediction during the second exposure. However, they still overpredicted pain associated with a different activity. Low-catastrophizing patients did not overpredict at all. Further, a questionnaire study in 85 chronic LBP patients (Goubert et al. 2005a) showed that high-catastrophizing and fearful patients were reluctant to generalize spontaneously occurring corrective experiences related to LBP in daily life situations toward other movements or situations. These findings suggest that the effect of exposure may be specific to the activity involved. Specifically, patients seem to be reluctant to change their general belief that back-stressing movements hurt and harm. In line with current theorizing about how organisms learn to correct previously acquired attitudes or beliefs (Bouton and Swartzentruber 1991; Bouton 2000), patients may rather learn exceptions of this rule ("this particular movement is not dangerous, but all the others are").

How then might we facilitate better generalization of exposure effects? There are several possibilities, including conducting exposure therapy in several different contexts (Gunther et al. 1998; Mineka et al. 1999; Bouton 2000), varying the stimulus during exposure (Rowe and Craske 1998b), distributing exposure sessions rather widely over time (Rowe and Craske 1998a; Bouton 2000), and altering the underlying cognitive schema about pain and movement (Moseley 2002). It certainly is not easy; exposure to three different movements did not decrease the likelihood of overprediction of pain during a fourth movement (Goubert et al. 2005b). Thus, it seems that processes underlying generalization of exposure effects are complicated, and it appears to be very difficult to correct the general "rule," or in fact, misconception, that "movement hurts and harms" (Goubert et al. 2005b).

But why are these misconceptions so difficult to correct? A very plausible reason is that misconceptions or "myths" about back pain appear to be prevalent in the general population (Deyo 1998; Goubert et al. 2004). For example, a recent study in a community sample ($N = 1624$) showed that most individuals, even those who reported no back pain, had a strict biomedical view in which LBP was seen as a symptom of underlying tissue damage and in which medical diagnosis, medical treatment, and activity avoidance were considered the proper approach to management (Goubert et al. 2004). Thus, unhelpful attitudes toward back-stressing activities are not an "abnormal" characteristic specific to individuals suffering from chronic pain.

There are many potential sources of such misconceptions. First, they may be cultural beliefs that are verbally transmitted (see Goubert et al. 2004). Second, they may be transmitted via social imitation and learning; observing a person in pain who moves and then rubs their back or grimaces, may lead the observer to do likewise and to believe that back-stressing movements are harmful. Finally, a negative attitude toward back-stressing movements may also develop as a consequence of previous experiences, i.e., an occasional experience of back pain after performing a certain movement. However, the fact that the fewest misconceptions were found to exist in participants with mild LBP but without disability suggest that it is the interpretation and consequence of the back pain that may affirm or dispel certain misconceptions.

Regardless of the mechanisms associated with fear and avoidance, there seems to be reasonable evidence that exposure to activity is critical in confronting and overcoming such fear. However, it is noteworthy that inherent to such an approach are an increase in physical activity and a decrease in disability, which raises the possibility that such parameters may themselves be appropriate targets for management.

PHYSICAL ACTIVITY AND DISABILITY
IN CHRONIC LOW BACK PAIN

Rehabilitation programs have conventionally used a physical reconditioning approach to low back pain, probably because of the assumption that disuse and physical deconditioning cause the problem. Although the concept is intuitively sensible, we lack a solid scientific basis for the presence of disuse and physical deconditioning in chronic LBP. For example, Nielens and Plaghki (2001) found a significantly lower physical activity level in those with chronic LBP whereas others did not (Protas 1999; Verbunt et al. 2001). Similarly, Brennan et al. (1987), Davis et al. (1992), and van der Velde and Mierau (2000) reported lower cardiovascular capacity in chronic LBP patients than in controls, but Hurri et al. (1991), Kellett et al. (1991), and Wittink et al. (2000) did not.

How can we explain this discrepancy between different research findings regarding disuse and its role as a disabling factor in back pain? In answering this question, it is important to consider three important issues. First, it is important to establish which measurement methods were used to quantify physical activity level. Various methods can be used, ranging from assessment tools that are easy to administer and require little time (e.g., questionnaires and diaries) to highly sophisticated measurement methods based on physiological measurement that can only be applied in a specialized setting (e.g., the doubly labeled water technique; Verbunt et al. 2003). Furthermore, regarding questionnaires, early research findings of Schmidt (1985) and Linton (1985) showed that patients with chronic LBP have difficulty in judging their own physical performance (Linton 1985; Schmidt 1985). The validity of physical activity assessment based on self-report may thus be compromised. Measurement of physical activity via movement recording by accelerometry and energy expenditure by the doubly labeled water technique is not compromised by self-evaluation, and therefore is probably more valid. Second, it seems important to establish whether patients compare their activity level to that of other persons or to themselves at a different time. Although most studies evaluating disuse refer to between-subject differences (i.e., the activity level of patients versus controls in a cross-sectional design), patients seem to refer to within-subject changes in their evaluation of disability. Results from a study in subacute LBP indicate that patients, when evaluating their level of disability, relate their current activity level to their recollected activity level before their back pain started. The level of perceived disability was significantly associated with a decline in activities, whereas it was not associated with the patient's actual physical activity level (Verbunt et al. 2005). This finding could explain the unclear association between disability and physical activity discussed earlier (Verbunt et al. 2001). Third, any incongruity in physical activity outcome in chronic pain could also be based on the assumption that there are subgroups of activity-related behavior in patients with chronic LBP. Hasenbring (1994) referred to this phenomenon in a postulated avoidance-endurance model of pain chronicity. She hypothesized that there is a subgroup of patients who have a tendency to cope with pain using endurance strategies, who ignore the pain, and who, by their suppressive behavior, overload their muscles. According to Hasenbring, and supported by Van Houdenhove (2005) and Vlaeyen and Morley (2004), both coping strategies (disuse and overuse) eventually lead to chronicity of pain. However, the existence of such subgroups has yet to be demonstrated. In the field of both behavioral sciences and movement sciences, more research is needed to explain differences in activity-related behavior in chronic pain.

CONCLUSION

The relationship between pain, mind, and movement is complex, variable, and integral to our understanding of each separate domain. Research into each domain has implications for the others, and the lack of integration may have increased the barriers to recovery after acute pain and rehabilitation of chronic conditions and overlooked the opportunities of cross-domain treatments. We contend that a better understanding of mechanisms and subgroups of chronic pain will facilitate translational research in rehabilitation, which should in turn promote the development and testing of hypothesis-led, and activity-based, pain and movement rehabilitation.

REFERENCES

Bouton ME. A learning theory perspective on lapse, relapse, and the maintenance of behavior change. *Health Psychol* 2000; 19:57–63.

Bouton ME, Swartzentruber D. Sources of relapse after extinction in pavlovian and instrumental learning. *Clin Psychol Rev* 1991; 11:123–140.

Brennan GP, Ruhling RO, Hood RS, et al. Physical characteristics of patients with herniated intervertebral lumbar discs. *Spine* 1987; 12:699–702.

Davis VP, Fillingin RB, Doleys DM, Davis MP. Assessment of aerobic power in chronic pain patients before and after a multi-disciplinary treatment program. *Arch Phys Med Rehabil* 1992; 73:726–729.

Deyo RA. Low-back pain. *Sci Am* 1998; 279:29–33.

Goubert L, Francken G, Crombez G, Vansteenwegen D, Lysens R. Exposure to physical movement in chronic back pain patients : no evidence for generalization across different movements. *Behav Res Ther* 2002; 40:415–429.

Goubert L, Crombez G, De Bourdeaudhuij I. Low back pain, disability and back pain myths in a community sample: prevalence and interrelationships. *Eur J Pain* 2004; 8:385–394.

Goubert L, Crombez G, Danneels L. The reluctance to generalise corrective experiences in chronic low back pain patients: a questionnaire study of dysfunctional cognitions. *Behav Res Ther* 2005a; 43:1055–1067.

Goubert L, Crombez G, Lysens R. Effects of varied-stimulus exposure on overpredictions of pain and behavioural performance in low back pain patients. *Behav Res Ther* 2005b; 43:1347–1361.

Gunther LM, Denniston JC, Miller RR. Conducting exposure treatment in multiple contexts can prevent relapse. *Behav Res Ther* 1998; 36:75–91.

Hasenbring M, Marienfeld G, Kuhlendahl D, Soyka D. Risk factors of chronicity in lumbar disc patients. A prospective investigation of biologic, psychological, and social predictors of therapy outcome. *Spine* 1994; 19–24:2759–2765.

Hodges PW, Moseley GL. Pain and motor control of the lumbopelvic region: effect and possible mechanisms. *J Electromyogr Kinesiol* 2003; 13:361–370.

Hodges PW, Moseley GL, Gabrielsson A, Gandevia SC. Experimental muscle pain changes feedforward postural responses of the trunk muscles. *Exp Brain Res* 2003; 151:262–271.

Hurri H, Mellin G, Korhonen O, et al. Aerobic capacity among chronic low back pain patients, *J Spinal Disord* 1991; 4:34–38.

Kellett KM, Kellett DA, Nordholm LA. Effects of an exercise program on sick leave due to back pain. *Phys Ther* 1991; 71:283–290.

Lee CE, Simmonds MJ. The role of fear-avoidance belief and pain distribution in walking performance of individuals with low back pain. Paper presented at: American Pain Society, Baltimore, March, 2002.

Lee CE, Simmonds MJ, Novy DM, Jones SC. Functional self-efficacy, perceived gait ability and perceived exertion in walking performance. *Physiother Theory Pract* 2002a; 18:193–203.

Lee CE, Simmonds MJ, Etnyre BR, Morris GS, Jones SC. Ground reaction forces pattern of walking in individuals with and without low back pain. Paper presented at: International Society for the Study of the Lumbar Spine. Cleveland, May, 2002b.

Linton SJ. The relationship between activity and chronic back pain. *Pain* 1985; 21:289–294.

Mineka S, Mystkowski JL, Hladek D, Rodriguez BI. The effects of changing contexts on return of fear following exposure therapy for spider fear. *J Consult Clin Psychol* 1999; 67:599–604.

Moseley GL. Combined physiotherapy and education is effective for chronic low back pain. A randomised controlled trial. *Aus J Physiother* 2002; 48:297–302.

Moseley GL. Joining forces—combining cognition-targeted motor control training with group or individual pain physiology education: a successful treatment for chronic low back pain. *J Man Manip Ther* 2003; 11:88–94.

Moseley GL. Evidence for a direct relationship between cognitive and physical change during an education intervention in people with chronic low back pain. *Eur J Pain* 2004a; 8:39–45.

Moseley GL. Graded motor imagery is effective for long-standing complex regional pain syndrome. *Pain* 2004b; 108:192–198.

Moseley GL. Widespread brain activity during an abdominal task markedly reduced after pain physiology education—fMRI evaluation of a single patient with chronic low back pain. *Aust J Physiother* 2005a; 51:49–52.

Moseley GL. Is successful rehabilitation of complex regional pain syndrome due to sustained attention to the affected limb? A randomised clinical trial. *Pain* 2005b; 114:54–61.

Moseley GL, Hodges PW. Are the changes in postural control associated with low back pain caused by pain interference? *Clin J Pain* 2005; 21:323–329.

Moseley GL, Nicholas MK, Hodges PW. Does anticipation of back pain predispose to back trouble? *Brain* 2004a; 127:2339–2347.

Moseley GL, Nicholas MK, Hodges PW. A randomized controlled trial of intensive neurophysiology education in chronic low back pain. *Clin J Pain* 2004b; 20:324–330.

Nielens H, Plaghki L. Cardiorespiratory fitness, physical activity level, and chronic pain: are men more affected than women? *Clin J Pain* 2001; 17:129–137.

Philips HC. Avoidance behaviour and its role in sustaining chronic pain. *Behav Res Ther* 1987; 25:273–279.

Protas EJ. Physical activity and low back pain. In: Mitchell M (Ed). *Pain 1999—An Updated Review: Refresher Course Syllabus*. Seattle: IASP Press, 1999, pp 145–152.

Rowe MK, Craske MG. Effects of an expanding-spaced versus massed exposure schedule on fear reduction and return of fear. *Behav Res Ther* 1998a; 36:701–717.

Rowe MK, Craske MG. Effects of varied-stimulus exposure training on fear reduction and return of fear. *Behav Res Ther* 1998b; 36:719–734.

Schmidt AJ. Performance level of chronic low back pain patients in different treadmill test conditions. *J Psychosom Res* 1985; 29:639–645.

Simmonds MJ. Physical function in patients with cancer. Psychometric characteristics and clinical usefulness of a physical performance test battery. *J Pain Symptom Manage* 2002; 24:404–414.

Simmonds MJ, Rebelo V. Self-selected speed of movement during a repeated sit-to-stand task in individuals with and without LBP. Paper presented at: 4th Congress of European Federation of the International Association for the Study of Pain Chapters, Prague, September 2–6, 2003a.

Simmonds MJ, Rebelo V. Increasing preferred speed of movement in individuals with low back pain. Paper presented at: WCPT 14th International Congress, Barcelona, 2003b.

Simmonds MJ, Olson S, Novy D, et al. Physical performance tests: are they psychometrically sound and clinically useful for patients with low back pain? *Spine* 1998; 23:2412–2421.

Simmonds MJ, Novy DM, Sandoval R. The influence of pain and fatigue on physical performance and health status in ambulatory patients with HIV. *Clin J Pain* 2005; 21:200–206.

van der Velde G, Mierau D. The effect of exercise on percentile rank aerobic capacity, pain, and self-rated disability in patients with chronic low back pain: a retrospective chart review. *Arch Phys Med Rehabil* 2000; 81:1457–1463.

van Dieen JH, Kingma I, van der Bug JCE. Evidence for a role of antagonistic cocontraction in controlling trunk stiffness during lifting. *J Biomech* 2003; 36:1829–1836.

van Houdenhove B. Premorbid "overactive" lifestyle and stress-related pain/fatigue syndromes. *J Psychosom Res* 2005; 58:389–390.

Verbunt J, Westerterp K, van der Heijden G, et al. Physical activity in daily life in patients with chronic low back pain. *Arch Phys Med Rehabil* 2001; 82:726–730.

Verbunt J, Seelen H, Vlaeyen J, et al. Disuse and deconditioning in chronic low back pain; concepts and hypotheses on contributing mechanisms. *Eur J Pain* 2003; 7:7–21.

Verbunt JA, Sieben JM, Seelen HA, et al. Decline in physical activity, disability and pain-related fear in sub-acute low back pain. *Eur J Pain* 2005; 9:417–425.

Vlaeyen JWS, Linton SJ. Fear-avoidance and its consequences in chronic musculoskeletal pain: a state of the art. *Pain* 2000; 85:317–332.

Vlaeyen JW, Morley S. Active despite pain: the putative role of stop-rules and current mood. *Pain* 2004; 110:512–516.

Von Korff M, Saunders K. The course of back pain in primary care. *Spine* 1996; 21:2833–2839.

Wittink H, Hoskins MT, Wagner A, Sukiennik A, Rogers W. Deconditioning in patients with chronic low back pain. Fact or fiction? *Spine* 2000; 25:2221–2228.

Correspondence to: Maureen J. Simmonds, PhD, School of Physical and Occupational Therapy, McGill University, 3654 Promenade Sir William Osler, Montreal, PQ, Canada H3G 1Y5. Email: maureen.simmonds@mcgill.ca.

Proceedings of the 11th World Congress on Pain, edited by Herta Flor, Eija Kalso, and Jonathan O. Dostrovsky, IASP Press, Seattle, © 2006.

70

Goals for Rehabilitation of Patients with Chronic Pain

Jenny Strong,[a] Scott Presnell,[b] and Chris Henriksson[c]

[a]School of Health and Rehabilitation Sciences, The University of Queensland, Brisbane, Queensland, Australia; [b]Caulfield Pain Management and Research Centre, Melbourne, Victoria, Australia; [c]Section of Occupational Therapy, Department of Neuroscience and Locomotion, Linkoping University, Linkoping, Sweden

The rehabilitation of patients with chronic pain is an important and complex process that requires considerable resources. For all concerned, it is important that the best outcomes be gained from rehabilitation. But what exactly are the best outcomes, and whose goals should be paramount in the rehabilitation process? In this chapter, we argue that it is the patient who should determine the goals of rehabilitation. The patient lives with chronic pain, such that pain is conceptually woven into his or her daily experience. It is not adequate to say that a good rehabilitation outcome has been achieved when patients stop verbalizing pain complaints, or when they can walk 50 meters.

This chapter considers the person with chronic pain and his or her experience of life with that pain and argues the importance of the patient's perceptions in the pain assessment process. By listening to each individual's narrative, the health practitioner can begin to understand and work with the patient on rehabilitation that is meaningful for him or her. The World Health Organization's 2001 volume, *International Classification of Functioning, Disability and Health* (ICF), provides a framework for a patient-centered, participative model of health. This framework is a model for health practitioners to use as a basis for their work with pain patients. Application of this model begins with understanding the patient's pain experience and continues with deciding upon the goals of the rehabilitation program, and then making rehabilitation efforts to enhance the person's participation in work. Functional goal setting is a tool that can be useful in pain rehabilitation. Thus, the rehabilitation agenda is moved to the workplace, given the importance of work in the lives of adult patients. Using a model of fibromyalgia in women, this chapter illustrates the importance of work participation and highlights the challenges faced by workers with pain. Studies referred to in the chapter span a variety of chronic pain conditions, including neuropathic pain secondary to human immunodeficiency virus (HIV), fibromyalgia, and chronic back pain.

UNDERSTANDING THE PATIENT'S EXPERIENCE

Chronic pain represents something of an anomaly within the structure of biomedical knowledge, defying objective investigation and classification because it is embedded in the subjective experience of the individual rather than in the body (Honkasalo 1998). The conceptualization of chronic pain as a multidimensional, subjective experience rather than as a directly observable event creates an immediate operational paradox for the health practitioner. If the experience of the individual is to form the basis upon which we determine the relative effectiveness of a given intervention, then it follows that we are primarily concerned with constructs that are inherently specific to the individual rather than necessarily generally applicable. Further, we might reasonably expect that the description, and more specifically, the interpretation of symptoms, will be highly personal and enmeshed with the individual's broader life story. Examining narrative accounts of living with chronic pain, that is indeed what we find (Presnell 2004).

Fundamental to a better understanding of what it is like to live with chronic pain is an examination of the narrative construction of the illness experience by individuals who are—in a very real and direct sense—*living* their symptoms. How individuals experience, appraise, and ultimately make sense of the events that are occurring in their bodies is of direct relevance to facilitating the process of rehabilitation and determining the impact and outcome of intervention. It is through a complex and ongoing dialogue between the individual and the symptoms that meaning ultimately emerges from experience, and it is only through a structured consideration of this dialogue that the clinician can attempt to influence the personal world of the individual with pain.

The description of experience as being *like* some comparative event— whether tangible or notional—is a fundamental mode of sharing human understanding (Sontag 1989). In chronic pain, the use of analogy has been promoted as the best means of achieving some degree of intersubjective understanding (Schott 2004). Pain resists objectification precisely because it provides no referential context (Scarry 1985). Little wonder then that the individual attempting a description turns, not just to analogy, but to an analogy that is conceptually grounded in individual experience. The following statements from patients living with chronic HIV-associated peripheral neuropathic pain provide an insight into the processes by which symptoms are experienced, evaluated, and imbued with meaning (Presnell 2004).

"My feet feel as if they're full of Coca-Cola."

"Sometimes the best way to describe it [is that] it's as if my skin from my knees down to my feet has all been removed, shrunk, and then put back."

Even where referents from the real world are used to convey experience, it is in fact the story that is imbued with the meaning, and the story is not reducible to an analysis of its constituent words.

"If you imagine you had been sort of walking on a shingle beach, right, and you'd spent an afternoon, I don't know, playing volleyball or something on that sort of surface and you came back and you thought to yourself: 'Well, what I really want is a foot bath.' It's that sort of level of intensity."

The use of analogy appears to be both common and complex (Presnell 2004). Not only does analogy appear to be how pain description occurs in the "real world" (i.e., outside the context of the clinical assessment), but also it is highly specific and highly individual. Williams et al. (2000) found that respondents actively reframed scale endpoints to better reflect individual experience, suggesting that responses served more as a surrogate for experience than as a direct representation. Hence, for someone who has not been free of pain for years, a "no pain" anchor may be re-interpreted as the least pain the patient can remember. Symptoms cannot be divorced from the individual who experiences them, and experiences derive meaning only from their relationship to the individual's broader life. This latter point is fundamental when conceptualizing a goal for rehabilitation of individuals with chronic pain—gains or losses are only meaningful in terms of how important they are to the individual.

The consequences of chronic pain are subjectively experienced as events in the ongoing story of one's life and cannot be understood in isolation. A problem in mobility is not just experienced as a problem in mobility—it is difficulty doing the shopping, meeting friends for a drink, going away for the weekend, getting from the desk to the photocopier, navigating from the table to the bathroom in a crowded restaurant. If it is the individual in pain who defines the nature of the experience, then it is to the individual that we must return in order to determine the impact of an intervention.

Incorporating a consideration of the individual narrative into our approach to the assessment of pain and the determination of treatment outcome requires us to look beyond the general and to the specific. It compels us to allow the voice of the individual to take priority over the voice of his or her pain.

A FRAMEWORK FOR GOAL SETTING

The ICF provides a useful framework within which to focus on the goals of rehabilitation. The ICF model conceptualizes the functional aspects of health, moving from an impairment-focused or deficit-focused framework to a participative one. Against the background of contextual personal and environmental factors, the impact of the health condition is considered in terms of the interaction between body structures and functions, activities, and participation (World Health Organization 2001; Gibson and Strong 2003). The ICF particularly directs health practitioners to be clear as to the level at which they are measuring outcomes. Are they confining their outcome assessment to body structures and impairment-based systems, such as passive range of motion or allodynia, or are they considering activity limitations, restrictions in participating in activities of daily living, and life roles? (Unsworth 2000). How can health practitioners best target assessments directed at levels of activity and participation? We argue that health practitioners should focus primarily on activity and participation, and not on the more traditional dimensions of body structure and function, in order to ensure that the patients, and their participation in life, are central to their rehabilitation efforts. These are the outcomes that are of most salience to patients and to insurers, and surely to health practitioners.

Goal setting is an important part of rehabilitation. Yet setting functional goals is not inherently easy. For a patient who has been beset by ongoing, unrelenting pain and concomitant suffering, the only immediate goal might be "to get rid of my pain." Most often, people with chronic pain may need assistance to think of life goals beyond the elimination of pain. In addition to interviews, the use of a specific goal-setting tool to tap into the activity and participation dimensions of a patient's life can help to frame the rehabilitation process. The Canadian Occupational Performance Measure (COPM) is one such tool (Law et al. 1990). It measures self-perceived change in goal attainment over time, using individually meaningful criteria, making it ideal for use with patients with chronic pain. The COPM is reliable, valid, and sensitive to change, and has good utility (McColl et al. 2000). It is a sensitive outcome measure for people with chronic pain (Carpenter et al. 2001).

The COPM utilizes a semi-structured interview format. Patients are guided through discussion on any perceived difficulties in the areas of activities of daily living, work, and leisure, and then choose three to five of the most important areas of decreased perceived performance and rate their current performance and satisfaction in these areas. Goals are then set, with a follow-up interview to assess goal attainment.

Redman et al. (2003) evaluated the impact of introducing the COPM to an existing multidisciplinary pain program through a randomized, time-limited trial whereby patients admitted to the program were assigned to either the COPM (treatment) or normal (control) condition. Thirty-two patients with a mean age of 49.0 years (SD = 12.4) participated in the study. At the completion of data collection, there were 26 complete data sets. Pain duration averaged 13.4 years (SD = 9.9). The gender split was 53% women and 43% men. Most had completed primary school (28%) or junior high school (34.4%). Nearly half were unemployed (43.8%). The most common cause of pain was work-related (31.3%), followed by motor vehicle accidents (15.6%). The most common pain sites were the back (62%) and head (42%).

A repeated-measures ANOVA examining the difference in Pain Self-Efficacy Questionnaire scores (Nicholas 1994) from admission to discharge and between treatment and control groups found a significant difference (F = 22.07, df = 24; $P < 0.0001$). Self-efficacy ratings were higher at discharge for the group that received the individual goal setting. Additionally, results illustrated a greater change in the self-efficacy of the COPM goal-setting group from admission to discharge. There was no pre-existing difference between the groups on self-efficacy before the COPM was administered.

The results of this study suggested that helping patients to take control over the goal-setting process in their pain rehabilitation program resulted in improved self-efficacy. Such improvements were not found in other patients who did not participate in the individualized goal-setting process. From the patient's perspective, the use of the COPM provides the opportunity to consider goals beyond pain reduction and to take control in choosing participation priorities. This skill is useful in fostering positive coping skills that can be generalized. One patient stated that he had learned the skill of "working to an action plan and achieving [goals]." Another commented: "This activity made me aware of activities of daily living that are important to me and which ones I spent a lot of energy on but aren't that important" (Redman et al. 2003).

For patients with the goal of returning to work, Gibson and Strong (2003) provided a framework for using the ICF for practitioners in work rehabilitation. They suggested that functional capacity evaluation that is based on observing a patient perform the physical demands of work can be classified as an evaluation of activity and activity limitations. Moreover, based on the person's performance of the activities (i.e., the physical demands of work), the health practitioner will make predictions about the person's capacity to participate in work activities and make recommendations for dealing with restrictions that the person may have in performing these work activities. The practitioner should consider contextual factors such as self-efficacy that may affect the person's performance when participating in work roles, as well as environmental factors such as specific physical demands of the workplace (Gibson and Strong 1997, 1998).

WORK PARTICIPATION

Fibromyalgia (FM), a chronic musculoskeletal pain condition with severe constant pain both in motion and at rest, is used as a model to examine the effect of pain on work performance. Work disability has consistently been reported as a consequence of FM (see, for example, Henriksson et al. 2005). Interview studies ($n = 80$) have shown that women with FM consider work outside home to be important to provide structure to the day, to provide feelings of achievement and value, and to strengthen self-confidence. Most women with FM wished to continue working (Henriksson 1995; Liedberg and Henriksson 2002).

When evaluating work disability, each of the three levels of the ICF must be considered. At the level of body structures, one must consider *individual capacity,* for example pain, fatigue, muscle power and endurance, and cognitive functions. At the personal level, the patient's *work performance* should be assessed, for example, applying knowledge, handling stress, lifting and carrying, and social competence. At the societal level, environmental factors often play a larger role than body and personal factors in the patient's *participation* in society and ability to maintain a work role. Thus, work functioning must always be considered in relation to a specific social context (Sandqvist and Henriksson 2004).

Chronic pain may also be associated with other symptoms that affect work performance, such as fatigue, memory and concentration difficulties, depression, and anxiety (White et al. 1999; Henriksson and Liedberg 2000). The impact of pain on muscular function (Bengtsson 2002), especially on endurance, influences performance; most patients report pronounced difficulties in activities involving static and repetitive work or endurance, for example walking, standing, carrying and lifting, climbing stairs, and working with elevated arms (Waylonis et al. 1994; Henriksson and Liedberg 2000). Variations in symptoms and thus also in activity performance are substantial, not only between individuals but also for the same individual at different times. Pain, tiredness, and stiffness rated on 0–100 mm visual analogue scales twice a day over a week showed daily variations of up to 90 mm. Patients report that they have "normal" days and days when they "can't do anything." Variations in the ability to perform make planning difficult and are experienced as a loss of control. Symptoms and activity limitations affect all areas of life. More time and effort are needed for all daily activities such as personal care, housework, recreational activities, and transportation. Limitations in activity performance, variations in severity of symptoms, and the extra time needed disrupt previous habits and roles; new functional habits and roles must be established that are adjusted to the new situation.

Participation in work is also to a large extent influenced by environmental factors in the patient's life situation, such as caring for small children and elderly relatives, receiving support from one's spouse, experiencing satisfaction in work, and commuting distance between home and work (Liedberg and Henriksson 2002). When assessing work functioning, the practitioner must consider the patient's total life situation. In addition to the total activity burden, a number of factors in society are important for a successful return to work, such as the conditions on the labor market, legislation affecting the workplace such as occupational health and safety requirements, and rehabilitation resources (Liedberg and Henriksson 2002).

In all assessments, the patient should be involved, and his or her opinion should be considered. Many patients can continue to work after consultation, sometimes after adequate adaptations in the workplace, modification of work tasks, or a change from full-time to part-time status. Other patients have difficulties in coping and may need interventions such as information, education, cognitive therapy, or more comprehensive rehabilitation to learn to manage the symptoms and consequences of their pain condition, and to improve their physical condition, self-esteem, and belief in their abilities to be able to return to work. Some patients will not be able to return to gainful employment and need to find other meaningful activities in order to obtain a healthy lifestyle with optimal physical activity, social contacts, and cognitive stimulation. The activity should preferably be regular, involve light activity and interaction with others, and be pursued in an environment other than their own home. Activities will vary depending on interest and availability. Some examples are choir singing, art classes or groups, literature discussion groups, light gardening, walking with others on a regular basis, church activities, spending time with children or elderly lonely people reading books, doing errands, or learning new skills such as computer use.

Before the patient returns to work, an assessment of the physical and psychosocial environment should be performed. If possible, the worker should be given some control; to be able to take a short rest and change work position and work pace could lessen stress and be an important factor for managing a work task. Stressful work tasks with sudden demands increase the pain level. Some patients are sensitive to cold or draughty environments and to changes in temperature such as walking between cold storage areas and a warm working area, or changes from outdoor to inside work tasks. Variations in severity of symptoms and disability must be considered.

Interventions must be introduced at the right time in the patient's change process. A model describing the change process, based on interview studies of people with chronic pain, indicates that timing is important for the success of rehabilitation (see Table I). In an early phase, the pain condition is seen

Table I
The adjustment process in chronic pain

Stage I	Stage II	Stage III	Maintenance
Present:	*Present:*	*Present:*	*Living with Pain:*
Feeling ill, having anxiety and worry over pain. Chaos. Self-deception. Struggles to restore daily life. Expects a cure and expects everything to be as before.	Sorrow and loss. Starting to understand. One day at a time. Gradual adjustment, learning new coping strategies, gradually taking control.	Starting to feel in control, can manage life roles and daily activities. Self-confidence improves.	A new "normal life." A good life in spite of the pain. Competence in handling changes.
Past and Future:	*Past and Future:*	*Past and Future:*	*Past and Future:*
Past—when I was well. Future—intact, as before.	Past—picture fading. Future—uncertain and threatening.	Past—new experiences. Future—changed but feels natural.	Past—before and after the pain began. Future—able to manage.

Source: Adapted from Gullacksen (2004).

as only a short episode. The patient expects a "cure," after which life will go back to normal. In the next phase, the patient is focused on managing the daily problems; the past is not given much thought, and the future is threatening. In the third phase, the patient learns to manage, adjustment is ongoing, and habits and roles are slowly changing to accommodate limitations. The patient has insight into the fact that the future will be different. In the maintenance phase, the patient has learned to deal with problems in daily life, has confidence in his or her ability to cope, and is prepared for changes in the future. The patient may pass to and fro between the different phases during the adjustment process. This model tells us that there is a need to consider how far the patient has come and how the life situation is experienced. The question of work should be raised early only to support and advise the patient on suitable changes that can be easily made. New, more radical, changes may not be possible until the patient has gained insight into the necessity of change.

Our studies on over 600 women with FM show that a large proportion (40–50%) continue working, about 25–30% stop working due to FM, and another 25% have other reasons for not working. Those working have usually needed some adjustments in work conditions such as a decrease in the number of work hours, doing work that is less stressful, or working when the symptoms are less pronounced. Changes in the workplace may also be needed, such as technical aids, adjustable seating, rearrangement of tools, and changes in tasks or procedures that can decrease or eliminate the more demanding elements.

In other cases a transfer to other duties, a change of employer, or retraining into another occupation may be the solution. Factors that increase pain should be avoided, for example working in the same position for longer periods, heavy and frequent lifting and carrying, repetitive movements, static work such as holding and stabilizing tools and static positions of the extremities or head, stressful situations, and cold and draughty work environments.

CONCLUSIONS

It is important in pain rehabilitation for the goals of the patient to be understood and used as the benchmark in determining outcome success. It is no longer appropriate or desirable to focus only on impairment-based goals. First, we must try to understand more about the patients, their pain experience, and their life goals. There is growing evidence for the power of narrative when working with patients with pain. Rehabilitation goals should be developed in collaboration with the patient.

REFERENCES

Bengtsson A. Editorial: the muscle in fibromyalgia. *Rheumatology* 2002; 41:721–724.

Carpenter L, Baker A, Tyldesley B. The use of the Canadian Occupational Performance Measure as an outcome of a pain management program. *Can J Occup Ther* 2001; 68:16–22.

Gibson L, Strong J. A review of functional capacity evaluation practice. *Work* 1997; 9:3–11.

Gibson L, Strong J. Assessment of psychosocial factors in functional capacity evaluation of clients with chronic back pain. *Br J Occup Ther* 1998; 61:399–404.

Gibson L, Strong J. A conceptual framework of functional capacity evaluation for occupational therapy in work rehabilitation. *Aust Occup Ther J* 2003; 50:64–71.

Gullacksen AC. The life adjustment process in chronic pain: psychosocial assessment and clinical implications. *Pain Res Manag* 2004; 9:145–153.

Henriksson C. Living with continuous muscular pain: patient perspectives. Part II: Strategies for daily life. *Scand J Caring Sci* 1995; 9:77–86.

Henriksson C, Liedberg G. Factors of importance for work disability in women with fibromyalgia. *J Rheum* 2000; 27:171–176.

Henriksson CM, Liedberg GM, Gerdle B. Women with fibromyalgia: work and rehabilitation. *Disabil Rehabil* 2005; 27:685–695.

Honkasalo ML. Space and embodied experience: rethinking the body in pain. *Body and Society* 1998; 4:35–57.

Law M, Baptiste S, McColl M, et al. The Canadian Occupational Performance Measure: An outcome measure for occupational therapy. *Can J Occup Ther* 1990; 57:82–87.

Liedberg GM, Henriksson CM. Factors of importance for work disability in women with fibromyalgia—an interview study. *Arthritis Care Res* 2002; 47:266–274.

McColl M, Paterson M, Davies D, Doubt L, Law M. Validity and community utility of the Canadian Occupational Performance Measure. *Can J Occup Ther* 2000; 67:22–30.

Nicholas M. *Pain Self-Efficacy Questionnaire (PSEQ): Preliminary Report,*. Sydney: University of Sydney Pain Management and Research Centre, Royal North Shore Hospital, 1994.

Presnell S. Whatever the individual says it is: a phenomenological analysis of chronic pain in people with human immunodeficiency virus-associated distal symmetrical polyneuropathy. Unpublished PhD Thesis: University of Queensland: St Lucia, 2004.

Redman C, Strong J, Sharry R, Cramond T. A randomized study of goal-setting in a multidisciplinary pain centre. Paper presented at: Australian and New Zealand Pain Societies Combined Annual Scientific Meeting, Christchurch, 2003.

Sandqvist JL, Henriksson CM. Work functioning—a conceptual framework. *Work* 2004; 23:147–157.

Scarry E. *The Body in Pain.* Oxford: Oxford University Press, 1985.

Schott GD. Communicating the experience of pain: the role of analogy. *Pain* 2004; 108:209–212.

Sontag S. *Aids and its Metaphors.* London: Penguin, 1989.

Unsworth C. Measuring of outcome of occupational therapy: tools and resources. *Aust Occup Ther J* 2000; 47:147–158.

Waylonis GW, Ronan PG, Gordon C. A profile of fibromyalgia in occupational environment. *Am J Phys Med Rehabil* 1994; 73:112–115.

White KP, Speechley M, Harth M, Ostbye T. Comparing self-reported function and work disability in 100 community cases of fibromyalgia syndrome versus controls in London, Ontario. *Arthritis Rheum* 1999; 42:76–83.

Williams AC, Davies HTW, Chadury Y. Simple pain rating scales hide complex idiosyncratic meanings. *Pain* 2000; 85:457–463.

World Health Organization. *The International Classification of Functioning, Disability and Health (ICF).* Geneva: World Health Organization, 2001. Available at: www.who.int.

Correspondence to: Jenny Strong, PhD, MOccThy, Visiting Professor, School of Social Work and Applied Human Sciences, The University of Queensland, Brisbane, Queensland 4072, Australia. Email: j.strong@uq.edu.au.

Proceedings of the 11th World Congress on Pain,
edited by Herta Flor, Eija Kalso, and Jonathan O.
Dostrovsky, IASP Press, Seattle, © 2006.

71

Risk-Factor-Targeted Psychological Interventions for Pain-Related Disability

Michael J.L. Sullivan,[a] Steven Linton,[b]
and William S. Shaw[c]

*[a]Department of Psychology, University of Montreal, Montreal, Quebec, Canada;
[b]Department of Behavioral, Social, and Legal Sciences—Psychology, Örebro
University, Örebro, Sweden; [c]Liberty Mutual Center for Disability Research,
Hopkinton, Massachusetts, USA*

Considerable research has accumulated over the past decade highlighting the importance of psychosocial risk factors for prolonged pain-related disability (Waddell and Waddell 2000; Shaw et al. 2002; Waddell et al. 2003; Linton 2005). Emerging from this body of research has been a call for more concerted efforts to develop effective means of identifying individuals at risk for the development of chronic pain and disability (Linton 2002; Linton et al. 2005b). There has been increasing recognition that effective secondary prevention of pain-related disability will require the development of interventions that specifically target risk factors for prolonged pain and disability (Shaw and Feuerstein 2004; Sullivan et al. 2005a).

In this chapter we review recent research on psychosocial risk factors for pain-related disability. We describe different approaches to the assessment of psychosocial risk for prolonged disability and address challenges to the implementation of risk detection methods in clinical practice. We also present recent efforts to develop risk-factor-targeted interventions aimed at reducing the probability that individuals identified as "at risk" will follow a trajectory of persistent pain and disability. Finally, we discuss directions for future research.

PSYCHOSOCIAL RISK FACTORS FOR
PROLONGED PAIN AND DISABILITY

Persistent pain consequent to injury remains one of the most significant and costly health challenges facing the working-age population (Frank et al. 1996; Waddell 1998). Musculoskeletal conditions involving the spine, such as soft-tissue injuries to the back or neck, represent the single largest category of injury contributing to absenteeism from work. Although the majority of soft tissue injuries to the back recover without complication within weeks of injury, a significant proportion of individuals will continue to experience symptoms of persistent pain and high levels of pain-related disability; many will remain permanently occupationally disabled (Spitzer et al. 1987; Waddell et al. 2003). One of the challenges in the area of occupational rehabilitation has been to discern the variables that distinguish between individuals who return to work and those who remain disabled as a result of an occupational back injury.

Over the past two decades, considerable research has accumulated indicating that medical variables cannot fully account for presenting symptoms of pain and disability (Fordyce 1995; Gatchel et al. 1995; Waddell 1998). Biopsychosocial models suggest that a complete understanding of pain experience and pain-related outcomes will require consideration of physical, psychological, and social factors (Feuerstein 1991; Turk 1996; Waddell 1998). The ultimate goal of research in this area is to contribute to the development of more effective clinical interventions for individuals who suffer from pain-related disability.

The identification of risk factors for work disability is considered an essential first step toward the development of effective interventions aimed at preventing prolonged pain-related disability. Although extensive research on psychosocial risk factors for pain and disability (e.g., Shaw et al. 2002; Waddell et al. 2003) has been invaluable in advancing knowledge about factors that might contribute to chronicity, the interpretation of the literature and its implications for clinical practice are not always clear. Risk factor analyses have been conducted in relation to a variety of outcomes (e.g., pain, disability, work absence), and implicit assumptions concerning the equivalence among these outcomes may not be tenable. Methodological issues limit the interpretability of research that has been conducted to date (Linton et al. 2005b), and these limitations have adversely affected the potential for developing effective tools for the identification of individuals at risk.

Numerous investigations have been conducted addressing the role of psychosocial factors in the prediction of prolonged pain and disability associated with work-related musculoskeletal conditions. Research indicates that initial levels of perceived pain and perceived functional disability are predictive of prolonged work disability (Schultz et al. 2004). Pain-related fears can be significant determinants of disability associated with back pain (Gheldof and al. 2005), high levels of pain catastrophizing contribute to more severe disability in injured workers (Sullivan et al. 1998; Picavet et al. 2002; Linton 2005), and low levels of functional self-efficacy and low expectancies for return to work have been associated with prolonged work disability (Kaivanto et al. 1995; Lackner et al. 1996). Depressive symptoms associated with musculoskeletal disorders may also increase the risk for prolonged work disability (Sullivan and Stanish 2003; Vowles et al. 2004).

Screening instruments have been developed in an effort to facilitate the identification of individuals at risk for prolonged pain and disability (Linton and Hallden 1998; Feuerstein et al. 2000; Waddell et al. 2003; Schultz and Crook 2004; Boersma and Linton 2005). A challenge to the development of effective screening tools has been to balance the need for comprehensiveness with the reality of time and resource constraints of typical clinical practice. Given the multitude of psychosocial risk factors identified to date, comprehensive assessment of each domain of risk would not be possible, or even desirable, thus initial screening should aim simply to identify individuals at risk. Subsequently a more in-depth follow up assessment could be conducted to specify the domains of risk that might need to be targeted in treatment.

A significant obstacle to successful identification of individuals at risk for chronicity involves the incorporation of screening instruments into the primary care setting. Risk factor identification in clinical practice is more likely to be based on intuition rather than systematic evaluation, although clinicians' intuitive understanding of risk factors for chronicity is at odds with research evidence (Overmeer et al. 2004). Thus, known risk factors for chronicity are likely to go undetected during routine primary care. Health care professionals often become aware of psychological factors in pain and disability only after chronicity has developed and the client has become resistant to treatment.

The Örebro Musculoskeletal Pain Screening Questionnaire was developed to assist health care providers in assessing psychosocial risk for prolonged pain and disability (Linton and Hallden 1998). The instrument consists of 25 items (Table I) and can be self-administered by the patient while waiting to see a health care professional. This screening instrument was found to have satisfactory test-retest reliability (0.83) and validity in a sample of 142 patients where the outcome was duration of work absence. Hurley et al. (2000) investigated the predictive ability of the instrument with regard to return to work after physical therapy. They reported that 80% of patients who obtained a total score above 112 on the screening measure did not return to work at the end of treatment. Linton and Boersma (2003) reported the results of a prospective study showing that the Örebro Musculoskeletal Pain Screening Questionnaire was a good predictor of future function and work absence, but did not predict future pain.

Table I
The Örebro Screening Questionnaire for problematic back pain

1. What year were you born?
2. Are you male or female?
3. What is your current employment status?
4. Where were you born?
5. Where do you have pain?
6. How many days of work have you missed (sick leave) because of pain during the past 12 months?
7. How many weeks have you suffered from your current pain problem?
8. Is your work heavy or monotonous?
9. How would you rate the pain you have had during the past week?
10. In the past 3 months, on average, how intense was your pain?
11. How often would you say that you have experienced pain episodes on average, during the past 3 months?
12. Based on all things you do to cope or deal with your pain on an average day, how much are you able to decrease it?
13. How tense or anxious have you felt in the past week?
14. How much have you been bothered by feeling depressed in the past week?
15. In your view, how large is the risk that your current pain may become persistent (may not go away)?
16. In your estimation, what are the chances that you will be working in 6 months?
17. If you take into consideration your work routines, management, salary, promotion possibilities, and work mates, how satisfied are you with your job?

Beliefs:
18. Physical activity makes my pain worse.
19. An increase in pain is an indication that I should stop what I am doing until the pain decreases.
20. I should not do my normal work with my present pain.
21. I can do light work for an hour.
22. I can walk for an hour.
23. I can do ordinary household chores.
24. I can do the weekly shopping.
25. I can sleep at night.

Source: Linton and Hallden (1998).

Research to date suggests that the Örebro Musculoskeletal Pain Screening Questionnaire is a useful instrument for identifying individuals at risk for prolonged pain-related disability and work absence (Boersma and Linton 2005). As with all screening measures, appropriate caution must be brought to bear in the interpretation of scores. Despite the questionnaire's apparent predictive value, decisions based only on questionnaire results may lead to misclassification of a certain number of patients. Nevertheless, the research at least shows that the questionnaire is likely to be more reliable than clinical intuition in its ability to identify patients at risk.

PSYCHOLOGICAL RISK-FACTOR-TARGETED INTERVENTIONS

Only recently has risk factor research been used as a basis for the development of early interventions aimed at minimizing the risk of chronic pain-related disability. Although psychological interventions have been included as an integral component of many tertiary care multidisciplinary pain management programs, psychological treatment has been under-represented in secondary prevention programs for occupational injury. Even when psychological interventions have been included as part of secondary prevention programs, few appear to have been specifically designed to target psychological risk factors for chronicity.

Promising results have emerged from recently developed programs targeting psychological risk factors for prolonged pain and disability. These programs have been designed to address specifically the cognitive (e.g., pain catastrophizing, pain beliefs), behavioral (e.g., activity avoidance) or emotional (e.g., fear) barriers to recovery. Compared to traditional approaches, these programs focus less on the management of pain symptoms and more on the management of pain-related disability.

Linton et al. (2005a) selected participants with short-term back pain in a primary care setting who had "at risk" profiles on a screening instrument and then provided a cognitive-behavioral group intervention designed to address these risk factors. Participants ($n = 185$) were randomly assigned to (1) standardized, guideline-based treatment as usual; (2) cognitive-behavioral therapy (alone); or (3) the combination of cognitive-behavioral and physical therapy (assessment plus exercise). The results showed that, for work absenteeism, the two groups receiving cognitive-behavioral interventions had fewer days off work for back pain during the 12-month follow-up than did the guideline-based treatment-as-usual group. The risk for developing long-term sick disability leave was more than five fold higher in the guideline-based treatment-as-usual group than in the other two groups receiving the cognitive-behavioral intervention (Linton et al. 2005a).

Other investigations have also pointed to the potential benefit of psychosocial risk-factor-targeted interventions for pain-related disability. A program of intervention developed by Vlaeyen and his colleagues (2003) proceeds from the perspective that disability develops as a function of high levels of pain-related fears. Individuals are selected for the treatment program on the basis of a screening procedure designed to detect high levels of such fears. Individuals are gradually exposed to the movements that are associated with fear with an approach similar to that which would be used for an individual who suffered from a phobic condition. A recent clinical trial has shown that this type of intervention can be effective in reducing levels of fear, pain, and pain-related disability (George et al. 2003).

Community-based intervention programs, such as the Pain-Disability Prevention (PDP) program, have also been developed to specifically target psychosocial risk factors (Sullivan and Stanish 2003). The PDP program was first implemented in 2001 in Nova Scotia, Canada, as part of a community-based approach to the management of pain-related occupational disability. Psychologists in communities across the province were trained to provide the intervention. By adding a psychosocial risk-factor-targeted intervention to existing community-based treatment services such as medical management and physiotherapy, the goal was to establish "virtual" multidisciplinary treatment teams at the level of the community. The primary objective of the intervention program was to facilitate return to work by maximizing activity involvement and reducing psychosocial barriers to rehabilitation progress.

Individuals are considered as possible candidates for the PDP program if they obtain elevated scores on risk factors addressed by the intervention program (pain catastrophizing, fear of movement/re-injury, perceived disability, and depression). The program is a standardized 10-week intervention that uses structured activity scheduling and graded activity involvement to target risk factors such as fear of movement/re-injury and perceived disability. Thought monitoring and cognitive restructuring strategies are used to target catastrophic thinking and depression (detailed information about the program can be obtained at www.pdp-pgap.com). A preliminary outcome study using a historical control group demonstrated a 60% return-to-work rate in the PDP-treated sample compared to 18% in the treatment-as-usual control (Sullivan and Stanish 2003). A recent study showed that, in a sample of 215 injured workers who completed the PDP program, treatment-related reductions in pain catastrophizing significantly predicted return to work (Sullivan et al. 2005b).

Preliminary results on the implementation of the PDP program indicate that it is feasible to establish a regional network of psychologists who can deliver a standardized activity mobilization intervention for injured workers. Our experience also suggests that the majority of injured workers considered as candidates for the program are willing to participate in psychological treatment. The findings indicate promising return-to-work rates for a population at high risk for prolonged disability. The adoption of a psychology-driven, community-based model of secondary prevention for pain-related disability may prove to be a cost-effective approach to the management of one of the most costly population health problems facing industrialized countries.

MANAGING PSYCHOSOCIAL RISK
FACTORS IN THE WORKPLACE

Intervention approaches for the management of disability associated with musculoskeletal conditions have typically involved a combination of medical management and physical rehabilitation, with psychological services sometimes considered in more complex cases. The assumption underlying this approach is that once the pathology responsible for pain and disability has been effectively treated, the patient should return to work without complication. It is becoming clearer, however, that interventions focusing exclusively on the treatment of the individual are limited in their impact on facilitating re-integration into the workplace. Psychosocial risk factors for prolonged work disability exist not only within the individual, but within the workplace as well. The workplace can also be described in terms of a psychosocial risk profile (Linton 2004). Investigations have revealed that psychosocial features of the workplace such as supervisor attitudes toward work disability, co-worker support, and willingness to accommodate are significant determinants of the probability of return to work (Shaw et al. 2002, 2003).

Only recently have intervention programs targeting workplace psychosocial risk factors been implemented with the goal of preventing prolonged work disability. Some evidence is emerging that return-to-work rates can be facilitated by interventions targeting supervisor attitudes and co-worker support (Shaw and Feuerstein 2004). Similarly, workplace accommodations such as ergonomic and modified work interventions can improve return-to-work rates (Loisel et al. 1997). Return-to-work rates might also be enhanced when rehabilitation treatment is provided within the work milieu (Loisel and Durand 2005). A number of reports suggest that training case managers in problem solving can facilitate the implementation of appropriate work accommodations (Shaw and Feuerstein 2004). Pransky et al. (2002) reported promising results of a pilot study involving a support and guidance intervention aimed at increasing employers' involvement in facilitating the return-to-work process.

In a recent study, occupational health nurses and case managers from a workers' compensation system were trained to provide early intervention to back-injured workers at elevated risk for disability (Schultz and Crook 2004). The intervention involved an individual session of motivational interviewing and return-to-work planning with the worker. The intervention also included phone communication with the worker's family physician, a workplace visit, focused case management, and follow-up with the worker and employer after the return to work. The preliminary outcomes have been positive with respect to duration of disability when compared to conventional treatment (Schultz and Crook 2004).

Shaw et al. (2005) reported the results of an outcome study in which individuals at risk for chronicity were selected for participation in one of four different treatment programs. Of primary interest was determining the added impact of a workplace transition program when combined with a multidisciplinary functional restoration program. Cost-effectiveness analyses revealed that the provision of risk-targeted early intervention yielded three-fold reductions in disability costs associated with occupational low back pain. Adding a workplace transition component further improved the efficacy and cost effectiveness of treatment for patients with occupational low back pain-related risk factors for delayed recovery and return to work.

New workplace-based initiatives are being developed to examine how interventions that have traditionally been considered outside of the psychosocial domain might be improving return to work through their influence on psychosocial risk factors. These initiatives will help define the potential benefits of incorporating psychosocial intervention techniques within ergonomic, physical therapy, or case management approaches in order to maximize their impact (Shaw et al. 2001, 2003; Feuerstein et al. 2003).

SUMMARY

Traditional approaches to the management of pain-related disability have tended to focus to a significant degree on pain reduction, and pain severity has been considered as a central outcome variable. As a result, many of the interventions included in pain management programs have included palliative strategies aimed at minimizing pain and tension. While analgesics, ultrasound, transcutaneous electrical nerve stimulation, or relaxation training can reduce physical and emotional distress, these approaches do not appear to have a significant impact on return-to-work potential (Fordyce 1995; Waddell 1998).

It is possible that effective secondary prevention of pain-related disability may be determined not by the degree to which pain can be reduced, but by the degree to which barriers to work re-entry can be minimized. Pain itself may not be the most important barrier. The key to success may lie in shifting emphasis away from the goal of managing or reducing pain and toward the identification and elimination of psychosocial and workplace factors that contribute to the development and maintenance of disability (Linton et al. 2005b; Pransky et al. 2005; Sullivan et al. 2005a).

The past decade has witnessed tremendous advances with respect to knowledge about factors that can contribute to prolonged pain-related disability. The development of effective screening tools has permitted better early identification of individuals at risk for chronicity. The development and implementation of psychosocial risk-factor-targeted interventions should provide additional resources to prevent a trajectory of prolonged pain and disability in individuals identified as being at risk. New approaches to targeted workplace psychosocial risk factors are also yielding promising results. Research conducted to date suggests that effective secondary prevention of work disability will require the use of screening tools for identifying individuals at risk, as well as the implementation of interventions that concurrently target both worker-related and workplace psychosocial risk factors.

ACKNOWLEDGMENTS

Research described in this chapter was supported by funding provided by the Canadian Institutes of Health Research, the Örebro County Council, and the Liberty Mutual Center for Disability Research.

REFERENCES

Boersma K, Linton SJ. Screening to identify patients at risk: profiles for psychosocial risk factors for early intervention. *Clin J Pain* 2005; 21:38–43.

Feuerstein M. A multidisciplinary approach to the prevention, evaluation, and management of work disability. *J Occup Rehabil* 1991; 1:5–12.

Feuerstein M, Huang G, Haufler A, Miller J. Development of a screen for predicting clinical outcomes in patients with work-related upper extremity disorders. *J Occup Environ Med* 2000; 42:749–761.

Feuerstein M, Huang GD, Ortiz JM, Integrated case management for work-related upper extremity disorders: impact of patient satisfaction on health and work status. *J Occup Environ Med* 2003; 45:803–812.

Fordyce WE. *Back Pain in the Workplace.* Seattle: IASP Press, 1995.

Frank JW, Brooker AS, DeMaio SE, et al. Disability resulting from occupational low back pain. Part II: What do we know about secondary prevention? A review of the scientific evidence on prevention after disability begins. *Spine* 1996; 21(24):2918–2929.

Gatchel R, Polatin P, Mayer R. The dominant role of psychosocial risk factors in the development of chronic low back pain. *Spine* 1995; 20:2701–2709.

George S, Fritz J, Bialosky JE, Donald DA. The effect of fear-avoidance-based physical therapy intervention for acute low back pain: results of a randomized controlled trial. *Spine* 2003; 28:2551–2560.

Gheldof EL, Vinck J, Vlaeyen JW, Hidding A, Crombez G. The differential role of pain, work characteristics and pain-related fear in explaining back pain and sick leave in occupational settings. *Pain* 2005; 113:71–81.

Hurley D, Dusoir T, McDonough S, et al. Biopsychosocial screening questionnaire for patients with low back pain: preliminary report of utility in physiotherapy practice in Northern Ireland. *Clin J Pain* 2000; 16:214–228.

Kaivanto K, Estlander A, Moneta G. Isokinetic performance in low back pain patients: the predictive power of the Self-Efficacy Scale. *J Occup Rehabil* 1995; 5:87–99.

Lackner J, Carosella A, Feuerstein M. Pain expectancies, pain, and functional self-efficacy as determinants of disability in patients with chronic low back disorders. *J Consult Clin Psychol* 1996; 64:212–220.

Linton SJ. Early identification and intervention in the prevention of musculoskeletal pain. *Am J Ind Med* 2002; 41:433–442.

Linton SJ. Environment and learning factors in the development of chronic pain and disability. In: Price D, Bushnell M (Eds). Psychological Methods of Pain Control: Basic Science and Clinical Perspectives. Seattle: IASP Press, 2004, pp 143–167.

Linton SJ. Do psychological factors increase the risk for back pain in the general population in both a cross-sectional and prospective analysis? Eur J Pain 2005a; 9(4):355–361.

Linton SJ. Do psychological factors increase the risk for back pain in the general population in both a cross-sectional and prospective analysis? Eur J Pain 2005b; 9(4):355–361.

Linton SJ, Boersma K. Early identification of patients at risk of developing a persistent back problem: the predictive validity of the Orebro Musculoskeletal Pain Questionnaire. *Clin J Pain* 2003; 19: 80–86.

Linton SJ, Hallden K. Can we screen for problematic back pain? A screening questionnaire for predicting outcome in acute and subacute back pain. *Clin J Pain* 1998; 14:209–216.

Linton SJ, Boersma K, Jansson M, Svard L, Botvalde M. The effects of cognitive-behavioral and physical therapy preventive interventions in pain-related sick leave: a randomized controlled trial. *Clin J Pain* 2005a; 21:109–119.

Linton SJ, Gross D, Schultz I, et al. Prognosis and the identification of workers risking disability: research issues and directions for future research. *J Occup Rehabil* 2005b; 15:459–474.

Loisel P, Durand M. Working with the employer: the Sherbrooke Model. In: Schultz I, Gatchel R (Eds). *Handbook of Complex Occupational Disability Claims: Early Risk Identification, Intervention, and Prevention.* New York: Springer, 2005.

Loisel P, Abenhaim L, Durand M, Esdaile J. A population-based randomized clinical trial on back pain management. *Spine* 1997; 22:2911–2918.

Overmeer T, Linton SJ, Boersma K. Do physical therapists recognize established risk factors? Swedish physical therapists evaluation in comparison to guidelines. *Physiotherapy* 2004; 90:35–41.

Picavet HS, Vlaeyen JW, Schouten JS. Pain catastrophizing and kinesiophobia: predictors of chronic low back pain. *Am J Epidemiol* 2002; 156(11):1028–1034.

Pransky G, Robertson M, Moon S. Stress and work-related upper-extremity disorders: Implications for prevention and management. *Am J Ind Med* 2002; 41:443–455.

Pransky G, Gatchel R, Linton SJ, Loisel P. Improving return to work research. *J Occup Rehabil* 2005; 15: 453–457.

Schultz IZ, Crook J. Application of a Risk-for-Disability Questionnaire in the identification of subacute low back injured workers who require early intervention. *J Pain* 2004; 4:8.

Schultz IZ, Crook J, Meloche GR, et al. Psychosocial factors predictive of occupational low back disability: towards development of a return-to-work model. *Pain* 2004; 107:77–85.

Shaw W, Feuerstein M. Generating workplace accommodations: lessons learned from the Integrated Case Management study. *J Occup Rehabil* 2004; 14:207–216.

Shaw W, Feuerstein M, Huang G. Secondary prevention and the workplace. In: Linton S (Ed). *New Avenues for the Prevention of Chronic Musculoskeletal Pain and Disability.* Amsterdam: Elsevier, 2002.

Shaw W, Feuerstein M, Miller V, Wood P. Identifying barriers to recovery from work-related upper extremity disorders: use of a collaborative problem-solving technique. *AAOHN J* 2003; 51:337–346.

Shaw W, Pransky G, Patterson W, Winters T. Early disability risk factors for low back pain assessed at outpatient occupational health clinics. *Spine* 2005; 30: 572–580.

Spitzer W, LeBlanc F, Dupuis M. A scientific approach to the assessment and management of activity-related spinal disorders: a monograph for clinicians. *Spine* 1987; 12(Suppl 75):S3–S59.

Sullivan MJL, Stanish WD. Psychologically based occupational rehabilitation: the Pain-Disability Prevention Program. *Clin J Pain* 2003; 19:97–104.

Sullivan MJL, Stanish W, Waite H, Sullivan M, Tripp DA. Catastrophizing, pain, and disability in patients with soft-tissue injuries. *Pain* 1998; 77:253–260.

Sullivan MJL, Feuerstein M, Gatchel R, Linton SJ, Pransky G. Integrating psychological and behavioral interventions to achieve optimal rehabilitation outcomes. *J Occup Rehabil* 2005a; 15:475–489.

Sullivan MJL, Ward L, Tripp D, et al. Secondary prevention of work disability: community-based psychosocial intervention for musculoskeletal disorders. *J Occup Rehabil* 2005b; 15:377–392.

Turk D. Biopsychosocial perspective on chronic pain. In: Gatchel R, Turk D (Eds). *Psychological Approaches to Pain Management.* New York: Guilford, 1996.

Vowles K, Gross R, Sorrell J. Predicting work status following interdisciplinary treatment for chronic pain. *Eur J Pain* 2004; 8:351–358.

Waddell G. *The Back Pain Revolution.* London: Churchill Livingstone, 1998.

Waddell G, Waddell H. Social influences on neck and back pain. In: Nachemson A, Jonsson E (Eds). *Neck and Back Pain: The Scientific Evidence of Causes, Diagnosis and Treatment.* New York: Lippincott Williams and Wilkins, 2000.

Waddell G, Burton A, Main C. *Screening to Identify People at Risk of Long-term Incapacity for Work.* London: Royal Society of Medicine Press, 2003.

Correspondence to: Michael J.L. Sullivan, PhD, Department of Psychology, University of Montreal, CP 6128 Succ. Centre Ville, Montreal, Quebec, Canada H3C 3J7. Email: michael.jl.sullivan@umontreal.ca.

Proceedings of the 11th World Congress on Pain,
edited by Herta Flor, Eija Kalso, and Jonathan O.
Dostrovsky, IASP Press, Seattle, © 2006.

72

Improving Physical Activity in Elderly Individuals with Chronic Low Back Pain

Heinz-Dieter Basler,[a] Helmut Bertalanffy,[b] Sabine Quint,[a] Axel Wilke,[c] and Udo Wolf[d]

*[a]Institute for Medical Psychology, [b]Department of Neurosurgery,
[c]Department of Orthopedics, and [d]Department of Physiotherapy,
Philipps University of Marburg, Marburg, Germany*

Systematic reviews and randomized controlled trials provide strong evidence that, over time, participation in regular physical activity reduces pain and enhances the functional capacity of older adults with persistent pain (American Geriatric Association 2002). Compliance, however, is often low (Allison and Keller 1997). We performed a study to evaluate the effect of motivation-oriented counseling in addition to physiotherapy on activity and function in a sample of older patients with chronic low back pain. Counseling strategies were based on the transtheoretical model and on the technique of motivational interviewing (Rollnick et al. 1999). We expected a better outcome in patients who participated in a combined program of physiotherapy and motivational counseling compared with those who only underwent physiotherapy.

METHODS

STUDY DESIGN

In a prospective controlled trial, elderly individuals with chronic low back pain were randomized to two groups in a blinded fashion. The study was approved by the ethics committee of the faculty of medicine at the University of Marburg. Patients were stratified according to their age and their readiness to resume physical activity, assessed as described below, in order to avoid confounding variables (Riebe et al. 2005). Patients in the active experimental group participated in physiotherapy and counseling, whereas control patients received physiotherapy and placebo "ultrasound" treatment. Inclusion criteria were a minimum age of 65 years, a diagnosis of chronic low back pain, and pain at the time of inclusion. Exclusion criteria were red flags and a diagnosis of dementia.

Patients were recruited from the departments of orthopedics and neurosurgery at the university hospital in Marburg. After receiving a medical examination, those who provided informed consent received an assessment by both a physiotherapist and a psychologist based on a published and evaluated structured pain interview for the elderly (Basler et al. 2001). Three assessments were conducted—the first before treatment, the second just after termination of treatment 6–7 weeks later, and the third at the 6-month follow-up. Primary outcome measures were physical activity, functional capacity, and range of motion.

SUBJECTS

A total of 170 individuals participated in the study, of whom 152 provided data at the follow-up (73 from the experimental group and 79 from the control group; the dropout rate was about 10%). Dropouts discontinued participation in the study mainly for medical reasons. At the follow-up, an additional 5% of patients did not return their activity diaries. Prior to treatment, due to a software problem with the ultrasound device, the data of 25 patients were not recorded accurately. Thus, the number of individuals with complete data at follow-up differed dependent on the outcome variable (see Table I). The average age

Table I
Statistics of the principal outcome variables

Variable	Group	t_1 Mean (SD)	t_2 Mean (SD)	t_3 Mean (SD)	Main Effect Group*	Main Effect Time*	Interaction Effect*
Mean duration of physical activity (minutes/day)	EG $n = 69$	14.0 (17.0)	29.1 (14.4)	29.5 (24.7)	$F_{1,136} = 2.05$, n.s., $\eta^2 = 0.015$	$F_{2,135} = 37.59, P < 0.01, \eta^2 = 0.358$	$F_{2,135} = 0.56$, n.s., $\eta^2 = 0.008$
	CG $n = 69$	13.3 (14.7)	25.0 (16.4)	25.6 (20.0)			
Functional capacity (% normal function)	EG $n = 73$	68.3 (19.3)	75.3 (16.1)	74.1 (20.7)	$F_{1,150} = 2.84$, n.s., $\eta^2 = 0.019$	$F_{2,149} = 15.01$, $P < 0.01, \eta^2 = 0.168$	$F_{2,149} = 1.15$, n.s., $\eta^2 = 0.015$
	CG $n = 79$	65.7 (18.8)	69.8 (17.6)	68.4 (19.5)			
Range of motion (degrees)	EG $n = 64$	22.9 (9.8)	24.1 (9.1)	23.5 (9.3)	$F_{1,125} = 1.12$, n.s., $\eta^2 = 0.009$	$F_{2,124} = 0.89$, n.s., $\eta^2 = 0.006$	$F_{2,124} = 1.32$, n.s., $\eta^2 = 0.021$
	CG $n = 63$	22.1 (9.6)	21.7 (9.5)	21.6 (9.1)			

Abbreviations and symbols: EG = experimental group, CG = control group; t_1 = before treatment, t_2 = after treatment, t_3 = 6-month follow-up; η^2 = effect size (> 0.01 small effect, < 0.06 average effect, < 0.14 large effect).
* Analysis of variance.

of the sample was 70.1 years (SD = 4.1 years, range 65–83 years); 64% of subjects were female. The principal diagnoses were spondylosis (50.5%) and osteochondrosis (21.5%).

ASSESSMENT INSTRUMENTS

Prior to treatment, we used an algorithm to allocate the patients to different stages of readiness for physical activity (Schumann et al. 2003; Basler et al. 2004), defined as pre-contemplation (PC), contemplation (C), preparation (P), action (A), and maintenance (M) in accordance with the transtheoretical model of change. Allocation to the stages depended on patients' self-reported readiness to carry out the target behavior, which was a minimum of 30 minutes of physical activity per day that included unsupervised stretching, strengthening, and endurance exercises. After each assessment, patients filled out a 7-day activity diary that included illustrations of the desired activities in order to facilitate the recording process.

Functional capacity was assessed by the Hannover Functional Disability Scale, a published instrument with good psychometric properties (Kohlmann and Raspe 1996). This scale measures activities of daily living, such as the ability to wash one's hair or to put on socks on one's own. Scores are transformed to values that indicate a percentage of normal function. A value of more than 80% indicates normal capacity. Data from different studies show that this scale has internal consistency of $\alpha = 0.90$ and retest-reliability of at least $r = 0.75$.

Range of motion was measured by ultrasound topometry utilizing the CMS 20S device offered by Zebris. This system depicts posture and movement in three-dimensional space. Patients are requested to bend forward while ultrasound signals measure the location of predefined reference points on the body. The data are automatically stored for subsequent computation.

TREATMENT

Over a period of 5 weeks, both groups received 10 physiotherapy sessions, each of 20 minutes' duration. Each session started with stretching exercises, followed by physiotherapy treatment tailored to the specific needs of the patient. Depending on the initial evaluation, the treatment aimed at improving the length, strength, endurance, and/or coordination of muscles of the torso and lower limbs. Sessions included homework assignments that were individualized for every patient and allowed for personal preferences. Special emphasis was placed on activities of daily living. Verbal instructions were complemented by written material in order to facilitate adherence to the assignments at home.

In addition, patients in the active group individually attended a standardized counseling procedure of 10 minutes' duration prior to every physiotherapy treatment. The program addressed readiness for change and integrated some of the relevant processes of change, such as by presenting information about chronic back pain and about the beneficial effects of physical activity. The program aimed to increase patients' self-efficacy and to positively influence their decision-making process. Additionally, the program was intended to enhance commitment to the desired behavioral changes through self-reinforcement and reinforcement by the therapist, to increase the patient's use of social support, and to help the patient to deal constructively with relapses.

In order to control for the additional attention given to the experimental group, the control group participated in placebo "ultrasound" therapy with an inactivated device. This procedure also lasted for 10 minutes. While the physiotherapists passed the device over painful areas of the patient's body, they were free to talk to the patient about any topic.

Four experienced physiotherapists participated in the study after completing an introductory class. Two therapists worked with the experimental group and two with the control group. Only the therapists in the experimental group, however, received information about the experimental treatment. They participated in an 8-hour class about the transtheoretical model, which included trial counseling sessions. They also recorded how they conducted the sessions and marked any deviations from the treatment plan. We inspected these recordings regularly and supervised the physiotherapists in order to encourage adherence to the treatment protocol.

HYPOTHESES AND DATA ANALYSIS

We expected that patients receiving the experimental intervention would spend more time engaging in physical activity compared to the control patients. Given the fact that physical activity corresponds with functional capacity in older adults (Riebe et al. 2005), we also expected better function in the experimental group at the follow-up assessment.

Calculation of the sample size relied on the assumption that effect sizes would be in the middle range and that the percentage of dropouts at follow-up would be 15%. Statistical procedures were χ^2 tests, t tests for independent samples, and analyses of variance, with level of significance assumed at 5% and statistical power at 80%.

RESULTS

Stratification for age and stage of readiness for change as possible confounding variables resulted in an equal distribution of these variables in the experimental and control group. The mean age in the experimental group was 70.1 years (SD = 4.2; N = 86) and in the control group 70.6 years (SD = 4.6; N = 84). These differences were not significant (t = 0.488, df = 168). The distribution of stage of readiness for change in the experimental group revealed that prior to treatment, 12.8% of the sample could be assigned to PC, 35.9% to C, 44.9% to P, 1.3% to A, and 5.1% to M. Respective values in the control group were 7.4% for PC, 35.8% for C, 44.4% for P, 4.9% for A, and 7.4% for M. Differences were insignificant (χ^2 = 0.529, df = 4).

Table I shows the distribution of the outcome variables over time. A significant main effect time indicates that both the experimental group and the control group showed an improvement in physical activity and self-reported functional capacity. Effect sizes were large. The interaction effect, however, remained insignificant. Consequently, motivational training did not result in a better outcome compared with placebo ultrasound treatment. Range of motion remained unchanged throughout the observation period. Consequently, our assumptions had to be rejected.

DISCUSSION

Ten minutes of motivational counseling provided by physiotherapists prior to every physiotherapy session failed to show better results than a placebo "ultrasound" treatment. The difference of 5 minutes of physical activity between the two groups at the follow-up assessment in favor of the experimental group was not statistically significant. The increase in physical activity and self-reported function cannot be attributed to the basic physiotherapy training due to the lack of an untreated control group. These results are not in accordance with those of a randomized controlled study conducted previously in the same setting (Friedrich et al. 1998). In that study, physiotherapists offered an activity program to low back pain patients that was similar to our own to both the experimental and the control group. In addition, the experimental group received motivational training. At the 1-year follow-up, no difference was found between the motivation group and the control group with regard to exercise adherence. Despite this finding, the effects of training were beneficial with respect to disability and pain intensity. Five years later, the motivation group was superior to the control group with regard to disability, pain intensity, and ability to work (Friedrich et al. 2005). Friedrich's team worked with a younger age group than our study and integrated the motivation training into the physiotherapy sessions, which may have contributed to the favorable results. Nevertheless, it remains unclear why this study resulted in reduced disability and pain levels, if this effect cannot be attributed to increased long-term adherence.

Obviously, in our study, the differences between the experimental and the control treatment were not large enough to have an impact on the outcome. Although the control therapists were not trained in motivational counseling, treatment diffusion cannot be excluded. Experimental and control therapists worked in the same department and communicated with each other. Moreover, the control therapists were allowed to talk to the patients during the placebo procedure. When questioned, they admitted the inclusion of motivational aspects either at that time or later on during the exercise part of the session. Unlike the experimental therapists, however, they did not use a structured and theory-based approach.

Pretest effects may be a further explanation for our negative findings. During every assessment, the attention of the patients was focused on physical activity. This focus may also have increased patients' adherence to the homework assignments. While our study controlled for nonspecific treatment effects by including a placebo treatment, it lacked sufficient control of treatment diffusion. In summary, the study does not encourage incorporation of a motivation program based on the transtheoretical model into physiotherapy treatment for elderly individuals with chronic low back pain.

ACKNOWLEDGMENTS

This study was funded by the Deutsche Forschungsgemeinschaft (BA 793/6-1,6-2).

REFERENCES

Allison M, Keller C. Physical activity in the elderly: benefits and intervention strategies. *Nurse Pract* 1997; 22:53–58.

American Geriatric Association. The management of persistent pain in older persons. *J Am Geriatr Soc* 2002; 50:205–224.

Basler HD, Bloem R, Casser HR, et al. Ein strukturiertes Schmerzinterview für geriatrische Patienten [A structured pain interview for geriatric patients]. *Schmerz* 2001; 15:164–171.

Basler H D, Quint S, Wolf U. Entscheidungsbalance und körperliche Aktivität bei Rückenschmerz im Alter—eine Studie im Rahmen des Transtheoretischen Modells [Decisional balance and bodily activities for back pain in the elderly: a study within the framework of the transtheoretical model]. *Z Med Psychol* 2004; 13:147–154.

Friedrich F, Gittler G, Halberstadt Y, et al. Combined exercise and motivation program: effect on the compliance and level of disability of patients with chronic low back pain: a randomized controlled trial. *Arch Phys Med Rehab* 1998; 79:475–487.

Friedrich M, Gittler G, Arendasy M, Friedrich KS. Long-term effect of a combined exercise and motivational program on the level of disability of patients with chronic low back pain. *Spine* 2005; 30:995–1000.

Kohlmann T, Raspe H. Hannover Functional Questionnaire in ambulatory diagnosis of functional disability caused by backache. *Rehabilitation* 1996; 35:1–8.

Riebe D, Garber CE, Rossi JS, Greaney ML, et al. Physical activity, physical function, and stages of change in older adults. *Am J Health Behav* 2005; 29:70–80.

Rollnick S, Mason P, Butler C. *Health Behaviour Change: A Guide for Practitioners*. Edinburgh: Churchill Livingstone, 1999.

Schumann A, Estabrooks PA, Nigg CR, Hill J. Validation of the stages of change with mild, moderate, and strenuous physical activity behaviour, intentions, and self-efficacy. *Int J Sports Med* 2003; 24:363–365.

Correspondence to: Heinz-Dieter Basler, PhD, Institute for Medical Psychology, Philipps University of Marburg, Bunsenstr. 3, Marburg 35037, Germany. Email: basler@med.uni-marburg.de.

Proceedings of the 11th World Congress on Pain,
edited by Herta Flor, Eija Kalso, and Jonathan O.
Dostrovsky, IASP Press, Seattle, © 2006.

73

Passive Joint Movement Produces Local and Widespread Hypoalgesic Effects in Subjects with Knee Osteoarthritis

Penny Moss,[a] Kathleen Sluka,[b]
and Anthony Wright[a]

*[a]School of Physiotherapy, Curtin University of Technology, Perth,
Western Australia, Australia; [b]Physical Therapy and Rehabilitation Science,
University of Iowa, Iowa City, Iowa, USA*

Physiotherapists and other health professionals make extensive use of passive joint movement to treat painful musculoskeletal conditions. Although the scientific literature has begun to characterize the hypoalgesic effects of spinal manual therapy, there is little experimental evidence to substantiate the effectiveness of peripheral joint mobilization techniques.

A number of studies have demonstrated that cervical spine mobilization reduces hyperalgesia in the upper limb (Wright 2002). Evidence is also emerging that upper-limb peripheral joint mobilization has a similar hypoalgesic effect (Vicenzino et al. 2001; Paungmali et al. 2003). However, evidence concerning the effects of joint mobilization in the lower limb is scarce and contradictory. Collins et al. (2004) found no change in pressure pain threshold (PPT) following mobilization-with-movement of a subacute ankle injury. In contrast, Yeo and Wright (2004) demonstrated an immediate improvement in PPT following accessory mobilization of similarly injured ankles (Yeo and Wright 2004). Further experimental evidence for the effects of lower-limb joint mobilization is needed.

Various mechanisms have been proposed to explain how the hypoalgesic effects of passive joint mobilization may be mediated. Although the effects may be the result of mechanically stimulated changes to the local chemical environment in joints (Sambajon et al. 2003), it has also been hypothesized that joint mobilization may activate descending pain modulation systems (Wright 2002). Evidence in support of this hypothesis comes from human studies showing that joint mobilization produces a rapid multi-system response, involving immediate pain reduction, sympathetic nervous system excitation, and alterations in motor function (Vicenzino et al. 1998; Sterling et al. 2001; Wright 2002; Paungmali et al. 2003). Recent studies using a rat model of articular pain have shown that the analgesia produced by joint mobilization involves serotonin and norepinephrine receptors in the spinal cord (Skyba et al. 2003). In addition, animal models have demonstrated reversal of hyperalgesia distal to the mobilized joint, suggesting relatively widespread analgesic changes (Sluka and Wright 2001). This distal hypoalgesic effect in the lower limb has yet to be investigated in human subjects.

This chapter describes a study designed to investigate the initial effects on pain of mobilization of a lower limb joint. The study sought to explore in humans the animal model of mobilization-induced antihyperalgesia demonstrated by Sluka and Wright (2001). The aim was to investigate whether mobilization of a chronically painful knee joint would produce immediate hypoalgesia both at the knee and at the ipsilateral heel. A secondary aim was to explore the initial effects of joint mobilization on motor function. Methodology was similar to that used in previous studies (Sluka and Wright 2001). The study employed a double-blind, controlled, repeated-measures design.

METHODS

Thirty-eight community-dwelling, ambulatory volunteers with knee osteoarthritis were recruited (mean age 65 years, 4 months). Subjects needed to experience mild to moderate knee pain and fulfill the American College of Rheumatology classification for knee osteoarthritis (Altman et al. 1986). Volunteers were excluded if they had recently undergone lower-limb surgery, had coexisting inflammatory or neurological conditions, experienced altered sensation around their knee, or exhibited cognitive difficulties. Ethical approval was obtained from the Curtin University Human Research Ethics Committee and the Royal Perth Hospital Human Ethics Committee. All participants provided written informed consent.

OUTCOME MEASURES (DEPENDENT VARIABLES)

All dependent variables were measured immediately before and after each experimental condition. Pressure pain threshold (PPT) was used as the primary pain-related outcome measure. The 1-cm^2 probe of a hand-held digital algometer was applied to the most tender point on the medial aspect of the affected knee. Pressure was increased at a rate of 40 kPa/second. Subjects were instructed to activate a button when the sensation of pressure had clearly become painful.

The same procedure was followed on the ipsilateral heel. All measures were taken in triplicate and averaged.

A 3-meter timed "up-and-go" walk test (TUG) (Podsiadlo and Richardson 1991) was used to measure the time taken to stand from a standard armless chair, briskly walk to a 3-meter mark, turn around, and return and sit down again. The test has demonstrated high inter- and intrarater reliability, with an intraclass correlation coefficient (ICC) of 0.99, in elderly arthritic populations (Podsiadlo and Richardson 1991; McMeeken et al. 1999). A lap-timer stopwatch was used to record sit-to-stand time as well as total time (Wall et al. 2000).

EXPERIMENTAL CONDITIONS (INDEPENDENT VARIABLES)

All subjects experienced each experimental condition in random order over three sessions, separated by at least 48 hours in order to control for carry-over effects (Vicenzino et al. 1998). Each condition was applied for three sets of 3 minutes, interspersed with 30-second rests. All interactions, procedures, timing, and positioning were identical for each condition and were strictly standardized. For all conditions, the subject was in a comfortable supine position, with the knees supported. The treatment consisted of a pain-free, large-amplitude, oscillatory anteroposterior glide of the tibia on the femur (Maitland 1990). The manual contact control condition precisely reproduced this hand positioning without applying any movement. The no-contact control condition reproduced all interactions, procedure timing, and positioning, without applying any manual contact. In order to improve subject blinding and reduce potential interactions, relaxing music was played and subjects were asked to close their eyes during procedures. Subjects were advised that the experiment was investigating the effects of manual contact and joint positioning.

MAIN PROCEDURES

Subjects were requested to continue with their normal medications throughout the study. At the first session, preliminary data about knee pain, chronicity, comorbidities, medications, and functional status were collected, together with scores on the Western Ontario and McMaster Universities (WOMAC) function subscale (Bellamy et al. 1988). A brief physical examination evaluated knee joint range of movement and sensation. In the case of bilateral knee pain, the subject nominated the most painful side. Procedural order was standardized, with the researcher first administering the TUG test, followed by heel and knee PPT measurements. On completion of baseline testing, a physiotherapist experienced in manipulation applied the experimental condition according to a pre-assigned randomization schedule. Immediately following the procedure, PPT and TUG measurements were repeated by the researcher, who remained blind to the experimental condition. The extent of subject blinding was assessed through a short, self-administered, post-experiment questionnaire, similar to previous studies (Vicenzino et al. 1998).

RELIABILITY

Test-retest reliability was evaluated in a pilot study using five subjects who fulfilled the study inclusion/exclusion criteria. Test-retest reliability was calculated using ICC for mean PPT values measured before and after application of the no-contact control condition. Levels of intra-subject reliability were good for knee PPT: ICC = 0.94 (95% CI = 0.55–0.99) and for heel PPT: ICC = 0.94 (95% CI = 0.59–0.99). Reliability analyses for timed "up-and-go" (TUG) values showed lower, although adequate, reliability: total ICC = 0.79 (95% CI = 0.67–0.88); sit-to-stand ICC = 0.57 (95% CI = 0.40–0.76).

DATA MANAGEMENT AND ANALYSIS

Data were analyzed using the SPSS statistical package with the α (internal reliability) level set at $P < 0.05$. Both PPT and TUG values showed normal distribution and required no transformation. In order to allow meaningful comparison of results with previous studies, we used percentage change between pre- and post-condition values as the primary dependent variable. Repeated-measures analysis of covariance was used to analyze differences between percentage change in knee PPT, heel PPT, and "up-and-go" times, using pre-condition mean as the covariate (Committee for Proprietary Medicinal Products 2003).

Power analyses were performed using the Power and Precision statistical software package. A $1 - \beta$ value (statistical power) of 0.93 was calculated for the primary PPT measurements for a sample of 38 subjects. The secondary measure of TUG demonstrated a $1 - \beta$ value of 0.69.

RESULTS

When baseline data were analyzed for comparability, no significant difference was found between pre-condition PPT means for the three conditions ($F_{2,74} = 1.02$, $P = 0.365$). Analysis of the post-experiment questionnaire revealed that 71% of subjects were unable to identify the treatment condition correctly, thereby adequately fulfilling double-blind criteria. Removal of data from non-blinded subjects made no difference to the results.

SUBJECTS

Thirteen male and 25 female subjects completed the study (mean age 65 years, 4 months, standard deviation 11 years, range 40–87 years). Subjects demonstrated similar levels of disease chronicity to that reported in recent knee osteoarthritis studies (Bellamy et al. 2005; Bennell et al. 2005), with 47.4% reporting knee pain for at least 5 years. However, subjects in the current study reported relatively low levels of functional disability and pain, with mean WOMAC scores of 6.3/20 for pain and 21.5/68 for function, compared with 8.1/20 and 28/68 in one previous study (Bennell et al. 2005) and 11.7/20 and 39.9/68 in another (Bellamy et al. 2005).

PRESSURE PAIN THRESHOLD

As illustrated in Fig. 1, knee joint mobilization significantly increased knee PPT over and above manual contact and no-contact control conditions ($F_{2,74}$ = 5.26, $P = 0.008$). Knee PPT increased by a mean of 27.3% (SE = 3.14) following treatment, compared with a 6.4% increase (SE = 2.97) following the manual contact intervention and a reduction in PPT by 9.5% (SE = 5.50) following the no-contact intervention. A priori contrasts demonstrated that treatment differed significantly from both manual contact ($F_{1,37} = 7.55$, $P = 0.008$) and no-contact ($F_{1,37} = 7.81$, $P = 0.010$) control conditions. A similar pattern of results was demonstrated at the ipsilateral, nonpathological, heel. Knee mobilization treatment increased heel PPT by 15.3% (SE = 3.26), which was significantly greater than the effect of either manual contact (6.9% ± 3.29) or no-contact (–0.43 ± 2.23%) control interventions. Treatment differed significantly from

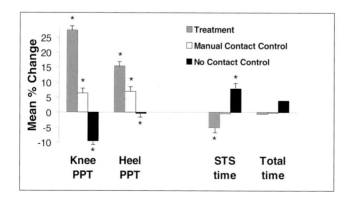

Fig. 1. Mean (± standard error) percentage change between pre and post condition measures for pressure pain threshold (PPT) at the knee and heel, and timed "up and go" test (sit-to-stand [STS] and total times). An asterisk (*) denotes a significant difference between conditions ($P < 0.005$).

both manual contact ($F_{1,37}$ = 6.02, P < 0.001) and no-contact ($F_{1,37}$ = 10.72, P < 0.019) control conditions.

TIMED UP-AND-GO TEST

A similar trend was demonstrated in the TUG results (Fig. 1). Knee mobilization treatment produced the greatest improvement in sit-to-stand times, decreasing time taken by 5.06% (SE = 2.08%). Sit-to-stand time decreased only slightly following manual contact (a decrease of 0.35% ± 1.84%) and increased significantly (by 7.92% ± 1.67%) following no-contact control. The overall difference between interventions was significant ($F_{1,37}$ = 12.45, P < 0.001), although contrasts demonstrated that the difference between treatment and manual contact was not statistically significant ($F_{1,37}$ = 2.64, P = 0.061). Results for total time taken were less conclusive. Although treatment produced the greatest improvement in time, the difference was not statistically significant ($F_{2,74}$ = 3.75, P = 0.78).

DISCUSSION

This study established that 9 minutes of accessory mobilization of the tibiofemoral joint immediately increased knee PPT significantly more than either manual contact or no-contact control procedures, in subjects with mild to moderate pain from knee osteoarthritis. Mobilization increased knee PPT by 27.3%, compared with a 6.4% increase following manual contact, indicating appreciably reduced sensitivity to mechanical pain. This result corresponds with evidence from spinal mobilization studies (Vicenzino et al. 1998; Sterling et al. 2001), which demonstrated improvements in PPT of approximately 25% and 30%, respectively, following treatment. It also supports a similar pattern found following ankle joint mobilization, where joint mobilization increased PPT 23% more than a manual contact procedure (Yeo and Wright 2004). Thus, both peripheral and spinal mobilizations immediately reduce mechanical hyperalgesia more than control conditions.

In addition, this study demonstrated that knee joint mobilization has a significant and immediate effect on PPT at a distal ipsilateral site, thereby supporting the animal model of widespread mobilization-induced antihyperalgesia (Sluka and Wright 2001). In a pattern strikingly similar to that at the knee, heel PPT increased by 15.3%, compared with an increase of 6.9% for manual contact and a minimal reduction of 0.43% following no-contact control.

The finding that the hypoalgesic response is more widespread than just at the mobilized joint appears to support the notion that central mechanisms may be important in mediating the effect. Although it might be hypothesized that segmental pain inhibitory mechanisms may play a part, it has previously been demonstrated in rats that pharmacological blockade of spinal cord γ-aminobutyric acid and opioid receptors, which are involved in segmental inhibition, has no effect on the analgesia produced by knee joint mobilization (Skyba et al. 2003).

We have previously hypothesized that supraspinal pain inhibitory mechanisms are activated by manual therapy (Wright 1995, 2002). Activation of supraspinal pathways would be expected to produce a widespread analgesic response, including areas outside the site of injury, as has been demonstrated by the current study. The fact that the hypoalgesic response produced at the heel was in proportions similar to that at the treated knee (Fig. 1) also suggests the influence of similar inhibitory mechanisms. Evidence from the current study supports both the animal study of Sluka and Wright (2001) and previous studies of spinal mobilization (Vicenzino et al. 1998) that have shown that cervical spine mobilization reduces hyperalgesia at a distal site in the upper limb.

It has been proposed that immediate changes in motor activity following joint mobilization may be a further indication of a centrally mediated response (Wright 2002). The current study demonstrated a clear trend toward mobilization producing the greatest improvement in sit-to-stand times (Fig. 1). Although improvement in motor function may be secondary to pain reduction, reflecting reversal of reflex muscle inhibition, human studies have begun to demonstrate that mobilization produces immediate and concurrent changes in motor function, pain perception and autonomic nervous system function, suggesting activation of a central modulatory mechanism (Wright 2002).

CONCLUSION

This chapter has described a study whose aim was to investigate the initial effects on pain and function of lower-limb joint mobilization. The study has provided new experimental evidence to demonstrate that accessory mobilization of a human osteoarthritic knee joint has both an immediate local and a more widespread hypoalgesic effect, thereby supporting the response seen in previous animal studies (Sluka and Wright 2001). The technique also appears to have a positive effect on motor function.

REFERENCES

Altman R, Asch E, Bloch D, et al. Development of criteria for the classification and reporting of osteoarthritis. Classification of osteoarthritis of the knee. Diagnostic and Therapeutic Criteria Committee of the American Rheumatism Association. *Arthritis Rheum* 1986; 29:1039–1049.

Bellamy N, Buchanan W, Goldsmith C, Campbell J, Stitt L. Validation study of WOMAC: a health status instrument for measuring clinically-important patient relevant outcomes following total hip or knee arthroplasty in osteoarthritis. *J Rheumatol* 1988; 15:1833–1840.

Bellamy N, Bell MJ, Goldsmith CH, et al. Evaluation of WOMAC 20, 50, 70 response criteria in patients treated with hylan G-F 20 for knee osteoarthritis. *Ann Rheum Dis* 2005; 64:881–885.

Bennell KL, Hinman RS, Metcalf BR, et al. Efficacy of physiotherapy management of knee joint osteoarthritis: a randomised, double blind, placebo controlled trial. *Ann Rheum Dis* 2005; 64:906–912.

Collins N, Teyes P, Vicenzino B. The initial effects of a Mulligan's mobilization with movement technique on dorsiflexion and pain in subacute ankle sprains. *Man Ther* 2004; 9:77–82.

Committee for Proprietary Medicinal Products. The European Agency for the Evaluation of Medicinal Products. *Points to Consider on Adjustment for Baseline Covariates.* Available at: www.emea.eu.int. 2003.

Maitland G. *Peripheral Manipulation,* 3rd ed. London: Butterworth-Heinemann, 1990.

McMeeken J, Stillman B, Story I, Kent P, Smith J. The effects of knee extensor and flexor muscle training on the timed-up-and-go test in individuals with rheumatoid arthritis. *Physiother Res Int* 1999; 4:55–67.

Paungmali A, O'Leary S, Souvlis T, Vicenzino B. Hypoalgesic and sympathoexcitatory effects of mobilisation with movement for lateral epicondylalgia. *Phys Ther* 2003; 83:374–383.

Podsiadlo D, Richardson S. The timed "up and go": a test of basic functional mobility for frail elderly persons. *J Am Geriatr Soc* 1991; 39:142–148.

Sambajon VV, Cillo JE, Gassner RJ, Buckley MJ. The effects of mechanical strain on synovial fibroblasts. *J Oral Maxillofac Surg* 2003; 61:707–712.

Skyba DA, Radhakrishnan R, Rohlwing JJ, Wright A, Sluka KA. Joint manipulation reduces hyperalgesia by activation of monoamine receptors but not opioid or GABA receptors in the spinal cord. *Pain* 2003; 106:159–168.

Sluka K, Wright A. Knee joint mobilisation reduces secondary mechanical hyperalgesia induced by capsaicin injection into the ankle joint. *Eur J Pain* 2001; 5:81–87.

Sterling M, Jull G, Wright A. Cervical mobilisation: concurrent effects on pain, sympathetic nervous system activity and motor activity. *Man Ther* 2001; 6:72–81.

Vicenzino B, Collins D, Benson H, Wright A. An investigation of the interrelationship between manipulative therapy induced hypoalgesia and sympathoexcitation. *J Manipulative Physiol Ther* 1998; 21:448–453.

Vicenzino B, Paungmali A, Buratowski S, Wright A. Specific manipulative therapy treatment for chronic lateral epicondylalgia produces uniquely characteristic hypoalgesia. *Man Ther* 2001; 6:205–212.

Wall J, Bell C, Campbell S, Davis J. The timed up and go test revisited: measurement of the component parts. *J Rehabil Res Dev* 2000; 37:109–114.

Wright A. Hypoalgesia post-manipulative therapy: a review of a potential neurophysiological mechanism. *Man Ther* 1995; 1:11–16.

Wright A. Pain-relieving effects of cervical manual therapy. In: Grant R (Ed). *Physical Therapy of the Cervical and Thoracic Spine.* New York: Churchill-Livingstone, 2002, pp 217–238.

Yeo H, Wright A. Effects of performing a passive accessory mobilization technique for lateral ankle pain. Paper presented at: 5th National Congress of Singapore Physiotherapy Association, May 6–9, 2004.

Correspondence to: Penny Moss, MMPty, Lecturer, School of Physiotherapy, Curtin University of Technology, GPO Box U1987, Perth, WA 6845, Australia. Email: P.Moss@curtin.edu.au.

Proceedings of the 11th World Congress on Pain,
edited by Herta Flor, Eija Kalso, and Jonathan O.
Dostrovsky, IASP Press, Seattle, © 2006.

74

Weight Loss Reduces Pain in Obese Patients with Osteoarthritis in the Knee: A Randomized Trial

Henning Bliddal,[a] Arne Astrup,[b]
and Robin Christensen[a]

*[a]The Parker Institute, H.S. Frederiksberg Hospital, Frederiksberg, Denmark;
[b]Department of Human Nutrition, Royal Veterinary and Agricultural
University, Frederiksberg, Denmark*

The association between being overweight and developing osteoarthritis (OA) has been well documented (Felson et al. 1997). Furthermore, once joint problems have developed, the deterioration of joints may be halted by substantial weight loss (Felson et al. 1992). In most cases, OA is accompanied by pain and reduced function (Pham et al. 2003). OA-related pain may depend on both central and peripheral factors (Ordeberg 2004). Indeed, studies on nonpharmacological therapies indicate that information and addressing cognitive factors such as attention should be regarded as highly important in the management of OA patients (Rene et al. 1992). Nevertheless, peripheral factors may also be important. For example, there is evidence that inflammatory components may play a role in knee OA (D'Agostino et al. 2005). The cartilage in OA is susceptible to accelerated degeneration under the influence of proinflammatory cytokines (van den Berg 1999), and cytokines may play an important role in obesity as well (Sonnenberg et al. 2004). The cytokine influence in obesity is reversible, which makes intervention all the more promising (Ziccardi et al. 2002). It is thus quite possible that the effect of obesity on deterioration of osteoarthritic joints is of multifactorial origin and not just a matter of weight (Bray 2004). This chapter describes a study conducted to test the efficacy of substantial weight loss on pain and overall disease symptoms in obese patients with knee OA.

METHODS

Patients. We recruited overweight patients with a body mass index (BMI) of more than 28 kg/m^2 who were over 18 years of age and willing to lose weight. All had primary knee OA, diagnosed according to the American College of Rheumatology, with radiographic severity assessed at grade 2 or 3 on the Kellgren and Lawrence scale. Major exclusion criteria included a history or active presence of other rheumatic diseases, diabetes mellitus, or other endocrine disorders. The participants were asked not to change their medication during the study.

Treatment assignment. All the subjects were randomly assigned to either the active treatment group, consuming a powdered low-calorie diet of 800 kCal/day, or to a group, consuming a conventional low-calorie diet of approximately 1200 kCal/day. This group was defined as control, as they received ordinary state-of-the art instruction in weight loss. For every 16 patients included, randomization was performed in a stratified way, according to gender, BMI, and age, in order to ensure homogeneity between intervention groups. After patient allocation, all individuals entered the defined intention-to-treat (ITT) population, as recommended for improving the quality of parallel-group randomized trials (Moher et al. 2003).

Diet. The powdered low-calorie diet consisted of a nutritional powder dissolved in water, taken as six daily meals. This diet provided the recommended daily intake of high-quality protein (Astrup 1999). Patients receiving the powdered low-calorie diet met in groups of eight to receive nutritional instruction and behavioral therapy, from the same experienced dietician, at weekly 1.5-hour sessions for 8 weeks to reinforce and continuously stimulate the patients' motivation to lose weight and thus encourage a high degree of compliance.

The protocol for the conventional diet consisted of a thorough presentation of nutritional advice in a 2-hour session by the same dietician who instructed the group receiving the powdered diet. The dietician recommended ordinary foods in amounts that would provide the patients with approximately 1200 kCal/day. The control patients had no contact with the dietician after this initial dietary consultation. After this initial session, all the patients in the conventional low-calorie group received ideas for diet plans in a booklet providing a wealth of advice on how to lose weight.

Outcome measures. Changes in body weight were examined as an independent predictor of changes in the pain indices of knee OA. Symptoms of OA, as perceived by patients prior to the assessment, were monitored by the Western Ontario and McMaster Universities' (WOMAC) osteoarthritis index, a validated, disease-specific questionnaire addressing the severity of joint pain (five questions), stiffness (two questions), and limitation of physical function

(17 questions). The visual analogue scale (VAS) version of the index was used, with the patient assessing each question on a 100-mm VAS. The global three-dimensional total WOMAC index was calculated by the summation of all 24 components, with 2400 mm being the worst possible score (Bellamy et al. 1988; McConnell et al. 2001). The outcome variables that were considered for analysis were pain and patient global assessment (Pham et al. 2003).

The primary objective and outcome of this analysis were the changes in pain following a weight loss regime in a randomized clinical setting, with strict adherence to ITT as advocated by Moher et al. (2003).

Statistics. With $\alpha = 5\%$ (two-tailed) and with a statistical power of 90% and a desired effect size of 0.8, we calculated the sample size as 34 knee OA patients in each of the two groups. For practical reasons, participants were included 16 at a time, and we increased the sample size to 48 patients per group to allow a dropout rate of more than one in four. Data were analyzed based on the "baseline value carried forward" technique in the ITT population using analysis of covariance (ANCOVA), with the baseline value as covariate. Differences between the final group means and 95% confidence interval (CI) with the associated *P* values were calculated based on the General Linear Model (GLM) procedure. The SAS statistical package (version 8) was used for all statistical analyses. The standardized mean difference was used to calculate the clinical effect size, as previously recommended when reporting randomized controlled trials with a focus on treatment of knee OA (Jordan et al. 2003) calculations were performed with software provided by the Cochrane Collaboration (Rev-Man 4.2).

RESULTS

A total of 109 patients were screened prior to the enrolment of 96 participants in the study, and these were randomly assigned to receive a powdered low-calorie diet or a conventional low-calorie control diet. The 13 subjects who were not enrolled in the study were excluded for the following reasons: three patients had a BMI of less than 28 kg/m^2, two patients had hypothyroidism, one patient had previously undergone surgery in both knees, and seven patients decided to withdraw their consent before randomization and without further explanation. After the random allocation of 48 subjects to each group, four patients in the active treatment group and three patients in the control group decided, before entering the study, to withdraw without further explanation. Only patients introduced to the proposed randomized interventions were handled as an ITT population. Among the ITT patients who entered the study, three patients in the active treatment group withdrew because of noncompliance with the intervention regime, and one decided to have knee replacement surgery and did not turn up for therapy. In the control group, three withdrew due to lack of motivation, one withdrew due to a broken arm, and one was excluded due to the diagnosis of type 2 diabetes mellitus. Demographic and baseline characteristics for the 89 patients are presented in Table I. The average patient entering this trial was a 63-year-old woman (standard deviation [SD] = 11 years), with a BMI of 36 kg/m^2 (SD = 5 kg/m^2). According to the WOMAC pain index, the patients had a mild-to-moderate (38% of the maximum) degree of knee OA, as indicated by the average scores shown in Table I.

WEIGHT CHANGES FOLLOWING THE 8-WEEK INTERVENTION

There was a significant weight reduction in both groups ($P < 0.0001$). Of the 89 ITT patients those allocated either to the powdered low-calorie diet or the control group lost on average 8.9 kg (SE = 0.5 kg) (9.2%) or 2.9 kg (SE = 0.5 kg) (2.9%), respectively. The powdered low-calorie diet group showed a significantly higher weight loss than the control group, with a mean difference of 6.0 kg (95% CI = –7.5 to –4.5; $P < 0.0001$), corresponding to a difference of 6.2 percentage points (95% CI = 4.8 to 7.7%).

EFFICACY RESULTS

As presented in Fig. 1, there was a significant reduction in both pain and total WOMAC index, following 8 weeks of treatment with the powdered low-calorie diet ($P \leq 0.02$), whereas there was no difference compared with the baseline in the control group ($P \geq 0.26$). Calculating these ITT results into an effect size, we found that after a weight loss of 6.2% (4.8% to 7.7%), the effect on pain was a moderate reduction of 37 mm (67 to 7 mm; $P = 0.02$), corresponding to an effect size of 0.51 (95% CI = 0.09 to 0.93) in favor of the powdered low-calorie diet. The effect on the overall disease symptoms (WOMAC total index)

Table I

Baseline characteristics of the intention-to-treat patients,
by randomization group, independent of dropout

Outcome	Active Treatment Group ($N = 44$)	Control Group ($N = 45$)
Weight (kg)	95.8 ± 14.4	95.4 ± 14.4
WOMAC pain index (mm)	192.6 ± 104.4	187.8 ± 104.4
Total WOMAC index (mm)	956.3 ± 498.9	916.8 ± 498.9

Note: WOMAC = Western Ontario and McMaster Universities' osteoarthritis index. Pain index ranges from 0 to 500 mm; total index ranges from 0 to 2400 mm. Values are mean ± SD.

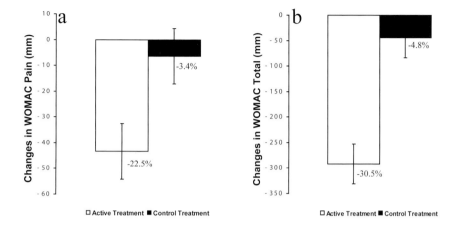

Fig. 1. Change in (a) pain index and (b) total index score on the Western Ontario and McMaster Universities' (WOMAC) osteoarthritis index following the 8-week dietary intervention period. Error bars indicate standard error.

was large reduction of 248 mm (358 to 138 mm; $P < 0.0001$), corresponding to an effect size of 0.94 (0.50 to 1.38).

As presented in Fig. 2, the percentage weight change predicted 18% of the variation in the changes in the WOMAC pain index ($R^2 = 0.178$), with a slope of 4.4 mm (SE = 1.0 mm) for each percentage point, corresponding to a 2.4% (1.3% to 3.4%) pain reduction following 1% weight loss. Thirty-seven percent of the variation in the changes in WOMAC total index ($R^2 = 0.370$) could be explained by body weight changes: 27.0 ± 3.8 mm for each percentage point, corresponding to a 2.9% (2.1% to 3.7%) reduction following 1% weight loss.

ADVERSE EVENTS

No serious adverse events were encountered during the 8-week intervention. No difference was noted in reports of changes in stools and gastrointestinal problems in the active and control groups.

DISCUSSION

The study demonstrated that an 8-week program yielding a substantial weight loss in obese patients with knee OA is accompanied by a statistically significant and clinically relevant reductions in pain and disease symptoms. The improvement in symptoms (WOMAC total index) following a moderate weight reduction, and accordingly the effect size, is much more pronounced

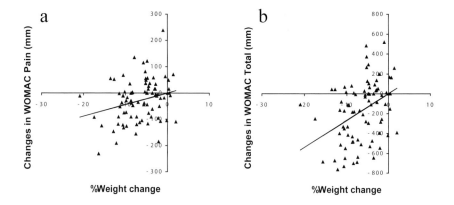

Fig. 2. The association between changes in the Western Ontario and McMaster Universities' (WOMAC) osteoarthritis index is scattered against the body weight changes (percentage weight change). (a) The percentage weight change predicted 18% of the variation in the changes in the WOMAC pain index, corresponding to a 2.4% pain reduction (95% CI = 1.3–3.4%) following 1% weight loss. (b) The percentage weight change predicted 37% of the variation in the changes in the WOMAC total index, corresponding to a 2.9% reduction (95% CI = 2.1–3.7%) following 1% weight loss.

than data reported after a 3-year intervention with glucosamine (Reginster et al. 2001): 0.94 vs. 0.32, respectively, and may be calculated to be as effective as knee alloplasty. It may be recommended that all obese patients be enrolled in such dietary programs, possibly before decisions are made of more invasive interventions. Obesity and osteoarthritis coexist in an increasing population of patients, and the two diseases intertwine in several ways. The growing public health focus on other obesity-related diseases should inspire clinicians to offer obese patients suffering from knee OA the same evidence-based weight-loss practices as seen in the prevention and treatment of type-2 diabetes mellitus. Accordingly, moderate weight loss of about 10% should be considered as the primary treatment in obese patients with knee OA.

ACKNOWLEDGMENTS

This study was supported by grants from the Oak Foundation and the Danish Rheumatism Association. The dietary intervention was sponsored by the manufacturers of Speasy®, Dansk Droge A/S. The authors are indebted to the dietician Lise Stigsgaard, the laboratory assistants Inger Wätjen, Jette Nielsen, Salomea Hirschorn, and Tove Riis Johannessen, and the database consultant Christian Cato Holm.

REFERENCES

Astrup A. Dietary approaches to reducing body weight. *Baillieres Best Pract Res Clin Endocrinol Metab* 1999; 13:109–120.

Bellamy N, Buchanan WW, Goldsmith CH, Campbell J, Stitt LW. Validation study of WOMAC: a health status instrument for measuring clinically important patient relevant outcomes to antirheumatic drug therapy in patients with osteoarthritis of the hip or knee. *J Rheumatol* 1988; 15:1833–1840.

Bray GA. Medical consequences of obesity. *J Clin Endocrinol Metab* 2004; 89:2583–2589.

D'Agostino MA, Conaghan P, Le Bars M, et al. Eular report on the use of ultrasonography in painful knee osteoarthritis part 1: prevalence of inflammation in osteoarthritis. *Ann Rheum Dis* 2005.

Felson DT, Zhang Y, Anthony JM, Naimark A, Anderson JJ. Weight loss reduces the risk for symptomatic knee osteoarthritis in women. The Framingham Study. *Ann Intern Med* 1992; 116:535–539.

Felson DT, Zhang Y, Hannan MT, et al. Risk factors for incident radiographic knee osteoarthritis in the elderly: the Framingham Study. *Arthritis Rheum* 1997; 40:728–733.

Jordan KM, Arden NK, Doherty M, et al. EULAR Recommendations 2003: an evidence based approach to the management of knee osteoarthritis: Report of a Task Force of the Standing Committee for International Clinical Studies Including Therapeutic Trials (ESCISIT). *Ann Rheum Dis* 2003; 62:1145–1155.

McConnell S, Kolopack P, Davis AM. The Western Ontario and McMaster Universities Osteoarthritis Index (WOMAC): a review of its utility and measurement properties. *Arthritis Rheum* 2001; 45:453–461.

Moher D, Schulz KF, Altman DG. The CONSORT statement: revised recommendations for improving the quality of reports of parallel-group randomised trials. *Clin Oral Investig* 2003; 7:2–7.

Ordeberg G. Characterization of joint pain in human OA. *Novartis Found Symp* 2004; 260:105–115.

Pham T, Van Der Heijde D, Lassere M, et al. Outcome variables for osteoarthritis clinical trials: The OMERACT-OARSI set of responder criteria. *J Rheumatol* 2003; 30:1648–1654.

Reginster JY, Deroisy R, Rovati LC, et al. Long-term effects of glucosamine sulphate on osteoarthritis progression: a randomised, placebo-controlled clinical trial. *Lancet* 2001; 357:251–256.

Rene J, Weinberger M, Mazzuca SA, Brandt KD, Katz BP. Reduction of joint pain in patients with knee osteoarthritis who have received monthly telephone calls from lay personnel and whose medical treatment regimens have remained stable. *Arthritis Rheum* 1992; 35:511–515.

Sonnenberg GE, Krakower GR, Kissebah AH. A novel pathway to the manifestations of metabolic syndrome. *Obes Res* 2004; 12:180–186.

van den Berg WB. The role of cytokines and growth factors in cartilage destruction in osteoarthritis and rheumatoid arthritis. *Zeitschrift fur Rheumatologie* 1999; 58:136–141.

Ziccardi P, Nappo F, Giugliano G, et al. Reduction of inflammatory cytokine concentrations and improvement of endothelial functions in obese women after weight loss over one year. *Circulation* 2002; 105:804–809.

Correspondence to: Professor Henning Bliddal, DMSc, MD, The Parker Institute, Frederiksberg Hospital, DK-2000 F, Denmark. Tel: 45-38164151; Fax: 45-38164159; email: henning.bliddal@fh.hosp.dk.

Proceedings of the 11th World Congress on Pain,
edited by Herta Flor, Eija Kalso, and Jonathan O.
Dostrovsky, IASP Press, Seattle, © 2006.

75

Recent Insights into Analgesic Mechanisms of Acupuncture and TENS

Kathleen A. Sluka,[a] Gen-Cheng Wu,[b] and Jin Mo Chung[c]

[a]Graduate Program in Physical Therapy and Rehabilitation Sciences, University of Iowa, Iowa City, Iowa, USA; [b]Department of Integrative Medicine, Shanghai Medical College, Fudan University, Shanghai, China; [c]Department of Neuroscience and Cell Biology, University of Texas Medical Branch, Galveston, Texas, USA

Acupuncture and transcutaneous electrical nerve stimulation (TENS) are two nonpharmacological treatments for pain with shared underlying mechanisms. Recently, these two treatments have been studied extensively, and significant progress has been made toward unveiling their underlying mechanisms. This chapter discusses two particular research efforts including basic acupuncture and TENS research in animal models.

THE SPINAL ORPHANIN FQ SYSTEM IN ELECTROACUPUNCTURE ANALGESIA IN NEUROPATHIC RATS

Clinical and experimental studies show that electroacupuncture plays its analgesic role by activating the endogenous pain-modulating systems, including the opioid system. Orphanin FQ/nociceptin (OFQ), a member of the opioid family that was discovered in 1995, is a 17-amino-acid peptide (FGGFTGARK-SARKLANQ) that acts as an endogenous ligand of the opioid receptor ORL1 (Meunier et al. 1995; Reinscheid et al. 1995). In pain modulation, the roles of supraspinal OFQ and spinal OFQ are different. Substantial evidence indicates that spinal OFQ produces analgesia and potentiates morphine analgesia. In contrast, supraspinal OFQ induces hyperalgesia and antagonizes morphine analgesia (Darland et al. 1998).

Electroacupuncture has a potent analgesic effect in patients with neuropathic pain (George et al. 1998). Wu and colleagues conducted a study to investigate the role of spinal OFQ in an animal model of neuropathic pain and to determine its role in electroacupuncture analgesia in the spinal dorsal horn (Wu et al., unpublished data).

Chronic constriction injury (CCI) to the rat sciatic nerve induces hyperalgesia (Bennett and Xie 1988), as measured by a decrease in the ipsilateral paw-withdrawal latency to heat for at least 28 days. For electroacupuncture treatment, two acupoints were selected: "Huan-Tiao" (GB-30, located near the hip joint, on the inferior borders of the gluteus maximus and piriformis muscles, near the inferior gluteal cutaneous nerve and the sciatic nerve) and "Yang-Ling-Quan" (GB-34, located near the knee joint, anterior and inferior to the small head of the fibula, in the peroneus longus and brevis muscles, where the common peroneal nerve bifurcates into the superficial and deep peroneal nerves). Stimulation comprised alternating strings of dense and sparse frequencies (60 Hz for 1.05 s and 2 Hz for 2.85 s alternately, for 30 minutes). Intensity was adjusted to induce a slight motor twitch of the hindlimb (≤ 1 mA, 12 V). Previous studies demonstrated that one treatment with electroacupuncture immediately increased the paw-withdrawal latency to heat in rats with CCI. Further, repeated electroacupuncture produced a cumulative increase in the ipsilateral paw-withdrawal latency of rats with CCI (Yang et al. 2002).

First, to examine the role of OFQ on neuropathic pain, we examined the effects of intrathecal (i.t.) OFQ on hyperalgesia induced by CCI in rats. On the seventh day after CCI, 3, 10, or 30 µg of OFQ or saline was administered in rats with neuropathic pain, and changes in paw-withdrawal latency were observed after OFQ administration. The results showed that OFQ dose-dependently increases the paw-withdrawal latency to heat in rats with CCI, suggesting that i.t. OFQ reduces hyperalgesia induced by CCI.

To examine the role of OFQ on neuropathic pain, two sets of pharmacological blocking experiments were conducted on the 7th day after CCI. In experiment 1, the ORL1-receptor antagonist [Nphe[1]]nociceptin(1–13)NH$_2$ (10 µg, i.t.) and the OFQ blocker nocistatin (10 µg, i.t.) were tested on rats with neuropathic pain. Neither drug had a significant effect on hyperalgesia induced by CCI, but both reversed OFQ analgesia (Ma et al. 2003).

Next, the role of OFQ in mediating electroacupuncture analgesia was examined. On the seventh day after CCI, electroacupuncture for 30 minutes significantly reduced hyperalgesia. Pretreatment with either [Nphe[1]]nociceptin(1–13)NH$_2$ (10 µg, i.t.) or nocistatin (10 µg, i.t.) 5 minutes before electroacupuncture prevented the increase in paw-withdrawal latency produced by electroacupuncture (Fig. 1). Treatment of rats with CCI-induced hyperalgesia with electroacupuncture in combination with OFQ (10 µg, i.t.) caused an enhanced reduction in hyperalgesia.

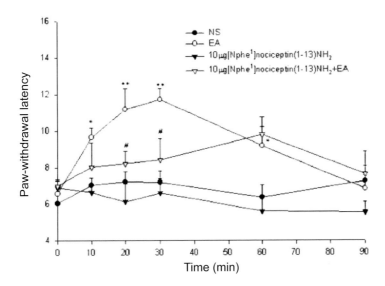

Fig. 1. Intrathecal injection of the ORL1-receptor antagonist [Nphe[1]]nociceptin(1–13)NH₂ blocked electroacupuncture (EA)-induced analgesia in rats with experimentally induced neuropathic pain. The graph shows paw-withdrawal latency to heat (PWL), in seconds. * P < 0.05, ** P < 0.01 vs. the normal saline (NS) control group; # P < 0.05 vs. the EA group.

In summary, intrathecal OFQ dose-dependently reduces hyperalgesia by activation of ORL1 receptors in the spinal cord. Blockade of ORL1 receptors in the spinal cord partly reversed electroacupuncture analgesia, and spinal OFQ enhanced electroacupuncture analgesia, indicating that spinal OFQ partially mediates the effects of electroacupuncture analgesia at the level of the spinal cord. Further study showed that prepro-OFQ mRNA, ORL1 mRNA, and OFQ immunoreactivity were expressed in the lumbar spinal dorsal horn of normal rats. Electroacupuncture treatment increased both prepro-OFQ and ORL1 mRNA expression and the number of OFQ immunoreactive cells in the lumbar spinal dorsal horn, suggesting the enhanced synthesis of OFQ. These results indicate that spinal OFQ and ORL1 receptors may be involved in neuropathic pain and in mediating electroacupuncture analgesia in rats.

MECHANISMS OF TENS ANALGESIA

The effects of TENS have been analyzed in several animal models of pain. TENS reduces acute pain responses, such as the tail flick (Woolf et al. 1980), and more persistent pain, such as hyperalgesia induced by inflammation (Sluka et al. 1998; Gopalkrishnan and Sluka 2000; King and Sluka 2001; Vance et al. 2006) or by nerve injury (Somers and Clemente 1998). In general, at intensities commonly utilized clinically, TENS activates large-diameter afferent fibers (Levin and Hui-chan 1993; Radhakrishnan and Sluka 2005). However, TENS must reduce hyperalgesia by activating deep tissue afferents, given that blockade of deep tissue afferents prevented the antihyperalgesia produced by TENS, but blockade of cutaneous afferents had no effect (Radhakrishnan and Sluka 2005).

Our data over the last several years points to a frequency-dependent difference in mechanisms in an animal model of inflammatory joint pain. We show that TENS delivered at low frequency (4 Hz) utilizes different neuropharmacological mechanisms than TENS delivered at high frequency (100 Hz). The antihyperalgesia produced by low-frequency TENS is prevented by blockade of μ-opioid receptors in the spinal cord and rostral ventromedial medulla, by blockade of serotonin receptors (5-HT$_2$ and 5-HT$_3$) in the spinal cord, and by blockade of acetylcholine receptors (M1 and M3) in the spinal cord (Sluka et al. 1999; Kalra et al. 2001; Radhakrishnan and Sluka 2003; Radhakrishnan et al. 2003). On the other hand, the reduction in hyperalgesia by low-frequency TENS in not prevented by blockade of δ-opioid, κ-opioid, M2-muscarinic, nicotinic, or α_2-noradrenergic receptors in the spinal cord, or by blockade of δ-opioid receptors supraspinally (Sluka et al. 1999; Kalra et al. 2001; Radhakrishnan et al. 2003; Radhakrishnan and Sluka 2003). In parallel, there is an increased release of serotonin, but not of norepinephrine, in the spinal cord dorsal horn during application of low-frequency TENS (Sodhi et al. 2003).

The reduction in hyperalgesia produced by high-frequency TENS in animals with joint inflammation is prevented by blockade of δ-opioid receptors in the spinal cord and the rostral ventromedial medulla, and of acetylcholine receptors (M1 and M3) in the spinal cord (Sluka et al. 1999; Kalra et al. 2001; Radhakrishnan et al. 2003; Radhakrishnan and Sluka 2003). The reduction in hyperalgesia is not prevented by blockade of μ-opioid, κ-opioid, M2-muscarinic, nicotinic, serotonergic, or noradrenergic receptors in the spinal cord, or by blockade of μ-opioid receptors supraspinally (Sluka et al. 1999; Kalra et al. 2001; Radhakrishnan et al. 2003; Radhakrishnan and Sluka 2003). High-frequency TENS also increases concentrations of γ-aminobutyric acid (Lisi et al. 2005) and reduces glutamate (Sluka et al. 2006) in the dorsal horn of the spinal cord. The reduction in glutamate by high-frequency TENS is prevented by blockade of δ-opioid receptors spinally.

These data show that different frequencies of TENS utilize different central neuronal mechanisms to reduce hyperalgesia. However, part of the inhibition of TENS is peripheral (King et al. 2005). Blockade of peripheral noradrenergic receptors in the knee joint attenuates the antihyperalgesia produced by TENS.

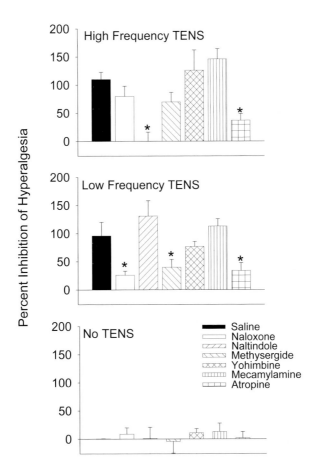

Fig. 2. Knee joints of rats were inflamed with 3% kaolin and carrageenan, and transcutaneous electrical nerve stimulation (TENS) was applied 4 hours after induction of inflammation. Paw-withdrawal latency to heat was measured before and after inflammation, and after treatment with TENS + drug or saline as control. Prior to treatment with TENS, rats were intrathecally administered antagonists to specific receptors: μ-opioid (open bars, naloxone), δ-opioid (right diagonal, naltrindole), serotonin (left diagonal, methysergide), noradrenergic (hatched, yohimbine), nicotinic (vertical, mecamylamine), and muscarinic (cross, atropine). Data were converted to percentage inhibition of hyperalgesia, with 100% representing a full reversal of hyperalgesia, 0% representing no change in hyperalgesia. Values greater than 100% are above baseline. There was a full reversal (approximately 100%) of hyperalgesia with TENS (saline, closed bars). High-frequency TENS antihyperalgesia was prevented by blockade of δ-opioid and muscarinic receptors in the spinal cord. Low-frequency TENS antihyperalgesia was prevented by blockade of μ-opioid, serotonergic, and muscarinic receptors in the spinal cord. Asterisks (*) denote statistical significance compared to saline.

Further, the antihyperalgesia produced by TENS is reduced in mice with a genetic mutation of the α_{2A} noradrenergic receptors. Thus, peripheral α_{2A} receptors in the knee joint must partially mediate the antihyperalgesic effects of both low- and high-frequency TENS.

Understanding these mechanisms and differences in frequencies should help to refine the selection of patients receiving TENS. For example, low-frequency TENS is less effective in morphine-tolerant rats (Sluka et al. 2000), and repeated application of TENS produces tolerance (Chandran and Sluka 2003). Further, combining pharmaceutical treatments with TENS could enhance its efficacy. We previously showed that morphine or clonidine enhances the reduction in hyperalgesia obtained with either low- or high-frequency TENS (Sluka et al. 2000; Sluka and Chandran 2002). Future studies should be designed to continue to address the basic science mechanisms behind TENS antihyperalgesia, and clinical studies should confirm and expand these results.

CONCLUSIONS

During the last several years, a great deal of progress has been made toward unveiling mechanisms of analgesia produced by acupuncture and TENS. Animal studies of the basic mechanisms of acupuncture analgesia have focused on molecular mechanisms in the brain that play critical roles in mediating acupuncture analgesia. One example would be the opioid OFQ; this chapter has shown that spinal OFQ seems to have an important role in acupuncture analgesia. Research in TENS mechanisms has also focused on critical brain structures and molecular mechanisms. One example discussed in this chapter is a differential activation of brain sites and release of neurotransmitters by different frequencies of TENS.

We are far from having a complete understanding of how acupuncture and TENS work. However, modern scientific tools allow us to unveil the mystery one step at a time. We need to continuously watch and encourage further development of research in these topics. Someday in the near future, we should be able to maximize these therapeutic regimes for the benefit of many pain patients who suffer unnecessarily.

ACKNOWLEDGMENTS

This work is supported in part by NIH grants R01 AT01474 (J.M. Chung) and K02 AR02201 (K.A. Sluka), and by a grant from the Arthritis Foundation (K.A. Sluka) and by the NSFC (30070948) from China.

REFERENCES

Bennett GJ, Xie YK. A peripheral mononeuropathy in rat that produces disorders of pain sensation like those seen in man. *Pain* 1988; 33:87–107.

Chandran P, Sluka KA. Development of opioid tolerance with repeated TENS administration. *Pain* 2003; 102:195–201.

Darland T, Heinricher MM, Grandy DK. Orphanin FQ/nociceptin: a role in pain and analgesia, but so much more. *Trends Neurosci* 1998; 21:215–221.

George AU, Han SP, Han JS. Electroacupuncture. Mechanisms and clinical application. *Biol Psychiatry* 1998; 44:129–138.

Gopalkrishnan P, Sluka KA. Effect of varying frequency, intensity and pulse duration of TENS on primary hyperalgesia in inflamed rats. *Arch Phys Med Rehabil* 2000; 81:984–990.

Kalra A Urban MO, Sluka KA. Blockade of opioid receptors in rostral ventral medulla prevents antihyperalgesia produced by transcutaneous electrical nerve stimulation (TENS). *J Pharmacol Exp Ther* 2001; 298:257–263.

King EW, Sluka KA. The effect of varying frequency and intensity of transcutaneous electrical nerve stimulation on secondary mechanical hyperalgesia in an animal model of inflammation. *J Pain* 2001; 2:128–133.

King EW, Audette KA, Athman GA, et al. Transcutaneous electrical nerve stimulation activates peripherally located alpha-2A adrenergic receptors. *Pain* 2005; 115:364–373.

Levin M F, Hui-Chan CW. Conventional and acupuncture-like transcutaneous electrical nerve stimulation excite similar afferent fibers. *Arch Phys Med Rehabil* 1993; 74:54–60.

Lisi TL, Vance CGT, Sluka KA. High frequency TENS reduces glutamate release and low frequency increases GABA release in the spinal dorsal horn. Paper presented at: Combined Sections Meeting, APTA, New Orleans, February 23–27, 2005.

Ma F, Xie H, Dong ZQ, Wang Y, Wu G. Effect of intrathecal administration of nocistatin on orphanin FQ/nociceptin analgesia in the nerve injury rat. *Brain Res* 2003; 988:189–192.

Meunier JC, Mollereau C, Tool L, Suaudeau C, et al. Isolation and structure of the endogenous agonist of opioid receptor-like ORL1 receptor. *Nature* 1995; 377:532–535.

Radhakrishnan R, Sluka KA. Role of spinal cholinergic receptors in TENS-induced antihyperalgesia. *Neuropharmacology* 2003; 45:1111–1119.

Radhakrishnan R, Sluka KA. Deep tissue afferents, but not cutaneous afferents, mediate TENS-induced antihyperalgesia. *J Pain* 2005; 6:673–680.

Radhakrishnan R, King EW, Dickman J, et al. Blockade of spinal 5-HT receptor subtypes prevents low, but not high, frequency TENS-induced antihyperalgesia in rats. *Pain* 2003; 5:205–213.

Reinscheid RK, Nothacker HP, Bourson A, et al. Orphanin FQ: a neuropeptide that actives an opioid like G protein-coupled receptor. *Science* 1995; 270:792–794.

Sluka KA. Systemic morphine in combination with TENS produces an increased analgesia in rats with acute inflammation. *J Pain* 2000; 1:204–211.

Sluka KA, Chandran P. Systemic administration of clonidine in combination with TENS produces an increased antihyperalgesia in rats. *Pain* 2002; 100:183–190.

Sluka KA, Bailey K, Bogush J, Olson R, Ricketts A. Treatment with either high or low frequency TENS reduces the secondary hyperalgesia observed after injection of kaolin and carrageenan into the knee joint. *Pain* 1998; 77:97–102.

Sluka KA, Deacon M, Stibal A, Strissel S, Terpstra A. Spinal blockade of opioid receptors prevents the analgesia produced by TENS in arthritic rats. *J Pharmacol Exp Ther* 1999; 289:840–846.

Sluka KA, Judge MA, McColley MM, Reveiz PM, Taylor BM. Low frequency TENS is less effective than high frequency TENS at reducing inflammation induced hyperalgesia in morphine tolerant rats. *Eur J Pain* 2000; 4:185–193.

Sluka KA, Vance CGT, Lisi TL. High, but not low, frequency transcutaneous electrical nerve stimulation (TENS) reduces aspartate and glutamate release in the spinal cord dorsal horn. *J Neurochem* 2006; 95:1794–1801.

Sodhi SK, Lisi TL, Westlund K, Sluka KA. Low-frequency TENS increases serotonin (5-HT) in dorsal horn of inflamed rats. Paper presented at: American Pain Society 22nd Annual Scientific Meeting, 2003.

Somers DL, Clemente FR. High-frequency transcutaneous electrical nerve stimulation alters thermal but not mechanical allodynia following chronic constriction injury of the rat sciatic nerve. *Arch Phys Med Rehabil* 1998; 79:1370–1376.

Vance CG, Radhakrishnan R, Skyba DA, Sluka KA. Effects of TENS on acute and chronic primary hyperalgesia induced by knee joint inflammation in rats. Paper presented at: Combined Sections Meeting, APTA, San Diego, 2006.

Woolf CJ, Mitchell D, Barrett GD. Antinociceptive effect of peripheral segmental electrical stimulation in the rat. *Pain* 1980; 8:237–252.

Yang XH, Wang YQ, Gao X, Wu GC. Effects of electroacupuncture on hyperalgesia score of neuropathic pain rats. *Acupunct Res* 2002; 27:60–63.

Correspondence to: Prof. Jin Mo Chung, PhD, Department of Neuroscience and Cell Biology, University of Texas Medical Branch, 301 University Boulevard, Galveston, TX 77555-1069, USA. Fax: 409-772-4687; email: jmchung@utmb.edu.

Index